Prescription for Natural Cures

Prescription for Natural Cures

REVISED 3rd EDITION

A Self-Care Guide for Treating Health Problems
with Natural Remedies Including Diet, Nutrition,
Supplements, and Other Holistic Methods

MARK STENGLER, N.M.D.

JAMES F. BALCH, M.D.

ROBIN YOUNG BALCH, N.D.

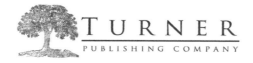
TURNER
PUBLISHING COMPANY

Turner Publishing Company 4507 Charlotte Avenue • Suite 100 • Nashville, Tennessee 37209
www.turnerpublishing.com

The Library of Congress has cataloged the earlier edition as follows:
Library of Congress Cataloging-in-Publication Data
Balch, James F., date.
Prescription for natural cures : a self-care guide for treating diseases and health problems with natural remedies including diet and nutrition, herbal medicine, nutritional supplements, bodywork, and more / James F. Balch, Mark Stengler.
p. cm.
Includes bibliographical references and index.
ISBN 0-471-49088-1 (paper : alk. paper)
1. Naturopathy—Popular works. 2. Alternative medicine—Popular works. 3. Self-care, Health.
I. Stengler, Mark. II. Title.
RZ440.B285 2004
615.5'35—dc22
2004005669

Project Credits
Cover Design: Maddie Cothren
Interior Design: Mallory Collins

9781630260903

Manufactured in the United States of America

9 8 7 Third Edition 21

Contents

Part One: Conditions

Contents

Part Two: The Essentials of Natural Medicine

Part Three: Appendix

Preface

It has been twelve years since the original version of *Prescription for Natural Cures* was published. The response has been overwhelming, with more than 500,000 copies sold. Many readers and patients have told us that this resource has helped to guide them and their loved ones to better health.

In this 3rd revised edition, we have added the newest research on natural medicine. The field of natural and integrative medicine continues to explode, with scientific discoveries and validation occurring at a rapid rate.

Once again we have also greatly expanded the number of conditions covered so that more people can benefit from this book. We have included emerging conditions such as Lyme disease and genetic mutations such as MTHFR. We have added nineteen new conditions to this edition to better help you and your loved ones. In addition, the nutrition section has been updated to include important information on artificial sweeteners, GMO foods, and the new USDA alternative to the Food Pyramid.

God has designed the human body to interact most precisely, efficiently, and safely with live foods, nutrients, and healing agents found in nature. Today an increasing number of conventional doctors are embracing holistic medicine due to its efficacy, scientific basis, cost-effectiveness, and patient demand.

Prescription for Natural Cures combines almost ninety years of clinical experience among the three authors and draws on hundreds of scientific studies to bring our readers the best in holistic medicine.

Our goal is to provide safe, easy-to-use, clinically proven recommendations to prevent and recover from disease. We have empowered the reader and the practitioner to address the root causes of illness instead of merely suppressing the symptoms.

Acknowledgments

First, I must thank my Lord Jesus Christ, who thirty years ago transformed my mind about healing and wellness. In addition, I thank my wife, Robin Young Balch, a talented naturopathic doctor, whose research and encouragement spurred us toward publication of this book. We pray that "the multitudes" will benefit from the information contained herein.

—James F. Balch, M.D.

Special thanks to my wife, Angela, and to my kids for all their support. Also to my hard-working clinic staff at the Stengler Center for Integrative Medicine. A special acknowledgment to my mother, Mary. And to our Creator, Jesus Christ, the One referred to in the following passages: Genesis 1:1, Genesis 3:15, Isaiah 9:6, Isaiah 53, Daniel 9:25–26, Matthew 2:1, John 14:6, 1 Corinthians 15:3–5, John 14:6, and John 20:28.

—Mark Stengler, N.M.D.

I would like to thank my Lord Jesus Christ for the knowledge about healing. He has imparted it to my heart in order to guide our readers on a path to good health. It was a joyful blessing to collaborate with my husband, Dr. James Balch, and Dr. Mark Stengler to bring forth a compilation of natural cures for all who seek them.

—Robin Young Balch, N.D.

Our thanks to Jeff Herman for representing this book as our agent and to the staff at Turner Publishing for their enthusiasm in publishing the third edition of *Prescription for Natural Cures*.

—From all the authors

How to Use This Book

This book focuses on providing you with results. We have incorporated the best of what science and nature have to offer in the field of natural medicine.

The largest component of the book, Part One, includes entries for health conditions. They are listed in alphabetical order. For easy reference, the exact page number of the condition you are looking for is located both in the table of contents and in the index at the back of this book. For most conditions, we include the following information. Note that a few conditions don't include all six parts, and the parts don't necessarily appear in this order.

DESCRIPTION OF THE CONDITION

The important features of each condition are described in a thorough yet easy-to-understand manner. We provide details on how conventional, as well as holistic, doctors understand and approach these conditions. We mention why researchers believe the disease process is occurring. In many cases, we give our own explanation of why an imbalance or an illness may occur.

SYMPTOMS

A summary of the symptoms helps you to determine whether you have a specific condition. Of course, you should consult a health professional to obtain an accurate diagnosis.

ROOT CAUSES

This section provides a summary of the root causes for a condition and its initiating factor(s). This will help you focus on what is causing your health problem.

TESTING TECHNIQUES

We list the most important tests to help determine the root cause of your illness. This section will help you choose the best type of health care. The tests are commonly available through your local medical doctor or natural–health care provider. Please note: not every type of standard conventional test is listed for each condition, because we assume that these are part of your doctor's investigative procedure.

TREATMENT

The Treatment section has a comprehensive description of the following natural methods:

Diet. This section includes foods that are known to prevent or heal the condition. It also describes foods that can cause or worsen an illness. Detoxification is important for preventing and healing disease. This section gives helpful advice on improving a condition with detoxifying techniques.

SuperSeven Prescriptions. One aspect of this book that distinguishes it from other natural-healing reference books is the Super Seven Prescriptions section. Here, we prioritize the top seven prescriptions a person can use for each condition. We chose these prescriptions based on what has worked clinically, is backed by scientific research, and is readily available to the public. You can glance through the top seven prescriptions and get a feel for what most accurately fits your symptom picture. After reviewing the super seven, you can start by using the first choice and see how it affects your condition. Also, you can pick more than one, for an aggressive approach to help prevent or improve a condition.

Studies. For most of the conditions, we provide concise studies demonstrating the scientific validity of the supplements and diets we recommend.

General Recommendations. Since there are so many different choices of nutritional supplements, we also provide general recommendations. These include other fine choices of supplements that are commonly available for each condition.

Homeopathy. Homeopathy is a distinct field compared to other practices, and it often requires more detailed information. We include a section on the most important homeopathic remedies and how to choose one that best fits your profile.

Acupressure. Most conditions have specific acupressure-point recommendations that can be incorporated for faster, gentler healing.

Bodywork. Bodywork techniques, such as massage and reflexology, are recommended throughout the book for anyone interested in a comprehensive self-healing approach.

Aromatherapy. Aromatherapy has had a tremendous surge in popularity in the last decade. Included here are some of the more effective choices for each condition.

Stress Reduction. Research has proved, time and again, that most health conditions can be positively or negatively influenced by how you cope with stress. This section describes practical, well-tested techniques to reduce the effects of stress and improve your health.

Other Recommendations. The field of holistic medicine is vast. This section briefly describes potentially helpful holistic therapies for each condition that were not mentioned in previous sections.

REFERENCES

For the scientifically minded, there is a summarization of the studies that we quoted for each condition.

Part Two, "The Essentials of Natural Medicine," gives detailed, user-friendly information on the natural-healing tools and methods we recommend throughout the book. It contains helpful advice on the clinical use of diet and nutrition, fasting, herbal medicine, homeopathy, detoxification, aromatherapy, traditional Chinese medicine and acupressure, hydrotherapy, natural hormones, bodywork, exercise and stress reduction, and nutritional supplements.

Part Three contains a comprehensive glossary of unfamiliar medical terms as well as a Natural Health Care Resource Guide. This section describes the training and the holistic approach of individual practitioners, as well as contact information for a reliable referral.

PART ONE

Conditions

Abscesses and Boils

An abscess is an accumulation of pus that can occur anywhere in the body, including on the skin and inside organs and tissues. When an abscess forms around a hair follicle, it is known as a boil. Boils often surface on the buttocks, the underarms, the neck, and the face. They first begin as small, firm, and tender nodules that become red and swollen. Generally, boils do not spread. Within two to four days, a pustule usually forms in the center of the infected area. Then, several days later, it tends to rupture and drain the white- or yellow-colored pus. The abscess is called a *carbuncle* when the skin is red, painful, swollen, and warm, and it forms an elevated lump.

Abscesses can occur on anyone at any age. No one is immune to them. They are generally triggered by an impaired immune system, trauma, improper drainage of tissues, bacterial invasion, poor nutrition, and other factors. Skin abscesses tend to develop in places where tight clothing rubs against the skin, as well as around small puncture wounds or cuts. The infected area becomes tender, red, and swollen, and fever may be present.

Delayed or improper treatment can lead to a spreading of the infection. People with a compromised immune system, such as those with HIV/AIDS or diabetes, are more susceptible to a serious infection. Depending on the severity and the location of the infection, antibiotics may be required. In some cases, the abscess will be cut open and drained by your doctor. Consult your doctor about any skin abscess that appears on your face, contains red streaks, or is filled with fluids. See your dentist regarding any mouth abscesses. If antibiotics are required, ensure a quicker recovery by simultaneously using natural treatments. Make sure to consume friendly flora, which are found in yogurt or probiotic supplements, if you are taking antibiotics.

SYMPTOMS

Each of the following symptoms can appear on the face, the chest, or the back.

- Red spots, bumps, or white/yellow pustules, often inflamed and painful
- Swollen, red, and hot area around the lesion
- Fever

Testing Techniques

The following tests will help to assess possible reasons for chronic abscess or boil formation:

Immune system imbalance or disease—blood

Intestinal permeability—urine

Detoxification profile—urine or blood

Vitamin and mineral analysis (especially vitamins A, C, E, selenium, zinc, iron)—blood, urine

Digestive function and microbe/parasite/fungal testing—stool analysis

Anemia—blood test (CBC, iron, ferritin, % saturation)

Food and environmental allergies/sensitivities—blood, electrodermal

Blood sugar imbalance—blood

ROOT CAUSES

- Poor diet and food allergies or sensitivities
- Improper drainage of tissues' lymphatic congestion
- Bacterial invasion
- Impaired immune system

- Clothing rubbing against the skin
- Trauma
- Digestive malabsorption and toxicity
- Puncture wounds or cuts
- Poor hygiene

TREATMENT

Diet

Recommended Food

Dark-green or orange vegetables are especially helpful because they contain carotenoids, which help maintain and repair the skin. Eat them raw or lightly cooked to retain their nutrients and fiber.

A quarter cup of ground flaxseeds provides helpful essential fatty acids and plenty of fiber for proper elimination. Take with at least 8 ounces of clean, quality water.

Nuts and seeds, such as almonds, walnuts, and pumpkin seeds, are good sources of skin-healthy vitamin E and essential fatty acids.

Onions and garlic help to fight infection.

Quality protein sources are beans, peas, lentils, eggs, and fresh cold-water fish, such as salmon, mackerel, herring, and sardines. The latter are rich in omega-3 fatty acids.

Drink a glass of clean, quality water every two waking hours to flush toxins out of the body and maintain good general health.

If you must use antibiotics, be sure to eat some live, unsweetened yogurt every day. The yogurt will replace the "friendly" bacteria in your digestive tract, which are necessary for good health and which antibiotics destroy.

Fresh vegetable juices reduce toxins and aid in skin healing. Drink 12 ounces or more daily.

Food to Avoid

Eliminate processed grains, colas, sugar, and candy. These products suppress immune function.

Food allergies or sensitivities, such as an allergy to cow's milk, can be a root cause. See the Food Allergies section for more information.

Avoid saturated and hydrogenated fats, which worsen skin inflammation. Stay away from fried foods and solid fats, such as margarine, lard, and vegetable shortening.

Coffee and other caffeinated products may aggravate skin conditions. If they cause problems for you, cut them out and drink herbal teas instead.

People with carbohydrate sensitivity may notice skin improvement by reducing their carbohydrate intake and increasing their protein sources. This is because elevated levels of the blood sugar–regulating hormone insulin increase skin inflammation.

R℞ Super Seven Prescriptions—Abscesses and Boils

Super Prescription #1 Colloidal silver
Apply topically as a cream or 2 drops four times daily to reduce the infection. Colloidal silver has potent antimicrobial effects.

Super Prescription #2 Tea tree (*Melaleuca alternifolia*) oil
Apply topically as a cream or 10 drops diluted in a half ounce of water three times daily. Tea tree oil has antimicrobial effects and helps to draw the pus out.

Super Prescription #3 Echinacea (*Echinacea purpurea*) and goldenseal (*Hydrastis canadensis*)
Take 500 mg or 2 to 4 ml of tincture four times daily. Both herbs enhance immune function.

Super Prescription #4 Oregano oil (*Origanum vulgare*)
Take 500 mg in the capsule form four times daily, or take the liquid form as directed on the container. In diluted form it can be applied directly to the lesions as well. Oregano has powerful antibacterial properties. *Note*: Do not take internally if you are pregnant.

Super Prescription #5 Vitamin C with bioflavonoids
Take 1,000 mg three times daily. Vitamin C supports immune function, and bioflavonoids reduce skin inflammation.

Super Prescription #6 Burdock root (*Arctium lappa*)
Take 3 ml or 500 mg three times daily. Burdock root is used as a skin detoxifier.

Super Prescription #7 Zinc
Take 30 mg twice daily, along with 2 mg of copper. Zinc supports immune function and promotes skin healing.

The antimicrobial activity of oregano oil has been recognized for centuries. A test tube study at the Western University of Australia found that oregano oil had powerful antimicrobial activity against several types of bacteria, including *Staphylococcus aureus*, the bacteria commonly associated with skin infections.

General Recommendations

Vitamin E is required for a healthy immune system and healthy skin. Take 400 IU of a mixed complex twice daily.

Vitamin A supports immune function. Take 10,000 IU for ten days, and then stop.

Homeopathy

Pick the remedy below that best matches your symptoms. For acute abscesses and boils, take a 30C potency four times daily. For chronic abscesses and boils, take a 6x, 12x, 6C, 12C, or 30C twice daily for two weeks to see if there are any positive results. After you notice improvement, stop taking the remedy, unless symptoms return. Consultation with a homeopathic practitioner is advised.

Belladonna (*Atropa belladonna*) is used in the initial stages of an abscess or a boil, when there is a rapid onset characterized by redness, burning, throbbing, and swollen skin. Pus is not usually present. Symptoms are worse from touch or jarring and at midnight. A high fever may also be present.

Hepar Sulphuris is for abscesses that come to a head. The lesion is very sensitive and tender to touch, with a sharp, sticking pain. There may be a cheesy odor with the pus formation. Symptoms are worse in cold air or from cold applications and are better from warmth. This remedy helps to bring the pus out of the abscess or the boil.

Lachesis is used for boils with a purplish or dark-bluish color. Pustules may be bloody and very painful, with a burning sensation. Symptoms are worse at night; with touch, heat, and pressure; and on the left side of the body.

Mercurius Solubilis or Vivus is for burning and stinging pustular discharges. There is often a foul smell and swollen glands. Symptoms are worse at night. Warm applications may make the pain worse.

Silica (*Silicea*) is a great choice for abscesses or boils that do not discharge pus and that fail to heal. It is often used in addition to or following Hepar Sulphuris, to finish the suppuration. Warm compresses feel good on the lesions.

Acupressure

See pages 787–794 for information about pressure points and administering treatment.
- Spleen 10 (Sp10) clears heat from the blood.
- Large Intestine 4 (LI4) relieves fever and inmammation.

Bodywork

Reflexology

See pages 804–805 for information about reflexology areas and how to work them. Work the kidneys and the liver to detoxify the blood.

Hydrotherapy

Alternate a hot and a cold cloth over the affected area to help reduce pain and help expel pus, if the abscess is on the skin: thirty seconds hot, followed by thirty seconds cold, and alternate.

Aromatherapy

Thyme helps to draw the pus out. Add 1 drop to a hot compress, and apply twice daily to the skin abscess.

Stress Reduction

The effects of stress can worsen skin conditions. Techniques to reduce stress will ultimately help with skin health and appearance. Exercise, prayer, reading, and many other techniques can be used to reduce the effects of stress.

Other Recommendations

- A clay poultice applied topically will draw pus out of the lesion. Use under the direction of a practitioner.
- Do not squeeze a boil, and keep the area clean.
- Sunlight can inhibit bacterial growth. Get fifteen minutes of sunlight daily, but never allow the skin to burn.

REFERENCES

Hammer, K. A., C. F. Carson, and T. V. Riley. 1999. Antimicrobial activity of essential oils and other plant extracts. *Journal of Applied Microbiology* 86:985–90.

Acne

The familiar red and white pimples of acne are caused by pores that are blocked and often infected. Although acne is most common in adolescents (more than 80 percent of those between ages twelve and twenty-one are afflicted), it now appears with increasing frequency in adults.

Researchers have shown that adopting the typical American diet, high in sugar and processed foods, contributes to acne in cultures where acne was uncommon or unheard of.

As most people are aware, hormones play a significant role in acne. Normally, the body produces sebum, an oily lubricant, and secretes it through sebaceous glands to the skin. This lubricant is necessary to protect the skin from the elements and to keep it moist. During adolescence and other times of hormonal change, fluctuating hormones change this process and create several conditions that are likely to produce acne. For one, sebum production increases, and the oil, instead of passing harmlessly through the glands, hardens and clogs up the glandular canals. As a result, a red bump—a pimple—appears on the skin. Second, there is also increased production of keratin, a protective protein that covers the skin. Third, the same hormones cause an increase in the number of sebaceous glands, so there are more opportunities for acne to develop.

All of these factors can lead to clogged and infected pores, resulting in increased bacteria and yeast overgrowth on the skin. Overgrowth of these organisms causes skin inflammation. Superficial inflammation results in pustule formation and skin redness. Inflammation that occurs deeper in the skin can result in the formation of nodules and cysts and, possibly, scars.

One must also consider the role of food sensitivities, which can cause or worsen acne. These are discussed further in the Food to Avoid section. In addition, candida or yeast overgrowth can be an underlying cause of acne. This is most common after chronic antibiotic use, when "friendly bacteria" are destroyed, setting up the overgrowth of candida. Many people are on long-term antibiotic use for the treatment of acne, which sets up not only a further acne problem but potential digestive problems as well. Finally, nutritional deficiencies often need to be addressed to improve acne. Zinc, essential fatty acids, and other nutrients are crucial in preventing acne.

If you suffer from acne, be wary of the usual conventional treatments. Most prescription drugs for acne are either harsh topical lotions, which can cause dryness, redness, scaling, and sun sensitivity, or antibiotics, which disrupt the natural balance of intestinal flora and may give you yeast infections and diarrhea. Instead, try a natural treatment plan for acne that emphasizes dietary changes, detoxification, stress reduction, natural hormone balancing, and identification of possible food allergies.

CAUSES OF ACNE

Hormones can fluctuate at times other than adolescence, most notably during pregnancy, around the time of menses or menopause, and during periods of emotional stress.

Surprising Facts about Acne

A key hormone during male adolescence is testosterone. More important, there is greater activity of the enzyme 5-alpha reductase in the skin, which converts testosterone to a metabolite known as DHT (dihydrotestosterone). These hormones, as well as the delicate balance of estrogen and progesterone, along with stress hormones, play a role in female-adolescent, as well as in adult-female and -male, acne.

Oral contraceptives can also affect hormonal production. Acne can appear on babies as well. This is normal and goes away with time.

It would be a mistake, however, to attribute acne solely to fluctuating hormones. The second biggest contributor to acne is poor nutrition. Fat, sugar, and processed foods accelerate skin inflammation and acne. They also contribute to constipation, and thus the body responds by trying to expel the poisons through a different avenue—via the skin.

SYMPTOMS

Each of the following symptoms can appear on the face, the chest, or the back.

- Red spots, bumps, or pustules, sometimes inflamed and painful
- Whiteheads
- Blackheads
- Oily skin

ROOT CAUSES

- Genetics
- Hormonal fluctuation or imbalance
- Poor diet
- Emotional stress
- Nutritional deficiencies
- Poor digestion/toxic body system
- Food sensitivities
- Candida/yeast overgrowth
- Insulin resistance/elevated blood sugar levels

Testing Techniques

The following tests can be helpful in choosing a therapy that will be the most beneficial:

Stool or blood analysis for fungal overgrowth

Food allergies/sensitivities (see Food Allergies section)

Saliva hormone analysis for estrogen/progesterone/testosterone balance, cortisol, DHEA

Nutritional testing (blood/urine/hair) for nutritional deficiencies

Blood glucose testing

TREATMENT

Diet

Recommended Food

In general, acne sufferers should follow a simple diet of basic, unprocessed foods.

Dark-green or orange vegetables are especially helpful for their carotenoids, which help maintain and repair the skin. Eat them raw or lightly cooked to retain their nutrients and fiber.

A quarter cup of ground flaxseeds provides plenty of fiber for proper elimination, as well as helpful essential fatty acids. Take with at least 8 ounces of clean, quality water daily.

Nuts and seeds, such as almonds, walnuts, and pumpkin seeds, are good sources of skin-healthy vitamin E and essential fatty acids.

A study in the *American Journal of Clinical Nutrition* confirmed the benefits of a low-glycemic diet for improving acne vulgaris. A low-glycemic diet means the foods are less likely to increase glucose and insulin levels. The twelve-week study involved forty-three male acne patients fifteen to twenty-five years of age. The participants were put on a low-glycemic-load diet composed of 25 percent energy from protein and 45 percent from low-glycemic-index carbohydrates while the control group was on a typical American carbohydrate-rich diet. Acne lesion counts and severity were assessed during monthly visits, and insulin sensitivity was measured at baseline and at twelve weeks. Researchers found the total lesion counts in the low-glycemic group had decreased by twenty-two whereas the control group had a decrease of approximately twelve.

Quality protein sources are beans, peas, lentils, eggs, and fresh cold-water fish such as salmon, mackerel, herring, and sardines. The latter are rich in omega-3 fatty acids.

Meat products should be hormone- and antibiotic-free and limited.

Drink a glass of clean, quality water every two waking hours to flush toxins out of the body and to maintain good general health.

The Mediterranean diet, which is rich in plant foods and omega-3 fatty acids, has been shown to make people less prone to acne.

If you must use topical or oral antibiotics for acne, be sure to eat some live, unsweetened yogurt every day. Antibiotics destroy the "friendly" bacteria in your digestive tract, which are necessary for good health, and yogurt will replace them.

News about Acne Treatments

- Vitex (chasteberry) and saw palmetto (*Serenoa repens*) alleviate hormone-related acne.
- Homeopathic Silica (*Silicea*) reduces pus formation.
- Reducing simple carbohydrates in the diet decreases skin inflammation.

Food to Avoid

Eliminate junk and processed food, such as refined grains, colas, and candy. These products are a large source of toxins in the average diet.

Sugar encourages oil production and provides food for bacteria and yeast. Do not consume foods that contain added sugar. Avoid artificial sugar substitutes like saccharine or aspartame.

Although any food can conceivably result in an allergic response, by far the most frequent triggers are dairy, wheat, sugar, chocolate, and corn. Try the elimination diet described on page 316 to determine whether a food allergy is causing your problem, or see a natural–health care practitioner for testing.

- Saturated and hydrogenated fats are particularly difficult to digest, and they worsen acne. Stay away from fried foods and solid fats, such as margarine, lard, and vegetable shortening.
- An acidic internal environment encourages acne, so avoid alcohol, sugar, chocolate, fried foods, and soda, and limit meat products.
- Coffee and other caffeinated products may aggravate skin conditions. If they cause problems for you, cut them out and drink herbal teas instead.
- People with carbohydrate sensitivity may notice improvement in their skin by reducing their carbohydrate intake and increasing protein sources. This is because elevated levels of the blood sugar–regulating hormone insulin increase skin inflammation.
- Iodine may trigger acne. Dairy products and kelp products contain iodine.

℞ Super Seven Prescriptions—Acne

Super Prescription #1 Vitex (chasteberry)
Take 160 mg of a standardized Vitex extract (0.6 percent aucubin or 0.5 percent agnuside) or 40 drops of the tincture form daily.

Vitex (chasteberry) is an excellent hormone balancer to reduce acne formation and is effective for men and women. Use this super supplement or a hormone-balancing herbal formula for at least six weeks. If you see improvement, continue with the same dose as long as it remains effective. Do not use if you are on birth-control pills or are pregnant.

Super Prescription #2 Essential fatty acids

Take 1 to 2 tablespoons of flaxseed oil or 3 to 5 grams of fish oil daily.

Essential fatty acids, formulations that contain flaxseeds, fish, or a mixture of omega-3, 6, and 9 fatty acids, are helpful for acne and reduce skin inflammation. Take as directed on container. It may take four to eight weeks for improvements to be noticed.

Super Prescription #3 Zinc

Take 50 mg of zinc twice daily with meals for three months, and then reduce the dosage to 50 mg daily for long-term supplementation. It should be taken in conjunction with copper (3 to 5 mg).

Zinc is one of the best minerals to use for the treatment of acne. It works to reduce the buildup of DHT and promotes skin healing. It may take up to three months for benefits to occur. Do not use zinc sulfate, which is not readily absorbed.

Super Prescription #4 Burdock root *(Arctium lappa)*

Take 300 to 500 mg of the capsule form, 30 drops of tincture, or 1 cup of tea three times daily.

Burdock root works as a blood purifier and a detoxifier, and it improves elimination. It also has hormone-balancing properties. Take it for a minimum of eight weeks.

Super Prescription #5 Tea tree oil *(Melaleuca alternifolia)*

Apply a solution by dabbing it onto blemishes twice daily. It's available in many over-the-counter acne preparations.

A 5 percent solution of tea tree oil in diluted water acts similarly to benzoyl peroxide but without the drying side effects. Since tea tree oil is quite potent, test the solution on a small area of your skin first.

Super Prescription #6 Gugulipid

Gugulipid has been shown in research to reduce acne, particularly cystic acne. Take an extract containing 25 mg of guggulsterones, an active component, twice daily.

Super Prescription #7 Vitamin A

Vitamin A is helpful for the skin and has been shown in studies to reduce sebum production and keratin production. Take 5,000 IU to 10,000 IU or higher daily, under the guidance of a doctor. Research has shown that doses of 100,000 IU or higher are effective for acne; these dosages require a doctor's supervision.

The problem with vitamin A is that high dosages are needed to be effective for acne, and these may cause side effects. A way around this problem is to use a lower dosage, along with other nutrients that work synergistically for skin health, such as selenium, vitamin E, and zinc. Pregnant women or those trying to conceive should not use more than 5,000 IU daily.

A double-blind study of ninety-one people with moderately severe acne found that 90 mg of zinc significantly improved the acne more than a placebo did.

One study showed that a 5 percent tea tree oil gel extract was comparable to benzoyl peroxide in the treatment of mild to moderate acne. Tea tree oil users experienced fewer side effects (dryness, burning, redness, and itching).

General Recommendations

Saw palmetto (*Serenoa repens*) blocks excessive DHT production and is effective for both sexes. Take 160 mg of an 85 to 95 percent liposterolic standardized extract or 30 drops of tincture twice daily.

Dandelion root (*Taraxacum officinale*) supports your liver, which may be over-taxed with toxins. This herb is also a gentle laxative and can facilitate waste removal. Take 300 to 500 mg of the capsule form, 30 drops of tincture, or 1 cup of the tea three times daily.

Milk thistle (*Silybum marianum*) also supports liver detoxification. Find a product that's standardized for 70 to 85 percent silymarin content, and take 200 to 250 mg twice a day.

Passionflower (*Passiflora incarnata*) and hops (*Humulus lupulus*) are used when stress is contributing to your acne. Drink a cup of these calming teas whenever you need to wind down.

Vitamin E complex enhances the beneficial effects of selenium and vitamin A. Take 400 to 800 IU of mixed vitamin E complex with tocopherols and tocotrienols.

Selenium, a trace mineral, is helpful in reducing the inflammation of acne. Take 200 mcg daily. Multivitamins contain selenium, and many have a dosage that's close to 200 mcg.

Chromium helps with blood sugar regulation, which can be an important factor with acne. Take 200 to 400 mcg daily.

Vitamin B6 is useful for premenstrual acne. Take a 50 mg B-complex before and during premenstrual flare-ups.

Oregano oil (*Origanum vulgare*) destroys yeast overgrowth associated with acne formation. Take 500 mg twice daily or use a liquid form.

Natural progesterone cream is effective for premenstrual and menopausal acne. To improve premenstrual and premenopausal acne, apply 20 mg once daily for ten days before your expected menstrual flow. Menopausal women can apply 20 mg one to two times daily for three or all weeks of the month.

Colloidal silver gel has an antimicrobial action. Dab it onto pimples twice daily.

Chamomile (*Matricaria recutita*) has an anti-inflammatory property as well as a soothing effect on the nervous system.

Super-green-food supplements, such as chlorella, spirulina, or blends of green foods, support skin healing and detoxification. Take as directed on the container.

Topical niacinamide 4 percent gel was shown to be comparable to topical antibiotic therapy for acne.

A study in the *Journal of Dermatology* involved twenty patients with cystic acne. They received either tetracycline 500 mg or tablets of guggul (equivalent to 25 mg guggulsterone). Both were taken twice daily for three months. The percentage reduction in inflammatory lesions in the tetracycline group was 65.2 percent as compared to 68 percent in the guggul group. In addition, researchers observed that the patients with oily faces responded remarkably better to guggul.

Homeopathy

Use a combination acne formula or one of the following if it matches your symptoms. Use a 6x, 12x, 6C, or a 30C potency for two weeks. If there is improvement, discontinue using it.

Calcarea Sulphurica is for cystic acne or chronic acne where there is a yellow discharge.

Hepar Sulphuris (*Hepar sulphuris calcareum*) may provide relief if you have several pus-filled spots that are painful when touched, and if your skin lesions feel better with a warm compress.

Ledum palustre is helpful for pustular acne on the nose and the cheeks that feels better with cold applications.

Pulsatilla (*Pulsatilla pratensis*) is for acne associated with the hormonal changes of puberty, menstrual onset, or menopause.

Silica (*Silicea*) is for chronic white pustules.

Sulfur is for reddish, inflamed acne pustules that may be itchy or very sore. Heat or washing may cause a worsening of symptoms.

These formulas contain the most common homeopathic medicines for acne and skin health. In rare cases, your acne may initially worsen for a week and then begin to clear up. They are safe to use for all ages. Take as directed on the container.

Acupressure

See pages 787–794 for information about pressure points and administering treatment.

- Spleen 10 (Sp10) clears heat from the blood.
- Bladder 23 and 47 (B23 and B47), as well as Stomach 2 and 3 (St2 and St3), help clear acne.
- Bladder 10 (B10) can relieve stress that's related to acne.
- Large Intestine 4 (LI4) relieves constipation and depression.

Bodywork

Reflexology

See pages 804–805 for information about reflexology areas and how to work them.

Work the kidneys and the liver to detoxify the blood.

If acne is caused by a hormonal imbalance, work the endocrine glands.

To prevent constipation and speed the elimination of toxins, work the colon.

Hydrotherapy

Constitutional hydrotherapy improves digestion and detoxification. See pages 796–797 for instructions on how to use.

Aromatherapy

Lavender is calming to the emotions and the skin; it also fights bacterial infection. Apply it with a compress or put it in your bath.

Germanium will regulate the production of oil.

Bergamot is both an astringent and an antidepressant. When the skin improves, apply a lotion made with diluted water, lavender, and orange blossom to reduce scarring.

Stress Reduction

The effects of stress can throw the body into a state of imbalance. Stress can affect the skin by altering hormone levels and disrupting digestion and detoxification. People with acne generally feel more self-conscious about their looks. Techniques to reduce stress will ultimately help with skin health and appearance. Exercise, prayer, reading, and many other techniques can be used to reduce the effects of stress.

Sunlight can inhibit bacterial growth. Get fifteen minutes of sunlight, but never allow the skin to burn. Laser therapies available from doctors can be an effective way to reduce acne and treat existing scarring.

REFERENCES

Bassett, I. B., et al. 1990. A comparative study of tea tree oil versus benzoyl peroxide in the treatment of acne. *Medical Journal of Australia* 153:455–58.

Hillstrom, L., et al. 1977. Comparison of oral treatment with zinc sulfate and placebo in acne vulgaris. *British Journal of Dermatology* 97:679–84.

Smith R. N., et al. 2007. A low-glycemic-load diet improves symptoms in acne vulgaris patients: a randomized controlled trial. *Am J Clin Nutr* 86:107–15.

Thappa, D. M., and J. Dogra. 1994. Nodulocystic acne: oral gugulipid versus tetracycline. *J Dermatol* 21:729–31.

Adrenal Fatigue

Adrenal fatigue is one of the most underrated causes of ill health and disease in America and in other population groups around the world. Although it is no longer recognized by mainstream medicine it has become accepted by holistic doctors and practitioners as a real disorder.

This condition is characterized by the body's inability to cope with physical, emotional, and mental stresses the way a healthy mind and body are normally able to. This sets the stage for chronic fatigue, chronic infections, cognitive problems, imbalanced immune system, joint and muscle deterioration, and the inability to control inflammation.

Interestingly, the conventional establishment used to recognize adrenal fatigue under a different name, *hypoadrenia*. This medical term means underfunction or low-functioning adrenal glands. Now conventional medicine only recognizes Addison's disease, a disorder characterized by the adrenal glands' inability to produce enough of the stress hormone cortisol and often of the hormone aldosterone. This can lead to a breakdown of the body and even cause an acute health crisis.

Adrenal fatigue refers to low adrenal-gland functioning but is not as severe as Addison's disease. So at one end of the spectrum of adrenal-gland functioning you have Addison's disease and at the other end optimal adrenal function. The area in between could be referred to as some degree of adrenal fatigue.

The triangular-shaped adrenal glands, which are located on top of your kidneys, have two sections. The adrenal cortex is the outer part of the gland; it produces life-sustaining hormones such as cortisol, pregnenolone, and dehydroepiandrosterone (DHEA). These three hormones support the body's response to stress, and aldosterone helps regulate blood pressure. The glands' inner portion, known as the medulla, produces adrenaline and noradrenaline, which also help the body respond to stress.

Our experience treating tens of thousands of patients is that most people with chronic fatigue and chronic illness have some degree of adrenal fatigue. And by treating adrenal fatigue holistically one can achieve recovery more effectively. In some conditions it takes improved adrenal function to achieve any noticeable improvement at all.

SYMPTOMS

- Fatigue or exhaustion
- Light-headedness upon standing up
- Low blood pressure
- Mood swings, especially irritability
- Low libido
- Poor concentration
- Poor memory
- Frequent infections
- Low back pain

- Salt and/or sugar cravings
- Inability to lose or gain weight despite appropriate diet changes
- Poor response to any type of stress
- Blood sugar imbalance (low or high)
- Joint and muscle aches
- Slow reflexes

ROOT CAUSES

- Prolonged mental, emotional, or physical stress
- Nutrient deficiencies
- Sleep disorders
- Chronic illness
- Chronic infections
- Steroid medication

- Overexercising
- Surgical menopause
- Chronic pain
- Digestive illness
- Cholesterol that's too low
- Anemia

A randomized, double-blind, placebo-controlled study was conducted to investigate Ashwaganda's effects on reducing stress and anxiety in adults. Those taking Ashwagandha exhibited a significant reduction in scores on stress assessment testing compared to the placebo group. In addition, blood cortisol levels were significantly reduced. Adverse effects were mild and similar in both groups.

TREATMENT

Diet

Recommended Food

Consume smaller, more frequent, whole-food meals throughout the day. Consume adequate protein with meals, especially breakfast. Blood sugar fluctuations put more stress on the adrenal glands. Consume pH-balancing fruits and vegetables. These include potassium-rich foods such as apples, avocados, coconut milk, and water. Use salt such as sea salt or Celtic salt for good adrenal function. However, keep your intake of sodium below 2,000 mg daily. Consume good fats such as olive oil and coconut oil.

Foods to Avoid

Avoid sugars and refined carbohydrates, which cause blood sugar swings and stress the adrenal glands. Also avoid artificial sweeteners and preservatives.

℞ Super Seven Prescriptions—Adrenal Fatigue

Super Prescription #1 Ashwagandha
Take 250 mg of a standardized extract one to two times daily. This adaptogenic herb helps with the symptoms of adrenal fatigue including fatigue, anxiety, and insomnia. It also promotes DHEA and cortisol balance.

Super Prescription #2 Rhodiola
Take 300 mg daily of a 3 percent rosavins extract to support normal adrenal function.

Super Prescription #3 Licorice root

Take 500 mg two to three times daily to support low cortisol levels. Caution if you have high blood pressure.

Super Prescription #4 Adrenal glandular

Take one tablet or capsule three times daily to nourish your adrenal glands.

Super Prescription #5 Vitamin C

Take 1,000 mg two to three times daily to support adrenal hormone production.

Super Prescription #6 B-complex

Take 50 to 100 mg daily to support normal adrenal function.

Super Prescription #7 Eleutherococcus extract

Take 100 to 300 mg daily to support improvement of adrenal gland function.

General Recommendations

DHEA is available over the counter. Typical doses are 15 mg to 50 mg daily. Use under the guidance of your holistic doctor if your levels are low.

Pantothenic acid is a B vitamin that supports adrenal health. Take 500 mg one to two times daily.

Magnesium is often deficient in those with adrenal fatigue. Take 250 mg twice daily.

Maca root is a known adaptogen that supports adrenal function. Take 500 mg twice daily.

Stress Reduction

Since adrenal fatigue often occurs as the result of chronic stress it is imperative to incorporate daily stress-reducing techniques into your lifestyle.

Other Recommendations

- Acupuncture and Chinese herbal therapy offer benefits for those with adrenal fatigue. Consult with a qualified practitioner.
- Chiropractic improves nerve flow to the adrenal glands. Consult with a qualified practitioner.
- Homeopathic treatment individualized specifically for your symptoms is very effective. Consult with a qualified practitioner.
- Nutritional IV therapy utilizing nutrients such as B vitamins, minerals, and vitamin C is extremely helpful for those with adrenal fatigue. See a holistic doctor for treatment.
- Bioidentical hormone replacement from a holistic doctor is useful for those with severe adrenal fatigue .

REFERENCES

Biswajit, A., et al. 2008. A standardized withina sominifera extract signifincantly reduces stress-related parameters in chronically stressed humans: A double-blind, randomized, placebo-controlled study. *The Journal of the American Nutraceutical Association* 11(1):50–56.

A different double-blind, placebo-controlled trial involving Ashwagandha extract found those taking the supplement experienced a 79 percent reduction in fatigue. In addition, there were reductions in stress, anxiety, irritability, inability to concentrate, and forgetfulness. These factors did not change in the placebo group. Finally, serum cortisol levels decreased by 24.2 percent and DHEA levels increased by 32.2 percent for those supplementing Ashwagandha, demonstrating an adrenal-function benefit.

A double-blind crossover trial involved fifty-six young, healthy physicians who worked the night shift. Total fatigue index scores were significantly improved after two weeks of taking *Rhodiola rosea* extract. Mental-performance parameters were also improved in the treatment group. No side effects were reported.

Chandrasekhar, K., et al. 2012. A prospective, randomized, double-blind, placebo-controlled study of safety and efficacy of a high-concentration full-spectrum extract of ashwagandha root in reducing stress and anxiety in adults. *Indian Journal of Psychological Medicine* 34(3):255–62.

Darbinyan, V., et al. 2000. Rhodiola rosea in stress induced fatigue: a double blind cross-over study of a standardized extract SHR-5 with a repeated low-dose regimen on the mental performance of healthy physicians during night duty. *Phytomedicine* 7(5):365–71.

Aging

Aging is a natural process and not a disease. It is something we all will experience and, it is hoped, deal with in a positive manner. Ideally, numerous benefits attend old age: wisdom; the pleasure of watching your children, grandchildren, and great-grandchildren flourish; and having time to help others and to enjoy life fully.

But to many people, old age is synonymous with ill health and disability. That's too bad, because most of the diseases we associate with aging—arthritis and other painful conditions, heart disease, diabetes, cancer, digestive problems, frailty, depression, sexual dysfunction, and fatigue—are not an inevitable part of growing older. These so-called age-related disorders are mainly caused by lifestyle factors, such as diet, exposure to environmental toxins, lack of exercise, and stress, along with genetic susceptibilities. If you're young or middle-aged, you can prevent many problems by changing your habits now. If you're older and already experiencing health difficulties, it's not too late to bring balance and harmony to your bodily systems.

Normal aging occurs when old cells start dying at a faster rate than new ones are generated. Since the body's tissues have a smaller supply of cells to draw upon, they begin to degenerate and malfunction. This process happens to everyone; it's simply a natural part of life. It appears that our cells are preprogrammed to have a maximum life span. Yet the key is to prevent premature aging, wherein one ages faster than one's genetic programming would have ordained. In addition, most people will agree that quality of life is even more important than life span.

In recent years, we have come to understand more about the highly reactive kinds of atoms or molecules called free radicals. In many cases, free radicals assist the body by destroying invaders, producing energy, and helping to carry oxygen through the bloodstream. When they are present in overwhelming numbers, however, they attack healthy cells, sometimes destroying them or mutating their DNA. When cells die before their time or are damaged, the normal aging process is accelerated, and the body becomes vulnerable to life-threatening ailments such as cancer, arteriosclerosis, and many degenerative diseases.

Damage to the ends of chromosomes known as telomeres affects aging. Shortening of telomeres affects the ability of cells to replicate.

It is becoming more and more difficult to keep the number of free radicals in the body down to a healthy level. Many aspects of modern living, including unwholesome diet and exposure to pollution, tobacco smoke, environmental contaminants, and even the sun, put us in contact with more free radicals than any previous generation ever encountered. Luckily, nature has equipped us with the means to neutralize free radicals in our bodies. Substances called antioxidants accomplish the task, and they're found in many fruits and vegetables and in some herbs. A combination of healthful eating, combined with antioxidant supplements and wise living, can prevent excessive damage from free radicals.

In fact, poor diet and nutritional deficiencies—including overeating—are major causes of several age-related diseases. Studies on laboratory mice prove that a reduced-calorie diet significantly extended their lives. Research is starting to show that this is true for humans as well. In addition, diets that are high in fat and sugar lack many essential nutrients, fiber, and antioxidants. Poor diets also contribute to gastrointestinal disorders, which can inhibit the body's ability to absorb important vitamins and minerals. Sometimes, however, a good diet is not enough to keep deficiency at bay. As a result of normal or accelerated aging, older people are often simply less efficient at absorbing nutrients, even if they eat well. If you have reached old age, you will need to redouble your efforts to take in nutrients.

Aging is accelerated by a lack of exercise. If you don't regularly exercise, you increase your risk for almost every kind of disorder, including heart disease, diabetes, arthritis, and osteoporosis.

Hormone balance is a key to healthy aging. This is particularly true of the stress hormones such as cortisol and DHEA. A deficiency or an abnormal elevation of these hormones (particularly cortisol) accelerates aging and immune-system breakdown. In reality, all the hormones are important for healthy aging. Thyroid, estrogen, progesterone, and testosterone, as well as growth hormones, must be kept at balanced levels to slow the aging process. Researchers are finding that growth hormones may play a special role in slowing down the "aging clock."

It is also important to keep blood sugar levels in the normal range. Elevated levels of glucose lead to a process known as glycosylation. This contributes to a weak immune system and speeds up aging. An example of this process is diabetes.

Finally, the effects of stress appear to play a role in aging. People who experience prolonged periods of intense and unresolved stress are more likely to develop chronic diseases. One major stressor is loneliness. This has become a big problem with the elderly, who may lack companionship and stimulation. Many older people cut back on social obligations, intellectual activities, and sports and exercise. Giving up these essential activities has been linked to a shorter life span and an increased risk of disease. It is up to all of us, whatever our age, to create families and communities in which the elderly are welcome, active members.

SYMPTOMS

- Frequent illness or chronic disease
- Weight loss
- Painful conditions and stiffness
- Decreased sex drive
- Memory loss or impairment
- Poor skin and/or muscle tone
- Digestive problems
- Frailty

ROOT CAUSES

- Free-radical damage
- Poor digestion and detoxification
- Poor diet and nutritional deficiencies
- Lack of exercise
- Hormone imbalance
- Genetics
- Elevated blood sugar levels
- Environmental toxins
- Stress and isolation
- DNA damage

Testing Techniques

The following tests can give you an assessment of how well you're aging:

Telomere length—blood

Oxidative stress analysis—urine or blood

Antioxidant testing—urine, blood

Blood profile for cardiovascular, immune, and blood sugar markers (glucose, hemoglobin A1C, and insulin)

Stool analysis

Detoxification profile—urine

Hormone analysis by saliva, urine, or blood (estrogens, progesterone, testosterone, DHEA, cortisol, melatonin, IGF-1, thyroid panel)

Omega-3 analysis—blood

TREATMENT

Diet

Recommended Food

A 2014 study published in the *British Medical Journal* found that greater adherence to the Mediterranean diet was associated with greater telomere length, a biomarker of aging. Key components of this diet include vegetabeles, fruits, nuts, legumes, olive oil, fish, unrefined grains, and a low intake of dairy, meat, and poultry.

Make sure you get enough fiber. Whole grains, oats, flaxseeds, chia seeds, and raw vegetables can prevent constipation and will reduce toxins in the digestive tract.

Yogurt and other fermented sour products (sauerkraut, kefir) encourage healthful bacteria in the digestive system.

Deeply colored fruits and vegetables are packed with antioxidants such as carotenoids, the substances that neutralize free radicals.

Vitamin E and selenium work together to prevent many different diseases. To lower your risk of diseases that affect aging, such as cancer, heart disease, and arthritis, eat plenty of seeds, nuts, and vegetable oils.

Be sure to incorporate sufficient high-quality protein into your diet. Beans, soy products, nuts and seeds, fish, and lean chicken and turkey will give you energy.

Vitamin C helps fight free-radical damage, reduces cancer risk, and strengthens the immune system. Good dietary sources of vitamin C include citrus fruits, green leafy vegetables, red peppers, strawberries, tomatoes, asparagus, and avocados.

Garlic and onions also have antioxidant properties and improve circulation, so enjoy them freely.

Whether you're thirsty or not, drink a glass of clean, quality water every two waking hours. Dehydration is linked to kidney malfunction, malabsorption of nutrients, chronic constipation, weight gain, high cholesterol, fatigue, and headaches. It can also cause disorientation and memory loss.

The skins of red grapes reduce plaque in the walls of arteries. They also have antioxidant properties, so drink a glass of red grape juice or an occasional glass of red wine. Keeping the digestive tract clean is essential for preventing disease, especially if you've spent a lifetime consuming and breathing toxins. Fresh vegetable and fruit juices and "super green foods," such as chlorella and spirulina, are excellent. Supplements such as milk thistle (*Silybum marianum*) and many of the antioxidants support proper detoxification.

Food to Avoid

Reduce your total caloric intake while maintaining good nutrition. As you get older, your metabolism slows down, and you require fewer calories to support your activities. Also, studies on laboratory mice have shown that a reduced-calorie diet significantly extended their lives. You can reduce calories by cutting out processed and junk foods, alcohol, sugar, and white flour—but don't skimp on nutritious foods that will keep you healthy.

In addition to the previous suggestions, avoid red meat and processed foods, as well as any food made with additives and preservatives. These foods are all high in free radicals. What's more, they clog up your digestive tract and inhibit proper functioning. Avoid the trans fat that is often contained in packaged and fried foods and that damages cell DNA.

℞ Super Seven Prescriptions—Anti-Aging

Super Prescription #1 Resveratrol
Take 250 mg daily. May activate anti-aging genes in your cells. Also reduces cellular inflammation.

Super Prescription #2 Green tea
Green tea is a rich source of antioxidants and substances that assist detoxification. Drink the organic tea regularly (2 cups or more daily), or take 500 to 1,500 mg of the capsule form.

Super Prescription #3 Fish oil
Take 1,000 mg of EPA and DHA daily. Fish oil supports the health of genes involved in aging and improves telomere length.

Super Prescription #4 Ashwagandha
Ashwagandha supports stress-hormone balance, which is important for healthy aging. Take 125 to 250 mg of a 0.8 percent standardized extract.

Super Prescription #5 Super-green-food supplement
Take an organic super green food such as chlorella or spirulina or a mixture of these each day. Take as directed on the container.

Cardiologists at the University of California–San Francisco have found that heart disease patients with high intake of omega-3 fatty acids had a slower rate of shortening of telomeres, the tips of chromosomes, than patients with low intake of omega-3s. Telomeres usually shorten with age, and heart disease speeds this process. Omega-3 fatty acids have the unique effect of protecting telomeres.

Tea consumption has been associated with better telomere length. The highest intakes, three cups or 750 millilitres per day, was associated with significantly longer telomere lengths suggesting an anti-aging effect.

> **Super Prescription #6 High-potency multivitamin**
> Take a high-potency multivitamin and -mineral formula daily, as it will contain a strong base of the antioxidants and other nutrients that protect against aging.
>
> ---
>
> **Super Prescription #7 Glutathione**
> Take 250 mg of glutathione twice daily before meals for optimized DNA and free -radical protection. Topical glutathione is also a good option.

General Recommendations

Enzymes aid in the digestion of food and are essential for all the metabolic activity in the body. Take 1 or 2 capsules with each meal.

Garlic. Take 1 or 2 capsules of an aged garlic product daily. Garlic benefits the immune and cardiovascular systems. It also improves detoxification and has antioxidant properties.

Cordyceps sinensis is a revered fungus used in Chinese medicine as a supplement to combat fatigue and the aging process. Take 2 to 4 capsules daily.

Royal jelly, the substance produced by worker bees as the sole food for their queen, contains a wide range of nutrients. Take as directed on the container.

Alpha lipoic acid is one of the most important antioxidants in the body. Take 50 mg twice daily.

CoQ10 is a potent antioxidant and a nutrient involved in many aspects of cardiovascular function. Take 50 to 300 mg daily.

Reishi extract, revered in Chinese medicine, is made from the "mushroom of immortality." It improves liver and immune-system function. Take 2 to 4 capsules daily.

Panax ginseng is revered in Chinese medicine as an anti-aging herbal therapy. Take a standardized product containing 4 to 7 percent ginsenosides at 100 to 250 mg twice daily. Do not use if you have high blood pressure.

DHEA is a hormone that research shows is an accurate marker of aging. If your level is low, talk with your doctor about supplementation.

Ginger (*Zingiber oformone*) is indeed excellent for aiding the digestion; it also prevents blood clotting and has anti-inflammatory properties. Instead of drinking sugary ginger ale, try ginger tea, made by pouring boiling water over fresh ginger. You can also take 1 or 2 grams of a powdered capsule or a tablet, divided over the course of a day. Or you can use 1 to 3 ml of a ginger tincture three times daily.

Siberian ginseng (*Eleutherococcus senticosus*), like most types of ginseng, helps the body to adapt to mental and physical stress. Take 600 to 900 mg of a standardized product daily.

Ginkgo biloba can also be helpful. Take 60 to 120 mg twice daily of a standardized product that contains 24 percent flavone glycosides and 6 percent terpene lactones.

Homeopathy

See a homeopathic practitioner who can prescribe a remedy to strengthen your particular state of body and mind.

If you're an older person who has already developed an illness or a painful condition, you will find homeopathic suggestions listed under the specific disorder that's plaguing you.

A double-blind clinical trial studied the effects of 1,500 mg of *Panax ginseng* on forty-nine elderly people. This herb was found to improve coordination and reaction time, as well as to increase alertness and energy.

A study published in the *American Journal of Clinical Nutrition* found that multivitamin use was associated with longer telomeres in women.

Acupressure

See pages 787–794 for information about pressure points and administering treatment.

- Stomach 36 (St36) is a good point for keeping up health in general. It strengthens the entire body but gives particular support to the immune and digestive systems.

Bodywork

Bodywork is more important than ever in old age. Not only does it increase circulation and reduce aches and pains, it can supply significant emotional benefits to people who are deprived of nurturing physical contact. If you are isolated or depressed, or if your body has become rigid from lack of touch, you might find massage both relaxing and invigorating.

Reflexology

See pages 804–805 for information about reflexology areas and how to work them.

Work the entire foot to provide support for all the systems of the body.

If you want to concentrate on just a few areas, work the kidneys, the liver, and the colon to encourage detoxification.

Hydrotherapy

Hot and cold hydrotherapy is invigorating and stimulates blood flow to the brain. Try alternating hot and cold baths for the best effect.

Aromatherapy

If you feel tense or irritable or have trouble sleeping, lavender can help you relax. Try it in a bath or as an inhalant, or slip a lavender-filled sachet under your pillow.

If you are depressed, bergamot, clary sage, geranium, or rosemary can be uplifting.

A few drops of jasmine, ylang-ylang, sandalwood, or patchouli in a bath will reignite sexual desire.

Stress Reduction

Exercise, prayer, reading, yoga, positive mental imagery, and many other techniques should be used to reduce the effects of stress and aging.

Other Recommendations

- Keep moving. Regular exercise plays a significant role in preventing heart disease, arthritis, osteoporosis, diabetes, and many other disorders. For maximum benefits, your exercise plan should include aerobic exercise (for your heart and lungs), weight lifting (to keep your bones strong), and stretching. It is never too late to start. People who begin exercise and weight-lifting programs as late as their nineties show marked improvement in their general health. If you're older, ill, or overweight, consult with your doctor before beginning an exercise plan.
- If you're having problems digesting your food, your body may not be producing sufficient enzymes. Take an enzyme supplement daily.

REFERENCES

Chan, R., et al. 2010. Chinese tea consumption is associated with longer telomere length in elderly Chinese men. *Br J Nutr* 103(1):107–13.

Crous-Bou, M., et al. 2014. Mediterranean diet and telomere length in Nurses' Health Study: population based cohort study. *British Medical Journal* 349:g6674.

Farzaneh-Far, R., et al. 2010. Association of marine omega-3 fatty acid levels with telomeric aging in patients with coronary heart disease. *Journal of the American Medical Association* 303:250–57.

Fulder, S., et al. 1984. A double blind clinical trial of panax ginseng in aged subjects. Presented at the Fourth International Ginseng Symposium, Daejon, South Korea.

Xu, Q., et al. 2009. Multivitamin use and telomere length in women. *Am J Clin Nutr* 89(6):1857–63.

AIDS and HIV

Although scientists have discovered several treatments that extend the life span of people with the virus, there is still no cure. More than 50 percent of new HIV infections occur in men who have sex with men. New HIV infections are also occurring more commonly in African Americans and Hispanics. However, HIV can infect anyone, regardless of race or sexual orientation.

HIV is transmitted via vaginal or anal sex or by blood-to-blood contact. It is vitally important for everyone to practice safe sex, preferably in the form of a monogamous relationship with an HIV-free partner, and to abstain from intravenous drug use. Don't rely solely on condoms to protect you, as they sometimes let HIV and other viruses pass through. Intravenous drug users are at a high risk: if you have an addiction, you should seek help, but at the very least you should never share needles with anyone.

The virus may also be passed from mother to child during birth or breastfeeding. It is possible to greatly reduce the chance of transmitting the disease during birth. Pregnant women should be tested for HIV as soon as possible, so that they and their unborn children can receive vital treatment. HIV is sometimes contracted by health care workers who are stuck with infected needles. Also, be aware that the virus cannot be transmitted through casual contact, such as coughing, sneezing, shaking hands, or dry kissing.

Like all viruses, once HIV has entered the body, it seeks to replicate itself. What makes HIV far deadlier than, say, a cold virus is that it takes a particularly aggressive tactic within the body: once it invades a cell, it reprograms that cell's genetic material. Normally, a cell will reproduce by dividing and creating a copy of itself. In this way, the body regenerates itself at the most basic level. But when cells that are invaded by HIV divide, they don't create copies of themselves—they create copies of the virus. Those copies then invade other healthy cells, so that, eventually, the virus cells far outnumber the healthy ones. To make matters worse, HIV attacks a particular kind of immune cell, called a Helper T-cell (these lymphocytes have a receptor protein called CD4+ in their outer membrane and so are also referred to as CD4+ lymphocytes). As more and more CD4+ cells are destroyed, the body's ability to fight off infections is dramatically weakened.

Most people do not notice any symptoms when HIV first invades the body. People with HIV will usually go for years without knowing it, unless they are tested for the disease. Before AIDS develops, many will begin to experience symptoms such as night sweats, fatigue, fevers, diarrhea, weight loss, enlarged lymph nodes, thrush, herpes, mouth ulcers, and bleeding gums. Later, as the number of T-cells continues to decrease, their bodies will be highly vulnerable to infection by viruses and bacteria. HIV-positive people might contract a variety of diseases that are otherwise rare, such as Kaposi's sarcoma (a kind of skin cancer characterized by raised purple welts), the Epstein-Barr virus (also known as chronic fatigue syndrome), neurological problems, eye infections (including cytomegalovirus, which can cause blindness), toxoplasmic encephalitis (a brain infection), and systemic candidiasis (yeast infection). Other infections are those we usually consider common, such as pneumonia and various respiratory ailments.

Acquired immunodeficiency syndrome (AIDS) is the most severe form of HIV infection. A person with HIV infection is considered to have AIDS when at least one complicating illness develops or the person's ability to defend against infection significantly declines, as measured by a low CD4+ lymphocyte count. Since the number of CD4+ lymphocytes in the blood helps to determine the ability of the immune system to protect the body from infections, it is a good measure of the degree of damage done by HIV infection. A healthy person has a CD4+ lymphocyte count of roughly 800 to 1,300 cells per microliter of blood. Typically, 40 to 60 percent of CD4+ lymphocytes are destroyed in the first few months of infection. After about six months, the CD4+ count stops falling so quickly, but it continues to decline. If the CD4+ count falls below about 200 cells per microliter of blood, the immune system is susceptible to severe, life-threatening infections.

It is important to note that while all people with AIDS are HIV-positive, not all people with HIV develop AIDS. Most HIV-positive people develop AIDS within eight to twelve years after first contracting the virus, but some develop it much faster, and many others still remain healthy decades after contracting HIV. It appears that people who are able to ward off full-blown AIDS are those whose immune systems are the strongest. Therefore, complementary therapies for HIV and AIDS work to bolster the ability of the immune system to fight infection.

If you contract HIV, you need to work with a doctor who knows about the latest treatments available for the disease. Antiviral medications have been largely successful in recent years. Holistic therapies can be used to augment conventional therapies.

SYMPTOMS

There are no symptoms during the early stages of HIV, except perhaps a fever when the virus first invades the body. As the virus continues to multiply, the following symptoms can occur:

- Night sweats
- Diarrhea
- Fatigue
- Weight loss
- Fevers

- Enlarged lymph nodes
- Thrush (mouth fungus)
- Herpes
- Mouth ulcers
- Bleeding gums

Several conditions are associated with full-blown AIDS. Following are some of the most common:

- Kaposi's sarcoma (a type of skin cancer characterized by raised purple welts)

- Epstein-Barr virus infection

Neurological problems:

- Eye problems (often related to cytomegalovirus, which can cause blindness)
- Pneumonia and other respiratory ailments

- Candidiasis
- Toxoplasmic encephalitis (a brain infection)
- Salmonella
- Cancer of various organs

ROOT CAUSES

- Anal or vaginal sex with an infected partner
- Transfusions of infected blood (in the United States, blood donations have been screened for HIV since 1985)

- Blood-to-blood contact with an infected person (such as from sharing needles for intravenous drug use)
- In the womb, at birth, or during breastfeeding

Testing Techniques

Diagnosis of HIV is done with the use of the following blood test:
    HIV ELISA Test
If this test is positive, it is confirmed with a more accurate test known as Western Blot. Also, the CD4+ count and the viral load are used to monitor progression of the disease.
It is also helpful to have:
    Oxidative stress analysis—urine or blood testing
    Antioxidant testing—urine, blood, or skin scanning
    Stool analysis
    Hormone analysis by saliva, urine, or blood (estrogens, progesterone, testosterone, DHEA, cortisol, melatonin, IGF-1, thyroid panel)

TREATMENT

Diet

To reduce the risk of toxins entering your body, food should be as clean and pure as possible. If you cook meat and poultry at home, reduce your risk of food poisoning by keeping preparation areas sanitary and by cooking at high-enough temperatures. Eat organic food, if it is available. If organic products are not an option, at least wash your food with pure water to get rid of pesticides and other toxins. A gluten-free diet is worth trying, especially if you have chronic diarrhea. Work with a nutritionist and avoid wheat, rye, barley, and oats.

Recommended Food

If you have HIV or AIDS, you absolutely must eat well. A good basic diet will include plenty of raw vegetables, seeds, nuts, grains, fresh fruit, and lean protein from quality sources. An adequate intake of calories is most important. Protein is particularly important to prevent weight loss and maintain optimal immune function. Try to consume 2.0 grams for every 2.2 pounds of body weight. A high-quality whey protein is helpful in attaining this goal.

Garlic and onions have natural antibiotic effects, so use them often.

To optimize immunity, include cruciferous vegetables (broccoli, cauliflower, cabbage, brussels sprouts, and others) in your diet.

Drink a glass of clean, quality water every two waking hours. Make sure the water is from a good source, to avoid bacteria and parasite infection.

The "good" bacteria in your digestive tract help fight infection, so maintain their presence by eating yogurt with live cultures, especially *Lactobacillus acidophilus* and *bifidus*. This is especially important if you are taking antibiotics, which kill the good bacteria along with the bad. If you cannot tolerate yogurt, take probiotic capsules.

If you have HIV, it is strongly advised that you invest in a good juicer. Live juices will help your weakened system absorb a maximum amount of nutrients. Drink several glasses daily of a variety of juices, especially those made from cruciferous and green vegetables, black radishes, cabbage, greens (such as wheatgrass), and carrots.

Food to Avoid

Do not consume raw eggs; unpasteurized milk, cheese, or cider; or rare meat. All these products can contain harmful bacteria. In people who have compromised immune systems, these bacteria can lead to septicemia, an extremely dangerous and often fatal condition.

Eliminate junk food, fried food, sugar, and alcohol, all of which suppress your immune system and tax your entire body.

Find out now if you have any food allergies or sensitivities, because they cause the immune system to attack itself. See the elimination diet on page 316 for further details.

℞ Super Seven Prescriptions—HIV/AIDS

Super Prescription #1 High-potency multivitamin
A daily base of vitamins and minerals supports a healthy immune system.

Super Prescription #2 Glutamine
Take 40 grams daily to prevent tissue wasting and to support muscle mass. It also promotes intestinal health and absorption.

Super Prescription #3 Coenzyme Q10
Take 200 mg daily to improve your immunity to this disease.

Super Prescription #4 Vitamin D3
Take 5,000 IU daily to support healthy immunity.

One clinical trial found that HIV-positive men who took a multivitamin and -mineral supplement had a slower onset of AIDS, as compared to men who did not take a supplement.

> **Super Prescription #5 *Saccharomyces boulardii***
> Take five billion colony-forming units daily to prevent HIV-associated diarrhea.
>
> **Super Prescription #6 Glutathione**
> Take 250 to 500 mg twice daily to support immunity and detoxification from the use of antiviral medications.
>
> **Super Prescription #7 DHEA**
> Take 50 to 500 mg daily under the supervision of a doctor to allay fatigue and support immunity.

A double-blind trial using the plant extract boxwood (SPV30) found that 990 mg per day could delay disease progression in HIV-infected patients (as measured by a decline in CD4+ cell counts).

General Recommendations

Take 5,000 IU daily of vitamin D with a meal. Vitamin D supports the immune system.

Enzymes aid in the digestion of food and are essential for all the metabolic activity in the body. Take 1 or 2 capsules with each meal.

L-glutathione is one of the most important antioxidants in the body. Take 500 mg twice daily.

Take 5,000 IU or more of vitamin A under your doctor's supervision. Vitamin A is important for healthy immunity.

Reishi (*Ganoderma lucidum*) extract improves liver and immune system function. Take 2 to 4 capsules daily.

Garlic (*Allium sativum*) supports immune function. Take an aged garlic supplement daily.

Milk thistle (*Silybum marianum*; 80 to 85 percent silymarin) supports liver function while you use pharmaceutical medications for HIV/AIDS. Take 250 to 300 mg three times daily.

Aloe (*Aloe vera*) has antiviral effects. Use a food-grade product, and take as directed on the container.

Selenium has antiviral effects. Take a daily dosage of 400 mcg.

Maitake (*Grifola frondosa*) supports immune function and has antiviral properties. Take 1 mg of the MD or D fraction per 2.2 pounds of body weight daily.

Turmeric (*Curcuma longa*; 90 to 95 percent curcumin) is shown in test tube studies to inhibit HIV infection. Take 500 mg three times daily.

Zinc supports immune function. Take a daily total of 30 to 50 mg.

Thyme extract supports healthy immunity. Take as directed on the container.

Super-green-food supplements supply a host of nutrients and antioxidants. Take an organic super-green-food supplement, such as chlorella or spirulina, as directed on the container, or eat a mixture of super green foods each day.

Take 25 grams daily of whey protein, or as directed by your doctor. It helps prevent tissue wasting and repairs the digestive tract.

Many studies have shown that people with HIV have a greater need for antioxidants. Take a combination antioxidant formula, as directed on the container.

Take 50 mg of vitamin B-complex twice daily. Many people with HIV have B-vitamin deficiencies, which can impair immune function.

Take 1,000 to 3,000 mg of vitamin C daily. It supports immune function.

Homeopathy

HIV and AIDS are complex disorders with many variables. A homeopathic practitioner can suggest a preparation that addresses your individual needs.

Acupressure

See pages 787–794 for information about pressure points and administering treatment.
- Conception Vessel 17 (CV17) helps the immune system and also eases depression and anxiety.
- To ease digestive problems and improve the absorption of nutrients, try Stomach 36 (St36).

Bodywork

Massage

A lymphatic massage, especially with the oils listed in the Aromatherapy section further on, will drain toxins from your body. Massage, in general, can help relieve stress, depression, and fatigue. Consult with your doctor before treatment.

Reflexology

See pages 804–805 for information about reflexology areas and how to work them.
Work the liver point to support this critical organ of the immune system.
If you are constipated or experience diarrhea, massage the area corresponding to the colon.

Hydrotherapy

Hot and cold hydrotherapy promotes healing and energy and also combats stress.
See Constitutional Hydrotherapy on pages 795–796.

Aromatherapy

Add juniper to a carrier oil, and use in a lymphatic massage. Juniper helps break down toxins that have built up in fatty deposits.
Several oils have antibacterial properties, especially tea tree and eucalyptus. These oils can be used in any form but are highly recommended for use in lymphatic massage.
To lift your spirits, use lavender or geranium oils in any form.

Stress Reduction

General Stress-Reduction Therapies

A diagnosis of HIV can be devastating. You need someone you can talk to as you work through the initial shock and then face each successive challenge. Although family and friends are always a welcome source of strength, you may also want to recruit the help of a professional who has experience working with people suffering from a difficult illness. A religious adviser, a psychotherapist, or a support-group leader can offer you invaluable advice and help.

In a world of expensive and invasive medical treatments, meditation and positive mental imagery can come as a relief. All you need is some private space and a comfortable place to sit. As you become skilled at meditation, you'll find that you can use its calming techniques whenever necessary, even if you're ill and bedridden.

Other Recommendations

- Intravenous nutrient therapy supplies high levels of nutrients that support good immune health.
- Get plenty of rest and fresh air.
- Regular exercise will counteract stress and help keep you healthy, but don't overdo it. A daily morning walk is a good idea. Weightlifting helps to maintain muscle mass.
- Try to get early morning sunlight on your skin, but make sure to stay away from harsh or bright sun. People with HIV have a heightened vulnerability to skin cancer.

REFERENCES

Durant, J., et al. 1998. Efficacy and safety of Buxus sempervirens L. preparations (SPV30) in HIV-infected asymptomatic patients: a multicentre, randomized, double-blind, placebo-controlled trial. *Phytomedicine* 5:1–10.

Ince, S. 1993. Vitamin supplements may help delay onset of AIDS. *Medical Tribune* 9:18.

"HIV in the United States: Still a Deadly but Preventable Disease." Centers for Disease Control and Prevention. www.cdc.gov/features/worldaidsday/.

Alcoholism. See Substance Abuse

Allergies. See also Asthma and Food Allergies

An allergic reaction occurs when the immune system misinterprets a normally non-toxic substance, such as grass, pollen, a detergent, or a certain food, as a harmful invader. The immune system then responds to this perceived threat, called an allergen, by releasing substances called histamines. Histamines produce a wide range of bodily reactions, including respiratory and nasal congestion, increased mucus production, skin rashes and welts, and headache. In the case of an actual threat to the body, in the form of, say, a flu virus, these reactions would form an important line of defense against the invader, helping to trap it and expel it, and encouraging you to rest and recover. But during the false alarm of an allergic response, the body overreacts to an otherwise harmless agent.

Most allergens are found either in the environment or in food. (For information about allergic reactions to food, see Food Allergies.) Environmental allergens include pollen (reactions to pollen are often called hay fever), mold, animal dander, dust, feathers, insect venom, certain cosmetics and household products, and metals. When the environmental allergens are removed or make their seasonal disappearance, the body returns to normal. If the allergens are not removed, the immune system will continue its artificially high state of alert. In these cases, the allergic response can develop into chronic allergic rhinitis, in which the nasal passages remain persistently inflamed.

Why some people develop allergies to certain substances and others do not remains unclear. It does seem that certain allergic responses, such as hay fever, have a genetic basis. An excess accumulation of mucus in the body, which attracts and stores the irritant, also contributes to or causes allergic responses. In addition, stress and a generally depressed immune system may contribute to the severity of allergies.

CAUSES

- Allergies happen when the immune system attacks a harmless substance. Common triggers for allergies include mold; dust; tree, grass, or flower pollen; animal dander; feathers; insect venom, especially from bee stings; metal, particularly nickel; household chemicals; and some cosmetics
- An excess of mucus, caused by a poor diet
- Stress, which depresses the immune system

SYMPTOMS

Allergic responses can produce any one or a combination of several of the following symptoms:

- Nasal congestion
- Headache
- Sneezing
- Fatigue
- Coughing
- Fluid retention
- Red, itchy, or watery eyes
- Swelling of the throat and the tongue
- Wheezing
- Sore throat
- Hives, rashes, eczema, or other skin eruptions

Caution: If you experience difficulty breathing or develop hives that spread rapidly, get emergency help at once. Allergic reactions like these can quickly be fatal. If you know you have severe reactions to certain substances, talk to your doctor about emergency adrenaline kits you can keep on hand.

ROOT CAUSES

- Genetics
- Poor digestion
- Nutritional deficiencies
- Lack of exposure to germs and allergens when a child
- Limited diet (in cases of food sensitivities, a lack of variety in the diet)

Testing Techniques

Blood IgG4 and IgE food and environmental panels

Skin-scratch allergy testing

Electrodermal testing for sensitivities

TREATMENT

Diet

If you have allergies, dietary therapy should include strategies for mucus reduction, elimination of allergenic pathogens, and general immune support.

Recommended Food

Base your diet on non–mucus forming foods: whole grains (although gluten sensitivity is common), fresh vegetables and fruits, cold-pressed oils, and raw seeds and nuts. (Many people with environmental allergies also have reactions to nuts, so monitor your reactions carefully.)

To keep your immune system healthy, make sure to get enough lean protein. Seafood and tofu are good sources that don't encourage mucus production.

Drink six to eight 8-ounce glasses of clean, quality water a day to thin mucus secretions.

Flaxseeds and flaxseed oil can reduce inflammation. Take 2 tablespoons every day.

Fresh vegetable juices improve detoxification, which indirectly helps an overactive immune system. A 3-day vegetable-juice fast can help reduce some allergy symptoms.

Food to Avoid

Eliminating foods that cause mucus should be a priority for any allergy sufferer. Mucus-forming foods include all dairy products, fried and processed foods, refined flours, chocolate, and eggs.

The immune response stresses your digestive system, so place as few additional burdens on it as possible. Cut down on bad fats and oils such as margarine. Instead focus on healthier oils such as coconut, olive, and macadamia nut.

Many people with environmental allergies also suffer from food allergies. See the Food Allergies section and follow the elimination diet there to ensure that certain foods aren't making your environmental allergies worse.

Wheat is the unsuspected culprit behind many allergies, including those characterized by sneezing and itching. Try eliminating wheat during the seasons that usually coincide with your allergic responses.

A randomized, double-blind study involving the use of freeze-dried nettles and people who had hay fever found that after one week of use, 58 percent of participants had a reduction in their sneezing and itching.

℞ Super Seven Prescriptions—Allergies

Super Prescription #1 Homeopathy
Take a combination allergy homeopathic remedy, as directed on the container, or read the description under Homeopathy in this section to pick a single remedy.

Super Prescription # 2 Butterbur
Take a standardized product that contains 8 to 16 mg of petasin per dose three to four times daily.

Super Prescription #3 Stinging nettles (*Urtica dioica*)
Take 300 to 500 mg daily. Studies show that it is effective for hay fever.

Super Prescription #4 Methylsulfonylmethane (MSM)
Take 3,000 to 5,000 mg daily. It reduces allergic and inflammatory responses.

Super Prescription #5 Quercitin
Take 1,000 mg three times daily. It has a natural antihistamine effect.

Super Prescription #6 Eyebright (*Euphrasia officinalis*)
Take 1 capsule three times daily or apply as a solution to irritated eyes by adding 3 to 5 drops of eyebright tincture to an ounce of contact lens (saline) solution in a disposable cup. Rinse each eye with a separate cup and toss the cups after use. Do this once or twice a day to relieve irritated eyes and remove redness.

Super Prescription #7 Vitamin C
Take 1,000 mg three to five times daily (reduce the dosage if diarrhea occurs). It has a natural antihistamine effect.

General Recommendations

Take 1 to 2 tablespoons of flaxseed oil or 3 grams of fish oil daily. They reduce inflammatory responses associated with allergies.

Thyme extract has been shown to calm the immune response to allergies. Take as directed on the container.

Probiotics reduce the potential for allergies. Take a product containing at least four billion organisms of *Lactobacillus acidophilus* and *bifidus*.

Nasal saline irrigation of both nostrils daily will reduce nasal and sinus symptoms related to allergies.

Protease enzymes decrease allergic and inflammatory responses. Take 2 capsules twice daily on an empty stomach or as directed on the container.

Digestive enzymes assist in the digestion of food and reduce the likelihood of food sensitivities. Take 1 or 2 capsules with meals.

Betaine hydrochloride assists in the digestion of food and reduces the likelihood of food sensitivities. Take 1 or 2 capsules with meals.

A randomized, double-blind study of 330 participants with hay fever compared the efficacy of butterbur to the medication Allegra and a placebo. Both treatments were superior to the placebo and comparable to each other. An additional study demonstrated butterbur to be as effective as the popular antihistamine drug Zyrtec.

Homeopathy

Pick the remedy that best matches your symptoms. Take 2 pellets of 30C potency twice daily. Should the first three days pass without any sign of improvement, you're probably taking the wrong remedy. Stop using the current one, and switch to something else. When you first notice improvement, stop taking the remedy unless your symptoms begin to return.

Allium Cepa is good for burning, watery eyes and a runny nose. Sneezing is common, and your symptoms feel better in the open air.

Arsenicum Album is for people with burning eyes and a runny nose that doesn't stop, causing the skin under the nose to get red and excoriated. This remedy is effective for the highly sensitive person with many allergies.

Euphrasia is for red, burning, tearing eyes.

Histaminum is for non–life threatening allergy symptoms that come on quickly.

Lycopodium (*Lycopodium clavatum*) is for people who have right-sided nasal and throat symptoms. Bloating after meals is common.

Natrum Muriaticum is for people who sneeze from the sun. They often get cold sores and crave salty foods.

Nux Vomica (*Strychnos nux vomica*) is also for people with diverse allergy symptoms,but those who benefit from this remedy tend to crave sweets, tobacco, and other stimulants. They often wake up sneezing.

Pulsatilla (*Pulsatilla pratensis*) is for people whose allergies are worse in a warm room and who crave the open air. Their nasal passages often get congested at night.

Sabadilla is for people who suffer from many repeated sneezes in a row and a runny nose.

Silica (*Silicea*) will help if your allergies manifest as upper respiratory problems that develop into infections and if you often feel fatigued and low in stamina.

Acupressure

See pages 787–794 for information about pressure points and administering treatment.
- Large Intestine 4 (LI4) relieves headaches and sneezing.
- For fatigue, swollen eyes, and headache, use Bladder 10 (B10).
- Triple Warmer 5 (TW5) fortifies the immune system.
- Stomach 36 (St36) is a good all-over toner and promotes balance within the body.

Bodywork

Massage

A percussive massage will help break up mucus. Percussive motions are best used on people who are relatively strong and healthy. If you are frail, thin, or elderly, check with your massage therapist about the suitability of this treatment for you.

A lymphatic drainage massage will carry mucus away from the body.

Reflexology

See pages 804–805 for information about reflexology areas and how to work them. Working the big toes and the inside of the heels helps abate allergic reactions. Work the adrenals, the sinus, and the lungs.

Hydrotherapy

Hot baths induce sweat, which carries toxins out along with it. And if you're congested, a steamy bath feels just plain wonderful. If you want a more powerful release of toxins, add Epsom salts to the water.

A wet compress will help draw out chest congestion. You can add ginger or cayenne for increased strength.

Aromatherapy

If you suffer from plant allergies, use caution when trying aromatherapy oils.

Several essential oils are excellent at loosening mucus. Try any combination of the following in a steam inhalant or a bath or diffused into the air: eucalyptus, peppermint, lemon balm, and tea tree.

Both lavender and chamomile are good stress relievers, in any form. If you're suffering from allergies, however, they may be of most help when combined with steam, so use them in a steam inhalant or a hot bath.

Other Recommendations

- Exercise to expel toxins, balance the immune system, and reduce stress.
- Don't smoke or expose yourself to secondhand smoke.
- Avoid or reduce exposure to allergy triggers. If you have mold or dust allergies, keep your house extremely clean and dry. A dehumidifier in the basement is a good idea, as are air filters and feather-free pillows and comforters. If you have a wood- or coal-burning fireplace or stove, you may need to find an alternate source of heat. In extreme cases, you may have to rid your home of any item that's likely to collect dust, including upholstered furniture, rugs, and curtains. A HEPA (high-energy particulate air) filter is highly recommended, especially in the bedroom at night.
- Xylitol nasal spray reduces allergy symptoms. Follow directions on the container.
- Consider desensitization treatments from a natural–health care practitioner.
- Intravenous vitamin C can help reduce acute and chronic allergy symptoms.

REFERENCES

Mittman, P. 1990. Randomized, double-blind study of freeze-dried Urtica dioica in the treatment of allergic rhinitis. *Planta Medica* 56:44–47.

Schapowal, A., and Petasites Study Group. 2005. Treating intermittent allergic rhinitis: A prospective, randomized, placebo and antihistamine-controlled study of butterbur extract Ze 339. *Phytotherapy Research* 19:530–37.

Schapowal, A., and Petasites Study Group. 2002. Randomised controlled trial of butterbur and cetirizine for treating seasonal allergic rhinitis. *British Medical Journal* 324:144–46.

Alzheimer's Disease

Alzheimer's disease is a progressive brain disorder that begins with memory loss and eventually leads to dementia and death. In the United States it affects more than five million people with the majority of those affected over the age of sixty. It is a leading cause of death, and the rates are rising with the aging population. It is almost twice as common in African Americans age seventy-one years and older than in whites.

Alzheimer's disease targets a part of the brain called the hippocampus, which is the seat of memory and intellect. In a person with Alzheimer's, the neurons in the hippocampus become entangled. The resulting formations, often called plaques, result in the loss of brain nerve cells, especially those that make new memories and retrieve old ones. Impairment in memory, cognition, and behavior characterizes the symptoms of Alzheimer's. It is not known whether these plaques cause Alzheimer's or whether they are a by-product of Alzheimer's. Furthermore, the entangled, twisted fibers build up inside nerve cells and disrupt function.

In the beginning stages of the disease, people will experience some mild memory problems. They may struggle with complex tasks like planning a party or balancing a checkbook. As the disease progresses, it becomes increasingly difficult to remember events that occurred very recently—say, the day before, or even just a few hours prior to the present time. Memory loss at this point looks more and more like dementia: affected people may not recognize others close to them or be able to recall appropriate words. Eventually, complete dementia sets in.

The Alzheimer's Association (Alz.org) gives ten early signs and symptoms of Alzheimer's: memory loss that disrupts life; challenges in planning or solving problems; difficulty completing familiar tasks at home, at work, or at leisure; confusion with time or place; trouble understanding visual images and spatial relationships; new problems with words in speaking or writing; misplacing things and losing the ability to retrace steps; decreased or poor judgment; withdrawal from work or social activities; and changes in mood and personality.

Although researchers are not yet sure what causes Alzheimer's, it is likely that several factors may play a role in the disease.

One area to consider is an elevation of the methionine metabolite homocysteine. A two-year trial at Oxford University followed 156 people, seventy years and older, who showed signs of cognitive impairment (a precursor to Alzheimer's) and elevated levels of the protein metabolite known as homocysteine. Patients were given vitamins B6, B12, and folic acid. They had MRI scans of their brains done to check for shrinkage and blood levels of homocysteine both at the beginning of and at the end of the trial. The study revealed that B vitamins reduce brain shrinkage in the areas of the brain associated with Alzheimer's by up to 90 percent and slash homocysteine levels. Elevated homocysteine levels are known to cause inflammation of the brain.

There's some evidence that Alzheimer's may actually be caused by the herpes simplex virus 1 (HSV1), the same virus that causes fever blisters or cold sores on the face or mouth. Research shows that HSV1 also can infect the brain and that flare-ups of HSV1 in the brain may be a primary cause of the brain damage associated with Alzheimer's. This means that it may be possible to stave off Alzheimer's by taking steps to suppress the virus, including consuming nutritional supplements that keep the virus from replicating. In a 2010 study published in *PLOS ONE*, Harvard researchers and other colleagues demonstrated that beta-amyloid could have a protective role, functioning in the immune system as an antimicrobial, attacking and destroying bacteria and viruses in the brain. This research is ongoing. Other research suggests that other causes of infection such as *Treponemas* and *Borrelia burgdorferi* may result in chronic inflammation and brain-cell destruction.

Common prescription drugs may be a factor. Research published in the *British Medical Journal* suggests a link between the use of brain-calming drugs known as benzodiazepines and an increased risk for Alzheimer's disease by up to 51 percent. This commonly prescribed class of medications for insomnia and anxiety includes medications such as Xanax, Valium, Klonopin, Ativan (lorazepam), Restoril, and others.

Genetics can be a cause but it accounts for a smaller number of cases. Most appear to be noninherited.

Although there is distressingly little that conventional medicine can do for Alzheimer's sufferers, it is very important to see a doctor if you think you may have the disease. One reason is that many elderly people take several different medications at once, and these combinations often result in memory loss, confusion, or even dementia—side effects that can easily be mistaken for symptoms of Alzheimer's. The first step for anyone suffering from memory problems should be a rigorous examination of prescription and other drugs. Furthermore, the symptoms of Alzheimer's mimic those of several other disorders that are quite treatable; many people who believe they have Alzheimer's are actually suffering from depression, hypothyroidism, B12 or folic acid deficiency, or other conditions. Only after your doctor has ruled out all other possibilities will he or she make a diagnosis of Alzheimer's. If you do have Alzheimer's, it's important to work with a good specialist. Although there's no cure, there are ways to help you improve your health, comfort, and independence.

There are no known cures for Alzheimer's, but conventional medicine recommends medications that alter the neurotransmitters acetylcholine and glutamate. Other medications are used to treat other symptoms such as depression and sleep disorders. Natural therapies should be employed to prevent or help slow down the disease and to improve life quality.

SYMPTOMS

Alzheimer's is a progressive disease. Its symptoms are listed here in the order in which they usually occur.

- Memory problems
- Confusion and disorientation
- Mood swings
- Depression
- Paranoia
- Inability to manage basic or familiar tasks
- Inappropriate behavior
- Hallucinations and delusions
- Episodes of violence and rage or childlike passivity
- Dementia
- Loss of judgment

Testing Techniques

Conventional testing, such as a CT scan, an MRI, a PET scan, and an electroencephalogram, as well as psychological testing and routine blood work, are standard. Additional helpful testing includes :

Toxic metal testing for elements toxic to brain tissue, such as aluminum, mercury, lead, arsenic, and others. The best test is a toxic element challenge urinalysis. The patient takes a chelating agent such as DMSA or DMPS, which pulls toxic metals out of tissue storage. Urine is then collected and tested.

Oxidative stress analysis—urine or blood testing

Antioxidant testing—urine, blood, or skin scanning

Stool analysis

Hormone analysis by saliva, urine, or blood (estrogens, progesterone, testosterone, DHEA, cortisol, melatonin, IGF-1, thyroid panel)

Blood work for nutritional deficiencies: B12, folate, vitamin D, omega-3 levels

ROOT CAUSES

- Advancing age
- Family history and genetics
- Insulin resistance/diabetes
- High blood pressure
- Obesity
- Chronic inflammation
- Brain injury
- Elevated lipids
- Chronic infections
- Toxic metals (especially lead and aluminum)
- Nutrient deficiencies (especially vitamin D, folate, B12)
- Omega-3 fatty acid deficiencies
- Hormone imbalance (especially chronic elevation of the stress hormone cortisol)

TREATMENT

Diet

Recommended Food

Eat a wholesome diet of basic, unprocessed foods. Because conventionally grown foods often contain toxins, buy organic whenever possible. If organic food is unavailable or too expensive, wash your food thoroughly before eating. The Mediterranean diet, rich in fruits, vegetables, legumes, fish, and olive oil, is associated with a decreased risk of developing Alzheimer's disease.

The antioxidant vitamins A, C, and E will combat damage from free radicals. Fresh fruits and vegetables are among the best sources of antioxidants, so have a couple of servings at every meal. For vitamin E, add wheat germ to salads, cereals, or juices. Nuts and seeds are other good sources of this vital nutrient.

The consumption of fish is very important. Salmon, halibut, cod, sole, and others are healthful sources of DHA, an essential fatty acid involved in brain function.

Use turmeric as a spice when preparing meals as it has anti-inflammatory effects on the brain.

Drink organic green tea to improve antioxidant status for the brain.

Many people with Alzheimer's are found to be deficient in zinc. To boost your intake, snack on pumpkin seeds regularly.

To improve circulation, increase energy levels, and detoxify your body, drink a glass of clean, quality water every two waking hours.

Eat plenty of fiber to keep toxins moving through your digestive tract and to prevent them from taking up residence in your body. Whole grains, oats, and raw or lightly cooked vegetables are good sources of fiber that are also nutritionally dense.

If you're older, your digestive system may not be able to absorb nutrients as well as it used to. Fresh fruit and vegetable juices are easily absorbable and packed with the vitamins you need, so have several glasses daily.

Food to Avoid

There is emerging evidence that elevated blood sugar levels as seen in diabetes are associated with an increased risk of Alzheimer's disease. Avoid all forms of refined carbohydrates such as white breads, white rice, cookies, crackers, soda pop, and undiluted fruit juice.

It may surprise you to learn that many foods, especially baked goods, contain aluminum. Read all food labels carefully. Choose nonaluminum baking powder, and avoid pickling salts. You will also need to avoid food cooked in aluminum pots and pans, as well as beverages that come in aluminum cans.

Avoid trans fats found in packaged, fast foods, and fried foods.

℞ Super Seven Prescriptions—Alzheimer's disease

Super Prescription #1 Citicoline
Take 250 to 500 mg twice daily. Research has shown benefit in early stage Alzheimer's disease.

Super Prescription #2 Acetyl-L-carnitine
Take 1,000 mg three times daily. It improves brain cell communication and memory.

Super Prescription #3 DHA
DHA is the primary component of the cell membranes of neurons. It also promotes nerve transmission in the central nervous system and protects the mitochondria (energy warehouse of cells). Studies have shown that low levels of serum DHA are a risk factor for Alzheimer's disease. Take 1,000 mg daily. It can be in taken in addition to EPA, found in fish oil.

Super Prescription #4 Turmeric extract
Take 1,500 mg daily of standardized turmeric extract. It may prevent or reduce amyloid plaque formation in the brain.

Super Prescription #5 Vitamin D3
Take 5,000 IU daily. Reduces brain inflammation and may prevent amyloid plaque formation.

Super Prescription #6 Phosphatidylserine

Take 300 mg daily. This naturally occurring phospholipid improves brain cell communication and memory and has shown benefits for early-stage Alzheimer's disease.

Super Prescription #7 Vitamin B12

Take 50 mcg to 200 mcg of the oral form or a sublingual form. Vitamin B12 deficiency mimics the symptoms of Alzheimer's disease and memory loss.

General Recommendations

In one study of nineteen people with Alzheimer's, 1,000 mg of citicoline was taken daily for thirty days. The supplement significantly improved the cognitive function for those with early-onset Alzheimer's and overall there was a trend of improvement in all the participants. Another study of people between fifty-seven and eighty-seven years old who had been diagnosed with Alzheimer's disease found that 1,000 mg daily of citicoline resulted in improved mental function, particularly for those who were suffering with early onset of the disease. This study *also* found improved blood flow in one of the main brain arteries.

Huperzine extract has been shown to increase acetylcholine levels in the brain and to improve memory in people with this disease. Take a product standardized to contain 0.2 mg of huperzine A daily.

Vitamin E complex (mixed tocopherals and tocotrienols). Studies show that it slows cognitive decline for those with this disease. Take 2,000 IU of mixed vitamin E daily.

Jellyfish extract supports brain function and health. Preliminary studies show that it helps memory for those with this disease. Take 10 to 20 mg daily of a standardized extract of jellyfish.

Phosphatidylcholine: take 2,000 to 3,000 mg daily to support the neurotransmitter acetylcholine, which supports memory.

Glutathione protects against brain cell oxidative damage. Take 250 mg twice daily.

Lemon balm extract has been shown to reduce agitation and improve symptoms of Alzheimer's disease when taken daily for four months. Take 60 drops daily or as directed on the label.

Vinpocetine improves circulation to the brain and may help with memory. Take 5 to 10 mg three times daily.

Alpha GPC may improve cognitive function for those with this disease. Take 1,200 mg daily.

Medium-chain triglycerides provide brain fuel. Take 20 grams one to three times daily or as directed by a doctor.

Alpha lipoic acid may be helpful for some people with this disease. Take 300 mg three times daily.

Ashwagandha (*Withania somniferum*) is used as a brain tonic in Ayurvedic medicine. It reduces stress hormone levels. Take 250 mg of a standardized extract daily.

Panax ginseng improves memory and balances stress hormone levels. Take a standardized product containing 4 to 7 percent ginsenosides at 100 to 250 mg twice daily. Do not use it if you have high blood pressure.

Lion's Mane is used in Asian medicine for poor memory. Take 2,000 to 3,000 mg daily.

DMAE helps the body produce acetylcholine for memory, and it also has antioxidant properties. Take 600 mg daily.

An antioxidant formula should contain a wide range of antioxidants, such as selenium, carotenoids, vitamin C, and others.

Chlorella speeds up the detoxification of toxic metals that may be causing free-radical damage. Take as directed on the container.

NADH has been shown to improve mental function and halt progression of the disease in one clinical trial. Take 10 mg daily.

Vitamin B1 has been shown to improve mental function in people with Alzheimer's disease. Take 300 mg daily.

DHA supplies essential fatty acids for proper brain function. Take a fish oil supplement that contains a daily dosage of 1,000 mg of DHA.

Ginkgo biloba (24 percent flavone glycosides) improves circulation to the brain, improves memory, and has antioxidant benefits. Take 120 mg two to three times daily.

DHEA is a hormone that helps cognitive function. Take 5 mg to 25 mg daily.

Homeopathy

Although homeopathy cannot cure Alzheimer's, it can reduce or alleviate many of its symptoms. Consult with a licensed homeopath for a constitutional remedy. In the meantime, here are a few temporary suggestions.

Alumina can clear confusion and reduce memory impairment. The person often suffers from constipation. Take 30C daily for three or four days, and see if improvement occurs within a week.

Lycopodium (*Lycopodium clavatum*) can help if you're fearful and have trouble recalling words. Take 30C two times daily for two weeks.

Acupressure

See pages 787–794 for information about pressure points and administering treatment.

- Stomach 36 (St36) tones the entire body, while improving the absorption of nutrients into the bloodstream.
- Governing Vessel 24.5 (GV24.5) is easy to reach (it's at the center of the forehead, between the eyebrows), and it strengthens both memory and concentration.
- To relieve anxiety or nervous tension, work Pericardium 6 (P6).
- Lung 1 (Lu1) will ease depression and encourage deep, slow breathing.

Bodywork

Reflexology

See pages 804–805 for information about reflexology areas and how to work them.

To detoxify cells and tissues, work the area corresponding to the lymph system.

Encourage blood flow to the brain by working the heart point.

Work the lungs to oxygenate the blood.

Other Bodywork Recommendations

Hot and cold hydrotherapy is invigorating and stimulates blood flow to the brain. Try alternating hot and cold baths for the best effect.

Aromatherapy

Juniper helps break down toxins that reside within fatty deposits. Add it to your bath or use it during a lymphatic massage.

Several clinical trials have found that supplementation of acetyl-L-carnitine delays the progression of Alzheimer's disease, improves memory, and improves overall performance in some people with Alzheimer's disease.

One placebo-controlled trial found that 58 percent of people with Alzheimer's disease had significant improvement in memory, as well as in mental and behavioral function, from taking 200 mcg of huperzine A twice a day for eight weeks. This was considered a statistically significant improvement, compared to the 36 percent who responded to placebo.

Researchers from Columbia University Medical Center in New York City found that as little as one additional gram of omega-3 fatty acids added to the daily diet could help prevent or delay onset of Alzheimer's disease. In the study, 1,219 people aged sixty-five or older with no diagnosis of dementia recorded their daily dietary intake for an average of 1.2 years. The people who consumed the most omega-3 fatty acids demonstrated the lowest blood levels of beta-amyloid, an undesirable protein associated with Alzheimer's disease and other memory problems. Specifically, people who consumed more than one additional gram of omega-3 per day than the average consumption reported by the group showed 20 percent to 30 percent lower blood beta-amyloid levels.

Black pepper will stimulate digestion, which can improve the absorption of nutrients. Dilute it in some carrier oil, and rub directly onto the abdomen.

The changing mood states of people with Alzheimer's may sometimes call for relaxing oils; at other times, oils with a stimulating effect are in order. Oils that have relaxing, calming properties include lavender and melissa. To rouse the mind and raise the spirits, try geranium, jasmine, neroli, bergamot, or rose.

Stress Reduction

A diagnosis of Alzheimer's is an extremely stressful event, especially when you are still quite capable and aware of the challenges to come. During these early stages, it's vital that you find stress-reduction techniques that work for you; they will increase the quality—and perhaps even the quantity—of the time you have left.

General Stress-Reduction Therapies

Alzheimer's can make you feel alone, even if you're supported by a loving family. Join a support group of other people who have Alzheimer's, to share your feelings. (You may also want to encourage your loved ones to attend a support group of their own. They're coping with the shock, too.)

Meditation and prayer will help you manage stress and will also keep your mind and memory functioning at their optimum level for as long as possible.

Other Recommendations

- Regular exercise will keep blood flowing to the brain. A daily walk in the morning sunlight can also do wonders for your spirits.
- If you're trying to prevent Alzheimer's, keep yourself active and learning. A lack of mental engagement may be connected to loss of brain function.
- Avoid sources of aluminum and mercury. Some food sources of aluminum were listed earlier, but you must also read the labels on antacids, diarrhea medications, buffered aspirin, deodorants, and douches. You may want to consider having dental fillings that are composed of a silver-mercury amalgam replaced with a nontoxic substance.
- Simple routines are quite helpful to many people in the early and middle stages of Alzheimer's. Make a schedule for your day, and plan to perform more complicated tasks during the hours when you usually feel your best.
- Although it is very difficult to face the inevitable, many people with Alzheimer's feel much better when they plan ahead. If you work out your legal and financial arrangements now, and discuss your wishes for the future with your family, you may find that you can enjoy a stronger sense of peace and well-being.
- If you are the caregiver of a person who has Alzheimer's, you probably need some help. Contact local support groups to find low-cost assistance with transportation, meals, and even day care for the elderly.

REFERENCES

Billioti de Gage, S., Y. Moride, T. Ducruet, et al. 2014. Benzodiazepine use and risk of Alzheimer's disease: case-control study. *The BMJ* 349:g5205.

Caamaño, J., et al. 1994. Effects of CDP-choline on cognition and cerebral hemodynamics in patients with Alzheimer's disease. *Methods Find Exp Clin Pharmacol* 16(3):211–18.

Douaud, G., et al. 2013. Preventing Alzheimer's disease-related gray matter atrophy by B-vitamin treatment. *PNAS* published ahead of print May 20, 2013.

Franco-Maside, A., et al. 1994. Brain mapping activity and mental performance after chronic treatment with CDP-choline in Alzheimer's disease. *Methods Find Exp Clin Pharmacol* 16(8):597–607.

Gu, Y., et al. 2012. Nutrient intake and plasma β-amyloid. *Neurology* 79(19):2011.

Leong, C. C., N. I. Syed, and F. L. Lorscheider. 2001. Retrograde degeneration of neurite membrane structural integrity of nerve growth cones following in vitro exposure to mercury. *Neuroreport* 12(4):733–37.

Maurer, K., et al. 1997. Clinical efficacy of Ginkgo biloba special extract EGb 761 in dementia of the Alzheimer's type. *Journal of Psychiatric Research* 31:645–55.

Moir, R. D., et al. 2010. The Alzheimer's disease-associated amyloid beta protein is an antimicrobial peptide, *PLOS ONE*. (2010).

Morris, M. C., et al. 2003. Consumption of fish and n-3 fatty acids and risk of incident Alzheimer disease. *Archives of Neurology* 60(7):940–46.

Pettegrew, J. W., W. E. Klunk, K. Panchalingam, et al. 1995. Clinical and neurochemical effects of acetyl-Lcarnitine in Alzheimer's disease. *Neurobiological Aging* 16:1–4.

Rai, G., G. Wright, L. Scott, et al. 1990. Double-blind, placebo controlled study of acetyl-L-carnitine in patients with Alzheimer's dementia. *Current Medical Research and Opinion* 11:638–47.

Salvioli, G., and M. Neri. 1994. L-acetylcarnitine treatment of mental decline in the elderly. *Drugs under Experimental and Clinical Research* 20:169–76.

Sano, M., K. Bell, L. Cote, et al. 1992. Double-blind parallel design pilot study of acetyl levocarnitine in patients with Alzheimer's disease. *Archives of Neurology* 49:1137–41.

Xu, S. S., Z. X. Gao, Z. Weng, et al. 1995. Efficacy of tablet huperzine-A on memory, cognition, and behavior in Alzheimer's disease. *Chung Kuo Yao Li Hsueh Pao* 16:391–95.

The herb *ginkgo biloba* has been shown to be helpful for people with early-stage Alzheimer's disease. It has been approved for the treatment of this disease by the German government. A study done in 1994, involving forty patients who had early-stage Alzheimer's disease, found that 240 mg of *ginkgo biloba* extract taken daily for three months produced measurable improvements in memory, attention, and mood. In addition, three other double-blind studies have demonstrated that ginkgo is helpful for the early stages of the disease.

Anemia

Over three million Americans suffer from anemia, making it the most common blood disorder. It is more common in the very young, menstruating women with heavy menses, and the elderly. Every cell in the human body gets a large portion of its energy from oxygen. In a healthy person, cells receive an adequate supply of oxygen, thanks to a substance called hemoglobin, which transports oxygen through the blood. Without sufficient hemoglobin, the cells don't get enough oxygen; without enough oxygen, the brain, the muscles, and all the other tissues begin to slow down. The anemic person feels weak and tired at first and then may experience several other symptoms, including headaches, difficulty concentrating, fainting, and a series of illnesses that are the result of a suppressed immune system.

The body needs iron to produce the necessary amount of hemoglobin, which is the oxygen-carrying portion of red blood cells. Iron deficiency can be the result of bleeding, poor diet, and absorption problems. The most common cause of anemia is blood loss. Blood loss for any reason, including surgery, trauma, gum disease, hemorrhoids, polyps, cancer of the colon, bleeding ulcers, and heavy menstrual periods, can produce an anemic state. So can an increase in the body's need for iron, which usually happens during pregnancy. Iron deficiency can also be caused by an inability to absorb certain nutrients, as can happen with folic acid and vitamin B12. In rarer cases, deficiencies of vitamins A, B2, B6, zinc, and C, as well as of copper, may lead to anemia. The elderly often lose their ability to absorb these nutrients, as do people with certain digestive disorders like Crohn's disease or ulcerative colitis. Usually, iron deficiency is caused by a combination of these factors.

In rare cases, anemia is the result of a hereditary blood disorder, in which red blood cells are destroyed prematurely. Thalassemia, sickle-cell disease, and spherocytosis are all very serious and sometimes fatal forms of anemia; people with these diseases must be under lifelong medical care. Anemia can also be caused by an inability to absorb any vitamin B12 at all. This condition can easily be treated with sublingual B12, with regular injections of vitamin B12, or by improving stomach acid levels.

If you suspect that you have anemia, it's important that you see a doctor for an accurate diagnosis. The symptoms of anemia can mimic those of other disorders, so you'll need to get a thorough evaluation. If you are diagnosed with anemia, don't let your doctor stop there. Make sure he or she explains the specific cause of your problem so that you'll know how to address any underlying disorders and prevent a recurrence.

SYMPTOMS

- Fatigue
- Weakness
- Shortness of breath after mild exertion
- Headaches
- Dizziness or fainting
- Difficulty concentrating
- Pale skin, lips, and nail beds
- Cold extremities
- Frequent illnesses
- Cessation of menstruation

ROOT CAUSES

- A poor diet, especially one that's deficient in iron, folic acid, or vitamin B12. This category includes eating disorders, such as anorexia nervosa and bulimia nervosa
- Blood loss (most often from menstruation, surgery, digestive diseases, or injury)
- Chronic blood loss (commonly from bleeding ulcers, colon disorders, gum disease, or bleeding hemorrhoids)
- Pregnancy
- Inherited blood disorders
- An inability to absorb vitamin B12
- Poor digestion and absorption—particularly due to low stomach acid, or celiac disease

---

Testing Techniques

- Blood testing—complete blood count (CBC), iron, ferritin (iron stores), B12, folate
- Occult blood stool test
- Endoscopy
- Colonoscopy
- Celiac blood test

TREATMENT

Diet

Dietary changes along with supplementation are of utmost importance for the anemic person to help improve red blood cell formation.

Recommended Food

If you have iron-deficiency anemia then plan your meals so that you get plenty of iron. Rich sources include beef and chicken liver; however, these should only be consumed if organic. Cooked beef, sardines, and turkey also contain high amounts of iron. Other good options include cooked beans, tofu, spinach, sesame seeds, squash seeds, leeks, cashews, cherries, strawberries, dried fruits, figs, kelp, and eggs.

Blackstrap molasses is rich in iron, so take a spoonful of it every day. Black-strap molasses can usually be found next to the pancake syrup at your grocery store. Make sure to read the label carefully, as you don't want molasses that's been sulfured.

Brewer's yeast is a good source of iron, folic acid, and B12, so add 1 tablespoon to cereals, salads, or juices daily.

Vitamin C will help your body absorb and retain iron. When you're eating foods that are high in iron, have some citrus fruits alongside them or take supplemental vitamin C.

Cook your food in cast-iron pots and pans. The food will absorb some of the mineral from the cookware. This strategy is especially helpful for vegetarians, who may have difficulty meeting iron requirements.

Also note that protein deficiency contributes to anemia since it is required for the formation of hemoglobin, the oxygen-containing component of red blood cells.

If you have a digestive disorder that prevents you from absorbing food properly, juice the vegetables that are suggested here and drink several glasses daily. Juices don't require as much digestive work from the stomach and the intestines, and their nutrients are easily passed into the bloodstream.

Food to Avoid

Sodas, dairy products, coffee, and black tea are iron blockers. Eliminate them from your diet.

Iron is removed from your body through the bowels, so take fiber supplements separately from iron sources.

Avoid cow's milk, which may cause hidden bleeding in the intestinal tract. This is particularly true with children.

Many young women—and, increasingly, men—become anemic as a result of following fad diets. If you truly need to lose weight, don't starve yourself; instead, restrict your consumption of fats and sugars, while eating lots of foods with high nutritional density, such as vegetables, fruits, soy products, and whole grains. For further weight loss suggestions, see Obesity.

℞ Super Seven Prescriptions—Anemia

Super Prescription #1 Iron
Take 50 to 100 mg of a well-absorbed form of iron, such as iron glycinate, citrate, gluconate, or fumarate, one to three times daily. Also, iron chelate is generally well absorbed. Avoid the use of iron sulfate (ferrous sulfate), which is poorly absorbed and can cause digestive upset. *Note*: Supplement iron only if you have iron-deficiency anemia or low iron stores as diagnosed by your doctor.

Super Prescription #2 B12
Take 1,000 to 2,000 mcg of B12 daily, preferably in the methylcobalamin form. Sublingual is very absorbable, or your doctor may use the injection form to start. *Note*: Supplement this higher dose of B12 if your doctor has diagnosed a B12 deficiency.

Super Prescription #3 Folate
Take 800 to 1,200 mcg of folic acid daily. Sublingual is very absorbable, or your doctor may use the injection form to start. *Note*: Supplement this higher dose of folic acid if your doctor has diagnosed a folate deficiency.

Super Prescription #4 Homeopathic Ferrum phosphoricum
Take 5 pellets of the 3x or 6x potency three times daily. This homeopathic remedy improves iron utilization in the cells.

Super Prescription #5 Taurine
Take 1,000 mg daily on an empty stomach. Research in women has shown it improves iron-deficiency anemia.

Super Prescription #6 Yellow dock (*Rumex crispus*)
Take 1 capsule or 20 drops of the tincture form with each meal. It contains iron and improves iron absorption.

Super Prescription #7 Vitamin C
Take 250 to 500 mg with each dose of iron. It provides an acidic environment for enhanced iron absorption.

General Recommendations

Gentian root (*Gentiana lutea*) increases stomach acid for improved absorption. Take a 300 mg capsule or 20 drops of tincture at the beginning of each meal.

Spirulina has been shown to help improve anemia by stimulating the bone marrow production of red blood cells. Take 2,000 mg daily.

Vitamin B6 deficiency can cause anemia. 25 to 50 mg may be helpful, particularly the activated B6 form known as pyridoxal 5 phosphate.

Betaine hydrochloride increases stomach acid. Take 1 to 3 capsules with each meal.

Dandelion (*Taraxacum officinale*), in addition to having a high iron content, cleanses the blood and detoxifies the liver. Choose a product made from dandelion root, and take 3 to 5 grams or 5 to 10 cc daily.

Nettle leaves (*Urtica dioica*) are used for anemia because they have a rich nutritional content. Take 300 mg two or three times daily, or use 2 to 4 cc of a tincture three times daily.

Ashwagandha (*Withania somniferum*) has been shown in human studies to increase red blood cell count. Take 250 mg of a standardized extract daily.

Dong quai is a traditional Chinese blood builder. Take 500 mg twice daily for one month.

Dessicated spleen and bone marrow formulas have been traditionally used to treat anemia. Take as directed on the label.

Homeopathy

Select the appropriate remedy from the following list, and take 30C two times daily for two or three weeks.

Calcarea Phosphorica is for anemia in schoolchildren or chronic anemia in adults. It has been shown in animal studies to stimulate the bone marrow to produce blood cells more effectively.

China Officinalis will improve anemic conditions that are a result of blood loss or illness.

Natrum Muriaticum is for anemia that's accompanied by headaches and constipation.

Acupressure

See pages 787–794 for information about pressure points and administering treatment.

- Improve your strength and energy, along with your ability to absorb nutrients from food, by working Stomach 36 (St36).
- For tension, work Lung 1 (Lu1) and Pericardium 6 (P6).
- If you have a headache, use Large Intestine 4 (LI4).

Bodywork

Massage

While massage won't address any of the causes of anemia, it's an effective way to improve your circulation and increase your energy level. A full-body massage is probably the best choice, but there are easy home-care techniques you can use to relieve headaches or to warm up cold extremities.

Forty-year-old Jessica had been anemic for almost a year when she presented to the clinic. While she knew she was anemic she could not tolerate the iron her medical doctor had prescribed. She was switched to iron glycinate, which she tolerated well, and within two months her anemia was cured.

Reflexology

See pages 804–805 for information about reflexology areas and how to work them. Work the spleen to encourage the manufacture and the recycling of hemoglobin. To aid circulation, blood formation, and detoxification, stimulate the liver.

Aromatherapy

Eucalyptus, ginger, black pepper, and rosemary all improve poor circulation. Add any of these oils—or, if you prefer, a combination of them—to a bath. You can also dilute them in a carrier oil and use in a massage.

For an uplifting effect, try geranium or jasmine oils. Use them in any preparation you like, but for a long-lasting effect, you might like to add a few drops to a diffuser and let the scent envelop your room or office.

REFERENCES

Chamorro, G., et al. 2002. Update on the pharmacology of spirulina (Arthrospira), an unconventional food. *Archivos Latinoamericanos de Nutricion* 52(3):232–40.

Zhang, C., et al. 1994. The effects of polysaccharide and phycocyanin from spirulina platensis variety on peripheral blood and hematopoietic system of bone marrow in mice. Second Asia Pacific Conference on Alga Biotechnology, April 25–27, p. 58.

Angina. See Cardiovascular Disease

Anorexia Nervosa. See Eating Disorders

Anxiety

Anxiety is a very common psychiatric disorder. Many people with anxiety experience physical symptoms that range from mild to severe. The three classifications of anxiety include anxiety disorder, obsessive-compulsive disorder and other related disorders, and trauma and stress or related disorders. The most common anxiety disorder is social phobia, where one fears being in certain social situations.

Anxiety becomes a troublesome response when it is inappropriate to the circumstances we encounter or interferes with normal daily activities. When a meeting, a deadline, or a family problem sets us on edge, our bodies signal "danger"—but physical action is rarely appropriate. Instead, we endure the unpleasant sensation of a rapid heartbeat and tensed muscles, often while having to smile at the "opponent" who sits across the desk or the dinner table. We are all able to handle occasional bouts of unreleased anxiety, but if the anxiety doesn't go away, or if it recurs frequently, it can lead to serious health problems. People who are exposed to prolonged anxiety—those who are going through a divorce, for example, or who are subject to intense pressures at work—often suffer from high blood pressure, insomnia, digestive problems, skin disorders, mood swings, depression, and many other conditions. The effects of anxiety can also make any existing health problems much worse. Sometimes people feel the symptoms of anxiety even when they're not facing a serious challenge or danger.

People with anxiety disorders are vulnerable to the same health problems as anyone else with prolonged anxiety. They may also experience extreme states of nervousness and worry, called panic attacks. During a panic attack, the heart pounds and breathing becomes rapid or difficult. Sufferers may break into a cold sweat, experience tingling in the extremities, or feel dizzy and weak. Although panic attacks rarely last long—they can take anywhere from a few seconds to half an hour—they are quite frightening. People may feel certain that they are having a heart attack or a stroke or may simply feel overwhelmed by intense terror.

There are three main classes of medications used to treat anxiety. They include antidepressants such as fluoxetine (Prozac), sertraline (Zoloft), escitalopram (Lexapro), paroxetine (Paxil), citalopram (Celexa), and venlafaxine (Effexor). Another common category are the benzodiazepines such as clonazepam (Klonopin), lorazepam (Ativan), alprazolam (Xanax), and buspirone (Buspar). Lastly there are beta-blockers, which are commonly used to treat cardiovascular conditions such as high blood pressure but are also used to reduce anxiety. A common one is propranolol (Inderal). Of course, all these medications have potential side effects that range from headaches, dizziness, poor memory, and insomnia to weakness. These drugs are not supposed to be taken on a long-term basis.

If you suffer from prolonged anxiety, whether as a result of an anxiety disorder or from a major unresolved source of tension, you can take certain steps to ease your symptoms, as described in this chapter.

As you employ these complementary healing strategies, it's also important to rule out any underlying physical causes. Disorders like low blood sugar, hormone imbalance, heart problems (mitral valve prolapse), and clinical depression can lead to the symptoms of anxiety, as can nutritional deficiencies. Certain substances can also create anxiety or make it worse. Caffeine is perhaps the most notorious tension-inducing chemical, but sugar, food allergens, nicotine, alcohol, environmental toxins and allergens, and other substances can be just as potent.

SYMPTOMS

- Constant worry
- Restlessness and tension
- Trembling
- Sweating
- Heart palpitations
- Weakness or tiredness
- Lump in the throat
- Diarrhea
- Feeling powerless
- Feeling of impending doom
- Dizziness

- Sleep disturbance
- Appetite changes
- Rapid pulse or high blood pressure
- Muscle tension
- Chest pains
- Hyperventilation
- Panic attacks
- Difficulty concentrating
- Headache

ROOT CAUSES

- Stress
- Caffeine
- Sugar
- Nicotine
- Alcohol and street drugs
- Prescription medications
- Disturbed sleep
- Food allergies

- Environmental toxins
- Poor nutrition
- Thyroid problems
- Mitral valve prolapse
- Low blood sugar
- Depression
- Adrenal disorders
- Neurotransmitter imbalance

Testing Techniques

The following tests can give you an assessment of possible metabolic reasons for your anxiety:

Hormone analysis by saliva, urine, or blood (estrogens, progesterone, DHEA, cortisol, thyroid panel). DHEA and cortisol are of particular importance.

Fasting blood sugar

Food allergy/sensitivity testing

Neurotransmitter testing—urine, blood

TREATMENT

Diet

Some foods can create anxiety, and others soothe it. If you're a victim of prolonged or frequent tension, a good diet can significantly—and sometimes completely—alleviate your symptoms.

Recommended Food

An anxiety-healing diet starts with a good base of nutrients. Plan well-rounded meals of basic, clean, natural foods. Some people with anxiety have their symptoms triggered by blood sugar drops. Do not skip meals, and consume adequate protein and healthy fats.

Complex carbohydrates contain serotonin, a neurotransmitter that has a calming effect on the brain. Have some whole grains, like brown rice or oats, at every meal.

Make sure you get enough B vitamins by increasing your intake of brewer's yeast, brown rice, and leafy green vegetables.

Calcium and magnesium calm the body. Good sources include sea vegetables, green leafy vegetables (except spinach), soybeans, nuts, molasses, salmon, oysters, sardines (with the bones), broccoli, and unsweetened cultured yogurt.

Food to Avoid

Caffeine and alcohol cause anxiety or the symptoms of anxiety. Wean yourself off of black tea, coffee, and alcohol, even if they seem to comfort you when you're stressed. Ultimately, these substances put a further strain on your system.

Refined sugars are another enemy of anxious people. Whole fruits and naturally sweet products are fine in moderation, but candy, cake, cookies, refined flour products, and soft drinks will cause your blood sugar to spike and then plummet. The resulting low levels of blood sugar produce feelings of irritability, tension, and depression.

A response to food allergies can lead to trembling, dry mouth, heart palpitations, misbehaving bowels, and other symptoms that mimic anxiety. See Food Allergies to learn more, and use the elimination diet presented there to identify any problematic foods.

If you suffer from anxiety, chances are that you're short on B vitamins and magnesium. Since refined flour and processed foods deplete your body of these nutrients, cut them out of your diet.

℞ Super Seven Prescriptions—Anxiety

Super Prescription #1 GABA
Take 250 to 500 mg three times daily on an empty stomach. GABA calms the brain for most users. Do not combine with antianxiety medications.

Super Prescription #2 5-hydroxytryptophan (5-HTP)
Take 100 mg three times daily on an empty stomach. Note that 5-HTP increases serotonin levels, which have a calming effect on the mind. *Note*: Do not take in conjunction with a pharmaceutical antidepressant or an antianxiety medication.

Super Prescription # 3 Inositol
Take 12 to 18 grams daily in divided doses. Benefits may also be noticed at lower dosages such as 6 grams daily when combined with other supplements used to treat anxiety. Research shows it reduces anxiety and panic attacks.

Super Prescription #4 L-theanine
Take 200 to 250 mg twice daily. This amino acid has a calming effect.

Super Prescription #5 Kava (*Piper methysticum*)
Take 200 to 250 mg two to three times daily of a product standardized to 30 percent kava lactones. Kava can significantly relieve a panic attack, as well as the symptoms of generalized anxiety. If you're using a pharmaceutical tranquilizer, you should talk to your doctor about making the switch. Do not, under any circumstances, take kava at the same time you're taking a medication for anxiety, depression, or Parkinson's disease. Do not use kava while consuming alcohol or if you have elevated liver enzymes. This supplement should be used with a doctor's supervision.

Super Prescription #6 Calcium and magnesium
Take a combination of 500 mg of calcium and 250 mg of magnesium twice daily. These minerals help calm the nervous system.

Super Prescription #7 Passionflower (*Passiflora incarnata*)
Take 250 mg or 0.5 ml two to three times daily. Passionflower relaxes a person without causing sedation.

A double-blind, controlled, cross-over trial published in the *Journal of Clinical Psychopharmacology* demonstrated that 18 grams of inositol daily for one month reduced the number of panic attacks from six to seven weekly to two or three. This is significant since only 70 percent of patients with panic attacks respond to conventional therapies

General Recommendations

B vitamins help combat the effects of stress and will balance your brain chemicals. Take a 50 mg complex one to two times daily. Vitamin B6 is especially important.

Valerian (*Valeriana ofelp comb*) is a strong nerve relaxer and is especially helpful for insomnia caused by anxiety. Take 300 mg or 0.5 to 1.0 ml two to three times daily.

Saint-John's-wort (*Hypericum perforatum*) can lift anxiety that's accompanied by depression. Take 300 mg three times daily. If you're on medication for depression or anxiety, talk to your doctor before switching to an herbal preparation.

Ashwagandha (*Withania somniferum*) helps balance stress-hormone levels and reduce tension. Take 250 mg of an extract daily.

Chromium balances blood sugar levels. Take 200 mcg two to three times daily.

Inositol has been shown in studies to be helpful for panic attacks. Take 4 grams three times daily.

Chamomile (*Matricaria recutita*) and oatstraw (*Avena sativa*) are proven herbal nerve relaxers. They can be taken as a tea or in supplement form.

Fish oil is important for the long-term treatment of anxiety. Take 2,000 mg of EPA and DHA combined daily.

Homeopathy

Pick the remedy that best matches your symptoms. Take 2 pellets of 30C potency twice daily to prevent or reduce anxiety. Should the first three days pass without any sign of improvement, you're probably taking the wrong remedy. Stop using the current one, and switch to something else. After you first notice improvement, stop taking the remedy, unless symptoms begin to return. For acute anxiety or a panic attack, take a 30C potency every fifteen minutes for up to 6 doses. After improvement is noticed, stop taking the remedy, unless symptoms return.

Aconitum Napellus is for acute panic attacks, especially those that make you feel as if you might die. You may experience shortness of breath, a sensation of impending doom, and heart palpitations.

Arsenicum Album is for anxiety and insecurity that are accompanied by a fast heartbeat, chills, and a disturbed appetite. People who benefit from this remedy are often obsessively tidy and organized.

Calcarea Carbonica is for symptoms of anxiety and a feeling of being overwhelmed. You are generally chilly and tire easily. Gelsemium (*Gelsemium sempervirens*) is effective for acute anxiety from stage fright or from being in crowds. Trembling and diarrhea often accompany anxiety.

Ignatia (*Ignatia amara*) is for when you feel moody, weepy, and brooding and may feel a lump in your throat. It is excellent for anxiety that results from an emotional trauma.

Kali Phosphoricum is for generalized anxiety, poor memory, and fatigue. Take a 6x potency three times daily.

Lycopodium (*Lycopodium clavatum*) will ease stage fright or social anxiety due to low confidence. You often crave sweets and have a digestive upset, such as gas and bloating.

Take pulsatilla for anxiety related to being alone.

Acupressure

See pages 787–794 for information about pressure points and administering treatment.

- For quick relief of anxiety, work Lung 1 (Lu1).
- Pericardium 6 (P6) is another good point for nervous tension. Because it's located on the wrist, you can easily work this point whenever you need quick relief—at the office, in meetings, or on a bus.
- For fear, work Bladder 23 (B23).
- For anxiety that leads to depression, work Conception Vessel 17 (CV17).

Bodywork

Massage

A regular full-body massage is a great way to relieve the tension that collects in your muscles. If you don't have the time or the money for a professional treatment, you or a loved one can easily perform some spot techniques at home. A neck, a shoulder, or a foot rub can help you unwind. Use any of the essential oils recommended under Aromatherapy in this section for an even more relaxing effect.

Reflexology

See pages 804–805 for information about reflexology areas and how to work them.

Work the areas corresponding to the diaphragm, all the glands, the heart, and the solar plexus.

Hydrotherapy

If you suffer from insomnia related to anxiety, it's important to draw blood away from your head before bedtime. Take a ten-minute hot foot bath to encourage the blood to move down and out toward your limbs.

Aromatherapy

Many essential oils have relaxing properties, but lavender, melissa, jasmine, and ylang-ylang are among the best for anxiety. Use them in a bath or a massage, or add some to a room diffuser for extended relief.

During a panic attack, inhale frankincense to encourage deep breathing.

If you have diarrhea, use chamomile, peppermint, lavender, and melissa to soothe gastric cramps. Add a few drops to a massage oil, and rub gently onto your abdomen.

Bergamot will restore a lost appetite. Try some in a room diffuser, or simply inhale deeply over the bottle.

Stress Reduction

If you suffer from anxiety, it's wise to have a repertoire of stress-reduction techniques you can call upon. Any of the techniques discussed in the Exercise and Stress Reduction chapter can help, but following are some specific suggestions.

General Stress-Reduction Therapies

Use prayer to alleviate and prevent anxiety. The Bible contains many scriptures that address anxiety.

It is also prudent to seek help from a counselor who specializes in anxiety disorder.

Positive mental imagery and meditation are useful. Whenever you feel your mind racing ahead to upcoming deadlines or unpleasant situations, try to bring it back to an awareness of the present. Focus for a moment on something beautiful: the sound of a singing bird, the color of the sky, the steam drifting up from your cup of tea.

Many people with anxiety have cold hands and feet, because the panic response pulls blood away from the extremities. Thermal biofeedback can help you use this symptom to your advantage. During a thermal biofeedback session, you'll be asked to try to warm your hands. As you learn this technique, you'll actually learn to control the nervous-system arousal mechanism that is set off by anxiety. Soon you'll be able to ward off a panic attack just by mentally warming your hands.

If you suffer from severe anxiety, consider EEG biofeedback. This form of bio-feedback can be expensive, but it does have an excellent track record of helping people calm their brainwaves.

Don't let stress management itself become a source of stress. You're not a failure if you have a panic attack or an episode of anxiety; no one can manage anxiety perfectly. Just keep practicing tension-relieving techniques daily, and try to accept whatever comes your way as best you can.

Other Recommendations

Regular exercise, prayer, deep breathing, and counseling will help reduce your susceptibility to anxiety. Acupuncture also helps people to relieve the effects of stress.

REFERENCES

Akhondzadeh, S. M., et al. 2001. Passionflower in the treatment of generalized anxiety: A pilot double-blind randomized controlled trial with oxazepam. *Journal of Clinical Pharmacy and Therapeutics* 26:363–67.

Lehmann, E. E., J. Kinzler, and J. Friedmann. 1996. Efficacy of a special kava (*Piper methysticum*) extract in patients with states of anxiety, tension and excited-ness of non-mental origin: A double-blind placebo-controlled study of four weeks treatment. *Phytomedicine* 3:113–19.

Palatnik, A., et al. 2001. Double-blind, controlled, crossover trial of inositol versus fluvoxamine for the treatment of panic disorder. *J Clin Psychopharmacol* 21(3):335–9.

Volz, H. P., and M. Kieser. 1997. Kava (*Piper methysticum*) extract WS 1490 versus placebo in anxiety disorders: A randomized placebo-controlled 25-week out patient trial. *Pharmacopsychiatry* 30:1–5.

Warnecke, G. 1991. Psychosomatic dysfunctions in the female climacteric. Clinical effectiveness and tolerance of kava (*Piper methysticum*) extract WS 1490. Fortschritte de medizin 119–22 [in German].

Arrhythmias

Incredibly, the heart beats around a hundred thousand times a day, and your heart's contractions need to be forceful enough to pump blood throughout the entire body. The electrical impulses that control those contractions need to fire steadily and regularly to keep everything in perfect working order. When they don't, the result is an irregular heartbeat, a condition known as an arrhythmia.

Although the condition is more common in those who have had damage to their heart muscle (such as from a heart attack or heart failure), there doesn't need to be a history of heart disease to experience an irregular heartbeat. An arrhythmia can strike anyone.

The electrical impulses in your heart follow a specific pathway from the upper to lower chambers, and any interruption in that pattern can lead to an arrhythmia. And while anyone can experience a random irregular heartbeat, when the arrhythmia is more than just temporary it can be a problem.

Not everyone with an arrhythmia experiences the same sort of irregularities in their heartbeat. If your heartbeat is too fast (more than a hundred beats per minute in adults) it's called tachycardia. If it beats too slow (fewer than sixty beats per minute) it's known as bradycardia. Some people have an erratic rhythm combining the two in no particular pattern.

The most common type of arrhythmia is called premature ventricular contraction (PVC). As the name implies, PVC occurs when one of the two *bottom* chambers of your heart contract prematurely. Similarly, premature atrial contraction (PAC), another common arrhythmia, occurs when one of the two *upper* chambers of your heart beat prematurely.

Atrial fibrillation, or A-Fib, is another common type of arrhythmia that occurs when there's an abnormal electrical impulse to the upper chambers of the heart, leading to a fast and irregular heartbeat. It can be continuous or come and go. A-Fib increases your risk of blood clots, stroke, and heart failure, so ongoing medical supervision is required. About 2.2 million Americans have the condition. It becomes more of a risk as you age, and it's fairly common among seniors. If you're forty or older your lifetime risk of developing A-Fib is over 25 percent.

Be aware that a number of pharmaceuticals can cause arrhythmias. If you're on a new medication and have developed an arrhythmia, make sure to discuss this with your doctor. A simple change in medication could resolve the problem.

Arrhythmias are very common as we age. But by addressing the root causes—and taking a holistic approach to treatment—you can achieve better heart control.

Common Types of Arrhythmias

- Atrial fibrillation: upper heart chambers contract irregularly
- Ventricular fibrillation and premature ventricular contractions: disorganized contraction of the lower chambers of the heart
- Bradycardia: slow heart rate
- Tachycardia: very fast heart rate
- Conduction disorders: heart does not beat normally
- Premature contraction: early heartbeat

SYMPTOMS

Most common is feeling like your heart is fluttering, pounding or skipping a beat. Other symptoms may include:

- Dizziness
- Fatigue
- Lightheadedness
- Fainting

- Shortness of breath
- Chest pain
- Rapid heartbeat
- Slow heartbeat

ROOT CAUSES

Medical conditions such as a congenital heart defect, current heart attack, scarring of heart tissue from a previous heart attack, structural changes to the heart tissue such as cardiomyopathy, mitral valve prolapse, coronary artery disease, high blood pressure, obstructive sleep apnea (breathing interrupted during sleep), diabetes, or an overactive or underactive thyroid gland can all serve as triggers for the condition. Other causes include:

- Caffeine
- Tobacco
- Alcohol
- Chocolate
- Cold and cough medications
- Appetite suppressants
- Asthma drugs
- Diuretics
- Psychotropic drugs (medications for mental illnesses)
- Beta-blockers for high blood pressure
- Recreational drugs, including cocaine, marijuana, and methamphetamines

- Drugs used to treat arrhythmias
- Nutritional deficiencies or imbalances, especially electrolyte imbalance
- Hormone imbalance, especially for menopausal women
- Food sensitivities
- Air pollution
- Stress
- Smoking
- Electrical shock
- Dietary supplements (although uncommon)

In a 2011 study published in the journal *Nutrition, Metabolism, and Cardiovascular Disease,* volunteers who didn't stick to an antioxidant-rich Mediterranean diet were more likely to have atrial fibrillation. In addition, those that did follow the diet religiously were much more likely to spontaneously convert back to normal rhythm. The diet appears to both ward off the condition as well as help to heal it.

Testing Techniques

The following tests may be performed based on your history and physical:

Electrocardiogram (EKG)—a noninvasive test that records your heart activity

Holter monitor—an EKG that's strapped to your chest and records your heart rhythm continuously for 24 hours a day to help pinpoint any abnormalities

Echocardiogram—an ultrasound of your heart to measure your heart size and the functioning of heart valves

Mineral analysis, especially potassium, sodium, chloride, calcium, magnesium—blood

Hormone testing (thyroid, cortisol, DHEA, estradiol, progesterone)—saliva, blood, or urine

Toxic metals—urine, blood, or hair

TREATMENT

Diet

Recommended Food

Anyone experiencing arrhythmias should make a switch to the heart-healthy Mediterranean diet. This style of eating is great for cardiovascular health in general, but research has also shown that the Mediterranean diet is especially beneficial for anyone with atrial fibrillation.

Cold-water fish and their omega-3 fatty acids stabilize heart electrical activity. Research in older people showed that those with higher levels of omega-3 fatty acids had a lower risk of atrial fibrillation.

Food sources of magnesium are important. Consume more magnesium from foods such as pumpkin seeds, spinach, quinoa, black beans, and navy beans.

If your potassium is low then good food sources include tomatoes, tomato juice, bananas, avocados, yogurt, and broccoli.

Foods to Avoid

Certain foods can play a role in this condition. If you and your doctor suspect that food triggers such as caffeine, alcohol, or chocolate may be behind *your* arrhythmia then you will need to eliminate the food from your diet entirely for at least a month to see if there's improvement.

℞ Super Seven Prescriptions—Arrhythmias

Super Prescription #1 Magnesium
Take 250 mg twice daily. Magnesium is one of the primary nutrients involved in heart contraction and the electrical activity of the heart. Low blood magnesium levels are associated with a higher risk of heart attacks.

Super Prescription #2 Coenzyme Q10 (CoQ10)
Take 200 to 400 mg daily. This nutrient supports normal heart contraction.

Super Prescription #3 Fish oil
Take 1,000 to 2,000 mg of the omega-3 fatty acids EPA and DHA combined. Research shows that fish and fish oil protect against arrhythmias.

Super Prescription #4 Hawthorn
Take 250 to 300 mg of an extract three times daily. This herb improves circulation and heart electrical activity.

Super Prescription #5 L-carnitine
Take 1,000 mg two to three times daily on an empty stomach. This nutrient stabilizes the cell membranes of heart muscle, which helps normalize electrical activity.

Super Prescription #6 Motherwort (*Leonorus cardiaca*)
Take 20 drops of the tincture form two to three times daily. This botanical has a historical use for treating heart palpitation symptoms. It is particularly useful for women in menopause who are experiencing arrhythmias.

One study found that oral magnesium supplementation of 3,000 mg daily improved symptoms in 93.3 percent of people with premature ventricular and supraventricular arrhythmias.

One large study analyzed blood plasma levels of omega-3 fatty acids in a group of more than 3,000 people without a history of atrial fibrillation. It was shown that older people with the higher levels of omega-3 fatty acids had a lower risk of atrial fibrillation.

Potassium has been shown to help people with diabetes reduce premature ventricular contractions. It not only helps with congestive heart failure but for people with this condition at a dose of 50 to 150 mg was associated with an improvement in signs and symptoms in the majority of patients. It also helps those who undergo heart bypass surgery reduce their risk of deadly ventricular fibrillation.

A meta-analysis of thirteen controlled trials found that L-carnitine supplementation in those who suffered a heart attack reduced all-cause mortality by 27 percent, ventricular arrhythmias by 65 percent, and the chest pain known as angina by 40 precent. In some of the studies L-carnitine was supplemented for up to a year, suggesting it had a long-term preventative effect.

Super Prescription #7 Potassium

This electrolyte is one of the most critical for maintaing normal heart rhythm. Since either a deficiency or an excess of potassium can cause arrhythmias, it is important to have your doctor test you before supplementing, especially higher doses.

General Recommendations

GABA can be effective for those who experience heart symptoms related to anxiety. Take 250 to 500 mg three times daily on an empty stomach. GABA calms the brain for most users. Do not combine with antianxiety medications.

Natural progesterone can help menopausal women who are experiencing heart palpitations. See the Menopause section for proper use.

Vitamin C has been shown to help prevent postoperative atrial fibrillation. Take 1,000 mg twice daily.

Vitamin E combined with vitamin C was shown in research to reduce the incidence of postoperative atrial fibrillation and other arrhythmias. Take 400 IU daily.

N-acetylcysteine (NAC) has also been shown in research to reduce the incidence of postoperative atrial fibrillation. Take 500 mg twice daily.

Other Recommendations

There's emerging evidence that some people are sensitive to the electromagnetic fields created by certain devices such as computers and Wi-Fi routers. Those individuals may develop arrhythmias as a result. Reduce your exposure as much as possible.

Acupuncture directly affects the electrical balance of your nervous system and heart, making it another excellent noninvasive choice for treating arrhythmias. Consult with an experienced acupuncturist in your area.

Spinal manipulation of the neck or thoracic spine can also improve electrical messages to the heart and normalize rhythm. Check with your local chiropractic, naturopathic, or osteopathic doctor to see if spinal manipulation might help you.

Bioidentical hormone replacement during menopause can eliminate heart arrhythmia symptoms for some women.

Intravenous magnesium by a holistic doctor can be of tremendous benefit in normalizing heart activity. One review of studies of those with atrial fibrillation found intravenous magnesium to achieve rate control or rhythm control in 86 percent of patients.

REFERENCES

Chello, M., P. Mastroroberto, R. Romano, et al. 1994. Protection by coenzyme Q10 from myocardial reperfusion injury during coronary artery bypass grafting. *The Annals of Thoracic Surgery* 58(5):1427–32.

DiNicolantonio, J. J., C. J. Lavie, H. Fares, et al. 2013. L-carnitine in the secondary prevention of cardiovascular disease: Systematic review and meta-analysis. *Mayo Clin Proc* 88(6):544–51.

Falco, C. N., C. Grupi, E. Sosa, et al. 2012. Successful improvement of frequency and symptoms of premature complexes after oral magnesium administration. *Arq Bras Cardiol* 480–87.

Fujioka, T., Y. Sakamoto, and G. Mimura. 1983. Clinical study of cardiac arrhythmias using a 24-hour continuous electrocardiographic recorder (5th report)–antiarrhythmic action of coenzyme Q10 in diabetics. *The Tohoku Journal of Experimental Medicine* 141 Suppl:453–63.

Mattioli, A. V., C. Miloro, S. Pennella, et al. 2013. Adherence to Mediterranean diet and intake of antioxidants influence spontaneous conversion of atrial fibrillation. *Nutr Metab Cardiovasc Dis* 23(2):115–21.

Onalan, O., et al. 2007. Meta-analysis of magnesium therapy for the acute management of rapid atrial fibrillation. *Am J Cardiol* 99(12):1726–732.

Wu, J. H., R. N. Lemaitre, I. B. King, et al. 2012. Association of plasma phospholipid long-chain omega-3 fatty acids with incident atrial fibrillation in older adults: the cardiovascular health study. *Circulation* 125(9):1084–93.

Arteriosclerosis. See Cardiovascular Disease

Arthritis

Arthritis is a degenerative joint disease that causes swelling and pain that can range from mild to excruciating. Although more than two hundred diseases are classified under the name "arthritis," most arthritic conditions fall into one of two categories: osteoarthritis and rheumatoid arthritis.

Osteoarthritis is by far the more common, afflicting more than fifty million Americans and 80 percent of people over fifty. The pain and the inflammation occur when the cartilage that protects the bones from rubbing against each other wears down. Not surprisingly, the disease usually appears in joints that do most of the body's hard work: the knees, the hips, the spine, and the hands. Although injury or the normal wear and tear of life often bring on cartilage damage, it can be made much worse by food allergies, poor diet, and mineral deposits in the joints. For some people, the effects of mental and emotional stress aggravate arthritis pain. Changes in the weather—usually rain and falling barometric pressure—often cause arthritis flare-ups.

Rheumatoid arthritis (RA) is quite another story. It is caused by an inappropriate immune reaction, in which white blood cells attack the cartilage in the joints; it can go on to destroy the bones themselves and even the muscles and the skin. It is often exceedingly painful and can cripple its sufferers. While osteoarthritis affects men and women equally, RA appears three times more frequently in women. It affects only 2 to 3 percent of the population and can occur at any age, even in childhood. The course of the disease is difficult to predict. It may disappear a few months after its appearance, or it may grow progressively worse. Experts disagree over the causes of RA, but it seems clear that genes, food allergies, bacterial or viral infection, stress, excess acid in the body, and the presence of certain antibodies in the blood all play a role. Many of the complementary therapies used for osteoarthritis are also effective in reducing the pain and slowing the spread of rheumatoid arthritis.

Underlying factors for both of these conditions may include poor digestive function (intestinal permeability), hormone imbalance, nutritional deficiencies, food allergies, and lifestyle factors.

SYMPTOMS OF OSTEOARTHRITIS

Symptoms usually come on gradually, progressing as follows:

- Morning stiffness
- Painful, swollen joints
- Restricted range of motion
- Deformity of joints (in some cases)

SYMPTOMS OF RHEUMATOID ARTHRITIS

- Inflammation, pain, tenderness, and discoloration in the joints, usually the shoulders, elbows, wrists, fingers, ankles, or toes
- Morning stiffness
- Lumps under the skin at the site of damaged joints
- Deformity of joints in long-term
- Fatigue, weight loss, weakness and occasionally fever
- Chronic infections

ROOT CAUSES OF OSTEOARTHRITIS

- Fractures or other injuries, even those that occurred early in life
- Food allergies
- A diet high in fats, animal products, and other foods that promote an internal acidic environment
- Excess of body fat, which places extra stress on joints
- Emotional stress
- Poor digestion heath (increased intestinal permeability, bacteria imbalance)
- Hormone imbalance
- Biomechanical imbalance (e.g., poor posture, abnormal foot arch)

ROOT CAUSES OF RHEUMATOID ARTHRITIS

No one is exactly sure what causes RA. It is likely multifactorial. Some probable causes include:

- Autoimmune malfunction
- Infection (mycoplasma, viral, fungal, Lyme disease, and others)
- Overgrowth of harmful bacteria in the digestive tract
- Food allergies
- Toxic metal accumulation
- Emotional stress
- Genetics

Canadian researchers examined the association between synthetic hormone replacement and a new diagnosis of arthritis. It was discovered that women who used synthetic hormones for five years or longer were twice as likely as nonusers to develop osteoarthritis. A separate study examining synthetic estrogen replacement therapy and arthritis found a 96 percent increased risk among women who used ERT for four to ten years.

Testing Techniques

The following tests can give you an assessment of possible metabolic reasons for arthritis:

Hormone analysis by saliva, urine, or blood (estrogens, progesterone, DHEA, cortisol, IGF-1, thyroid panel)

Fasting insulin levels—blood

Food allergy/sensitivity testing (including screening for celiac disease or gluten intolerance)

Intestinal permeability—urine test

Stool analysis—bacteria balance, parasites, fungal, food breakdown

Vitamin and mineral analysis—blood or urine

Toxic metal test—hair analysis or urine

Blood work—infections

TREATMENT

Diet

An effective diet will go a long way toward controlling arthritis for many people by providing nutrients that reduce inflammation and promote tissue pH balance.

Recommended Food

Flaxseeds and cold-water fish are high in essential fatty acids and have anti-inflammatory properties. Salmon and mackerel are good examples.

Eat lots of fiber in the form of raw vegetables and whole grains. It will help sweep away mineral and acid buildup and keep your digestive system free of harmful bacteria. Cruciferous vegetables such as broccoli and cauliflower also have anti-inflammatory properties.

Foods high in sulfur will help repair cartilage and bone. Try eating some asparagus, cabbage, garlic, or onion every day.

To keep cartilage lubricated and healthy, drink a glass of clean, quality water every two waking hours. Dehydration has been linked to arthritis pain.

Consume turmeric and ginger for their anti-inflammatory properties.

Food to Avoid

Consuming foods that promote tissue acidity in the body causes inflammation, which leads to pain. Avoid acid-promoting foods such as red meat, saturated fats, oils, fried foods, sugar, dairy products, refined carbohydrates, foods high in gluten (such as breads, pasta, and pastries), alcohol, excess salt, and caffeine. Although this list is long, arthritis sufferers who eliminate these foods often experience great relief. Food allergy or sensitivity testing helps to narrow down the group of offending foods (see the Food Allergies chapter).

Animal products generally worsen inflammation in the joints. Avoid all eggs, dairy, and meat, with the exception of fish, which contains anti-inflammatory oils.

Use the list on page 316 to determine whether you have food allergies. Allergies cause inflammation, and for people with RA, they also do further damage to the immune system and may increase the intestinal tract's vulnerability to bacteria.

The nightshade vegetables—tomatoes, potatoes, eggplant, and peppers—contain a substance called solanine, which can trigger allergic responses and pain in some arthritis sufferers. Eliminate these foods from your diet for a period of six weeks to see if there is improvement.

A randomized, double-blind study involving fifty-two women and men ages forty to seventy-five assessed the subjects' physical function, stiffness, and pain in the knees. A daily dose of 40 mg of undenatured collagen type II (UC-II) was compared to a daily dose of glucosamine (1,500 mg) and chondroitin (1,200 mg). Those receiving UC-II had more than twice the reduction in arthritis symptoms.

Turmeric extract was shown in a 2010 study to be very helpful for osteoarthritis. Fifty participants who were receiving conventional treatment from their doctor for osteoarthritis of the knees were divided into two groups. One group received 1,000 mg of a proprietary turmeric extract containing 200 mg of curcumin; the other received no additional treatment. After three months, those taking the supplement had a 58 percent decrease in pain and significantly increased their walking distance on a treadmill. Those in the control group had much less significant improvements.

Many studies have confirmed the efficacy of glucosamine sulfate for relieving osteoarthritis symptoms. A three-year, double-blind, placebo-controlled trial involving 212 people with knee osteoarthritis found that 1,500 mg of glucosamine sulfate taken daily significantly reduced symptoms. In addition, diagnostic images found that people supplementing glucosamine had no significant joint space loss, while those on placebo had joint deterioration.

Research has shown that turmeric supplemented at a dose of 500 mg four times daily was comparable to taking ibuprofen at a dose of 400 mg twice daily for reducing knee pain in people with osteoarthritis.

℞ Super Seven Prescriptions—Arthritis

Super Prescription #1 Collagen
Take 40 mg daily of undenatured collagen. It has been shown in a randomized, double-blind study involving fifty-two women and men to significantly help reduce symptoms for both osteoarthritis and rheumatoid arthritis.

Super Prescription #2 Turmeric
Take 500 mg one to three times daily. Turmeric has anti-inflammatory effects on the joints and muscles.

Super Prescription #3 Glucosamine sulfate
Take 1,500 mg daily. Many formulas combine it with 600 to 1,200 mg of chondroitin sulfate, a related compound that also reduces joint pain and rebuilds cartilage. Benefits are usually noticed within four to eight weeks. *Note*: Glucosamine and chondroitin sulfate are specific remedies for osteoarthritis.

Super Prescription #4 Methylsulfonylmethane (MSM)
Take 2,000 to 8,000 mg daily. MSM has natural anti-inflammatory benefits and contains the mineral sulfur, an integral component of cartilage. Reduce the dosage if diarrhea occurs.

Super Prescription #5 SAMe
Take 400 to 800 mg twice daily. This natural substance has been shown to be comparable in effectiveness to anti-inflammatory medications for osteoarthritis.

Super Prescription #6 Fish oil
Take a daily dosage of at least 1.8 mg of DHA and 1.2 mg of EPA. Fish oil contains a direct source of the omega-3 fatty acids that reduce joint inflammation and promote joint lubrication. This makes it a better choice than flaxseed oil, although flaxseeds are an option for vegetarians. Improvement may take up to twelve weeks of use.

Super Prescription #7 Bromelain
Take 500 mg three times daily between meals. Look for products standardized to 2,000 MCU (milk-clotting units) per 1,000 mg or 1,200 GDU (gelatin-dissolving units) per 1,000 mg. Bromelain has a natural anti-inflammatory effect. Protease enzyme products also have this benefit.

General Recommendations

Vitamin D acts as a natural anti-inflammatory. Take 2,000 to 5,000 IU daily with meals.

Many excellent herbs reduce inflammation. Devil's claw root (*Harpagophytum procumbens*), alfalfa (*Medicago sativa*), and yucca root (*Yucca schidigera*) capsules are among the best. Give these herbs at least two months to take effect. Recommended dosages are as follows:

Devil's claw (*Harpagophytum procumbens*) should not be taken if you have a history of gallstones, heartburn, or ulcers. Take 1,500 to 2,500 mg of the standardized powdered herb in capsule or tablet form daily, or use 1 to 2 ml of a tincture three times a day.

White willow (*Salix alba*) products that are standardized to contain 240 mg of salicin daily or 5 ml of the tincture form should be taken three times daily.

Alfalfa (*Medicago sativa*) comes in the form of capsules or tablets made from dried alfalfa leaves. Take 500 to 1,000 mg daily, or take 1 to 2 ml of a tincture three times daily.

Yucca root (*Yucca schidigera*) in the capsule form is taken in 1,000-mg doses twice daily.

Ginger (*Zingiber officinale*) is a popular choice for relief of both inflammation and pain. Pour boiling water over the grated root and drink the tea, or try adding fresh ginger to your meals. If you want something stronger, take 1 to 2 grams of dried powder in a capsule two or three times daily, or use 1 to 2 ml of a tincture three times daily.

Boswellia (*Boswellia serrata*) is taken in doses of 1,200 to 1,500 mg of standardized extract, containing 60 to 65 percent boswellic acids, two to three times daily.

Plant sterols and sterolin are more specifically used for rheumatoid arthritis, to calm down an overactive immune system. Take as directed on the container, between meals, three times daily.

DHEA: If your levels are low, work with a holistic doctor and start with 10 to 25 mg daily.

Evening primrose oil, black currant, or borage oil contain the essential fatty acid GLA, which reduces joint inflammation. Take up to 2.8 grams of GLA daily.

Cetyl myristoleate (CMO) is shown in preliminary studies to be helpful for arthritis. Take 540 mg daily.

Vitamin E is preferably taken via a vitamin E-complex with additional tocotrienols. If you are on blood-thinning medication, use a lower amount under your doctor's supervision. Take 800 to 1,200 IU daily.

Vitamin C: Take 1,000 two or three times daily.

Boron: Take 1 mg per day.

Niacinamide: Take 500 mg four times daily.

Plant enzymes: Take as directed on the container to improve food absorption.

Chlorella or spirulina are super green foods high in antioxidants and aid detoxification. Take as directed on the container.

DMSO (dimethyl sulfoxide) is a topical substance used for pain relief. Work with a doctor to use this substance.

Protease enzymes reduce inflammation. Take 1 or 2 capsules twice daily between meals.

A high-potency multivitamin that is rich in a blend of antioxidants will prevent joint-tissue destruction. Take as directed on the container.

Take betaine HCL or a bitter herb digestion formula. These supplements increase stomach acid and improve digestion. Take as directed on the container with each meal.

Apply cayenne (*Capsicum annuum*) cream to the affected area two to four times daily for symptomatic relief. Choose a cream standardized to between 0.025 and 0.075 percent capsaicin. Capsaicin depletes the nerves of substance P, a neurotransmitter that transmits pain messages.

A multicenter study conducted at different sites in multiple countries compared the effects of the common pain medication Celebrex (200 mg daily) to a glucosamine (1,500 mg) and chondroitin (1,200 mg) combination. The participants had knee osteoarthritis with moderate to severe pain. After six months of treatment the results between the two groups were comparable. Pain reduction was significant in both groups at 50 percent. Those taking the supplement formulation had 46.9 percent reduction in stiffness compared to 49.2 percent with Celebrex. Both groups had similar reductions in joint swelling.

Homeopathy

Pick the remedy that best matches your symptoms. Take 2 pellets of 30C potency twice daily. Should five days pass without any sign of improvement, you're probably taking the wrong remedy. Stop using the current one, and switch to something else. After you first notice improvement, stop taking the remedy, unless symptoms begin to return.

Apis (*Apis mellifica*) is for joints that are swollen and hot and having stinging pain that feels better with cool applications. It is more commonly used with rheumatoid arthritis.

Arnica (*Arnica montana*) is for bruising pain, especially for osteoarthritis arising from injuries.

Belladonna (*Atropa belladonna*) works on joints that are hot, red, and burning and that feel worse with motion. Pain and swelling may come on suddenly.

Bryonia (*Bryonia alba*) is for stitching pains and swollen, hot joints that are worse with any movement. People who benefit from bryonia tend to be irritable from the pain.

Calcarea Carbonica is for joint pains made worse from dampness and coldness. The person usually is overweight and chilly.

Calcarea Fluorica is for arthritis with enlarged joints or bone spurs, as well as for hypermobile joints.

Calcarea Phosphorica is for joint and bone pains that are made worse from cold and drafts of cold air. It's useful for arthritis that occurs from bone spurs, especially in the neck region.

Dulcamara is for arthritis that flares up from cold, damp weather.

Pulsatilla (*Pulsatilla pratensis*) is helpful if your pain wanders from joint to joint and if your symptoms improve in fresh, cool air or with cool applications.

Rhus Toxicodendron relieves arthritis that is worse in the cold and the damp or during long periods of inactivity. Stiffness is the main symptom, which improves with some movement and warmth.

Sulfur is for arthritis characterized by burning pains. Symptoms are better with cold applications.

Acupressure

Acupressure can be quite helpful in reducing or even eliminating arthritis pain. Because the suggested points may be very tender, be sure to press them firmly instead of massaging them. You may need to work the appropriate points two or three times a day for up to six months before you see complete results; afterward, reduce your practice to once daily. For more information about pressure points and administering treatment, see pages 787–794.

- To relieve arthritis in the hands, the wrists, the elbows, the shoulders, or the neck, use Large Intestine 4 (LI4).
- Large Intestine 11 (LI11) reduces pain and swelling in the elbow and the shoulder.
- For ankle pain, try Spleen 5 (Sp5) and Kidney 3 (K3).
- Stomach 36 (St36) supports the entire body, including the joints. In addition, it promotes the sense of well-being that arthritis sufferers sometimes lack.

Two significant studies were conducted at the University of Liege, Belgium, where researchers used digitial X-rays to precisely measure knee cartilage in patients with osteoarthritis. After taking 1,500 mg of glucosamine daily for three years, most patients had no loss of cartilage and many had increases in cartilage, along with significant reductions in pain. Meanwhile, patients taking placebos lost cartilage. In a follow-up analysis of fifteen human studies, the researchers reported that glucosamine increased joint cartilage, lessened pain, and improved knee mobility.

Bodywork

Massage

A light drainage massage of the areas surrounding an arthritic joint will reduce the buildup of lymphatic fluid.

Stress and tension can trigger painful episodes, especially for sufferers of RA. Regular massage will relax the body and the mind. It will also loosen muscles that have tightened in reaction to pain.

Reflexology

See pages 804–805 for information about reflexology areas and how to work them. Massage of the entire foot is best for relief of arthritis pain, with special attention to the region that corresponds to the painful area (i.e., shoulder, hands, or back).

Hydrotherapy

Soak in a hot bath with Epsom salts or mineral salts for at least twenty minutes. You'll eliminate toxins through sweat, and the salts will help replenish the body's mineral stores. Constitutional hydrotherapy is excellent (see the Hydrotherapy section for directions).

Aromatherapy

A number of different oils will reduce stress, so you should try several to see which ones work best for you. Some good choices are chamomile, jasmine, lavender, and rose. To assist in cleansing the joints of mineral and acid deposits, use juniper or lemon balm in a hot bath.

Chamomile, lavender, and peppermint all have anti-inflammatory properties. Use them in a bath, or combine them with a base oil and apply gently to the painful area. Lavender is an especially good choice for people with rheumatic pain.

Black pepper, ginger, and eucalyptus all stimulate blood flow around the joints and are invigorating in a bath.

Stress Reduction

Many doctors and other experts have noted that emotional stress and an inability to accept criticism seem to appear frequently in arthritis sufferers. In addition, arthritis itself can cause great tension, both muscular and emotional, and even depression.

General Stress-Reduction Therapies

Yoga works wonders for some people, as may tai chi or Pilates. Take a class with a qualified instructor, preferably one who has experience with arthritic clients.

Thermal biofeedback has produced good results for many arthritis sufferers. It teaches you to open up your blood vessels and stimulates warmth and nourishment to your hands and joints.

Other Recommendations

- Vitamin D from sunshine is crucial to bone health. Don't let arthritis pain keep you from getting out in the early morning sun every day.
- Arthritis sufferers often cut back on activity, but studies show that moderate exercise actually reduces pain and swelling. While you must avoid joint-pounding workouts like jogging or tennis, low- or no-impact exercises like swimming, aqua-aerobics, cycling, and walking are excellent choices.
- Chiropractic, acupuncture, prolotherapy, and laser therapies are all effective for arthritis.
- Natural injections using ozone, platelet-rich plasma, and stem cells are emerging as viable alternatives to conventional steroid injections for osteoarthritis relief and joint regeneration.

REFERENCES

Hochberg, M., et al. 2014. Combined chondroitin sulfate and glucosamine for painful knee osteoarthritis: a multicentre, randomised, double-blind, non-inferiority trial versus celecoxib. *Ann Rheum Dis* doi:10.1136/annrheumdis-2014-206792.

Kuptniratsaikul, V., S. Thanakhumtorn, P. Chinswangwatanakul, et al. 2009. Efficacy and safety of Curcuma domestica extracts in patients with knee osteoarthritis. *J Altern Complement Med* 15:891–7.

Pavelka, K., J. Gatterova, M. Olejarova, et al. 2002. Glucosamine sulfate use and delay of progression of knee osteoarthritis. *Archives of Internal Medicine* 162:2113–23.

Reginster, J. Y., R. Deroisy, L. C. Rovati, et al. 2001. Long-term effects of glucosamine sulphate on osteoarthritis progression: a randomised placebo-controlled clinical trial. *Lancet* 357:251–256 and 247–48.

Asthma

Approximately one in twelve people in the United States and an estimated three hundred million people worldwide suffer from this airway disorder. It is the most common chronic disease in childhood, affecting an estimated seven million children. Common symptoms include shortness of breath, chest pain or tightness, mucus production, wheezing, and coughing.

The increase in environmental allergens, food preservatives and contaminants, obesity, and elevated stress levels are thought to be reasons why asthma rates have risen among children.

Conventional medications such as inhalers are effective in managing asthma but they do not treat the actual triggers of asthma.

There are many different causes of asthma and the root cause(s) need to be treated to prevent flare-ups and to reduce one's susceptibility. Holistic approaches are very effective in treating the triggers of asthma.

If you are having an acute asthma attack or trouble with your long-term asthma control make sure to consult with a doctor.

SYMPTOMS

- Difficulty breathing
- Wheezing
- Coughing
- Tightness in the chest
- Loss of sleep due to coughing and blocked airways
- Increased heart rate
- Inflammation of the mucus linings
- Constriction of the muscles in the bronchial airways
- Increased mucus flow

ROOT CAUSES

Triggers that bring on an attack vary from person to person but most often include:

- Allergies, either environmental or food
- Pollution and irritants, including mold, dust, and others
- Infections (colds, flu, or other respiratory infections)
- Perinatal factors (maternal smoking and prenatal exposure to smoke are risks; breast-feeding is protective)
- Aspirin allergy
- Gastroesophageal reflux disease
- Sinusitis
- Obesity
- Cold air
- Heavy physical exertion
- Poor digestive function
- Hormone imbalance
- Emotional stress

Important: If you experience a severe asthma attack, get emergency help at once. Have someone call an ambulance or drive you to the hospital, where you will receive medication to open your air passages.

Testing Techniques

The following tests can give you an assessment of possible metabolic reasons for your asthma:

Food allergy/sensitivity testing—blood, electrodermal testing (see
    Food Allergies for more details)
Vitamin and mineral analysis—blood
Fungal and flora balance—stool analysis
Toxic metals—hair or urine analysis
Intestinal permeability—urine
Stress hormones DHEA and cortisol—saliva or urine
Omega-3 level—blood

TREATMENT

Diet

Diet often plays a role in many cases of asthma. Work on improving your diet and see if your susceptibility to asthma lessens. *Note*: Check with a pediatrician or a holistic doctor before eliminating any food group from a child's diet.

Recommended Food

Eat foods that don't promote mucus production: raw vegetables and fruits, seeds, whole grains, lean poultry, and fresh fish.

Carotenoids are antioxidants that have natural antioxidant and anti-inflammatory benefits. They are found in dark-green leafy vegetables and deep-yellow and orange vegetables.

Studies show that children who eat fish more than once a week have one-third the risk of developing asthma.

Garlic and onions have anti-inflammatory properties and are a savory addition to vegetable dishes.

A glass of clean, quality water every two waking hours will help keep your system cleansed and hydrated. Water is especially helpful after an asthma attack to break up mucus.

Ground flaxseeds are an excellent source of anti-inflammatory omega-3 fatty acids. For children over five years of age, use 1 to 2 teaspoons, and for adults, the dosage is 1 to 2 tablespoons daily.

Food to Avoid

It is most important to discover whether certain foods provoke allergic reactions. See the Food Allergies entry, especially the elimination diet on page 316.

Even if you don't have an allergy to dairy products, eliminate them from your diet. They encourage the production of mucus that plugs your airways. For the same reason, stay away from sugar, junk food, and fried and refined foods.

Do not eat foods that contain additives or preservatives. This means avoiding processed foods, dried or smoked foods, and salad bars, which are often sprayed with preservatives, such as tartrazine (yellow dye number 5), red dye, sulfites (as found in dried fruits), benzoates, and monosodium glutamate (MSG).

Never eat frozen or extremely cold foods, which can cause the muscles in your airways to tighten.

Keep pressure off your diaphragm by eating small meals and by avoiding foods that cause gas, such as beans and cruciferous vegetables (broccoli, cauliflower, and brussels sprouts are the most common offenders).

A randomized, placebo-controlled, double-blind study involving sixty subjects, ages six to eighteen, was conducted over a period of three months. Researchers found that those who took the supplement pycnogenol had significantly improved lung function and asthma symptoms compared to those who took a placebo. The study was published in the *Journal of Asthma*.

℞ Super Seven Prescriptions—Asthma

Super Prescription #1 Magnesium
Take 500 to 1,000 mg daily. Magnesium relaxes the bronchial muscles of the respiratory tract. Studies show that children with higher blood levels of magnesium have a lower risk of asthma.

Super Prescription #2 Pycnogenol
Take 1 mg per pound of body weight daily. This supplement has natural anti-inflammatory benefits for the respiratory system.

Super Prescription #3 Lycopene
Take 130 mg daily. It has been shown to be helpful for those affected by exercise-induced asthma.

Super Prescription #4 Choline

Take 1.5 to 3 grams daily. It has been shown to reduce the frequency and severity of asthma.

Super Prescription #5 Quercitin

Take 500 to 2,000 mg daily. Quercitin is useful for its anti-inflammatory and anti allergy benefits. Take 500 to 1,000 mg three times daily.

Super Prescription #6 Astragalus

A typical dose for children is 10 drops of the liquid form and for adults 20 to 30 drops or 500 mg of the capsule two to three times daily. Astragalus is used to strengthen the lungs and to prevent respiratory infections that can trigger asthma. Do not use if you have a fever.

Super Prescription #7 Essential fatty acids

Take 1 to 2 tablespoons of flaxseed oil or 4 to 8 grams of fish oil daily. Essential fatty acid formulations that contain flaxseed oil, fish oil, or a mixture of omega-3, -6, and -9 fatty acids are helpful for preventing asthma. Take as directed on the container. It may take four to eight weeks for you to notice an improvement.

General Recommendations

Vitamin B12 reduces the reaction to sulfites that causes asthma symptoms in some people, especially in children. Take 1,500 mcg orally or 400 mcg sublingually. The injectable form is also used by nutrition-oriented doctors.

Vitamin B6 has been found to be low in people who have asthma. In addition, asthma medications may lower B6 levels in the body. Take 100 to 200 mg daily.

N-acetylcysteine is a good antioxidant that also liquefies mucus in the bronchial tubes and the sinuses. Take 500 mg two or three times daily.

Betaine HCL is helpful for some people with asthma. This supplement increases stomach acid levels, which tend to be low in people with asthma. Take as directed on the container, with meals, or as directed by a doctor.

Ginkgo biloba has anti-inflammatory and antioxidant benefits for the lungs. A study using ginkgo extract found that it decreased asthma symptoms. Take 120 to 240 mg daily of an extract containing 24 percent flavone glycosides.

Mullein (*Verbascum thapsus*), licorice, and marshmallow (*Althea officinalis*) root have historically been used in the herbal treatment of asthma. Choose formulas that contain a combination of these herbs, and use as directed on the container.

Cordyceps is a medicinal mushroom used in Chinese medicine to reduce bronchial secretions, improve lung function, and energize the body. Take 800 mg twice daily of a standardized product.

Adrenal-support formulas are helpful in the prevention of asthma. They include herbs such as Panax ginseng, American ginseng, ashwagandha adrenal glandular, and pantothenic acid (vitamin B5). Take as directed by a nutrition-oriented doctor.

Magnesium relaxes the bronchial tubes and improves lung function. Take 250

A double-blind trial found that more than half of people with exercise-induced asthma had significantly fewer asthma symptoms after taking 30 mg of lycopene per day for one week, compared to when they took a placebo.

Several studies have shown an association between low vitamin D levels and asthma prevalence and symptoms in children. There have also been studies done with adults that show an association between decreased blood vitamin D levels and decreased lung function and response to asthma medications.

mg of magnesium two to four times daily. Reduce the dosage if loose stools occur. Nutrition-oriented doctors may also use magnesium intravenously for acute asthma.

Vitamin C lessens spasms of the bronchial passages and has anti allergy benefits. Take 1,000 mg two to four times daily. Reduce the dosage if loose stools occur. Use a nonacidic product, such as calcium ascorbate.

Antioxidants decrease inflammatory responses of the airways. Take an antioxidant formula as directed on the container.

Take a full-spectrum enzyme product with each meal to improve the absorption of nutrients and to decrease reactions to foods.

Intravenous nutrients are very effective for the management of acute and chronic asthma. Vitamin C, magnesium, molybdenum, B12, and B6 are key nutrients to receive.

Homeopathy

Many homeopathic remedies exist for asthma. The following suggestions are for use until you can consult with a qualified homeopath to find the remedy appropriate for your constitution. During an asthma attack, take 30C every ten or fifteen minutes until the symptoms subside. Long-term use of the proper homeopathic remedy can reduce your susceptibility to asthmatic attacks.

Aconitum Napellus is for attacks that start suddenly, especially after exposure to cold air, and that cause a great deal of fear or anxiety.

Arsenicum Album is for people with asthma who feel anxious, restless, and worse in the cold air and between midnight and 2 A.M. They feel better sitting up and when sipping warm drinks. This remedy is used for chronic and acute asthma.

Carbo Vegetabilis is for people who feel chilly and faint, yet better when being fanned or near a window. They may have a sensation of fullness in the upper abdomen and the chest and may feel relief from burping. They feel worse from talking, eating, or lying down.

Ipecacuanha is helpful when a lot of mucus formation causes coughing, gagging, and vomiting.

Kali Carbonicum is for asthma that is worse between 2 A.M. and 4 A.M. The person is usually chilly. Sitting up and leaning forward help to relieve symptoms.

Lachesis is for a feeling of constriction in the throat and the chest. Symptoms are better with fresh air. The person cannot stand any touching or pressure on the throat or the chest and tends to feel warm.

Medorrhinum is for chronic asthma, in which the person is prone to recurring respiratory tract infections, is usually very warm, and craves citrus fruit, especially oranges.

Natrum Sulphuricum is for asthma that comes on or is worse in cold, damp weather. Symptoms are often worse from 4 A.M. to 5 A.M.

Nux Vomica (*Strychnos nux vomica*) is for a constricted feeling in the chest and fullness in the stomach or stomach upset. Asthma symptoms are often worse upon awakening in the morning. Overindulging in food, especially alcohol, spicy foods, or sweets, can bring on symptoms. The person feels chilly and irritable.

Pulsatilla (*Pulsatilla pratensis*) is for asthma symptoms that are worse in the evening; in hot, stuffy rooms; or after eating fatty foods. The person often coughs up yellowish mucus, which may also cause gagging. The person desires fresh air and to be comforted by someone.

Acupressure

Acupressure is highly effective at increasing lung capacity and relaxing the muscles of the airways. Massage these points daily for best results. For more information about pressure points and administering treatment, see pages 787–794.

- Lung 1, 7, and 9 (Lu1, Lu7, and Lu9) relieve congestion and coughing due to asthma.
- Conception Vessel 17 (CV17) relieves tension in the chest.

Bodywork

Massage

A back massage will relax your bronchial muscles. A professional treatment is always nice, but you can ask a loved one to rub your back, if you like. And children enjoy receiving back massages from their parents, especially just before they go to bed. To break up congestion, get a cupping massage on your back or chest. Any kind of massage, especially with a calming essential oil, will dispel stress and anxiety.

Other Bodywork Recommendations

Osteopathic, acupuncture, and chiropractic treatments are useful for long-term treatment. Craniosacral therapy should also be highly considered, especially for children.

Reflexology

See pages 804–805 for information about reflexology areas and how to work them. Massage the points that correspond to the lungs, the diaphragm, and the adrenal glands.

Hydrotherapy

Hot baths and saunas are relaxing ways to sweat out toxins and mucus. Do not take a sauna if you have hypertensive cardiovascular disease.

Aromatherapy

Test separate oils for an allergic response before using any in a combination.

- Many oils open airways and loosen congestion. Try eucalyptus, lavender, tea tree, or a combination of these in a steam inhalation or a bath.
- Frankincense encourages deep, relaxed breathing. Do not use frankincense in a steam, as it can inflame the mucus membranes.
- Mix lavender oil in a base, and rub it directly on your chest to ease breathing and loosen congestion.

Stress Reduction

Anxiety can trigger an asthma attack, so keeping stress levels down is not a luxury, it is a necessity. Children in particular often feel helpless and fearful as a result of asthma; teaching them to manage stress can help them live normal lives that are not dictated by their disease.

General Stress-Reduction Therapies

Yoga and deep breathing will help train asthma sufferers to take deep, regular, and calm breaths. EEG biofeedback can teach you to control your brainwaves, and children, who love working with computers and machinery, respond especially well to this therapy.

Other Recommendations

- Mild to moderate exercise will increase your ability to take in oxygen, so get in a daily walk or other activity. Cold air can trigger an attack, though, so either wear a mask over your face and mouth during the cold months or exercise indoors.
- Perform deep-breathing exercises every day.
- Use a HEPA (high-energy particulate air) filter to clean the air in your room and home.
- Have the air vents in your house professionally cleaned each year.
- Wash all bedding in hot water one or two times weekly to remove dust and dust mites, which can trigger asthma. Use allergy-proof coverings for the mattress, the pillow covers, and the box spring.
- Vacuum twice weekly with a HEPA-filter vacuum. Consider removing carpets and rugs, especially in the bedroom, and replace with nontoxic wooden or laminate flooring.
- Avoid all sources of smoke.

REFERENCES

Black, P. N., and R. Scragg. 2005. Relationship between serum 25-hydroxy vitamin D and pulmonary function in the third national health and nutrition examination survey. *Chest* 128:3792–8. doi: 10.1378/chest.128.6.3792.

Brehm, J. M., B. Schuemann, A. L. Fuhlbrigge, et al. 2010. Serum vitamin D levels and severe asthma exacerbations in the Childhood Asthma Management Program study. *J Allergy Clin Immunol* 126:52–8.e5. doi: 10.1016/j.jaci.2010.03.043.

Chinellato, I., M. Piazza, M. Sandri, et al. 2011. Vitamin D serum levels and markers of asthma control in Italian children. *J Pediatr* 158:437–41. doi: 10.1016/j.jpeds.2010.08.043.

Chinellato, I., M. Piazza, M. Sandri, et al. 2011. Serum vitamin D levels and exercise-induced bronchoconstriction in children with asthma. *Eur Respir J* 37:1366–70. doi: 10.1183/09031936.00044710.

Guinot, P., C. Brambilla, J. Dunchier, et al. 1987. Effect of BN 52063, a specific PAFascether antagonist, on bronchial provocation test to allergens in asthmatic patients— a preliminary study. *Prostaglandins* 34:723–31.

Lau, B. H., et al. 2004. Pycnogenol as an adjunct in the management of childhood asthma. *Journal of Asthma* 41:825–32.

Li, F., et al. 2011. Vitamin D deficiency is associated with decreased lung function in Chinese adults with asthma. *Respiration* 81:469–75. doi: 10.1159/000322008.

Neuman, I., H. Nahum, and A. Ben-Amotz. 2000. Reduction of exercise-induced asthma oxidative stress by lycopene, a natural antioxidant. *Allergy* 55:1184–89.

Sutherland, E. R., E. Goleva, L. P. Jackson, et al. 2010. Vitamin D levels, lung function, and steroid response in adult asthma. *Am J Respir Crit Care Med* 181:699–704. doi: 10.1164/rccm.200911-1710OC.

Athlete's Foot

Athlete's foot, also known as tinea pedis, is a persistent and annoying fungal infection of the foot. It commonly occurs between the toes and the toenails but can also occur on other areas of the foot. The skin between the toes can appear red, cracked, and scaly. Sores and blisters can form on the soles of the feet and between the toes. The infected areas may burn or itch.

Moisture and warmth provide an environment for this fungus to thrive. Public or private showers, locker rooms, gym floors, and hotel bathrooms are common places for a person to contract this fungus. People with sweaty feet are more susceptible to getting athlete's foot. Some have a natural resistance to athlete's foot, while others must be more careful with hygiene. Changing into clean socks reduces the risk of reinfection.

We find that in many cases of chronic athlete's foot, there is an underlying systemic problem with candidiasis. For more effective therapy in these cases, it is important to have a systemic treatment to eradicate the fungus. See the Candidiasis section for detailed information.

Most cases of athlete's foot can be treated at home. However, complications can arise when a bacterial infection sets in along with the existing fungal infection. If your athlete's foot does not improve with natural treatment or gets worse, see a doctor for evaluation.

SYMPTOMS

- Burning, itching, and cracking between the toes and on other places of the foot
- Patches of dry skin
- Yellowish-brown toenails

ROOT CAUSES

- Prolonged or frequent use of antibiotics or corticosteroids, leading to a depletion of good bacteria that normally keep fungus in check
- Poor digestion and elimination
- Depressed immune system (e.g., diabetes)
- A high-sugar diet
- Poor hygiene (feet in a damp environment)

Testing Techniques

The following tests assess possible metabolic reasons for candidiasis, a potential underlying contributor to athlete's foot:

Candida levels—stool, blood (antibodies), or urine (yeast metabolites)
Intestinal permeability—urine test

TREATMENT

Diet

Recommended Food

For high-density nutrition and immune support, base your meals around fresh vegetables, whole grains, and quality sources of lean protein, such as beans, lentils, fish, and organic poultry.

To replace friendly bacteria, eat unsweetened yogurt daily. Make sure the brand you're using has live yogurt cultures. Sauerkraut and miso are other examples of foods that contain friendly bacteria.

Vegetable and green drinks will improve your resistance.

Drink eight glasses of clean, quality water a day to help flush out yeast toxins.

Consume 1 to 2 tablespoons of ground flaxseeds daily. Flaxseeds have antifungal properties.

Food to Avoid

Fungus feeds on sugar, so reduce or eliminate obvious sugars in the diet, such as refined carbohydrates including pastas, breads, crackers, cookies, sodas, fruit juice, and candies.

Avoid or reduce the use of fruits and fruit juices during the initial phase (first month) of treatment. It is especially important to avoid these foods between meals.

For severe toenail fungal infections, you can try the following home therapy. Please note that this therapy cannot be used if you have cuts or openings in the skin. Make sure the nails are trimmed as short as possible.

1. In a bucket, dilute 1 cup of bleach in 10 cups of water.
2. Dip the affected foot in the bucket for five seconds. Remove and towel dry.
3. Repeat this procedure every other day for four weeks. Make a new mixture each time.

You should notice that the skin dries out and flakes off. This is normal. You can apply tea tree (*Melaleuca alternifolia*) oil and calendula (*Calendula officinalis*) between treatments for better results.

℞ Super Seven Prescriptions—Athlete's Foot

Super Prescription #1 Tea tree (*Melaleuca alternifolia*) oil

Apply tea tree oil liquid directly to the fungal infection. For toenail fungus, trim the nails, wash the feet with soap (tea tree oil soap is a good choice), and apply as far under the nail as possible. Repeat daily for six to eight weeks or until the infection is cleared.

Super Prescription #2 Oregano oil (*Origanum vulgare*)

Take a 500 mg capsule or the liquid form (as directed on the container) orally, three times daily with meals. The tincture variety can also be applied topically. Oregano oil (*Origanum vulgare*) has a powerful antifungal effect, internally and externally.

Super Prescription #3 Garlic (*Allium sativum*)

Take 500 to 1,000 mg of aged garlic twice daily. Garlic fights fungal infections and also boosts immune strength.

Super Prescription #4 Grapefruit seed extract

Take 200 mg two or three times daily. Practitioners rely on this herb for its antifungal properties.

Super Prescription #5 Caprylic acid

Take 1,000 mg three times daily. This type of fatty acid has been shown in studies to have antifungal properties.

Super Prescription #6 Colloidal silver gel

Apply to affected area twice daily. This antimicrobial substance kills fungi.

Super Prescription #7 Probiotic

Take a product containing four billion active organisms, twice daily, thirty minutes after a meal. It supplies friendly bacteria such as *Lactobacillus acidophilus* and *bifidus*, which fight fungus and prevent its overgrowth.

General Recommendations

Calendula (*Calendula officinalis*) tincture or gel can be applied to the affected area between treatments of tea tree (*Melaleuca alternifolia*) oil. This herb has an antiseptic effect and promotes skin healing.

Thuja (*Thuja occidentalis*) oil has potent antifungal effects. Apply 2 drops to the affected area twice daily.

Pau d'arco (*Tabebuia avellanedae*) has strong antibacterial and antifungal properties. Drink several cups every day.

Wormwood (*Artemisia absinthium*), Oregon grape (*Berberis aquifolium*), and rosemary (*Rosmarinus officinalis*) all have antifungal properties. Take as part of a candida formula.

A high-potency multivitamin provides the many nutrients needed to support immune function. Take as directed on the container.

Vitamin C is used to enhance immune function. Take 1,000 mg two or three times daily.

Laser for nail fungus treatment is available from dermatologists. This natural treatment works by sending a series of tiny, painless pulses of energy into your nail. The laser pulses generate enough heat to kill the fungus, but many patients have no symptoms or a slight warming sensation and rarely burning pain. The treatment itself only takes five to ten minutes (depending on the size and thickness of the nail), but the benefits are long term. The nail with the dead fungus will grow out slowly over the next six to twelve months as it's replaced with your new, fungus-free nail. The treatment can be used for both fingernails and toenails.

One double-blind study reported in the *Australian Journal of Dermatology* looked at the effect of tea tree oil on people with a diagnosis of athlete's foot (tinea pedis). Patients applied the solution twice daily to affected areas for four weeks and were reviewed after two and four weeks of treatment. Fungal level was assessed by a culture of the skin and was found to be 64 percent cured in those applying a 50 percent tea tree oil, compared to 31 percent in the placebo group.

Homeopathy

Pick the remedy that best matches your symptoms in this section. Take a 6x, 12x, 6C, 12C, or 30C potency twice daily for two weeks to see if there are any positive improvements. After you notice improvement, stop taking the remedy, unless symptoms return. Consultation with a homeopathic practitioner is advised.

Graphites is helpful when there is cracked skin that oozes a thick, yellow fluid.

Silica (*Silicea*) is a good choice when there is profuse foot sweating and an offensive smell that excoriates feet.

Sulfur is the best choice for chronic athlete's foot when there is intense itching and burning of feet.

Thuja (*Thuja occidentalis*) is used when you have long-standing fungal infections of the skin that do not respond to other remedies.

Other Recommendations

- Expose your feet to the open air. Wear sandals or porous slippers around the home or outside (if the climate permits).
- Use cotton socks. If your feet perspire a lot, change socks twice daily.
- Wear waterproof slippers or sandals in locker rooms and showers.
- Make sure your feet are washed with soap daily.

REFERENCES

Satchell, A. C., A. Saurajen, C. Bell, and R. S. Barnetson. 2002. Treatment of inter-digital tinea pedis with 25% and 50% tea tree oil solution: A randomized, placebo-controlled, blinded study. *Australian Journal of Dermatology* 43(3):175–78.

Attention-Deficit/Hyperactivity Disorder

In the past, attention-deficit/hyperactivity disorder (ADHD) was known as attention-deficit disorder (ADD). But ADHD is the preferred term as it better defines the inattention and age-inappropriate impulsiveness. This condition typically manifests in children of early school years, and is more often seen in boys. These children generally have long-standing and ongoing difficulty controlling their behaviors and/or paying attention. It's estimated that between 3 percent and 5 percent of children have ADHD, or approximately two million children in the United States. In fact, ADHD is the most commonly diagnosed behavior disorder of childhood. ADHD has been shown to have long-term adverse effects on social-emotional development and school performance, as well as on vocational success when it continues into adulthood. The symptoms can vary; for example, boys may be more impulsive and hyperactive, while girls may tend to be more quiet and inattentive.

SYMPTOMS

Signs of hyperactivity:
- Is restless/squirmy, fidgety with hands and feet
- Is unable to sit quietly
- Runs, climbs, or leaves in situations when inappropriate
- Talks excessively

Signs of impulsivity:

- Blurts out answers
- Interrupts and/or intrudes on others
- Has difficulty waiting in line/ taking turns

Signs of inattention:

- Is easily distracted
- Gives little attention to detail, makes careless mistakes
- Has difficulty sustaining attention to tasks or at play
- Doesn't follow instructions carefully
- Has difficulty organizing tasks and activities
- Loses or forgets things consistently
- Skips from one incomplete task to another

Many parents instinctively believe that the problem is connected to their children's diet. They know that children can respond negatively to sugar or other foods, and they wonder if their child is simply suffering from an extreme version of this reaction. In most cases, these parents are absolutely correct. In the last few decades, sugars, preservatives, and colorings have been added to our food at an increasing rate. Too many children consume nothing but convenience foods, like hot dogs, fried chicken fingers, and highly sweetened fruit drinks and sodas. Since children's small bodies are especially vulnerable to additives in foods, it is not surprising that many of them have a toxic response.

Unfortunately, Western doctors have been trained to discount the importance of diet in hyperactive kids. Instead of nutritional therapy, they will often suggest medication to suppress the symptoms of ADHD. While medications may be necessary in some cases, parents should investigate holistic approaches to see how well their child responds as these approaches are nontoxic.

There are many underlying reasons why a child may have attention or behavior problems. Studies show that frequent ear infections and the regular use of antibiotics, as well as premature birth and family history, are associated with a greater likelihood of developing this disorder. Holistically speaking, causative factors include food additives and food allergies, environmental allergens, and heavy-metal toxicity (such as lead, mercury, and aluminum). A poorly functioning digestive system and increased intestinal permeability lead to an increase in metabolic toxins that disrupt brain chemistry. Nutritional deficiencies of essential fatty acids, B vitamins, and iron, magnesium, and other minerals appear to play a role. Finally, do not underestimate the role of emotional stress and its relationship to ADHD. The breakdown of the family unit in our culture places abnormal stresses on a child, which can result in attention and behavior changes.

If your child has ADHD, try the home-care suggestions outlined here for at least a month and optimally for three months. Some children settle down to a normal level of activity after just a few days without troublesome foods; others will need three or four weeks before the toxins are out of their bodies. Buying and preparing natural foods can be a challenge for busy parents, but your perseverance will be rewarded with a healthier child and a stronger family. Nutritional supplements can work extremely well for most children to correct underlying biochemical imbalances.

ROOT CAUSES

- A diet that's high in sugar and additives
- Food allergies/sensitivities
- Hypoglycemia
- Environmental toxins
- Nutritional deficiencies
- Poor digestion and absorption
- Emotional stresses
- Heavy-metal toxicity
- Neurotransmitter imbalance
- Genetics
- Emotional disturbances

Testing Techniques

The following tests can give you an assessment of possible metabolic reasons for ADHD:

    Food allergy/sensitivity testing—blood, electrodermal testing (see the Food Allergies section for more details)

    Neurotransmitter balance—urine or blood

    Vitamin and mineral analysis—blood

    Fungal and flora balance—stool analysis

    Toxic metals—hair or urine analysis

    Intestinal permeability—urine

    Blood sugar levels—fasting blood test

    Essential fatty acid levels—fasting blood test

    Amino acid levels—urine or fasting blood test

TREATMENT

Diet

Nutritional therapy should be an important component of the treatment of ADHD. The strategies described here will improve behavior and promote age-appropriate concentration and stability, and they will also help keep your child free of many other diet-related disorders. The same general recommendations hold true for adults with this condition.

Recommended Food

The best way to ensure that your child eats an additive-free diet is to buy only fresh foods and prepare them yourself. You don't need to prepare special meals for your child; instead, feed your entire family a whole-foods diet. Younger children will usually eat what everyone else is eat eating, especially if you can reserve a small portion for them before you season the meal to the taste of adult palates.

    B vitamins are healing to stressed-out nerves. Good sources include brown rice, brewer's yeast (which you can add to smoothies and yogurt), and leafy green vegetables.

    Tryptophan encourages the production of serotonin, a chemical that produces a sense of calm. Incorporate soy products, live unsweetened yogurt, whole grains, and organic turkey and chicken into meals and snacks. If your child has trouble sleeping, be sure to include some of these foods at dinner, and try a snack of turkey or chicken on whole-grain crackers before bedtime.

    Anyone with food sensitivities should drink lots of clean, quality water. Children over ten years of age should have a glass every two waking hours; children ten and under should drink half this amount.

Make sure to keep blood sugar levels balanced by avoiding simple sugars and refined carbohydrates and providing adequate protein with meals (nuts, legumes, lean poultry, and fish). Also, as much as possible, include vegetables with meals, as they slow down blood sugar release. Eating smaller, more frequent meals and snacks (every two to three hours) works well. Make sure that breakfast is not skipped, as it sets the biochemical balance for the rest of the day.

Regularly serve brain-healthy foods that are rich in essential fatty acids. Examples include fish (trout, salmon, halibut), nuts (walnuts, almonds), and ground flaxseeds (1 to 2 teaspoons for children and 1 to 2 tablespoons for adults).

We find that many kids and adults do better when they start the day with protein. One easy solution is 20 grams of a whey or rice protein shake mixed with almond or hemp-seed milk.

> ## Healthful Bean Dip
>
> Let your kids dip to their hearts' content.
>
> *Ingredients*
> - Black beans, cooked
> - Juice of 1 lime
> - 1 teaspoon cumin
> - ¼ cup fresh cilantro leaves
> - ½ clove minced garlic (optional)
>
> Combine all ingredients (leave out the garlic, if you like) in a food processor, and whirl until the consistency is smooth. For a fancy presentation and added nutrition, garnish with chopped tomato.

Food to Avoid

If your child suffers from ADHD, it's likely that he or she is allergic to at least one food product, if not several. Read the Food Allergies section in this book, and follow the elimination diet and testing techniques to determine which foods may be causing behavior problems. You may already suspect that a certain food is a trigger for your child, and you should target that product right away. You should also closely examine your child's consumption of the following, all of which are common allergens: wheat, dairy, corn, chocolate, peanuts, citrus, soy, food coloring, and preservatives.

- Do not feed your child anything with artificial colors, flavors, or preservatives. This means you'll have to eliminate fast food, as well as all junk and processed food. If you must buy canned or frozen products, read the labels carefully. Even items advertised as "all natural" may contain small amounts of additives.
- Sugar is famous for making children hyper, and, in fact, excess sucrose often leads to hypoglycemia, a factor in ADHD. Obviously, candy, sodas, and sweets are out of the question, but so are most store-bought fruit juices, which usually contain added sugar, and products made with white flour. If your child has been eating large quantities of refined sugar, you may see a dramatic difference in his or her behavior within just a few days of eliminating it.

A randomized, double-blind, placebo-controlled, crossover trial published in the journal *Lancet* tested whether the intake of artificial food color and additives affected childhood behavior. During the six-week trial, researchers gave 153 three-year-old and 144 eight- to nine-year-old children drinks with additives, colors, and a common preservative. These included sunset yellow, carmoisine, tartrazine, ponceau, quinolone yellow (E104), allura red (E129), and sodium benzoate. This combination is similar to what is found in commercial drink mixes and is equivalent to two servings of candy a day. Children in the placebo group received

A study involving twenty-one youths with ADHD, ages four to nineteen, found that daily supplementation of phosphatidylserine at dosages between 200 and 300 mg for four months benefited greater than 90 percent of cases. Attention and learning were the symptoms most improved.

a similar-looking and similar-tasting solution. Evaluation of the children was done by teachers, parents, and a computer test. Children in both age groups were significantly more hyperactive and had shorter attention spans from consuming the drink containing the additives. Symptoms of hyperactivity were present in some children within an hour of consuming the artificial additives.

℞ Super Seven Prescriptions—ADHD

Super Prescription #1 Fish oil
Take 2,000 mg or more of combined EPA and DHA daily. High-dose omega-3 supplementation has been shown to improve symptoms of ADHD and learning.

Super Prescription #2 Homeopathy
Pick the remedy that best matches your symptoms. Take a 6x, 12x, 6C, or 30C potency twice daily for two weeks to see if there are any positive improvements. After you notice improvement, stop taking the remedy, unless symptoms return. Consultation with a homeopathic practitioner is advised.

Super Prescription #3 Phosphatidylserine
Take 300 to 500 mg daily for three months. A maintenance dosage of 100 to 300 mg may be effective for some kids and adults. Phosphatidylserine is a naturally occurring substance found in high concentrations in brain cells; it helps brain cells function properly.

Super Prescription #4 Pycnogenol
Take 1 mg per 4.9 pounds of body weight per day.

Super Prescription #5 L-carnitine
Take 100 mg per 2.2 pounds of body weight daily. This has been shown to improve symptoms for boys with ADHD.

Super Prescription #6 High-potency multivitamin
Take as directed on the container. It provides a base of nutrients required for brain function.

Super Prescription #7 Calcium and magnesium complex
Take a combination of these two minerals, at a dosage of 500 mg of calcium and 250 mg of magnesium, twice daily. These two minerals relax the nervous system.

L-carnitine has been shown to help with ADHD. An eight-week, double-blind study resulted in improvement in 54 percent of boys compared to 13 percent for those taking placebo. L-carnitine significantly decreased the attention problems and aggressive behavior in boys with ADHD.

General Recommendations

Take a probiotic to maintain good bacteria levels in the digestive tract. Take as directed on the container.

Vitamin B6 is involved in the formation of serotonin, a neurotransmitter that has a calming effect. Give 100 mg daily to children five years or older. High doses of this vitamin are best used under the guidance of a nutrition-oriented doctor, along with a B-complex for balance.

Western Herbal

Ginkgo biloba carries oxygen and nutrients to the brain. Look for a product standardized to 24 percent flavone glycosides. People who are sixteen and older should take 60 to 120 mg twice a day. Give 30 to 60 mg twice a day to children ages ten through fifteen. Those under ten should be given 15 to 30 mg twice daily.

GABA is an amino acid that has a calming effect on the mind. Give 250 mg two or three times daily between meals.

Zinc deficiency can contribute to ADHD symptoms. Children ages two and older should get a daily total of 10 to 15 mg, along with 2 mg of copper.

B-complex vitamins supply all the B vitamins involved with brain function. Give a 50 mg B-complex daily.

Passionflower (*Passiflora incarnata*) can be effective in calming children with ADHD. Those sixteen years of age and older should take 100 to 200 mg twice a day. Children ages ten through fifteen should take 50 to 100 mg twice daily. Children under ten should be given 25 to 50 mg twice daily.

If your child is depressed, Saint-John's-wort (*Hypericum perforatum*) may help. Children ages ten through fifteen should take 50 to 150 mg twice a day. Children under ten should take 25 to 75 mg twice a day. Adolescents and young adults who are sixteen and older can take 100 to 300 mg twice a day.

A randomized, placebo-controlled, double-blind study involved sixty-one children who were given pycnogenol or a placebo. After one month, the children with ADHD who took pycnogenol were found to have a significant reduction of hyperactivity and improved attention, visual-motor coordination, and concentration.

Homeopathy

Pick the remedy that best matches your symptoms. Take a 6x, 12x, 6C, or 30C potency twice daily for two weeks to see if there are any positive results. After you notice improvement, stop taking the remedy, unless symptoms return. Consultation with a homeopathic practitioner is advised.

Anacardium Orientale is for children who tend to be cruel to animals and people. There is low self-esteem, and they are antisocial and absentminded. They often curse and swear.

Hyoscyamus Niger is for children who are very impulsive and violent, especially toward younger siblings. They are very talkative and sexually precocious.

Medorrhinum is for children who have major temper tantrums and are violent toward other kids. They have a hard time concentrating, are very warm, and crave oranges and ice.

Stramonium is for children who have many fears, such as of the dark or of animals. They have fits of anger and rage and destroy things. Night terrors are common.

Sulfur is for children who are curious, stubborn, and hyperactive. They are very warm, sweat easily, have a great thirst for cold drinks, and crave spicy foods.

Tarentula Hispanica is for children who are extremely hurried and restless. They are mischievous, destructive, and impulsive. They love music and dancing.

Tuberculinum is for children who are very stubborn, demanding, and impatient and get bored easily. They often have violent tempers and may hit other people and animals. They crave milk and smoked meats and are prone to respiratory infections.

A study in the *Journal of Alternative and Complementary Medicine* confirmed that vitamin-mineral supplementation modestly raises the nonverbal intelligence of some groups of schoolchildren.

Acupressure

Even young children can be taught acupressure techniques to practice when they feel upset. In fact, by teaching them to identify disquieting emotions and to take time out for a calming acupressure session, you'll give them a valuable life skill. For information about pressure points and administering treatment, see pages 787–794.

- Lung 1 (Lu1) releases tension and helps restore normal, deep breathing.
- If your child's hyperactivity seems to be triggered by frustration, teach him or her to press Conception Vessel 12 (CV12) while slowly repeating the point's descriptive name, Center of Power.

Bodywork

Massage
Young children—if you can persuade them to remain still long enough—enjoy soothing massages from their parents. Teenagers may prefer to have an appointment with a massage therapist; you can also show them the self-care techniques listed in the Bodywork chapter of this book.

Reflexology
See pages 804–805 for information about reflexology areas and how to work them.

Work the areas corresponding to the diaphragm and the solar plexus to encourage a sense of peace and stillness.

Other Bodywork Recommendations
Craniosacral therapy by a qualified practitioner is highly recommended to balance out the nervous system for people with ADHD.

Aromatherapy

Aromatherapy makes a relaxing complement to the other treatments suggested here. Use chamomile, lavender, or sandalwood to encourage serenity; try them in a bath or a massage, or add a few drops to a diffuser and let the pleasing scent waft through a room. These applications are especially helpful just before bedtime.

Stress Reduction

General Stress-Reduction Therapies
Although biofeedback may seem like the stress-reduction technique that's least likely to work for children, it is actually highly effective for kids with ADHD, many of whom enjoy the interaction with machines and computers. Of all the biofeedback techniques, EEG seems to work best for hyperactivity.

Consider signing up for a parent-and-child yoga class. Children usually have fun making the animal poses, and you'll both enjoy the lifelong health benefits of this ancient discipline.

Other Recommendations

- Encourage your child to play or exercise outside in the fresh air. Limit exposure to sedentary, passive activities, like watching television or playing video games.

- Consider buying an air filter to purify your household of environmental allergens that may contribute to nervous system irritation.
- Work with a counselor to help your child with behavior modification and learning styles. Every child is different and requires an individualized approach. Emotional counseling may be necessary for healing, especially in cases of broken families or abuse.

REFERENCES

Howard, A. L., et al. 2010. ADHD is associated with a "Western" dietary pattern in adolescents. *Journal of Attention Disorders*, published online July 14, 2010.

Kidd, P. 2000. Attention deficit/hyperactivity disorder (ADHD) in children: Rationale for its integrative management. *Alternative Medicine Review* 5(5): 402–28.

McCann, D., et al. 2007. Food additives and hyperactive behaviour in 3-year-old and 8/9-year-old children in the community: A randomised, double-blinded, placebo-controlled trial. *Lancet* 370:1560–67.

Richardson, A. J., et al. 2002. A randomized double-blind, placebo-controlled study of the effects of supplementation with highly unsaturated fatty acids on ADHD-related symptoms in children with specific learning difficulties. *Progress in Neuropsychopharmacology and Biological Psychiatry* 26:233–39.

Schoenthaler, S. J., I. D. Bier, K. Young, et al. 2000. The effect of vitamin-mineral supplementation on the intelligence of American schoolchildren: A randomized, double-blind, placebo-controlled trial. *Journal of Alternative and Complementary Medicine* 6(1): 19–29.

Trebaticka, J., et al. 2006. Treatment of ADHD with French maritime pine bark extract, Pycnogenol. *European Child and Adolescent Psychiatry* 15:329–35.

Van Oudheusden, L.J., and H. R. Scholte. 2002. Efficacy of carnitine in the treatment of children with attention-deficit hyperactivity disorder. *Prostaglandins Leukot Essent Fatty Acids* 67:33–8.

Autism

Autism is an increasingly common developmental disorder that occurs in early childhood. It is included in a group of developmental problems known as autism spectrum disorder (ASD). ASD involves a range of neurodevelopment disorders that affect a child's ability to interact and communicate with others.

Language, behavior, and social interaction are the three general areas that are affected in children who have autism. Symptoms vary from mild to severe in these categories and may be present in early infancy or may not appear until the child is a few years old. It is estimated that an average of one in ninety-one children in the United States has ASD.

Conventional medicine acknowledges that the exact causes of ASD are unknown, but it does admit that environmental causes may be a risk factor. It is the authors' opinion that conventional approaches to the prevention and treatment of ASD are woefully inadequate. Holistic doctors provide safe and often effective methods to help children with ASD.

It is reasonable to assume that the tremendous rise in ASD is related to environmental causes. Vaccines, toxic metals, chronic infections of the digestive or immune system, nutrient deficiencies, food sensitivities or allergies, environmental chemicals such as parabens and phthalates, and other factors may be involved.

SYMPTOMS

The National Institutes of Health describes how autism is diagnosed based on a number of symptoms. Early indicators include the following:

- No babbling or pointing by age one
- No single words by sixteen months or two-word phrases by age two
- No response to name
- Loss of language or social skills

- Poor eye contact
- Excessive lining up of toys or objects
- No smiling or social responsiveness

Later indicators include the following:

- Impaired ability to make friends with peers
- Impaired ability to initiate or sustain a conversation with others
- Absence or impairment of imaginative and social play
- Stereotyped, repetitive, or unusual use of language

- Restricted patterns of interest that are abnormal in intensity or focus
- Preoccupation with certain objects or subjects
- Inflexible adherence to specific routines or rituals

Testing Techniques

There is no metabolic test that is used to diagnose ASD. The following tests are helpful in identifying the contributing or root causes of ASD:

Nutrient analysis, especially vitamin D, vitamin B12, folate, essential fatty acids, zinc, vitamin B6, vitamin E, copper, glutathione, iron, lithium, and amino acids—blood and urine

Digestive function and microbe (fungi, parasite, bacteria) testing—stool analysis

Intestinal permeability—urine

Hormone testing (thyroid and others)—blood

Toxic metals—hair, urine

Toxic metal sensitivities—blood

Food sensitivities (especially gluten and casein)—blood, electrodermal, stool

Cholesterol deficiency (including total and apolipoprotein b)—blood

Inborn errors of metabolism—urine

Neurotransmitter balance—urine, blood

Genetic mutation of MTHFR gene—blood or saliva

ROOT CAUSES

There are various causes of ASD. Conventional medicine believes that the following are risk factors:

- Children with a parent or a sibling with ASD
- Certain medications taken during the mother's pregnancy, such as valproic acid and thalidomide
- Certain other medical conditions, particularly chromosomal disorders such as fragile X syndrome or Down syndrome

Holistic doctors and researchers strongly consider the following to be root causes, acknowledging that the causes are multifactorial and that they vary among individuals:

- Toxic metals (especially mercury, lead, and aluminum)
- Chronic infection (infection of the intestines, especially fungal; chronic viral infections)
- Chronic inflammation of the brain and the nervous system (often caused by vaccines, environmental chemicals, or chronic infections)
- Detoxification impairment
- Nutrient deficiencies
- Poor digestive function and malabsorption (leaky gut syndrome)
- Food allergies and sensitivities (especially gluten and casein)
- Inborn errors of metabolism (leading to cholesterol deficiency)
- Other environmental toxins (phthalates, parabens)
- Genetic factors such as MTHFR gene mutation and others

TREATMENT

All experts agree that the best approach to ASD is early diagnosis and treatment. However, natural and integrative approaches are the most effective. We highly recommend consultation with a doctor who is trained in holistic approaches to ASD. One very good resource is www.autismnow.org, which provides a list of DAN (Defeat Autism Now) practitioners. These health-care professionals are trained in a comprehensive, holistic approach to ASD.

Diet

Recommended Food

As much as possible, consume a diet of whole foods in their natural state. This should include vegetables, fruits, fish, legumes, nuts and seeds, and nongluten grains. Shakes made with protein and other nutrients can be helpful.

Food to Avoid

Many people with ASD benefit from a gluten-free (no rye, barley, wheat, and most oats) and casein-free (cow's-milk products) diet. Other food sensitivities may cause symptoms as well, which testing can identify. Avoid artificial dyes, colorings, sweeteners, and foods high in simple sugar.

℞ Super Seven Prescriptions—Autism

Super Prescription #1 Fish oil
Take 1,000 to 3,000 mg of EPA and DHA combined. Essential fatty acids are critical for normal brain function.

Super Prescription #2 Magnesium
Take 200 mg twice daily to provide nervous system support.

Super Prescription #3 Probiotic
Take as directed on the label. This provides beneficial intestinal bacteria that support healthy digestion and detoxification.

Super Prescription #4 Vitamin D
Take 2,000 to 5,000 IU daily with meals. Deficiency is common, and this nutrient is required for healthy brain and neurological function.

Super Prescription #5 Glutathione
Take 250 mg daily orally or as a transdermal application. This super antioxidant supports detoxification and improves cellular health.

Super Prescription #6 Vitamin B6
Take 20 to 50 mg daily. This B vitamin has been shown in several studies to be beneficial for those with autism.

Super Prescription #7 Multivitamin
Take an age-appropriate full-spectrum multivitamin and -mineral formula that is hypoallergenic.

General Recommendations

Calcium supports a healthy nervous system. Take 500 mg daily.

Coenzyme Q10 supports healthy brain function. Take 25 to 50 mg daily.

L-carnitine is important for nervous system health. Take 250 to 500 mg daily.

Digestive enzymes break food down and promote better absorption. This reduces the inflammatory response by the immune and nervous systems. Take 1 or 2 capsules with each meal. Children's formulas are available.

Methylfolate along with B12 can be helpful. Take as directed by a holistic doctor.

Homeopathy

See a practitioner trained in homeopathy for individualized treatment.

Bodywork

Reflexology

See pages 804–805 for information about reflexology areas and how to work them. Focus on the brain and spinal cord area.

Hydrotherapy

Constitutional hydrotherapy can be used to improve intestinal function related to ASD.

Other Recommendations

Several alternative therapies are available to help those with ASD. These include heavy-metal detoxification, antifungal and antiviral therapies, and hyperbaric oxygen therapy. See a qualified practitioner to guide you.

REFERENCES

National Institute of Neurological Disorders and Stroke, www.ninds.nih.gov/disorders/autism/detail_autism.htm.

Back Pain

If you're an American, you have an 80 percent chance of experiencing back pain at some point in your adult life. Back pain is one of the most common reasons for emergency room visits; in fact, it is the fourth most common ailment in our country.

A few years ago, it was generally believed that back pain was caused by the degeneration of one or more discs, the "shock absorbers" of the spine. This results in an impingement on and possible damage to the nerves that exit the spinal column. Today we know that almost all adults over forty have some disc deterioration; moreover, many people with degenerated discs don't feel any pain at all. While disc problems can be one cause of back pain, a more common cause is strained muscles. Stress, bad posture, and long periods of inactivity all weaken the back, making it vulnerable to pain from injury or exercise. When the back is very weak, even minor actions like twisting or coughing can trigger severe pain. Chronic back pain is frequently caused by muscular imbalance in the back, poor flexibility, spinal misalignment, and ligament or tendon injuries.

Although many cases of back pain have their roots in the muscles, other conditions can cause or contribute to pain. Pregnancy and obesity, which place stress on the muscles, are two common factors, as are arthritis, osteoporosis, and disorders of the kidney, the bladder, the pelvis, and the prostate. Constipation and other digestive disorders can also refer pain to the back area.

Proper lifting techniques are very important to prevent strain and injury of the back. This is especially true for people who have had previous back injuries.

Back pain does not automatically mean surgery and a lifetime of agony. It is now considered highly preventable and treatable with exercise, stretching, bodywork, supplements, and stress management. However, if you have pain that lasts for several weeks or extremely acute pain, contact your doctor so that he or she can check for underlying disorders that may be causing your pain. For example, certain kinds of back pain can signal a stroke, osteoporosis, or other serious medical conditions like cancer. If the pain radiates down your leg or is accompanied by numbness or loss of muscular, bowel, or bladder control, get medical help immediately.

SYMPTOMS

- Any kind of pain—sharp, lancing, dull, aching, gradual, sudden—usually in the lower or middle back

- Pain can radiate to the hips or the neck

ROOT CAUSES

- Inactivity, especially when punctuated by sudden exercise
- Poor posture and spinal misalignment
- Muscle strength and flexibility imbalances
- Sleeping on a poorly made mattress
- High heels
- Obesity
- Pregnancy

- Disorders of the kidney, the bladder, the prostate, or the pelvic region
- Arthritis
- Osteoporosis
- Emotional stress
- Premenstrual syndrome (PMS)
- Nutritional deficiencies
- Constipation
- Smoking

Testing Techniques

The following tests can give you an assessment of possible metabolic reasons for lower back pain:

Vitamin and mineral analysis—blood or urine

Diagnostic image of the spine

TREATMENT

Diet

Constipation, extra weight, and toxic buildup can aggravate back pain. Diet and detoxification therapies will help keep your body free of these stressors.

Recommended Food

Constipation makes back pain worse, so eat plenty of fiber, preferably in the form of vegetables.

Dehydration aggravates back pain. Drink a glass of clean, quality water every two waking hours. If you have an episode of back pain, drink a few glasses as soon as the pain starts.

Keep your bones well fed. Get protein from fish, soy products, and beans; for calcium, eat leafy greens, sea vegetables, nuts and seeds, and tofu.

Consume foods that are rich in essential fatty acids (salmon, mackerel, almonds, walnuts, and ground flaxseeds).

Food to Avoid

Stay away from products that are high in saturated fat and sugar, especially if you are overweight. Extra pounds on the waist and the hips means a heavier load on the back.

Avoid caffeine and alcohol products, which are known to worsen inflammation.

℞ Super Seven Prescriptions—Back Pain

Super Prescription #1 Methylsulfonylmethane (MSM)

Take 3,000 to 8,000 mg daily in divided doses. Reduce the dosage if diarrhea occurs. MSM alleviates muscle spasms and has natural anti-inflammatory effects.

Super Prescription #2 Devil's claw

Take a product standardized to daily doses of 50 to 100 mg harpagoside. This herbal extract has been shown to help with nonspecific low back pain.

Super Prescription #3 Calcium and magnesium

Twice daily, take a complex of these two minerals that contains 500 mg of calcium and 250 mg of magnesium. These minerals alleviate muscle spasms.

Super Prescription #4 Homeopathy

Pick the remedy that best matches your symptoms under Homeopathy in this section. For acute back pain, take a 30C potency four times daily. For chronic back pain, take twice daily for two weeks to see if there are any positive improvements. After you notice improvement, stop taking the remedy, unless symptoms return. Consultation with a homeopathic practitioner is advised.

Super Prescription #5 Bromelain

Take 500 mg three times daily between meals. Look for products standardized to 2,000 MCU (milk-clotting units) per 1,000 mg or 1,200 GDU (gelatin-dissolving units) per 1,000 mg. Bromelain has a natural anti-inflammatory effect. Protease enzyme products also have this benefit.

Super Prescription #6 White willow (*Salix alba*)

Take a product standardized to contain 240 mg of salicin daily or 5 ml of the tincture form three times daily. This herb reduces pain.

Super Prescription #7 Collagen

Take 40 mg daily of undenatured type 2 collagen to reduce back pain caused by osteoarthritis.

General Recommendations

Vitamin C reduces inflammation and strengthens connective tissue. Take 1,000 mg three times daily.

Pine bark or grapeseed extract reduces inflammation. Take 100 mg three times daily.

Ginger (*Zingiber officinale*) is a popular choice for relief of both inflammation and pain. Pour boiling water over the grated root and drink the tea, or try adding fresh ginger to your meals. If you want something stronger, take 1 to 2 grams of dried powder in capsule form, two or three times daily, or use 1 to 2 ml of a tincture three times daily.

Boswellia (*Boswellia serrata*): Take 1,200 to 1,500 mg of a standardized extract containing 60 to 65 percent boswellic acids two to three times daily.

Glucosamine sulfate: Take 1,500 mg daily to strengthen connective tissue.

DMSO (dimethyl sulfoxide) is a topical pain-relieving substance. Work with your doctor to use DMSO.

Many excellent herbs reduce inflammation. Devil's claw root (*Harpagophytum procumbens*), alfalfa (*Medicago sativa*), and yucca root (*Yucca schidigera*) capsules are among the best. Give these herbs at least two months to take effect. Recommended dosages are as follows:

Devil's claw should not be used if you have a history of gallstones, heartburn, or ulcers. Take 1,500 to 2,500 mg of the standardized powdered herb in capsule or tablet form daily, or use 1 to 2 ml of a tincture three times a day.

Arnica (*Arnica montana*) oil reduces pain and spasm. Rub this oil over the affected area twice daily.

Saint-John's-wort oil (*Hypericum oil*) reduces nerve pain. Rub over the affected area twice daily.

D-L phenylalanine is an amino acid used to reduce pain. Take 500 mg three times daily on an empty stomach.

Vitamins B1, B6, and B12 have been shown to reduce the amount of medication needed for back pain. Take 50 mg of B1 and B6 and 400 mcg of B12 three times daily. When using these individual B vitamins long term, make sure to also supplement a 50 mg B-complex for a balance of all the B vitamins.

Protease enzymes reduce inflammation. Take 1 or 2 capsules twice daily between meals or as directed on the container.

Apply cayenne (*Capsicum annuum*) cream to the affected area two to four times daily for symptomatic relief. Choose a cream standardized to between 0.025 and 0.075 percent capsaicin. Capsaicin depletes the nerves of substance P, a neurotransmitter that transmits pain messages.

Homeopathy

Pick the remedy that best matches your symptoms in this section. For acute back pain, take a 30C potency four times daily. For chronic back pain, take twice daily for two weeks to see if there are any positive improvements. After you notice results, stop taking the remedy, unless symptoms return. Consultation with a homeopathic practitioner is advised.

Aesculus is for lower back or sacral pain that is worse when you are sitting. The pain often radiates into the right hip.

Arnica (*Arnica montana*) is for an injury that leaves your back feeling bruised and sore and is helpful if you have difficulty moving around.

Bryonia (*Bryonia alba*) is for lower back pain and stiffness that feel worse with any movement and in cold, dry weather, and that feels better when the area is rubbed.

Calcarea Carbonica is for chronic lower back pain and weakness in overweight individuals who also are chilly. Symptoms are worse in the cold and in dampness.

Cimicifuga Racemosa is for a stiff and aching neck and back. Muscles feel bruised, but feel better with warmth. Also, it is used for menstrual cramps with lower back pain radiating to the thighs.

Ignatia (*Ignatia amara*) is for back spasms and cramping as the result of emotional stress.

Magnesia Phosphorica is for a muscle spasm in the back that feels better from warmth.

Nux Vomica (*Strychnos nux vomica*) is for back spasms and cramping, especially in the lower back. The person may also have constipation and feel chilly and irritable. The symptoms are worse from cold and feel better with warmth.

Rhus Toxicodendron is for a stiff lower back that is worse in the cold and the damp and feels better with movement. It is specific for a sprained back muscle or ligaments.

Ruta Graveolens is for pain near the neck or for lower back pain. The area of the injury feels lame, and the pain is worse at night. This remedy is useful for back sprains and strains.

Acupressure

Acupressure relieves back pain by stimulating blood flow, unblocking energy, and strengthening the internal organs. Some of the following points may be quite tender; if so, use a very light, continuous touch, instead of heavy pressure. In cases of severe pain or true disc damage, always consult a doctor before working these points. For more information about pressure points and administering treatment, see pages 787–794.

- For lower back pain, work Bladder 25, 31, and 40 (B25, B31, and B40).
- Bladder 20 (B20) is the point for pain in the middle back.
- Upper back pain can be eased by using Gallbladder 20 (GB20) and Governing Vessel 14 (GV14).
- For back pain accompanied or caused by tension, use Bladder 48 (B48).
- If you have arthritis as well as back pain, Bladder 54 (B54) is a good choice.

Bodywork

Complementary therapy for back pain should usually include some kind of bodywork. You may want to try several of the following methods until you find the combination that works best for you. For a thorough evaluation, check with an osteopathic doctor, a naturopathic doctor, a chiropractor, or a medical doctor. Then a course of treatment can be recommended.

Massage

Most people know instinctively that massage will relieve their back pain and tension, but many are held back by their inability to travel to a massage therapist or by fear of making the pain worse. Massage is so effective, it's worth taking extra steps to overcome any obstacles to treatment. Check around to find a licensed, experienced professional who knows how to work with different kinds of back pain. He or she may also be willing to come to your house if you're immobilized.

Reflexology

See pages 804–805 for information about reflexology areas and how to work them. Work the spine, the hips, and the tailbone area, all of which exist at the base of the heel.

Hydrotherapy

Hot water therapies are popular ways to treat backache and release stress. Although their relief is usually temporary, they feel wonderfully soothing and can get you mobile enough to receive other therapies.

To release spasms and tension, soak in a warm bath (90 to 100 degrees F). For an extra soothing effect, add any of the essential oils recommended under Aromatherapy in this section, or try a little mustard or ginger.

A hot water bottle is an old-fashioned remedy for back spasms, and it still works. Constitutional hydrotherapy is helpful. See the Hydrotherapy section for directions.

Other Bodywork Recommendations

For chronic or severe pain, a visit to a chiropractor or an osteopath is highly recommended. He or she will correct postural problems and manipulate your spine so that your body is balanced and aligned.

Pay attention to your posture. Stand up straight, with your pelvis tucked in. When seated, keep your back erect and your feet flat on the floor. If you have serious back problems, try postural methods such as Hellerwork or the Alexander technique, which seek to retrain the body so that it moves naturally, correctly, and painlessly. Contact a specialist for instruction.

The following exercise will often relieve lower-back pain:

1. Take your shoes off and stand against a wall so that your heels touch it.
2. Now adjust your posture so that your buttocks and shoulders also touch the wall.
3. Imagine that you are straightening the curvature of your spine, and try to make your entire back press flat against the wall. Take the stretch as far as you comfortably can, and hold it for twenty to thirty seconds.

Throw out your high heels. Most footwear companies now make beautiful shoes that aren't hard on your feet and back.

If you feel stiffness and pain in the middle of the night and in the morning but not during the rest of the day, your mattress may be the culprit. Find one that's firm and supportive. In addition, you should sleep with your knees bent. Placing a pillow between your knees may make you more comfortable.

Unless your health care provider recommends this, it is best to avoid bedrest with a back injury. Studies show that it often slows down recovery.

Laser therapy by a doctor can be very effective for back pain.

Orthotic support for foot arch problems can help back pain. Consult a podiatrist or a chiropractor.

Aromatherapy

- A massage with Idaho balsam or peppermint oils will help warm up muscles and dissolve cramps.
- To help relieve stress, try some of the many oils that have relaxing properties. Add geranium, jasmine, or lavender to a hot bath, or if you suffer from chronic tension, use a diffuser or a candle to release the scent throughout a room for long periods of time (just make sure you don't leave the flame unattended).
- If you tend to breathe shallowly in a crisis, use frankincense to encourage deep, relaxing breaths. Hold the vial directly under your nose and inhale.

Stress Reduction

General Stress-Reduction Therapies

Many people with back problems find that yoga eases their pain. Yoga releases emotional stress, as well as the physical tension that often deposits itself in the back; it also strengthens the spine and improves all-over flexibility. If you have or have had severe pain, take a class with an instructor who knows how to handle your condition.

If you have severe or chronic back pain, look into biofeedback. EMG biofeedback will help you identify just when you tense up your back muscles and will show you how to release them.

Many of the techniques mentioned throughout this section, such as massage, hot baths, and herbal treatments, treat stress as well as pain. Keep them in mind, and employ the ones you like best on a regular basis.

Other Recommendations

Regular exercise is the best way to prevent and treat back pain. While acute attacks may keep you in bed for a day or two, you should plan to get moving again as soon as possible. Gentle, nonjarring exercises such as walking, swimming, and cycling (with your back straight), are excellent choices. Whatever you do, do it consistently. Inactivity on the weekdays, punctuated by rigorous workouts on Saturday or Sunday, will only set up your back for injury.

REFERENCES

Bruggemann, G., C. O. Koehler, and E. M. Koch. 1990. Results of a double-blind study of diclofenac + vitamin B1, B6, B12 versus diclofenac in patients with acute pain of the lumbar vertebrae. A multicenter study. Klin Wochenschr 68:116–20 [in German].

Kuhlwein, A., H. J. Meyer, and C. O. Koehler. 1990. Reduced diclofenac administration by B vitamins: Results of a randomized double-blind study with reduced daily doses of diclofenac (75 mg diclofenac versus 75 mg diclofenac plus B vitamins) in acute lumbar vertebral syndromes. Klin Wochenschr 68:107–15 [in German].

Schwieger, G., H. Karl, and E. Schonhaber. 1990. Relapse prevention of painful vertebral syndromes in follow-up treatment with a combination of vitamins B1, B6, and B12. *Annals of the New York Academy of Science* 585:54–62.

Bad Breath (Halitosis)

If you've ever eaten garlic or onions—or stood next to someone who has—you know that certain foods reliably produce a sour or strong odor on the breath. These foods, usually ones that are pungent or spicy, contain foul-smelling sulfur compounds that are released not just into the mouth but into the bloodstream and the lungs as well. Even if you brush and gargle, you'll continue to exhale the sulfur with every breath until the food is fully metabolized, a process that can take up to twenty-four hours. This kind of food-induced bad breath can sometimes be socially troubling (especially if your companions have not eaten the same sulfur-producing food that you have), but it is in no way a health threat. If you enjoy eating spicy, strong food, complementary medicine offers some effective ways to mask the temporarily offensive result.

Persistent bad breath, on the other hand, is medically known as halitosis and is a symptom of an underlying problem. Many cases are warning signs of insufficient oral hygiene. If you do not clean your teeth after eating, bacteria will feed on the food particles left in your mouth and emit sulfur as a digestive by-product. Eventually, these bacteria will cause tooth decay and gum disease, disorders that, in turn, lead to even worse-smelling breath.

If regular brushing and flossing don't improve chronic bad breath, it's quite possible that you are suffering from a toxic body system. An improper diet and a poorly functioning digestive system can lead to the accumulation of toxins, which is reflected in bad breath. If you are constipated (as are many people who follow poor diets) and cannot eliminate the poisons via your bowels, the body may try to expel some of them every time you breathe out. A cleansing program, followed by dietary changes, should help get rid of the toxins and, with them, the cause of bad breath.

Also, an undetected infection such as tonsillitis or sinusitis can be the underlying cause of foul breath. These conditions may be the result of food or environmental allergens causing mucus formation and postnasal drip. Along these lines are chronic root canal infections, as well as teeth and mercury fillings that are decaying. The repeated use of antibiotics can wipe out the good flora in your mouth, which leads to the overgrowth of bad bacteria that cause bad breath.

Mouth breathing at night or sleep apnea may also be at the root of bad breath.

Smoking is another obvious method of poisoning your body, and the best way to clear up the breath it causes is to give up the habit.

In rare cases, halitosis is a symptom of a serious disease. If the suggestions listed here don't improve your breath, consult a holistic dentist first and then a doctor, if necessary. It is possible that you have a dental disorder or even a disease of the kidneys or the liver. Take chronic bad breath seriously, but do exercise some common sense. Our society places an unnaturally high priority on eliminating body odors, and many dentists have noted that otherwise healthy patients can become convinced their breath is offensive, when in fact it is perfectly normal. If your close friends and health professionals assure you that your breath is fine, it's probably wisest to trust them.

SYMPTOMS

- Unpleasant odor on the breath

ROOT CAUSES

- Pungent or spicy foods
- Inadequate dental hygiene
- Poor diet
- Constipation
- Smoking
- Tooth decay
- Gum disease
- Decaying mercury fillings
- Chronic infection in the mouth (especially root canals), throat,
- or sinuses
- Liver failure
- Kidney disease
- Diabetes
- Mouth breathing at night
- Sleep apnea
- Flora imbalance in the mouth and the respiratory tract

TREATMENT

Diet

Recommended Food

Base your meals on healthful sources of fiber. Whole grains, raw or lightly cooked fruits and vegetables, beans, and raw nuts and seeds will all improve your digestive system's ability to process food and expel toxins.

Drink a glass of clean, quality water every two waking hours. This will keep your digestive system regular and help eliminate poisons.

If you go to a diner or an old-fashioned restaurant, you may notice that a sprig of parsley accompanies your meal. The parsley is meant to be more than a garnish; it's a traditional breath freshener that really works. Parsley is high in chlorophyll, an agent that neutralizes odor in the bloodstream and the lungs. Other good sources of chlorophyll include green vegetables, watercress, and alfalfa. If you know you're going to eat a type of food that causes bad breath, you may want to incorporate some of these greens into your meal.

Vitamins A and C are necessary for good dental health. For vitamin A, consume green or orange vegetables like carrots, kale, squash, sweet potatoes, and spinach. Eat citrus fruits for vitamin C.

Cultured products, especially live, unsweetened yogurt, will encourage healthy bacteria to grow in the intestines and will improve digestion.

Food to Avoid

Avoid foods that take a long time to travel through the digestive system. Red meat, fried food, and processed food all linger in the system and cause both constipation and halitosis.

Mucus slows waste matter in its passage through the intestines. Cut down on mucus-forming foods like dairy products, refined flours, chocolate, and bananas.

Avoid foods that are high in refined sugar, which leads to tooth decay. Be especially wary of sticky treats like caramels or hard candies, which can lodge between your teeth and attract oral bacteria.

Foods that are most likely to cause temporary bad breath include garlic, onions, strong cheese, cured meats, and anchovies. If the resulting odor bothers you, limit or stop your consumption of these items.

℞ Super Seven Prescriptions—Bad Breath

Super Prescription #1 Chlorophyll
Take a teaspoonful of liquid chlorophyll after meals. Chlorella, alfalfa, and spirulina are also rich sources. Take as directed on the container.

Super Prescription #2 Xylitol
Use 4 to 12 grams of xylitol in natural gums, mints, toothpastes, or as a mouth rinse. This natural sweetener prevents the bacteria that cause bad breath from sticking to the mucosa of your mouth and teeth.

Super Prescription #3 Parsley

Take 5 drops of a liquid parsley extract after each meal to freshen your breath.

Super Prescription #4 Probiotic

Take a product containing at least four billion organisms. Mix it into water, swish it in your mouth, and swallow. It contains friendly bacteria that prevent the buildup of bacteria that cause bad breath, and it improves digestive function and elimination. Probiotics specific to gum health are available.

Super Prescription #5 Enzymes

Take a full-range enzyme with each meal to enhance the breakdown and the absorption of food.

Super Prescription #6 Bitter herbs

Take a digestion formula that contains bitter herbs, such as gentian, to improve overall digestive function. Take as directed on the container at the beginning of each meal.

Super Prescription #7 Milk thistle (*Silybum marianum*)

If you are frequently constipated, you probably need to detoxify your liver. Cleanse it with milk thistle extract. Choose a product standardized to 70 to 80 percent silymarin, and take 200 to 250 mg twice a day.

General Recommendations

Coenzyme Q10 is for people with active gum disease. Take 200 mg daily.

Cooled rosemary and peppermint tea makes a highly effective mouthwash.

Essential oil formulas used as mouth rinses are effective in reducing oral bacteria that cause bad breath.

Homeopathy

Pick the remedy that best matches your symptoms. Take a 6x, 12x, 6C, or 30C potency twice daily for two weeks to see if there are any positive results. After you notice improvement, stop taking the remedy, unless symptoms return.

Mercurius Solubilis is for offensive breath caused by tooth decay and accompanied by a yellow coating on the tongue and excessive salivation.

Nux Vomica (*Strychnos nux vomica*) is helpful if you have bad breath after drinking alcohol or have a history of constipation and/or heartburn.

Pulsatilla (*Pulsatilla pratensis*) is for sour breath caused by eating too much fatty food.

Acupressure

See pages 787–794 for information about pressure points and administering treatment.

- You can reduce the frequency of constipation by strengthening your colon. Use Large Intestine 11 (LI11) to achieve this goal.
- Stomach 36 (St36) tones your digestive system.

Aromatherapy

Essential oils are much more effective than commercial mouthwashes are at eliminating oral bacteria and neutralizing bad breath. To make your own mouthwash, add a few drops of peppermint or eucalyptus oil to clean, quality water.

Other Recommendations

- Brush after every meal, and floss your teeth before you go to bed. Many people who are assiduous brushers neglect flossing, but this step is vital to keep food particles out of the spaces between the teeth.
- Avoid toothpastes that are full of chemicals and artificial sweeteners. Natural toothpaste is now available at many drugstores and health food stores. You can also make your own with baking soda and hydrogen peroxide. Just before you brush, combine the two ingredients until they form a paste with a consistency that's to your liking. You should make a fresh mixture each time you brush your teeth.
- Commercial mouthwashes are just as bad as most toothpastes. They irritate the soft tissues of the mouth and can actually encourage bacterial growth. Instead, use a homemade mouthwash of water and essential oils, as previously recommended.
- Even if you keep your teeth scrupulously clean, see your holistic dentist for regular checkups. He or she can remove plaque and other buildup that you may not be able to reach and will also check for any early signs of decay.

Bee Stings

When a bumblebee or a honeybee attacks, it leaves its stinger and attached venom sac in the skin. In most cases, the sting creates only slight pain, swelling, and irritation. It is more of a nuisance than a concern. However, look for signs of an allergic reaction, such as swollen eyelids or hands, difficulty breathing or wheezing, dizziness, fainting, nausea, vomiting, and the appearance of a hive-like rash. For these symptoms, go immediately to the emergency room or your doctor's office. The bee sting can be fatal in people who are allergic to its venom.

Other insects, including fire ants, paper wasps, hornets, and yellow jackets, are capable of stinging, but they do not leave stingers in their victims.

TREATMENT

Diet

Recommended Food

Consume foods rich in omega-3 fatty acids that promote skin healing and reduce inflammation, such as fish (salmon, cod, mackerel). Ground flaxseeds, avocados, and wheat germ are also recommended.

Eat green, orange, and yellow vegetables at every meal. These foods are packed with vitamins A and C, which will speed your skin's recovery from the inflammation.

Food to Avoid

Sugar worsens the inflammatory response. Stay away from refined sugar products, including cookies, cakes, sweet baked goods, and sodas, and eat naturally occurring sugars, such as those found in fruit, in moderation.

℞ Super Seven Prescriptions—Bee Stings

Please note that these therapies do not replace conventional therapy for people who are having a severe allergic reaction to a bee sting.

Super Prescription #1 Homeopathic Apis (*Apis mellifica*)
Take a 30C potency every thirty minutes to reduce swelling and pain. The stinging or burning pain, along with great swelling, is reduced with cold applications.

Super Prescription #2 Homeopathic Carbolic Acid (*Carbolicum acidum*)
Take a 30C potency every five minutes to reduce severe reactions to a bee sting, while waiting to get conventional therapy with an epinephrine injection.

Super Prescription #3 Homeopathic Ledum (*Ledum palustre*)
Take a 30C potency every thirty minutes to reduce swelling and pain. The person has a bruising pain that feels better with cold applications.

Super Prescription #4 Quercitin
Take 500 mg three times daily. This flavonoid reduces inflammation of the skin.

Super Prescription #5 Super-green-food supplement
Take a super-green-food product, such as spirulina, chlorella, or a combination of greens, to reduce the inflammatory response. Take as directed on the container.

Super Prescription #6 Bach flower rescue remedy
This decreases anxiety and emotional upset. Take 10 drops four times daily.

Super Prescription #7 Vitamin C with bioflavonoids
Take 1,000 mg three times daily to reduce swelling and inflammation. *Note*: Reduce the dosage if loose stools occur.

Tips for Avoiding a Bee Sting

1. Wear light-colored, smooth-finished clothing.
2. Avoid perfumed soaps, shampoos, and deodorants. Don't wear cologne or perfume. Avoid bananas and banana-scented toiletries.
3. Wear clean clothing and bathe daily. Sweat angers bees.
4. Cover the body as much as possible with clothing.
5. Avoid flowering plants.
6. Check for new nests during the warmer hours of the day in July, August, and September. Bees are very active then.
7. Keep outside areas clean. Social wasps thrive in places where humans discard food, so clean up picnic tables, grills, and other outdoor eating areas.

8. If a single stinging insect is flying around, remain still or lie face down on the ground. The face is the most likely place for a bee or a wasp to sting. Swinging or swatting at an insect may cause it to sting.

9. If you are attacked by several stinging insects at the same time, run to get away from them. Bees release a chemical when they sting. This alerts other bees to the intruder. More bees often follow. Go indoors. Outdoors, a shaded area is better than an open area to get away from the insects.

10. If a bee comes inside your vehicle, stop the car slowly, and open all the windows.

What to Do If Someone Is Stung

1. Have someone stay with the victim to be sure that the person does not have an allergic reaction.
2. Wash the site with soap and water.
3. The stinger can be removed by wiping a four-inch gauze pad over the area or by scraping a fingernail or a credit card over the area. Never squeeze the stinger or use tweezers. It will cause more venom to go into the skin and will injure the muscle.
4. Apply ice to reduce the swelling.
5. Do not scratch the sting. This will cause the site to swell and itch more and will increase the chance of infection.
6. If the victim is having a severe allergic reaction, seek emergency medical attention.
7. Epinephrine is given by injection to stop allergic reaction.

Bladder Infection (Cystitis)

The uncomfortable and irritating symptoms of a bladder infection send American women to their doctors six to nine million times every year. Most of these women will be treated with a course of antibiotics, a strategy that kills the current infection but that leaves the bladder vulnerable to a future bacterial invasion. As a result, most of the women who see a doctor about a bladder infection will return; 10 to 20 percent of all women experience a bladder infection at least once over a twelve-month period.

When the bladder is infected, usually by bacteria, its interior walls become inflamed. This inflammation, medically known as cystitis, leads to a frequent and urgent need to urinate, although the urine produced may be scanty, and the bladder may not feel completely empty. There is usually pain or burning upon urination, and there may be cramping in the abdomen or the lower back, and fever.

Women suffer from bladder infections far more frequently than men do, mainly because of the female anatomy. In women, the urethra—the tube that conducts urine away from the bladder and out of the body—is very short, and its opening is in close proximity to both the anus and the vagina. It's relatively easy for vaginal or intestinal bacteria to travel to the opening to the urethra, make their way up the tube, and infect the bladder. Although bacteria are the cause of most infections, several other conditions put women at risk for this disorder. Frequent use of antibiotics is one of the most prevalent, since these medications destroy the "good" bacteria needed to fight infections. Anything else that weakens the immune system, such as stress or a poor diet, increases the likelihood of an infection. Pregnancy, sexual intercourse, and injury to the area are associated with a higher risk. Hormone imbalances can also contribute to an increased susceptibility. Menopause is a time when many women first start to experience bladder infections.

You should consult a doctor, as there is a possibility that the infection can spread to the kidneys. Your physician should monitor your progress and make sure the infection isn't traveling upward. And if you have recurring infections, your doctor should examine you for a structural abnormality in the urethra or the bladder that prevents urine from flowing properly. Should your doctor want to prescribe antibiotics, explain to him or her your desire for more conservative treatment and ask whether antibiotics are really necessary. (In some cases, they're needed to prevent a kidney infection.) If you are a man with a bladder infection, you may have a more serious condition. For more information, see the sections on prostate problems in this book.

SYMPTOMS

- Pain or burning upon urination
- Frequent need to urinate
- Scanty flow or dribbling
- Cramps in abdomen or lower back
- Nausea or vomiting
- Fever

TREATMENT

Diet

Recommended Food
Make sure that you're getting all the nutrients you need. Plan well-rounded, wholesome meals, made with basic foods that you prepare yourself.

One of the best strategies for fighting a bladder infection is to increase your urine output. Drink as much clean, quality water as you can stand. Try for one 6- to 8-ounce glass every waking hour.

Cranberry juice has long been a folk remedy for bladder infections, and now science helps us understand why: it appears that cranberry juice keeps bacteria from clinging to the linings of the bladder and the urethra. You can find unsweetened cranberry juice at most health food stores and many supermarkets. Drink several glasses a day.

Blueberry juice may help with expelling bacteria from the urinary tract. Drink 10 to 12 ounces.

Natural diuretics will help flush out the infection. Eat plenty of watermelon, celery, or parsley, or use them to make fresh juices.

Add some garlic to clear soups or other meals. It's a potent infection fighter.

If you must take antibiotics, eat a cup of unsweetened live yogurt or another cultured product every day that you're on antibiotics. These foods help return "good" bacteria to your body.

Food to Avoid

Sugar depresses the immune system and encourages the growth of bacteria. Avoid all refined sugars (including those in alcohol) while you're battling the infection, and restrict them once you've recovered.

During the course of the infection, stay away from salty, spicy, processed, or refined foods, as well as caffeine. All of these substances will further aggravate the problem.

Food allergies can cause recurring bladder infections. See the Food Allergies section and the accompanying elimination diet to determine whether a food is at the heart of your problem.

Many women who are frequent consumers of sodas (both sugary and diet) experience recurring bladder infections. Sodas, whether made from natural or artificial sweeteners, are never a good idea; if you are troubled by bladder infections, you now have another compelling reason to avoid sodas.

℞ Super Seven Prescriptions—Bladder Infection

Super Prescription #1 Uva ursi
Take a standardized capsule containing 250 mg of arbutin or 5 ml of the tincture form four times daily. Arbutin is a constituent in uva ursi that is converted in the body to a chemical called hydroquinone, which destroys bacteria.

Super Prescription #2 D-mannose
Take 500 mg four times daily. This substance prevents bacteria from being able to attach to the urinary tract and the bladder wall.

Super Prescription #3 Homeopathy
Pick the remedy that best matches your symptoms under Homeopathy in this section. For acute bladder infection, take a 30C potency four times daily. After you notice improvement, stop taking the remedy, unless symptoms return. Consultation with a homeopathic practitioner is advised.

Super Prescription #4 Echinacea (*Echinacea purpurea*) and goldenseal (*Hydrastis canadensis*)
Take 500 mg of the capsule form or 4 ml of the tincture four times daily. These herbs enhance immune function to combat infection.

Super Prescription #5 Cranberry (*Vaccinium macrocarpon*) extract
Take 400 to 500 mg twice daily of cranberry extract capsules. Cranberry prevents bacteria from adhering to the bladder wall. This herb is best used for the prevention of urinary tract infections but can also be used as part of a comprehensive protocol for acute infection.

Super Prescription #6 Oregano oil (*Origanum vulgare*)
Take 500 mg of the capsule form four times daily or as directed on the container. This botanical has powerful antibacterial and antiviral effects.

Super Prescription #7 Vitamin C
Take 1,000 mg four to five times daily. Vitamin C enhances immune function, inhibits the growth of E. coli, and makes the urine more acidic so that bacteria cannot grow as easily.

General Recommendations

Horsetail (*Equisetum arvense*) herb has a long history of use for urinary tract infections. Take 500 mg of the capsule or 2 ml of the tincture four times daily.

Oregano oil (*Origanum vulgare*) has powerful antibacterial and antiviral effects. Take 500 mg of the capsule form four times daily or as directed on the container.

Vitamin A enhances immune function. Take 25,000 to 50,000 IU daily for one week. Do not use if you are pregnant.

Probiotics contain friendly bacteria that prevent the overgrowth of harmful bacteria. It is especially important to take probiotics if you are using antibiotics. Take them at a separate time during the day, and continue daily use for two months. Take a product containing at least four billion organisms.

Homeopathy

Pick the remedy that best matches your symptoms in this section. For acute bladder infection, take a 30C potency four to six times daily. After you notice improvement, stop taking the remedy unless symptoms return. Consultation with a homeopathic practitioner is advised.

Aconitum Napellus is helpful for the very first two hours of a bladder infection. Urination feels hot, and the person feels anxious. A fever comes on quickly.

Apis (*Apis mellifica*) is good for sharp, stinging pains that feel better with cold compresses or cool drinks and feel worse with warm applications (such as a warm bath). There are often only small amounts of urine passed.

Belladonna (*Atropa belladonna*) is for burning in the urethra, with a feeling of great urgency and with bladder spasm. A high fever comes on quickly.

Cantharis is the homeopathic remedy of choice for bladder infections. Use it if you have a strong urge but produce very little urine. You may have burning and cutting pain upon urination, as well as cramps in your abdomen and lower back. Small tinges of blood may be present.

Mercurius Corrosivus is helpful when blood and pus are in the urine. The person feels great burning pains and spasm in the bladder.

Nux Vomica (*Strychnos nux vomica*) helps when there is a constant urge to urinate, with only small amounts being passed. The person feels chilly and irritable. Symptoms are better with warmth (a warm bath).

Sarsaparilla can be taken when there is burning pain at the end of urination. The person seems to urinate only when standing and not sitting.

Staphysagria is for the burning pains of a bladder infection that come on after sexual intercourse. It is also used for bladder infections that result from the use of a catheter.

Bodywork

Reflexology

Reflexology is helpful to prevent bladder infections, and you should see improvement after two or three treatments. For information about reflexology areas and how to work them, see pages 804–805.

Work the areas corresponding to the bladder, the kidneys, and the ureters.

A study reported in the *Journal of the American Medical Association* found that regular consumption of cranberry juice (10 ounces a day) significantly reduced the amount of bacteria and pus in the urine of elderly women. Another study found that cranberry capsule extract (400 mg twice daily) for three months significantly reduced the recurrence of urinary tract infections in women ages eighteen to forty-five who had a history of reoccurring infections.

Hydrotherapy

A hot sitz bath is a comforting and powerful therapy for bladder infections. Take it once or twice a day until you are healed. Add vinegar or garlic oil for an even stronger effect.

Constitutional hydrotherapy can also be used for an acute bladder infection.

Aromatherapy

- Bergamot, chamomile, and lavender all have gentle antiseptic qualities. Use them in a sitz bath. If you prefer, a regular hot bath is still an effective delivery system for these oils.
- Tea tree oil (*Melaleuca alternifolia*) is a potent infection fighter that also stimulates the immune system. It can be irritating to some people, so add just a few drops to a bath for your first use. If you do not have a reaction, you can add a few more.
- If you need to relieve stress, several oils can help you. See page 778 for information on oils. Here are some good ones to get you started: lavender, jasmine, rose, geranium, and bergamot.

Stress Reduction

General Stress-Reduction Therapies

Stress depletes the immune system and leaves you vulnerable to recurring infections. If you need to reduce the level of stress in your life, experiment with the different techniques described in the Exercise and Stress Reduction chapter until you find the ones that are best for you.

Other Recommendations

- Always empty your bladder when you feel the need. Delaying urination sets the stage for an infection.
- Empty your bladder prior to and, if possible, after sexual intercourse to reduce the likelihood of infection. It's a good idea for women to drink a big glass of water before and after intercourse.
- After swimming, immediately change out of your wet bathing suit and into dry clothes. Damp conditions are a breeding ground for bacteria.
- If you're prone to bladder infections, wear cotton underwear that lets the genital area breathe.
- After going to the toilet, always wipe from front to back. This reduces the chances that intestinal bacteria will travel to the urethra.
- Avoid products that may irritate the urethra or the vagina. Do not use powders, sanitary napkins, or tampons that are scented.
- A hot compress is very soothing to an irritated urinary tract. Lie down somewhere comfortable, and place the compress on your lower abdomen.
- For bladder infections that occur around menses or that began with menopausal changes, hormone balancing is likely the issue. See the chapters that correspond to your situation, such as PMS and Menopause.

REFERENCES

Avorn, J., M. Monane, and J. H. Gurwitz, et al. 1994. Reduction of bacteriuria and pyuria after ingestion of cranberry juice. *Journal of the American Medical Association* 271:751–54.

Walker, E. B., D. P. Barney, J. N. Mickelsen, et al. 1997. Cranberry concentrate: UTI prophylaxis. *Journal of Family Practice* 45:167–68 [letter].

Blood Clots

Blood clots are one of the biggest health risks for people over the age of fifty. They are among the most common causes of heart attacks and are the leading cause of stroke. In addition, blood clots are a common cause of death in people with cancer because the disease creates conditions in the blood vessels more favorable to clotting.

Here are some sobering statistics. It has been estimated that nine hundred thousand people in the United States are afflicted with deep vein thrombosis (DVT), blood clots in the deep veins of the body, (usually the legs), and pulmonary embolism (PE), blood clots in the lungs. Blood clots account for approximately three hundred thousand deaths per year. About 33 percent of those with a DVT or PE will suffer a recurrence within ten years, and up to 33 percent die within one month of diagnosis. Among those who have had a DVT, 50 percent will have long-term complications such as swelling, pain, and discoloration in the affected limb. Finally, up to 8 percent of the US population has one of several genetic risk factors that increase their risk for blood clots.

The key to preventing blood clots is severalfold. Your doctor can identify any genetic predispositions to blood clots with lab tests. If the tests indicate a susceptibility, the following preventative measures can greatly minimize risk: avoidance or limited use of drugs that predispose one to clots, proper diet, exercise, and targeted nutritional supplements.

Blood flows through our arteries and veins, supplying nutrients and oxygen to tissues and removing waste products from cells. As part of our God-given protective mechanism, blood clots occur when blood vessels become damaged. A cascade of clotting mechanisms stabilizes and repairs the damage so we do not bleed to death. For instance, when the lining of blood vessels is damaged it causes substances known as platelets to form an initial plug in the vessel wall. Platelets then release a chemical that summons a series of clotting factors. In the end a protein known as fibrin is produced that works to form a clot.

You may have heard of the medical term *thrombus*, another word for blood clot. In some cases thrombus (or the plural term, *thrombi*) continues to accumulate and travel throughout the circulatory system, cutting off blood supply to the heart arteries and leading to a heart attack, or affecting vessels in the brain, leading to a stroke, or in the lungs, leading to pulmonary embolism.

Approximately 80 percent of blood clots originate in the deep veins of the legs (DVT). This is particularly problematic for the elderly, among whom the incidence is fourfold that of the general population.. The incidence is also greatly increased for those who are hospitalized. Fortunately, most cases of DVT resolve spontaneously.

SYMPTOMS

Blood clots may produce no symptoms, or any of the following symptoms may occur:

- Pain, swelling, redness, and tenderness in the area where the clot is located
- Heart attack or stroke

ROOT CAUSES

Besides inherited conditions, which cause a small percentage of blood clots, here are other known risk factors:

- Abnormal lipids and plasma fibrinogen levels
- Age
- Antiphospholipid syndrome (when the immune system mistakenly attacks some of the normal proteins in your blood and leads to clot formation)
- Arteriosclerosis / atherosclerosis (plaque in the arteries) and high blood pressure
- Atrial fibrillation
- Being sedentary (particularly if immobilized three days or longer)
- Burns
- Cancer
- DVT in the past
- Elevated homocysteine
- Fracture or injury
- Genetic factors such as prothrombin mutation or factor V Leiden
- Pharmaceutical medications such as nonsteroidal anti-inflammatories (NSAIDs), oral contraceptives, hormone therapy drugs (especially synthetic versions), and some breast cancer medications
- Heart arrhythmias
- Heart attack
- Heart failure
- Increase in blood viscosity
- Inflammatory bowel disease
- IV drug abuse
- Lupus
- Long plane or car trips (greater than four hours)
- Nephrotic syndrome (type of kidney disease)
- Obesity
- Peripheral artery disease (narrowing of arteries, reducing blood flow to the limbs)
- Polycythemia vera (slow-growing blood cancer)
- Pregnancy
- Sepsis (blood infection)
- Smoking
- Surgery (especially major surgery in previous four weeks)
- Thyroid disorders

Testing Techniques

Blood clots are identified with diagnostic imaging and blood tests. For preventative purposes we also test other markers:

Genetic markers such as prothrombin mutation and factor V Leiden

Blood viscosity (hematocrit and RBC)—blood

Blood clotting (fibrinogen)—blood

Blood Viscosity and Clotting Prevention

The Edinburgh Artery Study involved 4,860 men between the ages of forty-five and fifty-nine and women between the ages of fifty-five and seventy-four. The researchers found that the 20 percent of study participants with the thickest and stickiest blood had the majority (55 percent) of the major cardiovascular events over a five-year period. Researchers found that the link between blood viscosity and cardiovascular events was at least as strong as that of diastolic blood pressure and LDL cholesterol, and stronger than that of smoking.

We frequently test patients' blood to check its viscosity. When your blood is "too thick" and does not flow well, it increases friction in the walls of the blood vessels, which contributes to inflammation, plaque deposits, high blood pressure, and blood clots. This type of blood work includes testing for a common blood marker known as hematocrit. It is part of a complete blood count (CBC) that is routinely ordered by doctors and refers to the proportion of your blood that is made up of red blood cells. The higher your hematocrit, the thicker your blood. Elevated hematocrit levels can be attributed to several factors, including dehydration. The simplest solutions include drinking more water and donating blood.

Another marker we test to identify general blood clot risk is fibrinogen. This is a type of protein that can be formed into a clot in response to a tissue or blood vessel injury. An elevation increases the risk of a stroke. When both LDL cholesterol and fibrinogen are elevated, the risk for coronary disease can increase sixfold.

TREATMENT

Diet

Recommended Food
One of the best ways to reduce your risk of stroke is to consume a Mediterranean-style diet with some modifications. This diet is rich in vegetables, fruit, fish, nuts, and olive oil and low in dairy, sweets, and meat. The one recommended change would be to drastically reduce intake of processed grains, which increase the risk of diabetes, obesity, and cardiovascular disease.

One study demonstrating the power of the Mediterranean diet is the REGARDS study, which was published in the journal *Stroke*. Researchers looked at the dietary patterns of over twenty thousand participants who had no history of a stroke. After adjusting for various risk factors they found that people who closely followed a Mediterranean diet had a 21 percent lower risk of getting a stroke. Of course, many other studies have shown the stroke-reducing effects of the Mediterranean diet. Another recent study found that people who followed the Mediterranean diet more closely were less likely to suffer from a stroke caused by a blood clot compared to people with the lowest adherence to the diet. The study involved more than one hundred thousand teachers in California who averaged fifty-two years of age. And previous research has also shown that consuming at least one serving of fish weekly reduces the risk of clot-related (ischemic) strokes in women by 27 percent.

Teas, including green tea, have been shown in several population studies to reduce the risk of stroke and to reduce platelet clumping. Another food to consider is pomegranate. Pomegranate juice reduces platelet clumping and makes a tasty treat. Additional foods to consider include turmeric, garlic, cayenne, and ginger, all of which confer a mild blood-thinning effect.

Food to Avoid

Avoid simple sugars, which cause elevated levels of cholesterol, triglycerides, C-reactive protein, insulin, and other markers that contribute to stroke risk.

Radically reduce your consumption of sodium. Packaged and processed foods are by far the highest source of sodium in the Western diet, so stay away from them. A high sodium intake, combined with a low potassium intake, increases your likelihood of having high blood pressure, which damages the blood vessel walls.

℞ Super Seven Prescriptions—Blood Clots

Super Prescription #1 Nattokinase
Take 5,000 to 20,000 fibrinolytic units (FUs) daily. It is best taken on an empty stomach.

Super Prescription #2 Fish oil
Take 1,000 mg of EPA and DHA combined to reduce blood-clotting tendencies.

Super Prescription #3 Pycnogenol
Take 100 to 200 mg daily. Pycnogenol inhibits platelet activity by stimulating the release of nitric oxide; it also improves circulation.

Super Prescription #4 Vitamin E
Take 400 to 800 IU of mixed vitamin E to protect against clots.

Super Prescription #5 Garlic
Take 250 to 500 mg of an extract daily to reduce clot formation and for overall cardiovascular health.

Super Prescription #6 Turmeric
Take 500 mg twice daily to prevent platelet aggregation and inflammation of the blood vessels.

Super Prescription # 7 Grapeseed extract
Take 100 mg daily to reduce clotting and improve circulation.

One study looked at the effects of pycnogenol on cigarette smokers who had increased platelet activity. The higher the dose of pycnogenol, the greater the reduction in platelet activity. Even a low dose of 25 mg demonstrated a significant effect on blood platelets. In another study pycnogenol was tested in a group of people at high risk for developing blood clots. These two hundred participants had previous problems with blood clots, varicose veins, severe obesity, sedentary lifestyle, or cardiovascular disease. The participants were in sedentary positions for prolonged periods of time during travel exceeding eight hours, a known risk factor for blood clots, especially in the lower legs. One group was given 200 mg of pycnogenol prior to departure and again after six hours plus 100 mg the following day. The other group was given a placebo. At the destination the participants were evaluated with an ultrasound. In those taking placebo, 5.15 percent experienced superficial vein thrombosis; in those taking pycnogenol, no blood clots were found.

A two-month study published in *Nutrition Research* demonstrated that nattokinase supplementation decreased clotting factors, including fibrinogen, factor VII, and factor VIII, between 7 and 19 percent. No adverse events were observed. In a separate study nattokinase was taken in conjunction with pycnogenol for their effectiveness in preventing deep vein thrombosis (DVT) in those on long flights. The study, published in the mainstream journal *Angiology*, involved 186 participants in flights traveling across the Atlantic Ocean. Ninety-two participants were shown exercises to reduce DVT while ninety-four participants were shown the same exercises and were also given a supplement containing pycnogenol and nattokinase. Both groups were evaluated for DVTs before and after their flights. Researchers found that there were no DVTs formed in the exercise and supplement group. Five participants in the exercise-only group developed DVTs.

OTHER RECOMMENDATIONS

Don't underestimate how important it is to get plenty of movement every day. If you work in front of a computer, make sure to get up and move around every one to two hours. If you are on a long plane flight, make sure to get up and walk around. At minimum, point your toes forward and backward for several repetitions every hour.

REFERENCES

Belcaro, G., et al. 2004. Prevention of venous thrombosis in long-haul flights with Pycnogenol. *Clin Appl Thromb Hemost* 10:373–77.

Centers for Disease Control and Prevention website. Accessed May 25, 2015 at http://www.cdc.gov/ncbddd/dvt/data.html.

Cesarone, M. R., G. Belcaro, A. N. Nicolaides, et al. 2003. Prevention of venous thrombosis in long-haul flights with Flite Tabs: the LONFLIT-FLITE randomized, controlled trial. *Angiology* 54(5):531–9.

Hsia, C.H., et al. 2009. Nattokinase decreases plasma levels of fibrinogen, factor VII, and factor VIII in human subjects. *Nutrition Research* 29(3):190–6. doi: 10.1016/j.nutres.2009.01.009.

Iso, H., K. M. Rexrode, M. J. Stampfer, et al. 2001. Intake of fish and omega-3 fatty acids and risk of stroke in women. *JAMA* 285:304–12.

Lowe, G. D., A. J. Lee, A. Rumley, et al. 1997. Blood viscosity and risk of cardiovascular events: the Edinburgh Artery Study. *Br J Haematol* 96:168–73.

National Blood Clot Alliance website. Blood Clot Statistics Vary–What to do About it? Alan P. Brownstein. Accessed May 25, 2015 at http://www.stoptheclot.org/news/article153.htm.

Putter, M., et al. 1999. Inhibition of smoking-induced platelet aggregation by aspirin and pycnogenol. *Thromb Res* 95:155–61.

Tsivquaolis, G., et al. 2015. Adherence to a Mediterranean diet and prediction of incident stroke. *Stroke* 46(3):780–5. doi: 10.1161/STROKEAHA.114.007894. Epub 2015 Jan 27.

Wright, Paul. 2015. American Stroke Association, news release, Feb 12.

Blood Pressure, High

As blood circulates through the body, it presses against the walls of the arteries. The force of this action is called blood pressure. When the pressure is too high, the arterial walls become distorted—they may narrow or thicken—and an extra burden of stress is placed on the heart.

Blood pressure may temporarily rise from exercise, stress, and emotions ranging from joy to anger. Usually, the pressure returns to normal once the situation has passed. In many people, however, blood pressure is high all the time. About one in three adults in the United States has high blood pressure (also known as hypertension), including almost half of those over the age of sixty-five. The disorder can lead to very serious conditions, including stroke, heart disease, diabetes, eye damage, and kidney problems, so it is considered one of the country's leading health problems.

Sometimes there are symptoms of high blood pressure. You may have unexplained headaches, nosebleeds, or spells of dizziness or sweating. But most of the time high blood pressure is completely asymptomatic, so it's vital that you have it checked regularly. The disorder can strike anyone at any age, but it is most common among the elderly, African Americans, and people of all races living in the southeastern United States. If you fall into any of these risk categories, or if you have a family history of hypertension, you should be doubly sure to have routine checks and to take preventative measures.

About 90 percent of all cases of high blood pressure are called primary or essential hypertension, meaning that there is no underlying disease and no obvious cause. Most likely, a cluster of lifestyle factors is to blame: diet, lack of exercise, stress, and smoking have all been linked to an increase in blood pressure. If another disease or condition—such as cardiovascular, kidney, adrenal, or thyroid disease—causes the problem, it is called secondary hypertension. A very small percentage of people suffer from malignant hypertension, in which blood pressure can suddenly soar to extremely dangerous levels.

Essential hypertension, as discussed, can often be controlled with home treatment, but if you have any kind of high blood pressure, you must be under the care of a doctor. Talk to him or her about the strategies you want to employ for wellness.

Secondary hypertension, as discussed, is elevated blood pressure that results from an underlying, identifiable, and often correctable cause. Only about 5 to 10 percent of hypertension cases are thought to result from secondary causes. Patients with secondary hypertension are treated by controlling or removing the underlying disease or pathology, although they may still require antihypertensive medication.

SYMPTOMS

High blood pressure does not usually produce symptoms. If, however, you experience any of the following, see a doctor:

- Recurring headaches
- Dizziness
- Unexplained sweating
- Nosebleeds
- Visual disturbances
- Shortness of breath
- Flushed cheeks
- Ringing in the ears

ROOT CAUSES

- A diet that's high in fat, sugar, and/or salt
- Use of alcohol or caffeine and other stimulants
- Smoking
- Obesity
- Inactivity
- Pregnancy or birth-control pills
- Underlying medical disorders
- Heavy-metal poisoning
- Stress

Testing Techniques

The following tests help assess possible metabolic reasons for high blood pressure:

    Vitamin and mineral analysis—blood or urine
    Food allergy testing—blood or electrodermal
    Toxic metals (lead, cadmium, etc.)—hair or urine

TREATMENT

Diet

The Western diet has a lot to do with hypertension. Following the suggestions here can make a real difference in your blood pressure and your overall wellness.

Recommended Food

A diet high in fiber is an excellent way to control or reverse high blood pressure. Your meals should be based around fresh, raw vegetables; soy products; whole grains, like oats; beans; nuts; and seeds.

Dehydration increases the risk of hypertension, so drink a glass of clean, quality water every two waking hours.

As you lower your intake of salt, you must also increase your consumption of potassium. A combination of excess sodium and a deficiency in potassium has been found in many people with hypertension.

Good sources of potassium include apples, avocados, asparagus, cabbage, oranges, tomatoes, bananas, kelp (*Ascophyllum nodosum*), and alfalfa.

Apples are superfoods for people with high blood pressure. Not only do they have high levels of potassium, they're also a good source of pectin, which is an excellent type of soluble fiber.

Onions, garlic, and parsley have been shown to bring down blood pressure. They also add flavor to vegetarian meals, so take advantage of their healing properties daily.

Celery has been shown in animal studies to reduce blood pressure. Consume up to four stalks a day.

Consume dark chocolate that contains a daily total of 213 to 500 mg of cocoa polyphenols. This has been shown to have a mild lowering effect on blood pressure.

Pomegranate juice has been shown to reduce blood pressure; consume 4 to 8 ounces daily.

Consume half a teaspoon of olive oil daily to reduce blood pressure.

Food to Avoid

Some people with high blood pressure benefit from restricting their intake of salt. Salt contains sodium, which causes water retention and increases the pressure

---

The DASH Diet

Consider following the well-studied DASH diet with your doctor's supervision. DASH stands for "Dietary Approaches to Stop Hypertension." The DASH diet has been shown to reduce blood pressure. It includes whole grains, poultry, fish, and nuts, and low amounts of fats, red meats, sweets, and sugared beverages. It is high in potassium, calcium, and magnesium, which help to lower blood pressure. Potassium is particularly important to reduce blood pressure.

inside the arteries. It is not enough to simply stop using table salt; you must also cut out high-sodium processed and packaged foods, as well as smoked meats and cheeses, which are loaded with sodium. Limit your sodium intake to less than 1,500 mg daily.

- Saturated, hydrogenated, and partially hydrogenated fats cause high blood pressure and place a terrible burden on your arteries and heart. Eliminate animal products, margarine, butter, shortening, and refined vegetable oils.
- Sugar is linked to hypertension. If you do not eat packaged or processed foods, you will eliminate the largest source of added sugar from your diet, but you should also avoid sugary baked goods and limit your intake of foods that are sweetened naturally.
- Overindulgence in caffeine is a cause of high blood pressure. Cut back on your intake of coffee, colas, chocolate, and caffeinated teas.
- Allow yourself no more than one alcoholic beverage a day.

When you have your blood pressure checked, the doctor or the nurse usually tells you the two numbers of your reading and whether you have cause for concern. But most health care professionals don't take the time to explain exactly what those numbers mean. Since this is one of the most important medical tests people receive on a regular basis, here's a quick analysis.

The first number is called the systolic pressure. It is measured when the heart beats and indicates the highest amount of pressure against the arterial walls. Between heartbeats, the heart is at rest and pressure drops to its lowest level. This low reading is called the diastolic pressure.

Sample blood pressure reading of 120/80
systolic pressure = 120
diastolic pressure = 80

Blood pressure varies with age and fluctuates many times over the course of a day; it often rises in a doctor's office, when many people feel nervous or tense. Blood pressure should be taken when you are calm and unstressed, and it is best to average a total of three readings, taken on different days. The consensus is that for most healthy adults, 120/80 is normal.

Readings are broken down into several categories:

Normal. Your blood pressure is normal if it's below 120/80 mm Hg.
Prehypertension. Prehypertension is a systolic pressure ranging from 120 to 139 mm Hg or a diastolic pressure ranging from 80 to 89 mm Hg.
Stage 1 hypertension. Stage 1 hypertension is a systolic pressure ranging from 140 to 159 mm Hg or a diastolic pressure ranging from 90 to 99 mm Hg.
Stage 2 hypertension. The most severe hypertension, stage 2 hypertension is a systolic pressure of 160 mm Hg or higher or a diastolic pressure of 100 mm Hg or higher.

R̸ Super Seven Prescriptions—High Blood Pressure

Super Prescription #1 Hawthorn (*Crataegus oxycanthae*)
Take 250 mg of a standardized extract three times daily. This herb dilates the artery walls and decreases blood pressure.

Super Prescription #2 Coenzyme Q10
Studies show that this nutrient reduces blood pressure. Take 100 mg two to three times daily.

Super Prescription #3 Calcium and magnesium
These minerals have been shown in studies to lower blood pressure. Take a combination of 500 mg of calcium and 250 mg of magnesium twice daily.

Super Prescription #4 Hibiscus
Take 1.25 grams in tea form, mixed in 240 ml of water, three times daily.

Super Prescription #5 Garlic (*Allium sativum*)
Several studies confirm garlic's ability to lower blood pressure. Take 600 mg twice daily of an aged garlic extract.

Super Prescription #6 Fish oil
Fish oil reduces blood pressure when taken on a long-term basis. Take 3,000 mg three times daily.

Super Prescription #7 Potassium
This mineral has been shown in repeated studies to lower blood pressure. Take as part of a salt-substitute product. Otherwise, use up to 2,000 mg under the supervision of a doctor. Do not use if you are taking a potassium-sparing diuretic medication or have kidney disease or serious heart disease.

A randomized, double-blind, placebo-controlled study of seventy-four people with type 2 diabetes found that 100 mg of coenzyme Q10 taken twice daily significantly lowered blood pressure over a period of twelve weeks. Other studies have also found CoQ10's blood pressure–lowering benefits.

A randomized, double-blind, placebo-controlled clinical trial published in the *Journal of Nutrition* was conducted on sixty-five prehypertensive and mildly hypertensive adults who were not taking blood pressure–lowering medications. Those who drank 1.25 grams of hibiscus tea brewed in 240 ml of water for six minutes three times daily significantly reduced systolic blood pressure by a mean of 7.2 mm Hg after six weeks of treatment.

A study published in the *American Journal of Hypertension* found that melatonin, a supplement typically taken to promote sleep, reduces nighttime blood pressure in women with hypertension. This randomized, double-blind study involved eighteen women, ages forty-seven to sixty-three, half with hypertension that was successfully controlled with ACE-inhibitor medication and half with normal blood pressure. For three weeks, participants took either 3 mg of time-released melatonin or a placebo one hour before going to bed. They were then switched to the other treatment for another three weeks. After taking melatonin for three weeks, 84 percent of the women had at least a 10 mm Hg (systolic and diastolic) decrease in nocturnal (nighttime) blood pressure, while only 39 percent experienced a decrease in nocturnal blood pressure after taking the placebo. No change was found in daytime blood pressure readings. The reduction in nighttime blood pressure was the greatest in the women with controlled hypertension. Previous studies have found similar results when men with untreated hypertension took melatonin.

General Recommendations

Vitamin C has mild lowering effects on blood pressure and helps the body to detoxify toxic metals, such as lead, which contribute to high blood pressure. Take 1,000 to 2,000 mg daily.

Passionflower (*Passiflora incarnata*) relaxes the nerves and is helpful for blood pressure that increases with stress. Take 250 mg or 0.5 ml two or three times daily.

Valerian (*Valeriana officinalis*) is a strong nerve relaxer and may indirectly lower blood pressure. Take 300 mg or 0.5 to 1.0 ml two or three times daily.

Chamomile (*Matricaria recutita*) and oatstraw (*Avena sativa*) are great herbal nerve relaxers. They can be taken as a tea throughout the day.

Taurine is an amino acid shown in research to lower blood pressure in humans and animals. Take up to 6 grams daily between meals.

Reishi (*Ganoderma lucidum*) extract should be taken in 500-mg doses three times daily for a blood pressure–lowering effect. Dandelion leaf (*Taraxacum officinale*) acts as a gentle, natural diuretic to lower blood pressure. Take 300 mg of the capsule form or 2 ml three times daily.

Vitamin D3 supplementation in those who have low levels has been shown to reduce blood pressure. Take 2,000 to 5,000 IU daily.

L-arginine at a dose of 6 grams daily can lower blood pressure.

Snakeroot is effective for those with moderate high blood pressure. Take under the guidance of a holistic doctor.

Pycnogenol supplementation can help reduce the amount of pharmaceutical medication needed to control blood pressure. Take 100 mg daily.

> Avoid the use of the herbs ephedra (*Ma huang*), Chinese ginseng (*Panax ginseng*), and large amounts of licorice (*Glycyrrhiza glabra*), as they may increase blood pressure.

Homeopathy

Argentum Nitricum is for elevated blood pressure that occurs with anxiety. Symptoms often come on from a stressful event or "stage fright." The person is usually very warm and has strong salt and sweet cravings.

Belladonna (*Atropa belladonna*) is for high blood pressure that comes on suddenly. The person has a flushed face and dilated pupils and feels a great deal of heat, although the hands and the feet are cold. Pounding headaches may occur, and the person is sensitive to light.

Glonoinum may be helpful for high blood pressure that's accompanied by a bursting headache and a flushed face. The person is worse from the heat and sun exposure or from consuming alcohol.

Lachesis is for a person who is very intense, who feels suspiciousness and jealousy, and who is very talkative. The person feels warm and is intolerant of anything touching the neck.

Natrum Muriaticum is for high blood pressure that begins after an emotional upset. The person desires to be alone and often experiences headaches, heart palpitations, and insomnia. There is a strong craving for salt, a great thirst, and an aversion to being in the sun.

Nux Vomica (*Strychnos nux vomica*) is for high blood pressure that occurs from the effects of stress. The person feels irritable and impatient and has a strong desire for stimulants such as coffee, as well as alcohol. The person is usually chilly and is prone to constipation.

Acupressure

See pages 787–794 for information about pressure points and administering treatment.

- Bladder 38 (B38) simultaneously lowers blood pressure and relieves nervous tension.
- If you tend to get heart palpitations when you're agitated, take some time out of a tense situation to work Pericardium 6 (P6). This spot is located at your wrist, so it's easy to use even in a public place like the office.
- People who feel chest tension when they're upset or worried should use Conception Vessel 17 (CV17).
- Encourage circulation to your heart and chest by working Heart 3 and 7 (H3 and H7).

Bodywork

Massage

Massage can be of great help to people with high blood pressure. It regulates the body's rhythms, improves circulation, and promotes relaxation, so make a regular appointment with a good therapist, if possible.

If stress makes your chest feel tight and full, try a neck massage to relieve tension and steady your heartbeat. You can do this yourself or have a loved one do it for you.

Reflexology

See pages 804–805 for information about reflexology areas and how to work them.

Work the areas corresponding to the thyroid, the kidneys, the solar plexus, and the pituitary and adrenal glands.

Hydrotherapy

Do not use saunas. The hot steam can make your blood pressure rise to dangerous levels.

Other Bodywork Recommendations

Acupuncture is helpful for high blood pressure, especially when the underlying cause is stress.

Osteopathic and craniosacral therapy can help normalize circulation.

Aromatherapy

Take advantage of the soothing effects of essential oils. Many oils will help you relax, but lavender, marjoram, and ylang-ylang are those most often used to calm the body and bring down blood pressure. You can use them in any preparation that suits you.

When used in a massage, juniper oil will help break down fatty deposits in your arteries and elsewhere in your body.

Stress Reduction

General Stress-Reduction Therapies

Meditation is a cheap, portable technique that can be used anywhere for a calming effect. You can practice meditation on a regular basis in a quiet room at home. If you feel your blood pressure rise while sitting at a stoplight, during a meeting, or while waiting for your teenager to come home, you can easily spend a few moments paying attention to your breath. Meditative breathing won't stop the stress, but it can help you take a few steps back and view the problem with detachment.

Stress can cause your body to constrict its blood vessels, making it harder for blood to get through and thus raising your blood pressure. Biofeedback can help you identify when you constrict your blood vessels, and it can train you to relax them.

Other Recommendations

- If you are obese, you must lose weight. The dietary suggestions in this section will help you take off the pounds safely, but if you'd like to learn more, see Obesity. Do not rely on stimulant diet products; they may contain additives that could make your condition worse.
- Moderate exercise is a reliable way to reduce blood pressure, but consult with your doctor before starting an exercise program. As a person with hypertension, you may have special needs that should be addressed.
- Do not smoke or expose yourself to secondhand smoke.
- If testing shows that you have high toxic-metal levels (such as lead, cadmium, and mercury), work with a doctor who is knowledgeable in chelation therapy. Chelation therapy, which reduces lead and other toxic metals in the body that cause high blood pressure, is effective. It improves circulation by improving nitric oxide levels and improving microcirculation.
- Deep breathing has been shown to reduce blood pressure. A small computerized device known as the Resperate, available from pharmacies, has been shown to reduce systolic blood pressure quite significantly. It monitors respiration and helps the user to breathe more slowly, which reduces blood pressure. The unit looks like a portable CD player— it has a headphone set and a sensor belt, which wraps around the chest or upper abdomen. Resperate is designed to slow your respiration rate from the average of twelve to nineteen breaths per minute to the hypertension-lowering rate of ten or fewer breaths per minute. The user listens to tones that guide his or her breathing rate. An average reduction in blood pressure is ten points for systolic pressure and five points for diastolic pressure. So far, eight clinical trials published in medical journals have confirmed its benefits.
- The Zona Plus Hypertension Relief Device has also been shown to significantly lower blood pressure. It involves squeezing a hand-held device.
- Intravenous magnesium administered by a doctor can be effective in reducing blood pressure spikes.

REFERENCES

Cagnacci, M., A. Cannoletta, F. Renzi et al. 2005. *American Journal of Hypertension* December.

Digiesi, V., F. Cantini, and B. Brodbeck. 1990. Effect of coenzyme Q10 on essential arterial hypertension. *Current Therapeutic Research* 47:841–45.

Hodgson, J. M., G. F. Watts, D. A. Playford, et al. 2002. Coenzyme Q10 improves blood pressure and glycemic control: A controlled trial in subjects with type 2 diabetes. *European Journal of Clinical Nutrition* 56(11):1137–42.

McKay, D. L., et al. 2010. Hibiscus Sabdariffa L. tea (tisane) lowers blood pressure in prehypertensive and mildly hypertensive adults. *Journal of Nutrition* 140:298–303.

Singh, R. B., M. A. Niaz, S. S. Rastogi, et al. 1999. Effect of hydrosoluble coenzyme Q10 on blood pressures and insulin resistance in hypertensive patients with coronary artery disease. *Journal of Human Hypertension* 13:203–8.

Bone Fractures

A bad fall, a hard blow, an automobile collision, a sports injury, or an underlying medical condition such as osteoporosis can result in a broken bone.

When a bone breaks, it triggers not only pain, swelling, bruising, and immobility but also trauma and shock throughout the entire body. Fractures located near joints are sometimes misidentified as simply bad sprains.

There are varying degrees of fractures. Here are definitions and causes for the main types:

1. *Partial* (incomplete): The break across the bone is incomplete.
2. *Complete*: The bone is broken in two pieces.
3. *Closed* (simple): The broken bone does not protrude through the skin.
4. *Open* (compound): The broken bone protrudes through the skin.
5. *Comminuted*: The bone is splintered at the broken area, and many smaller fragments of bone are found between the two main pieces.
6. *Greenstick*: This occurs only in children and is defined by having one side of the bone break and the other side just bend, often seen on the radius (forearm bone).
7. *Spiral*: A breaking force has twisted the bone apart.
8. *Transverse*: This occurs at right angles to the bone.
9. *Impacted*: One fragment is forcibly driven into the other.
10. *Colles'*: This is a fracture of the distal end of the radius (wrist), and the fragment is displaced posteriorly (behind).
11. *Pott's*: This is a fracture of the distal end of the fibula (lower portion of leg), with serious injury of the distal tibia articulation.
12. *Nondisplaced*: The correct anatomical alignment of the bone is maintained.
13. *Displaced*: The correct anatomical alignment of the bone is not maintained.
14. *Stress*: This is a partial fracture, resulting from the inability of the bone to withstand repeated stresses (such as doing aerobics on hard surfaces or running long distances for prolonged periods of time). Almost one-fourth of stress fractures occur in the fibula.
15. *Pathologic*: This fracture is a result of normal stress on a weakened bone. It occurs in such diseases as osteoporosis, neoplasia, osteomyelitis, and osteomalacia.

If you have had an accident in which you may have broken a bone, it is important to get immediate medical attention. For a more serious injury and if you have someone to help you, try to stay immobilized until medical personnel assess and move you. Otherwise, if you must move, it is important to have the fracture site immobilized with splinting materials. Even magazines or a towel can be used.

Once your fracture has been assessed and immobilized by medical personnel, it is very helpful to utilize the natural therapies outlined in this chapter. They can help to speed healing of the fracture and can reduce pain and swelling. Remember, our bones are living tissues that have the ability to repair themselves when damaged. They must be given the correct nutrients to do so. Many vitamins and minerals are required for healthy bones. Calcium is the obvious one, but magnesium; boron; silicon; strontium; vitamins D, C, and K; and others play important roles in bone metabolism.

SYMPTOMS

- Bone pain
- Swelling
- Bleeding

ROOT CAUSES

- Fall or injury
- Osteoporosis

Testing Techniques

The following tests help assess possible reasons for people whose bones fracture easily:

Hormone testing (thyroid, DHEA, cortisol, testosterone, IGF-1, estrogen, progesterone)—saliva, blood, or urine

Intestinal permeability—urine

Vitamin and mineral analysis (especially magnesium, calcium, vitamin K, vitamin D)—blood, hair

Toxic metals—urine or hair

Digestive function and microbe/parasite/candida testing—stool analysis

Food and environmental allergies/sensitivities—blood, electrodermal

Bone resorption (pyridinium and deoxypyridinium)—urine

TREATMENT

Diet

Recommended Food

Eat foods that are high in calcium and the other nutrients needed for calcium's assimilation. Sea vegetables, green leafy vegetables (except spinach), soybeans, nuts, molasses, salmon, oysters, sardines (with the bones), broccoli, and unsweetened cultured yogurt are all good sources.

Green vegetables, such as collard greens, kale, romaine lettuce, and others, are important for their vitamin K content, which helps with bone formation.

Fermented soy products, such as tofu and miso, are good for the bones. Essential fatty acids found in walnuts, almonds, flaxseeds, and fish are important for healthy bones.

Food to Avoid

Eliminate sugar, refined grains, and soda pop from your diet, as they contribute to bone loss.

High salt intake is linked to bone loss. Do not eat processed foods, which are usually loaded with salt, and never add conventional table salt to your meals.

Moderate your use of caffeine and alcohol, as they contribute to bone loss.

A study in the *American Journal of Clinical Nutrition* reported that a low intake of vitamin K was associated with an increased risk of hip fracture. The data from the study came from a review of the diets of over seventy-two thousand women. Studies have also shown that vitamin K supplementation improves bone density.

℞ Super Seven Prescriptions—Bone Fractures

Super Prescription #1 Homeopathic Symphytum (*Symphytum officinale*)
Take a 30C potency four times daily for two weeks. Symphytum is a specific remedy for healing bones and reducing fracture pain more quickly. Make sure to use Symphytum only after the fracture has been set, as it rapidly speeds knitting of the bone.

Super Prescription #2 Calcium
Take 500 to 600 mg twice daily in divided doses of well-absorbed calcium complexes, such as citrate, citrate-malate, chelate, or hydroxyapatite. Calcium is the main mineral that bone is composed of.

Super Prescription #3 Magnesium
Take 250 to 350 mg twice daily in divided doses. Magnesium is required for proper calcium metabolism and bone formation. Some researchers feel that it is as important as calcium. *Note*: Reduce the dosage if loose stools occur.

Super Prescription #4 Vitamin D
Take 800 IU daily for one month and then 400 IU daily. This vitamin improves intestinal calcium absorption and reduces the urinary excretion of calcium.

Super Prescription #5 Vitamin K
Take 5 mg daily for one month and then 100 to 500 mcg daily to finish bone healing. Vitamin K is needed to form the protein osteocalcin, a substance that attracts calcium into the bone matrix. Low levels of vitamin K are associated with osteoporosis and fractures. *Note*: Do not use if you are taking blood-thinning medications.

Super Prescription #6 High-potency multivitamin
This provides a base of the nutrients required for healthy bones. Take as directed on the container.

Super Prescription #7 Essential fatty acids
Take 4 grams of fish oil daily, along with 3,000 mg of evening primrose oil. Studies show that these essential fatty acids improve calcium absorption and deposition into the bone.

General Recommendations

Boron is a mineral that activates vitamin D for effective calcium metabolism. Take 3 to 5 mg daily.

Vitamin C is used to manufacture collagen, an important component of bones. Take 500 to 1,000 mg twice daily.

Silicon is a mineral that is involved in calcification and making collagen. Take 50 to 200 mg daily.

Zinc is required for enzymatic reactions that build bone. Take a daily total of 30 mg, along with 2 to 3 mg of copper.

Manganese helps with bone calcification. Take 15 to 30 mg daily.

A greens formula that contains super green foods, such as chlorella, spirulina, and others, has an alkalinizing effect and is rich in minerals. Take as directed on the container.

Soy protein powder has been shown to protect against bone loss. Take 40 grams daily; this amount contains 90 mg of isoflavones.

Strontium is a mineral that was shown to be helpful in increasing bone density when combined with calcium. Take 340 to 680 mg daily.

Homeopathy

Pick the remedy that best matches your symptoms described in this section. For acute fracture pain, take a 30C potency four times daily. For chronic fracture pain, take a 6x, 12x, 6C, 12C, or 30C potency twice daily for two weeks to see if there are any positive results. After you notice improvement, stop taking the remedy, unless symptoms return. Consultation with a homeopathic practitioner is advised.

Aconitum Napellus is used when people are in shock from a trauma. They are restless and fearful. Aconitum will help calm them down as they seek medical attention.

Arnica (*Arnica montana*) is the first remedy to give immediately after a fracture has occurred. This will help reduce pain, shock, and swelling. Give the highest potency available. Most health food stores carry a 30C potency; take it four times daily for two days.

Bryonia (*Bryonia alba*) is to be given during the first week of a fracture, when the slightest movement aggravates the pain. The person exhibits great irritability from the pain. Bryonia can be alternated with homeopathic Symphytum (*Symphytum officinale*).

Calcarea Carbonica is a remedy for people with signs of calcium imbalance, such as a slow-healing fracture, osteoporosis, aching bones, muscle cramps, and swollen joints. People requiring this remedy are generally chilly and flabby and feel worse in the cold and the dampness. They are easily fatigued and get overwhelmed. There is a craving for sweets, milk, and eggs.

Calcarea Phosphorica is a good remedy for fractures that are slow to heal. This remedy stimulates bone building.

Hypericum (*Hypericum perforatum*) is for crushing injuries that result in nerve damage. There are sharp, shooting pains. It is especially good for fractures of the coccyx (tailbone).

Phosphorus is a remedy for weak bones or fractures that heal slowly. People requiring this remedy tend to be tall and thin. There is a strong craving for ice-cold drinks. The person tends to be very social and suggestible.

Silica (*Silicea*) is for people who have poor bone density and tend to be very thin. People who need this remedy are often nervous, easily fatigued, and chilly and have low resistance to infection.

Symphytum (*Symphytum officinale*) is a specific remedy for healing and reducing fracture pain more quickly. Make sure to use it after a bone has been set.

Acupressure

See pages 787–794 for information about pressure points and administering treatment.

- To increase your ability to absorb nutrients (including calcium), work Stomach 36 (St36). With regular practice, your digestion will improve, and you'll find that you have more energy than before.
- If you have pain, work Large Intestine 4 (LI4). Do not use this point if you are pregnant.

Bodywork

Massage

Massage is a good wellness measure after the fracture has been set, to encourage blood flow and healing.

Acupuncture

Acupuncture is recommended to help relieve the pain and the swelling from a fracture.

Magnet Therapy

Magnets can be used by a knowledgeable practitioner to reduce fracture pain and stimulate healing.

Reflexology

See pages 804–805 for information about reflexology areas and how to work them.

Work the areas corresponding to the area of injury and the lymph area to reduce swelling.

Working the spine areas will help with the nerve endings of the fractured area.

Hydrotherapy

Alternate hot and cold towels over the opposite body part affected. For example, if the left arm is broken, alternate a hot towel (two minutes) with a cold towel (two minutes) over the right arm, repeat three times, and perform twice daily. There is a reflex action whereby circulation will be increased in the opposite body part, which increases nutrition to the healing bone.

Aromatherapy

Black pepper and rosemary both have warming qualities that soothe aching bones and joints. Use them in a massage, a lotion, or a bath.

Other Recommendations

- Start doing regular weight-bearing exercise once you have been instructed to by your doctor, as it stimulates bone healing.
- Don't smoke or expose yourself to secondhand smoke. Smoking makes bones brittle and weak.

REFERENCES

Feskanich, D., P. Weber, W. C. Willett, et al. 1999. Vitamin K intake and hip fractures in women: A prospective study. *American Journal of Clinical Nutrition* 69(1): 74–79.

Brittle Nails

Nails are made of skin cells hardened by a protein called keratin. The different parts of a fingernail include the following:

- Nail plate (the visible covering)
- Nail bed (the skin underneath the nail plate)
- Cuticle (the fold of skin at the base of the nail plate)
- Matrix (located under the cuticle)
- Lunula (the white, half-moon-shaped portion of the nail matrix)

Nails, with their hard shells, protect the tissue underneath and assist in manual dexterity. The health of fingernails mirrors the health of the body. Skin conditions such as psoriasis or fungal infections can cause the nail to become flaky and brittle. Fingernails are influenced by nutritional habits and digestive health. People who do not eat a healthy diet are prone to brittle or splitting nails.

SYMPTOMS

- Nails that break, peel, bend, split, or tear easily

ROOT CAUSES

- Poor diet, deficient in protein, vitamin A, biotin, vitamin B12, iron, sulfur, silica, calcium, essential fatty acids, or other nutrients
- Topical use of nail polish remover
- Poor digestion and absorption, possibly caused by deficiency in stomach acid, friendly flora, or enzymes
- Hormone deficiency, especially low thyroid

Testing Techniques

The following tests assess possible reasons for brittle nails:

Vitamin and mineral analysis—blood, urine

Essential fatty acids—blood

Total protein and amino acid analysis—blood or urine

Hormone testing (thyroid, DHEA, cortisol, testosterone, IGF-1, estrogen, progesterone)—saliva, blood, or urine

Intestinal permeability—urine

Digestive function and microbe/parasite/candida testing—stool analysis

Anemia blood test (CBC, iron, ferritin, percentage of saturation)

TREATMENT

Diet

Recommended Food

Quality protein sources, such as fish, legumes, nuts, and lean poultry, are important.

Foods rich in B vitamins, such as whole grains, should be increased. Other food sources of the B vitamin biotin are soybeans, eggs, cauliflower, and mushrooms. Another good source of B vitamins is nutritional brewer's yeast.

Sulfur-rich foods, such as broccoli, garlic, onions, and sea vegetables, should be included in the diet. So should silicon-rich foods like whole grains, bananas, raisins, beans, and lentils. Calcium-rich sources, such as carrots, broccoli, kale, and vegetable milks, are recommended.

One packet of gelatin daily is a home remedy that has been used throughout the years to improve nail health .

Food to Avoid

Decrease the consumption of simple sugars, alcohol, caffeine, and soda, which leach minerals out of the body.

℞ Super Seven Prescriptions—Brittle Nails

Super Prescription #1 Silicon
Take 10 mg daily for at least eight weeks. Research proves it benefits brittle nails. Silica extract is also effective.

Super Prescription #2 Biotin
Taking a dose of 300 to 3,000 mcg daily is effective for many people with brittle nails.

Super Prescription #3 MSM
Take 1,000 mg twice daily. One study found it to be effective for brittle nails. This supplement contains sulfur, a mineral involved in healthy nail formation.

Super Prescription #4 Essential fatty acids
Take a fish oil product containing 1,000 mg of EPA and DHA or 1 tablespoon of flaxseed or hempseed oil daily.

Super Prescription #5 Calcium
Take 500 mg daily, combined with 250 mg of magnesium and 1,000 IU of vitamin D.

Super Prescription #6 Collagen
Take a well-studied form of collagen as directed on the label. It is involved in the formation of nails.

Super Prescription #7 Digestive enzymes
Take 1 or 2 capsules with meals to enhance the absorption of the amino acids and nutrients necessary for nail health.

A study published in the *Archives of Dermatological Research* found that silicon was effective for brittle hair. Forty-eight women with fine hair were given 10 mg of silicon a day, in the form of choline-stabilized orthosilicic acid beadlets, or a placebo for nine months. Hair quality and tensile-strength properties were evaluated before and after treatment. Silicon supplementation had a positive effect on hair thickness and tensile strength, including elasticity and break load.

General Recommendations

Betaine hydrochloride improves the absorption of the amino acids and minerals necessary for nail health. Take 1 or 2 capsules with meals.

A high-potency multivitamin and mineral formula will provide a base of nutrients for healthy nails. Take as directed.

Probiotics improve the absorption of nutrients. Take as directed.

Homeopathy

Pick the remedy that best matches your symptoms as described below. Take a 6x, 12x, 6C, 12C, or 30C potency twice daily for two weeks to see if there are any positive improvements. After you notice improvement, stop taking the remedy unless your symptoms return. Consultation with a homeopathic practitioner is advised.

Calcarea Carbonica helps overweight people who tend to get chilly and have brittle nails.

Calcarea Phosphorica helps people with brittle nails who also have a tendency toward brittle bones.

Silica helps those with brittle nails who have absorption problems. White spots on nails may occur with this remedy.

Acupressure

Stomach 36 (St36) improves digestion and absorption.

Bodywork

Reflexology

Work on the areas of the foot that correspond to the stomach and the small intestine, as well as the hands or the feet, depending on which nails are affected. See pages 804–805 for more information about reflexology areas and how to work them.

Hydrotherapy

If poor digestion is present follow the constitutional hydrotherapy treatment on pages 795–796.

Aromatherapy

Apply 1 to 3 drops of myrrh, lemon, or frankincense oil to the base of the nails for thirty days.

Stress Reduction

The effects of stress can both worsen absorption and contribute to depletion of the nutrients that are required for nail healing. Any technique to reduce stress will ultimately help with skin health and appearance. Exercise, prayer, reading, meditation, and visualization are examples.

Other Recommendations

Do not use topical nail remover until the underlying causes of your brittle nails have been treated successfully.

REFERENCES

Hochman, L. G., et al. 1993. Brittle nails: Response to daily biotin supplementation. *Cutis* 51:303–5.

Wickett, R. R., et al. 2007. Effect of oral intake of choline-stabilized orthosilicic acid on hair tensile strength and morphology in women with fine hair. *Archives of Dermatological Research* 299:499–505.

Bronchitis

Acute bronchitis is the deep, wet, or dry cough that comes on and lingers after an infection, such as a cold, sinusitis, or the flu. The cough, which may start out dry and then turn productive, is the body's way of expelling infected mucus (phlegm) from the lungs. An episode of bronchitis may last for one to two weeks, and because a virus usually causes it, antibiotics may not be helpful. The best treatment is usually rest, combined with immune-enhancing natural therapies, as well as symptomatic therapy to calm the cough and promote removal of the mucus.

Chronic bronchitis develops in the continual presence of irritants, usually tobacco smoke, but also environmental allergies and damp, foggy weather; it sometimes results from food allergies. It often begins as a protracted case of acute bronchitis that returns every few months and, if the irritants are not removed, will develop into a constant cough, often accompanied by breathlessness and sometimes wheezing. The weakened condition of the lungs leaves the body vulnerable to infections like acute bronchitis, pneumonia, and emphysema. In its advanced stage, even minor colds can grow into deadly diseases. The best treatment is to eliminate the irritants that caused the condition. This is accomplished by identifying the offending allergens and removing them or reducing your body's sensitivity to them.

SYMPTOMS

Acute bronchitis

- A cough that may start out dry but that turns deep and productive, with thick clear or yellow mucus
- Usually follows a viral infection

Chronic bronchitis

- Long bouts of acute bronchitis that recur frequently
- A persistent, constant cough that's worse upon waking

- Breathlessness
- Wheezing

ROOT CAUSES

Acute bronchitis

- Food or environmental allergens causing excess mucus in the lungs

- Viral infection

Chronic bronchitis

- Smoking or exposure to second-hand smoke
- Food allergies
- Environmental irritants

(especially dust, pollen, animal dander, or mold)
- Cold, damp, foggy weather

Testing Techniques

The following test helps assess possible metabolic reasons for chronic bronchitis:
    Food and environmental allergy testing—blood or electrodermal

---

TREATMENT

Diet

Recommended Food

To thin mucus secretions, drink a glass of clean water every two waking hours. Homemade chicken soup also thins mucus. Add garlic or ginger for flavor and immune support.

To reduce phlegm, have some hot barley soup.

Onions are an old folk remedy and have anti-inflammatory properties, so eat them often.

If you have bacterial bronchitis and are taking antibiotics, consume nondairy sour products, such as kefir or sauerkraut, daily to replenish disease-fighting bacteria.

Food to Avoid

Eliminate foods that encourage mucus production: dairy products, chocolate, and bananas, as well as processed, refined, fried, and junk foods. Avoid simple sugars, as they suppress immune function.

℞ Super Seven Prescriptions—Bronchitis

Super Prescription #1 N-acetylcysteine (NAC)

NAC reduces the viscosity of phlegm so it is easier to expectorate. It's useful for acute and chronic bronchitis (especially for smokers and people with asthma or emphysema). Take 300 to 500 mg twice daily.

Super Prescription #2 Homeopathy

Use a combination cough remedy, as directed on the container, or pick the remedy that best matches your symptoms under Homeopathy in this section. For acute bronchitis, take a 30C potency four times daily. For chronic bronchitis, take twice daily for two weeks to see if there are any positive improvements. After you notice improvement, stop taking the remedy, unless symptoms return. Consultation with a homeopathic practitioner is advised.

Super Prescription #3 Ivy leaf

Take 25 drops twice daily or as directed on container. This reduces the symptoms of bronchitis.

Super Prescription #4 Echinacea (*Echinacea purpurea*) and goldenseal (*Hydrastis canadensis*)

Take 500 mg or 2 ml of this combination four times daily for acute bronchitis with a wet cough. Both herbs enhance immune function, and goldenseal works to dry up mucus.

Super Prescription #5 Mullein (*Verbascum thapsus*)

Take 500 mg of the capsule or 2 ml of the tincture four times daily. This herb promotes the discharge of mucus and has soothing/anti-inflammatory effects for the respiratory tract.

Super Prescription #6 Astragalus (*Astragalus membranaceus*)

Astragalus is an excellent treatment for chronic, as well as acute, bronchitis. It strengthens weak lungs and increases the body's general resistance to infection. Take 500 to 1,000 mg or 3.5 ml of a tincture two or three times daily. Do not take astragalus if you have a fever.

Super Prescription #7 Colloidal silver

Take ½ to 1 teaspoon, or as directed on the container, three times daily for five days. It has an antimicrobial effect, especially for bacteria.

General Recommendations

Garlic (*Allium sativum*) has antimicrobial effects. Take 300 to 600 mg of garlic extract twice daily.

Licorice (*Glycyrrhiza glabra*) reduces coughing, enhances immune function, and soothes the respiratory tract. Use caution when supplementing licorice if you have high blood pressure. It's best used short term under the guidance of a holistic doctor. Take 500 mg of the capsule or 1 ml of the tincture four times daily.

Bromelain has a natural anti-inflammatory effect and enhances the effectiveness of some antibiotics. Take 500 mg three times daily between meals or along with anti-biotic therapy. Look for products standardized to 2,000 MCU (milk-clotting units) per 1,000 mg or 1,200 GDU (gelatin-dissolving units) per 1,000 mg.

Vitamin A enhances immune function. Take 25,000 to 50,000 IU daily for five days.

Vitamin C enhances immune function for acute bronchitis and has antiallergy benefits for chronic bronchitis. It is particularly important for smokers. Take 500 to 1,000 mg three times daily.

Other useful herbs that can be found in respiratory formulas include horehound, pleurisy root, plantain, marshmallow, ginger, peppermint, and cherry bark.

Homeopathy

Antimonium Tartaricum is for a congested, wet cough that produces a rattling noise in the chest. The person has trouble expectorating and may find it hard to breathe at times. The person feels better in a cool room and with the windows open.

Arsenicum Album is for a cough with a burning pain that feels better from taking sips of warm drinks. The person feels anxious and restless and may be very fatigued. Symptoms are worse from midnight to 2 A.M.

Bryonia (*Bryonia alba*) will treat a dry cough that causes stitching pain in the throat or the chest and that is worse at night. Movement of any type feels worse. The person has a great thirst and prefers to be left alone.

Coccus Cacti is for a cough that produces stringy mucus. The person feels like constantly clearing the throat. Coughing often leads to vomiting.

Drosera is for a dry, barking cough that may end in gagging. The cough is worse when lying down and is also worse after midnight.

Hepar Sulphuris (*Hepar sulphuris calcareum*) is for a rattling, barking cough that comes on after exposure to dry, cold air. The person coughs when uncovered and feels chilly and irritable. There is often yellowish mucus.

Kali Bichromium is for a hoarse cough that produces thick, stringy, yellow mucus. The cough is worse from eating and drinking.

Phosphorous is for a dry, tickling cough that is worse in the cold air, with talking or laughing, and when lying on the left side. The person may have a burning sensation in the chest and feels better with cold drinks.

Pulsatilla (*Pulsatilla pratensis*) will clear up a cough with yellow or green phlegm that is looser in the morning and drier at night. The person has a low thirst and feels better near an open window. The cough is worse when the person lies down.

Rumex Crispus is for a dry cough that begins as soon as a person lies down. The person feels a tickling sensation in the throat that leads to a cough. The cough is worse in cold air.

Silica (*Silicea*) is for someone who seems to have bronchitis all winter long. The person has weak immunity and low stamina and feels chilly. Coughing up mucus takes a lot of effort.

Spongia Tosta helps when one has a dry, barking cough that is better after ingesting warm foods or liquids.

Sulfur is for bronchitis with burning pains that are better after having cold drinks. The person feels warm and desires a cool room. Sulfur is often used after a long bout of bronchitis, for complete recovery.

Acupressure

See pages 787–794 for information about pressure points and administering treatment.
- To relieve chest congestion, massage Kidney 27 (K27), Conception Vessel 22 (CV22), and Lung 1 and 7 (Lu1 and Lu7).
- If you have difficulty breathing and need to calm your emotions, use Bladder 38 (B38).

Bodywork

Massage

A back massage will break up excess phlegm. If you have chronic bronchitis, you might want to schedule regular sessions with a professional massage therapist. If you're generally a strong and healthy person, ask your therapist to use percussive motions, which are highly effective at releasing phlegm. People who suffer from an occasional bout of acute bronchitis might prefer to rely on a loved one to perform this task each evening.

Hydrotherapy

Sit in a hot, steamy bath or a sauna to thin mucus secretions and sweat out toxins. If you have hypertension, do not use saunas.

Constitutional hydrotherapy works well for acute and chronic bronchitis. Follow the directions for treatment on pages 795–796.

Aromatherapy

Add eucalyptus, peppermint, lemon balm, or tree tea oil to a hot bath or a steam inhalation to drain congestion. You can also add any of these oils to a base oil and rub it directly onto your chest.

Stress Reduction

General Stress-Reduction Therapies

Stress can weaken your immune system, leaving your lungs open to infection. If you're vulnerable to frequent bouts of bronchitis, or if you suffer from chronic bronchitis, experiment with the techniques in the Exercise and Stress Reduction chapter until you find ones you like. Practice them on a daily basis, or more often as needed.

Other Recommendations

- Rest, preferably in bed, while the illness is at its worst. When you feel better, move around to keep the infection from settling into your lungs, but continue to rest after periods of activity.
- Don't take a cough suppressant. The lungs need to expel phlegm to get healthy, and suppressants keep them from doing so. Consistent use of suppressants can lead to worse cases of acute bronchitis or even to chronic bronchitis or pneumonia.
- Encourage expectoration by applying warm compresses to your chest.

- Don't smoke or expose yourself to secondhand smoke.
- If you have chronic bronchitis and live in a damp, cold climate, you may have to move to another location that's dry and warm. You should have your doctor consider mold allergies as a possible cause of chronic bronchitis.
- People with chronic bronchitis need to keep their lungs as elastic and strong as possible. Exercise, breath deeply, and, if you enjoy music, take up a wind instrument.

Bruises

A bruise is an injury caused by a blow or a bump that does not cut the skin but breaks blood vessels underneath the skin. Blood seeps out of the vessels, producing the tell-tale black-and-blue discoloration, as well as swelling and soreness.

The deeper the bruise, or contusion, the longer it will take to heal. Leg bruises, for instance, can linger for up to four weeks because leg vessels have greater blood pressure than arm vessels.

Bruises also change in color, first starting off red, then becoming blackish-blue, and finally turning yellowish-green. The final color is a sign that the body has worked to remove the dead cells and tissues and replace them with healthy, new cells to restore color to the skin.

Falls, sprains, pinches, and suction can cause bruises. These are occupational hazards for active children who love to run, jump, bike, climb, or skate. People who are anemic or obese tend to bruise easily. Nutritional deficiencies of vitamin C, iron, vitamin K, bioflavonoids, and other nutrients can contribute to easy bruising. Sometimes, unexplained bruising can be a clue that a person's blood vessel walls are brittle or that a child has insufficient blood-clotting factors. Bruising can also signal the onset of serious illnesses such as leukemia or hemophilia.

Parents should have their child's bruise examined by a doctor if:
- The bruise is located on the head or near the eye.
- Bruising seems to show up without any apparent cause.
- A minor bump or blow creates a large bruise.
- Bruises are located in unusual places, such as the back, the calves, or the backs of the arms.
- The child has difficulty talking, walking, or seeing, or appears drowsy and dizzy.

People of all ages should see a doctor if a fever accompanies the bruising or for bruises that do not heal. Medications such as aspirin and other blood thinners like Coumadin can cause bruising. Check with your doctor if you use one or more of these medications to see if it is related to your bruising.

If your doctor has determined that your bruising occurs as the result of anemia, see the Anemia section for more information.

SYMPTOMS

- Red, black and blue, or yellowish skin discoloration

ROOT CAUSES

- Trauma to soft tissues
- Anemia
- Clotting disorders or other underlying medical conditions

Testing Techniques

The following tests help assess possible reasons for chronic bruising:

Immune system imbalance or disease—blood

Hormone testing (thyroid)—saliva, blood, or urine

Intestinal permeability—urine

Vitamin and mineral analysis (especially iron, B12, folic acid, vitamin C, and vitamin K)—blood

Digestive function and microbe/parasite/candida testing—stool analysis

Anemia—blood test (CBC, iron, ferritin, % saturation)

Food and environmental allergies/sensitivities—blood, electrodermal

---

TREATMENT

Diet

Recommended Food

Dark-green leafy vegetables provide many minerals that help heal bruising, such as vitamin C and vitamin K.

Citrus fruits, bell peppers, and other brightly colored vegetables and fruits provide bioflavonoids that help heal bruises.

Fish such as salmon, nuts like walnuts, and seeds such as flaxseeds provide essential fatty acids that are necessary for tissue repair.

Brussels sprouts, broccoli, potatoes, and many citrus fruits are good sources of vitamin C.

Food to Avoid

Reduce or eliminate sugars, as they interrupt the healing of tissue.

Avoid saturated, hydrogenated, and trans-fatty acids found in meat and packaged, processed foods, as they interfere with the healing of cells.

℞ Super Seven Prescriptions—Bruises

Super Prescription #1 Homeopathic Arnica (*Arnica montana*)
Take a 30C potency four times daily for five days. Arnica is a specific remedy for healing bruises and soft tissue injuries.

Super Prescription #2 Bromelain
Take 500 mg three times daily between meals. Look for products standardized to 2,000 MCU (milk-clotting units) per 1,000 mg or 1,200 GDU (gelatin-dissolving units) per 1,000 mg. Bromelain has a natural anti-inflammatory effect. Protease enzyme products also have this benefit.

In one early clinical trial, seventy-four boxers who regularly suffered bruising on the face, the lips, the ears, the chest, and the arms were given bromelain. When bromelain was given four times a day, all signs of bruising disappeared by the fourth day in fifty-eight of the boxers. In contrast, those in a control group receiving a placebo required seven to fourteen days before the bruises healed.

Super Prescription #3 Vitamin C

Take 500 to 1,000 mg three times daily. Vitamin C is used to manufacture collagen, the protein that holds blood vessels and connective tissue together. Vitamin C also improves wound healing.

Super Prescription #4 Bioflavonoids

Take a 500 mg complex three times daily. Bioflavonoids such as rutin and hesperedin act similarly to vitamin C and improve vitamin C's therapeutic effect.

Super Prescription #5 Arnica oil (*Arnica montana*)

Apply arnica oil topically over the area of the bruise twice daily. This herb in oil form has anti-inflammatory benefits. Do not use on broken skin.

Super Prescription #6 Vitamin K

Take 2 mg daily for two weeks for an acute bruise and 500 mcg daily to prevent bruising. Vitamin K is involved with the blood-clotting process. *Note*: Do not use if you are taking blood-thinning medications.

Super Prescription #7 High-potency multivitamin

This provides a base of the nutrients required for healthy blood vessels. Take as directed on the container.

General Recommendations

Essential fatty acids, as found in fish oil or flaxseed oil, are required for tissue healing. Take 3 grams of fish oil daily or 1 tablespoon of flaxseed oil. A greens formula that contains super green foods, such as chlorella, spirulina, and others, has an alkalinizing effect and is rich in nutrients such as vitamins K and C, which promote healing of the soft tissue. Take as directed on the container.

Maritime pine bark and grapeseed extract are rich sources of proanthocyandins, which promote tissue healing. Take 50 mg twice daily.

Homeopathy

Pick the remedy that best matches your symptoms in this section. For acute bruises, take a 30C potency four times daily. For chronic bruising, take a 6x, 12x, 6C, 12C, or 30C twice daily for two weeks to see if there are any positive results. After you notice improvement, stop taking the remedy, unless symptoms return. Consultation with a homeopathic practitioner is advised.

Arnica (*Arnica montana*) is for any injury to the soft tissues and will treat or prevent bruising. Arnica is generally the first remedy to use for bruising. It's also used for early-stage sprains and strains that result in bruising. The injury feels bruised and sore. Symptoms are worse from touch and motion and feel better with a cold compress and in the open air.

Bellis Perennis is for bruising of the deep and internal tissues, especially of the abdomen, the back, and the breasts. It is also used for bruises that do not respond to Arnica. Swelling and tumors may occur at the site of the injury. Symptoms are worse from cold bathing and touch. Improvements are noted from movement and rubbing the injury.

Ferrum Phosphoricum is the indicated remedy when bruising occurs as the result of anemia.

Hamamelis is a good choice when there is intense soreness associated with a bruise; it is especially good for injuries to the veins and for black eyes. One's symptoms are worse with pressure and cold applications.

Ledum (*Ledum palustre*) should be used for bruises that are a result of puncture wounds. It is also used for bruising that results from sprains and strains, such as a sprained ankle. Symptoms feel better with cold applications.

Ruta (*Ruta graveolens*) is useful for bruising of bone coverings, such as the shinbone, or from a cartilage or joint injury.

Sulphuricum Acidum is for large, red or black-blue, itchy bruises that do not heal, especially after using Arnica. The person feels weak from the injury.

Bodywork

Hydrotherapy

Ice the bruise for the first twenty-four hours, then alternate hot cloths (one minute) and cold cloths (one minute) over the affected area and repeat four times. Perform twice daily. This improves circulation to the injury site and speeds up healing.

Aromatherapy

Add 2 drops of lavender oil to a carrier oil, and rub over the bruise twice daily.

REFERENCES

Blonstein, J. L. 1960. Control of swelling in boxing injuries. *Practitioner* 185:78.

Bulimia. See Eating Disorders

Burns (Including Sunburn)

Few injuries are more frightening or painful than a serious burn. The skin may be burned from heat, steam, scalding liquids, the sun, chemicals, or electricity. Treatment is based on the type of burn, the severity of the burn, the location of the burn, and the source of the burn. Severe burns can destroy all skin layers and damage the underlying muscle and fat.

Heat burns can be caused by wet heat, such as scalding hot water, or dry heat, caused by a flame. These burns are classified by degree. A first-degree burn affects only the skin surface and is considered the most minor of all burns. The skin is usually red and slightly swollen. A second-degree burn affects the skin surface and the layer just beneath the skin surface. Blisters and swelling may occur. A third-degree burn, the most serious, results in white or blackened skin layers, is extremely painful, and involves all layers of the skin.

Chemical burns are caused by caustic substances that can be either acidic or alkaline. If the source of the burn is acidic, use water to wash the chemical off the wound. If the source of the burn is alkaline, it is vital not to wet the wound because that can cause further burning. Symptoms of chemical burns include redness of the skin, blistering, swelling, and peeling.

Electrical burns are caused by electric shock. It is important to realize that the body is electrically charged and that the heart functions on tiny pulses of electricity. Electrical burns have the potential to disrupt the heartbeat and cause cardiac and respiratory arrest. Be aware that severe electrical burns quite often do not display much damage on the surface layer of skin. The real damage is deeper in the layers underneath.

Consult your doctor about your burn under the following circumstances:

- All electrical burns
- Any burn located on the face, the mouth, the hands, or the genitals
- Any burn that covers more than 10 percent of the body or completely encircles an arm or a leg
- Any burn that blisters or turns the skin white
- Any burn that remains red or oozes longer than twenty-four hours and intensifies in pain

Natural therapies can be very effective in relieving the pain of minor burns and, to some degree, major burns (along with pain medicines). They are even more effective in promoting faster skin healing and may help in the prevention of secondary skin infections.

SYMPTOMS

- Burning sensation and damage of the skin

ROOT CAUSES

- Heat, chemicals, or electricity

TREATMENT

Diet

Recommended Food

Drink electrolyte drinks and plenty of water to replace lost fluids.

Citrus fruits, bell peppers, and other brightly colored vegetables and fruits provide bioflavonoids that help heal the skin.

Fish such as salmon, nuts like walnuts, and seeds such as flaxseeds provide essential fatty acids that are necessary for tissue repair.

Brussels sprouts, broccoli, potatoes, and many citrus fruits are good sources of vitamin C, which helps heal the skin.

Food to Avoid

Reduce or eliminate sugars, as they interrupt the healing of tissue.

℞ **Super Seven Prescriptions—Burns**

Super Prescription #1 Homeopathic Cantharis (*Cantharis vesicator*)
Take a 30C potency four to six times daily for acute burns, including sunburns. This remedy prevents or reduces blistering and burn pain.

Super Prescription #2 Aloe vera
Choose an aloe gel product (80 percent or higher) and apply to the burned area twice daily. Aloe has a soothing effect and may stimulate skin healing.

Super Prescription #3 L-glutamine
Take 500 to 1,000 mg three times daily on an empty stomach or in the intravenous form given by your doctor. L-glutamine is required for tissue healing and to prevent secondary infection that often occurs with burns.

Super Prescription #4 Zinc
Take 30 mg twice daily, along with 2 mg of copper. Zinc promotes skin healing.

Super Prescription #5 Calendula (*Calendula officinalis*)
This herb can be used topically in the liquid or gel form to help heal burns. Apply twice daily.

Super Prescription #6 Mixed carotenoids
Take 25,000 IU of a mixed carotenoid complex daily to protect against sunburns. Carotenoids help to absorb the UV rays of the sun.

Super Prescription #7 Antioxidant complex
Take a complex composed of antioxidants such as vitamins E, C, selenium, and others, which will neutralize free-radical damage that results from burns, including sunburns.

L-glutamine is proving to be a valuable supplement for burns. It is currently used orally and in intravenous methods to increase body levels of this healing nutrient. One study of people with burns serious enough to require hospitalization found that oral glutamine supplementation resulted in a shorter hospital stay.

General Recommendations

Topical creams that contain vitamins C and E, CoQ10, and carotenoids may be helpful in preventing sunburns. Apply as directed on the container.

Vitamin C promotes skin healing. Take 1,000 mg three times daily. Reduce the dosage if loose stools occur.

Vitamin E is a good antioxidant that helps with tissue healing. Take 400 IU daily. Vitamin E gel, cream, or oil can be applied topically for burn healing.

Propolis is a bee product that speeds healing of a burn and prevents secondary infections. It's available as a spray, a salve, or a tincture. Manuka honey, applied to burns, helps to speed healing and prevent infection. This is commonly done in countries such as New Zealand.

Colloidal silver is used topically to prevent secondary skin infections.

Homeopathy

Pick the remedy that best matches your symptoms described in this section. For acute burns, take a 30C potency four times daily. For chronic burn pain, take a 6x,

12x, 6C, 12C, or 30C potency twice daily for two weeks to see if there are any positive results. After you notice improvement, stop taking the remedy, unless symptoms return. Consultation with a homeopathic practitioner is advised.

Apis (*Apis mellifica*) is for burns characterized by stinging, burning pains that feel better from cool applications and worse from warmth. The skin is hot, dry, and puffy and may have small vesicles.

Arsenicum Album is for people with burning skin pain that is worse from cold and better from warm applications. They are restless, anxious, and weak. It is also for severe burns that turn blue or black.

Cantharis (*Cantharis vesicator*) is for intense scalding burns or sunburns. This remedy is used for any burn but particularly for second- or third-degree burns. Cold water gives relief to the pain.

Causticum is indicated for severe burns, especially caustic chemical burns, and for old burns that do not heal. Symptoms are worse from dry, cold drafts and better from warmth or damp weather.

Hypericum (*Hypericum perforatum*) is a remedy for burns that affect the nerves and cause a sharp, radiating nerve pain.

Phosphorus is a specific remedy for electrical shocks and burns.

Rhus Toxicodendron is a good choice when the skin has itching, burning vesicles. The person is restless. Symptoms feel better from applying hot water to the burn and feel worse in cold air.

Urtica Urens is a good remedy to use if Cantharis (*Cantharis vesicator*) is not helpful. The person experiences scalding, burning pain and fluid-filled blisters. It is mainly used for first- and second-degree burns.

Bodywork

Electrical acupuncture has been shown to reduce the pain associated with burns. See a qualified practitioner for treatment.

Other Bodywork Recommendations

Magnet therapy can be effective in reducing pain and stimulating skin healing. Use under the guidance of a knowledgeable practitioner.

Other Recommendations

Testosterone, growth hormone, and stem cell therapy may be helpful when used under an experienced doctor's guidance.

REFERENCES

Zhou, Y., Y. Sun, Z. Jiang, et al. 2002. The effects of glutamine dipeptide on the improvement of endotoxemia in severely burned patients. Zhonghua Shao Shang Za Zhi 18(6):343–45 [in Chinese].

Cancer

Almost all the cells in our bodies must be replaced on a regular basis. Some cells, like those that make up the intestinal lining, die out quickly and are replaced every few days. In other parts of the body, the cells live for years before they divide and form new ones. Under special circumstances, such as an injury or an illness, healthy new cells may grow more quickly than usual to replace those that are damaged. When the area is healed, the cell growth slows back down to its normal rate.

Normally, the genes that control the growth of cells automatically know when to start and stop the replication process. But when those genes are mutated—perhaps because of an inherited flaw or, more commonly, because of dietary and environmental factors—cells may begin to multiply and divide at an unusually fast rate. Eventually, these cells form a lump. Sometimes lumps are benign (meaning that they are non-cancerous and relatively harmless), as in the case of warts or uterine fibroids. Other growths, however, are malignant. They pull nutrients away from the healthy tissues that surround them, and they interfere with the body's normal functions, to a potentially life-threatening extent. If a tumor continues to grow, its cells may spread via the blood vessels or the lymphatic system to other parts of the body, where they form new tumors. Once this process, called metastasis, is underway, there is a risk of dying from the complications that can occur. Although many cancers can be treated successfully when caught early, the sad fact remains that they are the second-leading cause of death in the United States. Every minute, another person dies of some form of the disease.

The word *cancer* refers to the process of uncontrolled cell division, but, technically, it is not, in itself, the name of a specific disorder. Instead, cancer is an umbrella term that refers to more than one hundred different kinds of diseases, which are generally named according to the area where a tumor first appears. In men, prostate cancer is most common; in women, breast cancer is most frequent. But both of these cancers can be highly treatable when caught early. Lung cancer is common and one of the deadliest. Cancer also tends to strike the skin, the urinary tract, the colorectal region, and the female reproductive organs, although it can attack anywhere. It's beyond the scope of this book to discuss each individual type of cancer, but the suggestions here apply to anyone who is fighting off a tumor, wants to keep a cancer in remission, or hopes to avoid developing cancer in the first place. We also have recommendations on what to take if you are undergoing chemotherapy and/or radiation, to reduce side effects and optimize immune function and outcome.

Scientists classify cancers into four very broad categories listed below. If you're trying to communicate with your doctor or keep up with medical literature, it's helpful to understand the differences among them.

Carcinomas affect soft tissues in organs and glands, like the skin, the breasts, the lungs, and the pancreas.

Sarcomas, which are quite rare, occur in solid tissues, especially bone, muscle, and cartilage.

Lymphomas appear in the lymphatic system.

Leukemias are cancers of the tissues that form blood; these cancers are unusual in that they don't form hard tumors.

As with so many other chronic and deadly diseases, researchers have not been able to pinpoint the cause of uncontrolled, cancerous cell growth, despite decades of hard work and billions of dollars in funding. It's obvious that there isn't just one cause. We know, for example, that faulty genes play a role in some cancers—but most people with genetic flaws aren't doomed to develop cancer; they simply have a greater chance of doing so. Although a family history of cancer carries with it increased risk, most cancer researchers agree that as a sole cause, genetics is relatively insignificant, accounting for only 5 to 15 percent of cancers. It appears that most cancers are caused by largely controllable factors, such as nutrition, lifestyle, and environmental factors. One of the criticisms of conventional medicine in preventing and treating cancer is that diet, lifestyle, stress, and the ability to rid the body of environmental toxins rarely are addressed in a comprehensive fashion. Yet these factors are both most influential and most controllable in the prevention of cancer, and they play important roles in the recovery from cancer. To reduce the risk of developing cancer, we all need to reduce free-radical formation in the body, limit exposure to dietary and environmental sources of free radicals, and increase our intake of antioxidant nutrients.

We also know that environmental carcinogens like cigarette smoke, man-made food, and pollution can have a devastating effect on the body. These toxins encourage the formation of free radicals, and many experts now believe that these unbalanced molecules contribute to uncontrolled cell growth. People with strong immune systems and high levels of antioxidants—the substances that neutralize free radicals—are in a much better position to stave off tumor growth. But again, not everyone exposed to high levels of carcinogens or with a weakened immune system will necessarily suffer from cancer. An increasing amount of research is demonstrating how the effects of unresolved stress may be the root cause for some people. In all probability, a combination of several factors leads to this group of diseases.

There is a lot of evidence that viral or fungal infections may initiate cancer for some people with a susceptible immune system.

Since we can't control the genes we inherit (not yet, anyway), it's wise for people who are battling cancer or who want to prevent it to turn their attention to things we can control. First things first: Early detection is the key to successful treatment, so have regular checkups and cancer screenings, as are appropriate for your age, sex, and medical history. Learn the warning signs of cancer, and contact a doctor immediately if one shows up on your body. Aside from these common-sense strategies, you must do everything you can to support your immune system and increase your intake of antioxidants, while minimizing your exposure to environmental toxins. You should also cleanse your body by drinking lots of clean, quality water and eating plenty of fiber. Periodic fasts will further detoxify your system. Your liver is one of the most crucial organs for cancer defense; under normal conditions, it filters out toxins and helps them pass out of the body. But when unhealthful food, pollution, or other carcinogens overtax it, some of those toxins are reabsorbed into the body, where they may encourage cancerous growths. Good nutrition and a detoxification plan will support your liver, but you'll also want to give it a boost with cleansing herbs. And because unresolved stress can produce free radicals and lower immunity, it's also important to find measures that release tension and get your stress levels under control.

As most of us know, the conventional measures for treating cancer—chemotherapy, radiation, and surgical removal of the tumor or the affected organ—can be effective in some cases but also carry the risk of serious side effects, even death.

Integrative therapy, which blends conventional and natural treatments for optimal outcomes, is becoming more popular. Talk to your doctor, do your own research, and weigh the pros and cons of the different treatments available for your type of cancer. If you choose to undergo chemotherapy or other conventional treatments, try to find a doctor who is sympathetic to your desire to incorporate natural strategies into your healing process. Dietary changes, herbs, and other natural treatments can significantly reduce your discomfort and boost your ability to fight the disease.

SYMPTOMS

Cancers often grow for years, even decades, before they manifest in symptoms. Nevertheless, there are some early warning signs you should watch for. If you experience any of the following symptoms, don't panic. Most likely, you don't have cancer: the symptoms of cancerous growths are similar or identical to the symptoms of many other illnesses, often ones that are much less frightening. Nevertheless, you should see your doctor right away for an accurate diagnosis. If you do have a cancerous growth, the sooner you start treatment, the better your chances of sending the disease into permanent remission.

- A mole, a wart, or a blemish that changes in diameter, shape, color, or thickness
- A sore that doesn't heal within three weeks
- A lump or a swelling under the skin
- Thickening of the skin on any part of your body
- Chronic indigestion or difficulty swallowing
- A change in bowel or bladder habits
- Blood in the urine or the stool
- Rectal bleeding
- An unexplained vaginal discharge or bleeding between periods
- Recurring headaches
- An unexplained loss of weight or appetite
- An unexplained pain, especially in the bones
- A persistent low-grade fever
- Recurrent infections
- Hoarseness that lingers for more than a week
- A persistent cough or a cough that brings up blood
- Persistent fatigue, nausea, or vomiting

Testing Techniques

The following tests help assess possible reasons for cancer:

Immune system imbalance or disease—blood

Genetic defects—blood, saliva

Hormone testing (thyroid, DHEA, cortisol, testosterone, IGF-1, estrogen, progesterone)—saliva, blood, or urine

Intestinal permeability—urine

Detoxification profile—urine

Oxidative stress—urine or blood

Vitamin and mineral analysis (especially magnesium, B12, iron, and CoQ10)—blood

---

Digestive function and microbe/parasite/candida testing—stool analysis
Food and environmental allergies/sensitivities—blood, electrodermal
Blood-sugar and insulin balance—blood, stool
Toxic metals—blood, urine, or hair

ROOT CAUSES

There is no single cause of cancer, but the factors that are tied to a greater likelihood of developing cancer are listed as follows:

- Genetic flaws
- Environmental toxins, including pollution, toxic metals, and radiation
- A poor diet, especially one high in fat, additives, pesticides, and improperly prepared meats
- A toxic liver
- Viruses, fungi, and other stealth infections

- A weakened immune system
- Unresolved stress
- Poor digestion and detoxification
- Lack of exercise
- Nutritional deficiencies
- Certain medical therapies (such as synthetic hormone replacement, related to breast cancer)
- Tobacco use

TREATMENT

Diet

Dietary therapies for cancer seek to return your body to its natural state of balance and health. Focus on a diet of whole foods, as outlined in this chapter, which optimize immune function and detoxification.

Recommended Food

Wherever possible, eat clean, live foods. Look for food that's organically grown. If you're eating poultry, check the label to be sure the animal was not raised on antibiotics or other unnatural substances. When buying fish, ask whether the product comes from a clean water source.

When the liver processes toxins, cancer-promoting free radicals are produced in high quantities. Of all the antioxidants, glutathione is the best at counteracting the free radicals created during this process. Asparagus, avocados, broccoli, brussels sprouts, cabbage, and walnuts are all excellent sources of glutathione. Make it a priority to put one or more of these foods on your menu every day.

Eat as many raw vegetables and fruits as possible, especially those that have deep, rich colors. These foods are high in fiber, which helps flush toxins from your system, and they're potent sources of antioxidants. When you eat them raw, you will also retain their natural enzymes, which help you digest food and absorb the maximum amount of nutrients into your bloodstream.

For even more fiber, eat plenty of whole grains, including oats and brown rice.

Eat wheat germ, nuts, and seeds for their vitamin E content. Vitamin E is another powerful antioxidant.

Garlic, onions, and legumes will help keep your liver functioning at optimum capacity.

Fermented soy products, such as tofu, tempeh, and miso, appear to have anticancer properties, based on population studies. Consume these products three to four times weekly, unless you are sensitive to soy products. (But don't take isoflavone extracts. Their effects on the body are still unknown.)

If you're battling cancer, you don't need to be told how important it is to keep up your strength and energy. Eat lean protein from beans, eggs, tofu, poultry, or fish. People undergoing conventional cancer therapy require increased protein intake to prevent tissue wasting. A 2010 McGill University analysis conducted a review of thirty-one studies and found that fish consumption was associated with an impressive 63 percent reduction in the risk for late-stage or fatal prostate cancer.

Studies in Japan show that in areas where people drink green tea, there are significantly lower rates of stomach, esophageal, colon, skin, bladder, ovary, mouth, and liver cancer. It also acts as a mild stimulant of the immune system.

Tomatoes are high in lycopene, a substance that's been shown to prevent and even help counteract prostate cancer. Cooked tomatoes are higher in lycopene than raw ones.

Make sure to drink plenty of clean, quality water to promote healthy detoxification. Drinking freshly prepared vegetable and fruit juices is highly advised. Try to consume 8 to 10 ounces a day of a variety of juices. Great vegetable-juice choices include kale, collard greens, tomatoes, spinach, cucumber, cabbage, carrots, beets, barley green, wheat grass, and berries.

For extra fiber and cancer-fighting phytonutrients known as lignans, take 4 tablespoons of ground flaxseeds daily with 10 ounces of water.

Food to Avoid

Do not eat foods that don't come from nature. Processed food, junk food, and anything containing chemicals, additives, or dyes should be banished from your menu.

Make every effort to avoid foods that have been sprayed, waxed, or otherwise treated. If you absolutely cannot avoid eating these foods, at least be sure to remove their peels, skins, or outer layers and to wash the food thoroughly in clean, quality water before eating.

While there's no evidence that refined sugar directly causes cancer, we do know that too much of it significantly depresses your immune system and feeds cancer. A weak immune system may leave you vulnerable to cancer, and it can also sap your ability to handle aggressive cancer treatment. Do not eat products containing refined sugar. This includes sodas, candy, cakes, and cookies, as well as store-bought juices and many processed foods. You should also restrict your intake of natural sugars. Go easy on homemade fruit juices and baked goods sweetened with molasses or honey.

Saturated, hydrogenated, and partially hydrogenated fats are linked to most degenerative disorders, and cancer is no exception. High consumption of these "bad" fats (as opposed to the "good" essential fatty acids found in cold-pressed oils and some fish) has been strongly linked to several types of cancer, including breast, prostate, and colorectal cancers. Avoid red meat, margarine, shortening, and products made with these foods. Especially carcinogenic are meats that have been grilled, charcoal-broiled, cured, or smoked. If you're trying to prevent cancer and want to enjoy red meat as an occasional treat, it would be wise to stay away from meats prepared in any of these manners, including hot dogs, cold cuts, and luncheon meats, as well as most types of bacon, ham, and sausage.

Be wary of alcohol. Heavy use is linked to mouth and throat cancers and possibly to cancer of the stomach, the colon, and the rectum. If you're a healthy person trying to avoid cancer, limit yourself to a glass or two of wine per week. If you have cancer, it's best to avoid alcohol entirely, as it depletes much-needed nutrients from your body.

Work with a holistic doctor to incorporate detoxification into your program. Fresh juicing, especially vegetable juicing, should be done daily. Start with 8 ounces daily and work up to 24 ounces daily.

None of us can completely avoid exposure to toxins, no matter how well we eat or change our lifestyle habits, so a person hoping to avoid cancer would do well to practice regular short fasts. You do not need to undertake the longer fasts recommended for a person diagnosed with cancer. Try doing a three-day juice fast once a month, or fast one day out of every week. These should be done under medical supervision.

There is research that a low-carbohydrate diet, known as the ketogenic diet, can benefit someone battling cancer when adopted immediately before chemotherapy and radiation. Speak with a holistic doctor about how to incorporate this treatment. A team of researchers from University of California, Los Angeles (UCLA) and collaborators from Memorial Sloan-Kettering Cancer Center and Weil-Cornell Medical College showed that depriving cancer cells of glucose does indeed cause them to die. When you take away the glucose your body responds by creating free radicals that destroy the cell.

Cancer cells have a huge appetite for glucose, a simple sugar. Cancer cells require a by-product of glucose metabolism for energy. Normal cells can use fats as fuel in addition to glucose. In 1924, German medical doctor, physiologist, and Nobel Laureate Otto Warburg discovered that cancer cells are fueled by the metabolism of sugar inside cells. He published several works on this concept, including *The Metabolism of Tumours*.

℞ Super Seven Prescriptions—Cancer Treatment

Super Prescription #1 Fermented wheat germ extract

Take 9 to 12 grams daily (powder form). This has been shown to combat a variety of cancers.

Super Prescription #2 Coriolus versicolor (*Trametes versicolor*)

Take 1,000 mg three times daily of the PSP or PSK standardized extracts on an empty stomach. Coriolus contains polysaccharides that have been shown to enhance immune function. It is mainly used for esophageal, lung, stomach, and colon cancer. *Note*: It can be safely used in conjunction with conventional treatment (surgery, chemotherapy, and radiation).

Super Prescription #3 Maitake (*Grifola frondosa*)

Take 0.5 to 1 mg of the standardized MD or D fraction per kg of body weight per day in divided doses on an empty stomach. Maitake enhances immune cells that fight cancer. It was found to be most effective for breast, prostate, liver, and lung cancers. *Note*: It can be safely used in conjunction with conventional treatment (surgery, chemotherapy, and radiation).

Super Prescription #4 Proteolytic enzymes

Take a complex of proteolytic enzymes (dependent on the dose of the formula, take as directed on the container) three times daily between meals. Proteolytic enzymes have been shown to have numerous anticancer effects. *Note*: They can be safely used in conjunction with conventional treatment (surgery—except not three days before or after surgery—chemotherapy, and radiation).

Green tea contains a powerful group of antioxidants known as polyphenols that prevent free radicals (unstable molecules) from damaging cell DNA and tissues of the body. If you're undergoing chemotherapy or radiation, check with your oncologist about the most recent research on green tea to make sure it's compatible with your therapy. A Japanese study found that five or more cups of green tea a day could slash the risk of blood and lymph-based cancers by about 50 percent.

Sixty-six patients with colorectal cancer were given a specific fermented wheat germ extract (FWGE) at a dose of 9 grams daily for at least six months in addition to anticancer treatments, while 104 patients received only conventional anticancer treatments. Those who took FWGE had fewer disease-progression-related events compared to the control group. There was also an improvement in the overall survival of the patients taking FWGE.

Super Prescription #5 Curcumin

Take 400 mg of curcumin extract three times daily on an empty stomach. This extract from turmeric has many different anticancer effects. *Note*: It can be safely used in conjunction with conventional treatment (surgery, chemotherapy, and radiation).

Super Prescription #6 Green tea

Drink five or more cups of organic green tea daily. If you are sensitive to caffeine, there are many brands that have the caffeine removed. Or take 1,500 mg daily of the capsule form standardized to contain at least 80 to 90 percent polyphenols and 35 to 55 percent epigallocatechin 3 gallate (EGCG).

Super Prescription #7 Astragalus (*Astragalus membranaceus*)

Take 1,000 mg or 4 ml of the tincture three times daily. Astragalus enhances natural-killer and other immune cells that fight cancer. *Note*: It can be safely used in conjunction with conventional treatment (surgery, chemotherapy, and radiation).

Coriolus Alleviates Side Effects of Chemotherapy and Radiation

A study at the University of Shanghai examined whether coriolus polysaccharides (PSP) could lessen the side effects of chemotherapy or radiation. In this study, 650 people with cancer who were undergoing chemotherapy and radiation were given either PSP or a placebo, and their side effects were assessed. Researchers used twenty different criteria to assess adverse reactions and determined that people receiving PSP had markedly fewer side effects than did those receiving placebo.

℞ Super Seven Prescriptions—Cancer Prevention

Super Prescription #1 Vitamin D3

Take 5,000 IU or more daily depending on your blood vitamin D levels. A variety of studies have demonstrated a cancer-protective effect of vitamin D.

Super Prescription #2 Green tea (*Camellia sinensis*)

Drink three to five cups of organic green tea daily. *Note*: If you are sensitive to caffeine, there are many brands that have the caffeine removed. Or take 1,500 mg daily of the capsule form standardized to contain at least 80 to 90 percent polyphenols and 35 to 55 percent epigallocatechin-3 gallate (EGCG).

Super Prescription #3 Probiotic

Take a product containing at least twenty billion organisms of the friendly bacteria per daily dose. These good bacteria support immune function, digestion, and detoxification of carcinogenic matter.

Super Prescription #4 Glutathione

Take 250 to 500 mg twice daily on an empty stomach. Glutathione protects against cell DNA damage and aids in DNA repair. It also supports detoxification of the cells and improves immunity.

Super Prescription #5 Fish oil

Take a daily dose of 1,000 mg of combined DHA and EPA. These essential fatty acids support healthy cell structure.

Super Prescription #6 Modified citrus pectin

Studies suggest that MCP reduces the risk of metastasis in prostate cancer. Take 10 mg of the powder form three times daily. *Note*: Do not use if you are taking blood-thinning medications.

Super Prescription #7 High-potency multivitamin

Take a high-potency multivitamin and -mineral formula, as directed on the container. It provides a base of nutrients and antioxidants for immune health.

Dr. Bruce Hollis, from the Medical University of South Carolina, completed a sixty-day study on thirty-seven men who were scheduled to undergo prostate-removal surgery. Before having the surgery the men were given either 4,000 IU of vitamin D daily or a placebo for sixty days. When the glands were removed and examined Dr. Hollis and his team found that the tumors in the men who had received the vitamin D supplements had improved, while the tumors removed from the men who had received placebos had stayed the same or gotten worse. The vitamin D had significantly reduced several markers of cell inflammation. In addition, the nutrient had stimulated an inflammation-reducing protein called growth differentiation factor 15 or GDF-15. Research has shown that aggressive prostate cancers often make little to no GDF-15.

General Recommendations

IP6 (inositol hexaphosphate) has been shown in studies to be an effective immune booster. Take 4 to 8 grams of IP6. *Note*: It can be safely used in conjunction with conventional treatment (surgery, chemotherapy, and radiation).

Quercitin is a type of flavonoid that has been shown to inhibit tumor formation in test-tube studies. Take 400 mg three times daily on an empty stomach.

Fish oil is an important supplement, especially in preventing cachexia (tissue wasting). Take a product that contains a daily combined total dosage of 1,500 to 2,000 mg of DHA and EPA.

Whey protein provides valuable support to the immune system. It also increases the levels of the important antioxidant glutathione. Take 25 grams twice daily as part of a protein shake or a smoothie.

A greens drink containing super green foods, such as chlorella, spirulina, wheatgrass, and others, supports detoxification and offers an array of phytonutrients and antioxidants that promote healthy cells. Take daily as directed on the container.

Animal studies have shown that modified citrus pectin (MCP) may prevent or slow the spread of prostate cancer and melanoma cells to other organs. Human cell research shows that MCP attaches to galectin-3, an element found on the surface of most cells. MCP attaches to the galectin-3 and prevents the cell from attaching to other cells. Galectin-3 is overly abundant on many tumor cells and seems to help them spread. In a male study, MCP was shown to increase the doubling time of prostate-specific antigen (PSA), suggesting a protective effect against prostate cancer.

Probiotic supplements are important for optimal immune function and for digestion and detoxification. Take a product containing a daily total of at least four billion active organisms.

Colostrum is a good supplement to support the immune system. Take 500 mg three times daily.

Indole-3-carbinol supports the detoxification of cancerous estrogen metabolites. Take 300 to 400 mg daily.

Melatonin has been shown in several studies to be helpful as an adjunctive therapy for certain types of cancers. It activates immune cells and improves the action of chemotherapy drugs and radiation. Take 20 mg or more under the direction and the guidance of a doctor.

Milk thistle (*Silybum marianum*) will protect your liver during chemotherapy and radiation treatments. Find a product standardized for 70 to 80 percent silymarin content, and take 150 to 200 mg twice a day.

A high-potency multivitamin and -mineral formula provides a base of nutrients for immune support. Take as directed on the container.

A substance called carnosol, which is found in rosemary, has been found to inhibit cancer in laboratory animals. Take 2 to 3 grams twice a day, or use 2 to 3 cc of a tincture three times daily.

If you are undergoing radiation treatment or chemotherapy, drink fennel tea to reduce the side effects.

Garlic (*Allium sativum*) strengthens the immune system. Take 300 to 450 mg twice a day. Aged garlic extract is preferred.

Cat's claw (*Uña de gato*) stimulates the activity of white blood cells. Take 500 mg or 1 to 2 cc twice a day.

Pau d'arco (*Tabebuia avellanedae*) is another highly potent immune system enhancer. Take 100 mg or 0.5 to 1.0 ml three times daily.

Take 300 mg of echinacea (*Echinacea purpurea*) three times a day for its immune-boosting properties.

Take 5,000 to 10,000 mg or more of vitamin C in divided doses. One technique is to buildup to as high a dosage as you can tolerate. When diarrhea occurs, cut back on the dosage. Intravenous vitamin C can be administered in very therapeutic levels by a doctor who is trained in intravenous therapy.

If cancer treatment is making you nauseated, drink peppermint or ginger tea to soothe your stomach.

Homeopathy

Homeopathic treatment can be helpful for someone with cancer but requires a skilled homeopathic practitioner. The following remedies can be used safely to reduce the side effects of chemotherapy and radiation. Pick the remedy that best matches your symptoms described in this section. For acute symptoms, take a 30C potency four times daily. After you notice improvement, stop taking the remedy, unless symptoms return.

Cadmium Sulphuratum is used to prevent and treat fatigue, vomiting, and loss of hair.

Ipecacuanha (*Cephaelis ipecacuanha*) is for persistent nausea and vomiting when vomiting does not provide any relief from symptoms.

Nux Vomica is for symptoms of heartburn, reflux, constipation, and nausea. The person feels irritable and chilly.

Traditional Chinese Medicine

Many Chinese patent herbal remedies can strengthen your immune system and help you fight infection while undergoing conventional treatment. Consult a TCM practitioner for a combination that meets your individual needs.

Acupressure

See pages 787–794 for information about acupressure points and administering treatment.

- Liver 4 (LV4) is the point for general pain relief.
- Kidney 27 (K27), Bladder 23 (B23), Bladder 47 (B47), Conception Vessel 6 (CV6), and Stomach 36 (St36) all strengthen the immune system.

Bodywork

Massage

Massage won't cure cancer, but while you're undergoing conventional treatments, the compassionate touch of a massage therapist can be quite welcoming. Depending upon your individual need, you can ask for a relaxing massage or an invigorating one. Check with your doctor first before starting massage to make sure it's not a problem with your type of cancer.

Reflexology

See pages 804–805 for information about reflexology areas and how to work them. When time permits, work the whole foot to stimulate all areas of your body's defense and promote a general sense of well-being.

If you have a limited amount of time, focus on the region or the regions where the growth is located. You should also work the liver and the colon to facilitate detoxification.

Hydrotherapy

Many cancer patients have responded well to fever therapy, which stimulates the body's immune response in the same way that a fever does. It also pulls toxins from the body and expels them as you sweat. At the very least, hydrotherapy will help fight bacteria or viruses that may be trying to take advantage of your body's weakened state. Saunas also can be used. We recommend constitutional hydrotherapy, which you can do at home. See the Hydrotherapy chapter for directions.

Intravenous vitamin C is gaining acceptance as a complementary therapy based on an increasing number of studies. It can be used to enhance the quality of life for people with cancer (and other diseases). Two published studies have demonstrated this benefit. One found that IV vitamin C significantly reduced side effects caused by the cancer, chemotherapy, or radiation, including nausea, loss of appetite, fatigue, depression, sleep disorders, dizziness and bleeding. No side effects were documented.

Intravenous ozone therapy is used by doctors around the world for its ability to oxidize cancer cells and enhance immunity.

Aromatherapy

Juniper breaks down toxins that are hiding in fatty deposits. To bolster the detoxifying effects of a lymphatic massage, ask your massage therapist to use an oil mixed with a little juniper. You can also add a few drops of juniper to your bath.

If you are fatigued, use rose, geranium, or jasmine for an energy lift. You can employ these oils in almost any preparation, but for all-day relief, you may want to place a few drops in a diffuser and let the scent waft throughout your room.

Lavender and melissa are calming when you feel anxious and stressed. Warming oils like black pepper, rosemary, and ginger can help relieve pain. Add them to a bath, a compress, or a lotion.

Tea tree oil (*Melaleuca alternifolia*) is antibacterial, antifungal, and antiviral. When treatment has left you vulnerable to infection or if you're exposed to a contagious illness like the flu, take a hot bath and run a few drops of tea tree oil under the tap. (Add just two or three drops for your first use, as this oil can be irritating to some people.)

If cancer treatment leaves you feeling queasy or downright sick, you can use peppermint or ginger oils to calm your stomach. If your nausea is unpredictable, try carrying a vial around with you; place the vial under your nose and inhale deeply as needed. You can also make a lotion or a cream with either oil and rub it into your skin. The scent will stay with you and reduce your chances of feeling ill.

Stress Reduction

General Stress-Reduction Therapies

Stress is a carcinogen, just like radiation and pesticides. Reducing stress has an inhibiting effect on tumor growth; it will also improve the quality of your life during treatment. Support groups are an excellent way to handle stress and reduce tension.

One famous study of breast-cancer patients showed that women who discussed their problems in support groups lived a full two years longer than women who did not.

It's a good idea to supplement weekly sessions with daily stress-reducing exercise and other stress-reducing techniques. A variety of studies have shown that regular exercise reduces the risk of some cancers, including breast, colon, endometrium, advanced prostate, and possibly pancreatic.

Cancer also causes stress. In order to keep yourself in peak fighting condition, do everything you can to avoid tense situations, even those that you usually accept as a normal part of a full life. This is the time to unload a demanding project at work or to avoid your personal stress triggers, like crowded roads or difficult relatives.

Other Recommendations

- One of the most avoidable—but most prevalent—carcinogens is cigarette smoke. Everyone knows it causes lung cancer, but the free radicals produced by inhaling smoke may contribute to many other forms of the disease. Do not smoke, not even socially, and do not expose yourself to secondhand smoke.
- As much as possible, avoid radiation. Do not sit or stand close to television sets or microwave ovens (a distance of about eight feet is preferable). If you work on a computer, invest in a radiation screen. And limit X-rays to those that are absolutely necessary for your health.
- You must also avoid harsh chemicals. A good rule of thumb is to stay away

from any substance that releases fumes. Nail polish remover, hair spray, gasoline, household cleaners, and dry-cleaning solvent are all dangerous.

- Establish a healthy relationship with the sun. You need about fifteen minutes of sunshine a day to keep your body in proper working order, but sunburn and prolonged exposure can result in skin cancer. (The sun is, after all, a source of radiation.) Try to get your daily dose of sunlight in the early morning hours, when the rays are weak; if you must go out in broad daylight, wear protective clothing and use sunscreen.

- Radon is a radioactive gas that is strongly linked to lung cancer. It's usually found in the soil, but it may seep out, contaminating the air in your house and the water you drink. Radon cannot be detected with the senses, so you should buy a radon test kit and use it in your home. Should you have a radon problem, you can insulate your home by sealing up leaks.

- A sexually transmitted organism called human papilloma virus is a leading cause of cervical cancer, so do not engage in sexual intercourse with people whose sexual histories you do not know. Don't rely on condoms to protect you, as the virus can pass through them.

REFERENCES

Chen, Q., et al. 2005. Pharmacologic ascorbic acid concentrations selectively kill cancer cells: Action as a pro-drug to deliver hydrogen peroxide to tissues. *Proceedings of the National Academy of Sciences of the United States of America* 102:13604–9.

Guess, B.W., M. C. Scholz, S. B. Strum, et al. 2003. Modified citrus pectin (MCP) increases the prostate-specific antigen doubling time in men with prostate cancer: A phase II pilot study. *Prostate Cancer Prostatic Dis* 6(4):301–4.

Hollis, D. Vitamin D may keep low-grade prostate cancer from becoming aggressive. Accessed March 22, 105 at http://www.newswise.com/articles/vitamin-d-may-keep-low-grade-prostate-cancer-from-becoming-aggressive. 249th National Meeting & Exposition of the American Chemical Society (ACS).

Jakab, F., et al. 2003. A medical nutriment has supportive value in the treatment of colorectal cancer. *British Journal of Cancer* 89:465–69.

Mavlit, G., Y. Ishii, Y. Patt, et al. 1979. Local xenogenic graft-vs-host reaction: A practical assessment of T-cell function among cancer patients. *Journal of Immunology* 123(5):2185–88.

Naganuma, T., et al. Green tea consumption and hematologic malignancies in Japan—The ohsaki study. *American Journal of Epidemiology.* Published online ahead of print, doi:10.1093/aje/kwp187.

Nakachi, K., K. Suemasu, K. Suga, et al. 1998. Influence of drinking green tea on breast cancer malignancy among Japanese patients. *Japanese Journal of Cancer Research* 89(3):254–61.

Nanba, H. 1999. Presented at the 3rd International Conference on Mushroom Biology and Mushroom Products in Sydney, Australia.

Strum, S., et al. 1999. Modified citrus pectin slows PSA doubling time: A pilot clinical trial. Presentation: International Conference on Diet and Prevention of Cancer, Ampere, Finland. May 28–June 2.

Sun, Z., et al. 1999. The ameliorative effect of PSP on the toxic and side reaction of chemo and radiotherapy of cancers. In *Advanced Research in PSP*, ed. Q. Yang. Hong Kong: Hong Kong Association for Health Care Ltd.

Torisu, M., Y. Hayashi, T. Ishimitsu, et al. 1990. Significant prolongation of disease-free period gained by oral polysaccharide K (PSK) administration after curative surgical operation of colorectal cancer. *Cancer Immunology and Immunotherapy* 31(5):261–68.

Vollbracht, C., et al. 2011. Intravenous vitamin C administration improves quality of life in breast cancer patients during chemo-radiotherapy and aftercare: Results of a retrospective, multicentre, epidemiological cohort study in Germany. *In Vivo* 82:983–90.

Candidiasis (Thrush and Yeast Infection)

Candida albicans is one of the many types of fungi that live and grow inside most human bodies. Normally, candida causes no harm; our bodies are equipped with probiotic (or "friendly") bacteria and immune cells that keep it under control. However, some medications, high-sugar diets, allergies, and other factors can cause the friendly bacteria to die, leaving candida free to grow unchecked in parts or all of the body.

The medical name for this overgrowth is candidiasis, but most people know the condition as either thrush or a yeast infection. Thrush is marked by soft white patches in the oral cavity, around the anus, or on the skin. It most often appears in babies and in the elderly, but people with seriously compromised immune systems— such as those who have AIDS or who are undergoing chemotherapy—are also quite vulnerable. Many conventional doctors do not believe that such a condition exists except in cases of a seriously compromised immune system such as AIDS. Our view is different, and we find that many people with chronic fatigue or chronic digestive, neurological, autoimmune, or other chronic health conditions have problems with yeast overgrowth.

A vaginal yeast infection, by far the more common manifestation of candidiasis, causes burning, itching, and soreness in the vagina, along with a thick, sticky discharge. It's often the result of antibiotic use, poor diet, hormone imbalance, or a combination of these causes.

Sometimes the fungus spreads throughout the entire body in a condition known as systemic candidiasis. This disorder can produce any of a wide variety of symptoms and is often at the root of a persistent, mysterious illness. If you feel sick but are told by doctors that nothing is wrong, there's a good chance that you're actually suffering from systemic candidiasis. For people with dramatically weakened immune systems, systemic candidiasis is a grave threat, as the fungus can actually poison the blood.

Holistic treatments, which emphasize therapies that reduce the levels of candida to normal levels, are the best ways to resolve this condition. Depending on the person, several steps are often required for success in treating candida overgrowth. This requires treating the underlying cause(s). One of the obvious steps is to eliminate or cut down on simple sugars, alcohol, and so on, which feed yeast. Also, direct therapy that destroys candida works to assist the body in getting candida levels down to a controllable level. Common examples include oregano oil and garlic.

However, many chronic cases require a change in the biological terrain. By this, we mean the state and the health of the digestive tract, the organs of detoxification and elimination, the immune system, and hormone balance. In particular, one often needs to improve digestion and elimination. The by-products of poor digestion can form metabolites that can promote candida growth. Leaky gut syndrome, as the result of intestinal permeability, is often a root problem of chronic candida. It is also imperative to promote the growth of the friendly flora that inhabit the digestive tract and many other areas of the body. These good bacteria are an essential component of the immune system that keep yeast levels in check. Also, keep in mind that uncontrolled stress can alter flora balance and can suppress immune function. And finally, hormone balance is important, especially for women. The use of the birth-control pill or other forms of synthetic hormones may set the stage for candida overgrowth. Additionally, toxic metals such as mercury suppress healthy gut flora and suppress immunity.

In some cases, antifungal medications may be required. They, of course, should be used sparingly and with close supervision. They are not a magic bullet, and the root causes described in this chapter must still be addressed for long-term success.

There is evidence that fungal organisms such as candida may be a root cause of blood sugar disorders such as diabetes, a variety of digestive ailments, and possibly even cancer.

SYMPTOMS OF THRUSH

- White patches on the inside of the mouth
- Inflamed red patches on the skin
- Bad breath
- Heavily coated tongue
- Dry mouth

SYMPTOMS OF YEAST INFECTION

- Vaginal itching, pain, and burning
- Burning during urination
- Thick yellow discharge

SYMPTOMS OF SYSTEMATIC CANDIDIASIS

The list of symptoms that systematic candidiasis can cause is too long to print here, but following are some of the most common:

- Persistent fatigue
- Rectal itching
- Constipation
- Kidney and bladder infections
- Diarrhea
- Muscle pain
- Colitis
- Arthritis
- Abdominal pain
- Canker sores
- Congestion
- Cough
- Headaches
- Numbness or tingling in the limbs
- Poor memory and concentration
- Mood problems (depression, anxiety)
- Chronic skin rashes
- Genital or toenail fungus
- Allergies
- Blood sugar imbalance

ROOT CAUSES

- Prolonged or frequent use of antibiotics or corticosteroids, leading to a depletion of good bacteria
- Poor digestion and elimination
- A depressed immune system
- A high-sugar diet

- Allergies
- Stress
- Hormonal changes and birth-control pills
- Aging
- Mercury toxicity

Testing Techniques

The following tests help assess possible metabolic reasons for candidiasis:
    Candida levels—stool, blood (antibodies), or urine (yeast metabolites)
    Intestinal permeability—urine test

TREATMENT

Diet

Recommended Food

For high-density nutrition and immune support, base your meals around fresh vegetables, whole grains, and quality sources of lean protein, such as beans, lentils, fish, and organic poultry.

To replace friendly bacteria, eat unsweetened yogurt daily. Make sure the brand you're using has live yogurt cultures. Sauerkraut and miso are other examples of foods that contain friendly bacteria.

Vegetable and green drinks will improve your resistance. Drink eight glasses of clean, quality water a day to help flush yeast toxins out.

Consume 1 to 2 tablespoons of ground flaxseeds daily. Flaxseeds have antifungal properties.

Food to Avoid

The fungus that causes candidiasis feeds on sugar and yeast, so you must absolutely avoid all foods (especially alcohol) containing these substances during the initial phase of treatment.

Many people with candidiasis also have undiagnosed allergies. See the Food Allergies entry on pages 312–317 to determine whether you're one of them.

During the course of your infection, avoid foods with mold (aged cheese, nuts, and nut butters).

Bacteria Basics

Many cultured and sour products contain the friendly bacteria that will prevent candidiasis and many other infections. Yogurt can be an especially good source, but you need to shop carefully—many mass-produced yogurt products just don't have enough of the bacteria you need. When you're reading labels, look for one or more of these Latin names:

    Lactobacillus acidophilus
    Bifidobacterium bifidum
    Lactobacillus bulgaricus
    Streptococcus thermophilus

When buying yogurt, be sure the label or the container lists yogurt cultures that are "live," "living," or "active." And since sugar encourages the growth of *Candida albicans*, buy unsweetened yogurt only.

Avoid refined foods that are likely to be loaded with sugars. Avoid or reduce the use of fruits and fruit juices during the initial phase (first month) of treatment. It is especially important to avoid these foods between meals.

℞ Super Seven Prescriptions—Candidiasis

Super Prescription #1 Oregano (*Origanum vulgare*) oil
Take a 300 to 500 mg capsule or the liquid form (as directed on the container) three times daily with meals (to avoid digestive upset).

Super Prescription #2 Probiotic
Take a product containing at least twenty billion active organisms twice daily, thirty minutes after a meal. It supplies friendly bacteria, such as acidophilus and bifidus, which fight candida and prevent its overgrowth.

Super Prescription #3 Garlic (*Allium sativum*)
Take 500 to 1,000 mg of aged garlic twice daily. Garlic fights fungal infections and also boosts immune strength.

Super Prescription #4 Grapefruit seed extract
Take 200 mg two to three times daily. Practitioners rely on this herb for its anti candida properties.

Super Prescription #5 Caprylic acid
Take 1,000 mg three times daily. This type of fatty acid has been shown in studies to have antifungal properties.

Super Prescription #6 Gentian root (*Gentiana lutea*)
Take 250 mg or 0.5 to 1.0 ml at the beginning of each meal. It improves stomach acid levels and overall digestive function. It's often used with other bitter herbals.

Super Prescription #7 Echinacea (*Echinacea purpurea*) and goldenseal (*Hydrastis canadensis*) combination
Take 500 mg or 2 to 4 ml of tincture three times daily. Both herbs enhance immune function. Echinacea has been shown to have anti yeast effects.

A study compared the anti-candida effect of oregano oil to that of caprylic acid. Researchers found that oregano oil is over one hundred times more potent than caprylic acid against candida.

General Recommendations

Pau d'arco (*Tabebuia avellanedae*) has strong antibacterial and antifungal properties. No matter what kind of candida infection you have, drink several cups of this tea every day.

Peppermint (*Mentha piperita*) oil relieves the intestinal cramping often associated with candida. Studies also show that it has antifungal properties. Take 1 or 2 enteric-coated capsules or 0.2 ml of peppermint oil two or three times daily.

Wormwood (*Artemisia absinthium*), Oregon grape (*Berberis aquifolium*), and rosemary (*Rosmarinus officinalis*) all have antifungal properties. Take as part of a candida formula.

Tea tree oil (*Melaleuca alternifolia*) is mainly used topically for skin-related yeast infections. The tincture form can also be mixed in water (5 to 15 drops) and swished in the mouth for treating thrush.

A high-potency multivitamin provides the many nutrients used to support detoxification.

Vitamin C is used to enhance immune function. Take 1,000 mg two or three times daily.

Milk thistle (*Silybum marianum*), reishi (*Ganoderma lucidum*), and dandelion (*Taraxacum officinale*) are herbs used individually or in formulas to support liver and kidney detoxification while you undergo an anticandida program. Generally, you take 1 or 2 capsules with each meal or as directed on the container.

Betaine HCL, taken with meals, improves stomach acid levels and absorption. Take 1 or 2 capsules with meals.

Enzymes also support digestion when taken with meals. Protease enzymes, taken between meals, may have antifungal effects and reduce inflammation.

Colloidal silver kills candida. Take as directed on the label.

Homeopathy

See a qualified homeopathic practitioner for an individually prescribed remedy. For specific problems related to candida, see the corresponding sections in this book, such as AIDS, Constipation, Diarrhea, Headache, and so on. Otherwise, try the following recommendation:

Candida Albicans 6x, 12x, or 30x. This is a homeopathic preparation of candida that can be used to stimulate the immune system to target candida organisms. Take 2 pellets three times daily.

Acupressure

See pages 787–794 for information about acupressure points and administering treatment.

If candidiasis is accompanied by nervousness and stress, massage Large Intestine 4 (LI4) and Liver 3 (LV3).

Bodywork

Massage

Any massage, especially with one of the relaxing oils listed in Aromatherapy, below, is wonderful for reducing stress. If you have a yeast infection and prefer to remain clothed, try a shoulder, a head, or a foot rub. Lymphatic massage is particularly good to support detoxification for people undergoing treatment for chronic candida.

Reflexology

See pages 804–805 for information about reflexology areas and how to work them.

Work the areas that correspond to the location of your symptoms. For thrush, massage the head region. For a yeast infection, concentrate on the pelvic area. If you have systematic candidiasis, work the entire foot or the hand.

Aromatherapy

- To relax and reduce stress, try any of the following in a bath, in steam inhalation, or in a diffuser: chamomile, jasmine, lavender, or rose.
- Tea tree oil, peppermint, and myrrh all have a natural antifungal action. Use any one of them in a massage, a bath, or a compress. Tea tree oil can sometimes be irritating, so if you're adding it to a bath or a compress, use just a few drops.

Stress Reduction

General Stress-Reduction Therapies

High levels of stress have been implicated in candida infections. If you're prone to candidiasis, any stress-reduction technique is likely to help. Exercise, yoga, and prayer are very good.

Other Recommendations

- Whether you have thrush, a yeast infection, or systemic candidiasis, change your toothbrush monthly to avoid reinfecting yourself.
- For a yeast infection, wear cotton underwear and loose clothes to keep the area dry.
- If you have a yeast infection, you can apply live yogurt locally to replace probiotic bacteria. Spoon the yogurt onto a towel or a sanitary pad, or douche with yogurt and distilled water.
- Be aware that sexual intercourse can spread candida. Partners should both be treated if vaginitis is a chronic problem.

REFERENCES

Stiles, J. C. 1995. The inhibition of Candida albicans by oregano. *Journal of Applied Nutrition* 47:96–102.

Cardiovascular Disease

Numerous disorders fall under the broad category of heart and vascular disease. Here, discussion is restricted to arteriosclerosis, angina, and heart attack. For related subjects, see High Blood Pressure and Stroke.

According to the Centers for Disease Control and Prevention, more than one out of every four deaths in the United States is attributable to heart disease. Coronary heart disease is the most common form of heart disease.

Arteries transport blood from the heart and deliver it to other parts of the body. Arteriosclerosis occurs when the inside of the artery wall thickens, leaving a narrower passageway for the blood to travel through. This disorder is often called hardening of the arteries. Arteriosclerosis can affect the coronary arteries—the arteries that lead to the heart—and is usually caused by a buildup of fatty deposits within the arterial walls. This buildup is often the result of a poor diet, one that's high in bad fats and low in fiber. Most people who have arteriosclerosis are not aware of it, as it does not trigger symptoms in the body until later in the disease.

Unfortunately, when arteriosclerosis is left untreated, it just gets worse. Without treatment, the arteries will eventually become so constricted that adequate supplies of oxygenated blood can't reach the heart muscle. This oxygen deprivation may result in the chest pain known as angina. Angina is often a precursor to a heart attack.

In some ways, people with angina are lucky. Their pain usually leads to a diagnosis of cardiovascular disease, and they can then take several steps to slow or reverse their condition before it results in a trip to the emergency room or even death. But for many, a heart attack is the first outward sign of trouble; 25 percent of people who suffer heart attacks have never felt any previous symptoms. A heart attack—or myocardial infarction, as it's called by doctors—is brought on when blood flow to a section of the heart muscle is completely cut off, either because a clot has backed up behind a thickened artery, or because the artery itself has become so narrow that no blood at all can pass through. If you ever suspect that you are having a heart attack, you must receive emergency medical care at once. Instead of having someone drive you to a hospital (unless you are really close), call for an ambulance. Life-saving treatment for heart attacks requires special medical techniques and tools, and the sooner professionals arrive with their equipment, the greater your chances of survival.

Heart disease is so prevalent now, most people are surprised to hear that it was actually quite rare until the turn of the twentieth century. Our modern diet and way of life are at the root of most heart problems, and the best way to prevent or reverse heart disease is to change our habits. Because heart disease is caused by a variety of factors, it is best to include several kinds of therapies in your treatment or prevention plan. Eat well, exercise, manage stress, and identify and treat genetic susceptibilities that are known to bring on cardiovascular disease.

In recent years, researchers have found that chronic inflammation in the blood vessels is a central factor in the development of heart disease. This chronic inflammation leads to arterial wall damage and the resulting plaque formation. Although cholesterol levels have some importance, it appears that this substance is not the "villain" that it was once thought to be. While diet and lifestyle factors are root causes of chronic inflammation, there are also genetic reasons beyond inheriting a disposition to high cholesterol levels. They include one's levels of homocysteine, insulin, HDL and LDL particle sizes, damaged or oxidized LDL levels, stress-hormone imbalance, nutritional deficiencies, and hereditary factors. Fortunately, genetic susceptibilities can be reduced through natural therapies. Stealth or hidden infections in the body are also suspected of increasing the inflammatory response. Therefore, it is imperative that you are tested for these newer, more predictive markers of heart disease.

Finally, the impact of stress and negative emotions cannot be underrated as a cause of heart disease.

SYMPTOMS OF ARTERIOSCLEROSIS

There are usually no overt symptoms until later in the disease. See your doctor if you experience any of the following:

- Dizziness
- Fainting
- Leg pain that starts after walking a short distance and goes away with rest

SYMPTOMS OF ANGINA

- Mild to severe chest pain, often feeling like the heart is being squeezed
- Pain that feels worse after exercise or a heavy meal and better when resting
- Tightness in the chest

SYMPTOMS OF HEART ATTACK

If you have any of the following symptoms, call 911 immediately. Even if the symptoms pass, you need emergency medical attention.

- The classic symptoms are crushing or tight pain in the chest, which may extend to the arms, the back, the shoulders, the neck, or the jaw. The pain may be intense and severe, or it could be so mild that you might mistake it for indigestion.
- Women sometimes have heart attack symptoms that are different from the ones listed above. The pain may begin in the stomach or the jaw or as stabbing pains between the breasts. The symptoms in general may be more vague than for men.
- Other possible symptoms include profuse sweating, a drop in blood pressure, difficulty swallowing, dizziness or faintness, ringing in the ears, or, more rarely, nausea and vomiting.

ROOT CAUSES

- Poor diet, especially one that's high in fat and low in fiber and antioxidants
- Genetics
- Smoking
- High blood pressure
- Low levels of omega-3 fatty acids, vitamin K, magnesium, coenzyme Q10, and other nutrients
- Stress, depression, and anxiety
- Obesity
- Inactivity
- Diabetes and syndrome X
- Stealth infections
- Excess of toxic metals and other toxins such as air pollutants
- Elevated iron level

Testing Techniques

The following tests help assess possible metabolic reasons for cardiovascular disease. We have included both the historic markers and the new ones. These are all blood tests.

Historic Markers

Total cholesterol

Normal range is 165–200 mg/dL.

LDL cholesterol

Normal range is below 130 mg/dL.

HDL cholesterol
>   Normal range is 50 mg/dL or higher.

Triglycerides
>   Normal range is less than 150 mg/dL.

New Markers

Testing that measures LDL and HDL particle size and other cholesterol subtypes is very important.

C-reactive protein is a marker of inflammation in the body, including in the blood vessel walls. It is considered a predictor of heart disease.
>   Normal range is less than 1.0 mg/dL.

Homocysteine—Buildup of this toxic metabolite increases plaque formation in the artery walls. Genetics, low thyroid, B-vitamin deficiencies, and a diet high in animal protein increase the level.
>   Normal range is less than 10 micromol/L.

Lipoprotein(a) is a more specific cholesterol marker and a stronger risk factor than is LDL cholesterol.
>   Normal range is less than 32 mg/dL.

Fibrinogen plays an important role in blood clotting. Elevated levels increase the risk of stroke and coronary artery disease.
>   Normal range is 200–400 mg/dL.

Apolipoprotein B is a type of lipid that binds to LDL cholesterol and accelerates plaque formation.
>   Normal range is 55–125 mg/dL.

Apolipoprotein A-1 is found in HDL cholesterol and provides a protective effect against heart disease.
>   Normal range is 125–215 mg/dL.

The ratio between apolipoproteins B and A-1 is considered a good overall predictor of heart disease risk.
>   Normal range is 0.30–0.90.

Glucose—Diabetes predisposes one to early heart disease.
>   Normal range is between 80 and 110 mg/dL.

Insulin—Elevation of this hormone is seen with syndrome X, a condition characterized by rising blood sugar and insulin levels. Spiked insulin levels increase arterial inflammation, as well as triglyceride, cholesterol, and blood pressure levels. They also contribute to weight gain.
>   Normal range is between 4 and 15 micromol (fasting).

Iron—Excessive iron in the body produces free radicals and oxidative damage.
>   Normal range is less than 150 mg/dL.

Abnormal LDL density pattern.
>   Normal is pattern A.

Recent research has shown that measuring oxidized LDL, or damaged LDL cholesterol, is important. Oxidized LDL can lead to inflammation in your arteries. Inflammation attracts immune cells into your arteries, creating more inflammation, which leads to formation of plaque and loss of elasticity. The less flexible your arteries, the more apt they are to rupture. So not only do you build plaque more readily when your LDL becomes oxidized, your arteries become less flexible and and more prone to rupture and the formation of blood clots. Causes of oxidized LDL may include too few antioxidants in the diet, pollution exposure, and stress.

TREATMENT

The following therapies are recommended as ongoing support for your heart. They are not treatments for a heart attack. If you suspect that you're having a heart attack, get emergency medical help immediately.

Diet

When most people think of diets to prevent or reverse heart disease, they think of reducing cholesterol and fat. In reality, many other factors must be taken into account, such as an adequate intake of "good" fats, fiber, and antioxidants. A heart-healthy diet, in fact, is much like the basic wholesome eating plan this book suggests for almost everyone.

Recommended Food

A whole-foods, plant-based diet (with the addition of fish) has been shown to sweep away arterial plaque. Your meals should emphasize vegetables, fruits, and whole grains, with soy products, beans, and fish for protein. People who require a higher-protein diet can add more lean poultry to their menu.

Highly reactive molecules known as free radicals are closely linked to heart disease. Foods that contain antioxidants will help prevent damage caused by free radicals, so eat a wide variety of fruits and vegetables every day.

Essential fatty acids are "good" fats that actually protect the heart and help the rest of the body function smoothly. Essential fatty acids are found in cold-water fish like halibut, salmon, and mackerel; raw nuts (excluding peanuts); olive oil; and flaxseeds.

Eat lots of fiber. A whole-foods diet will automatically increase your fiber intake, but if you need more, include oat bran or flaxseeds with your meals.

Garlic and onions reduce levels of bad cholesterol and lower the blood pressure. They make excellent additions to low-fat meals, like vegetable stir-fries, clear soups, and bean dishes.

The skins of red or purple grapes help clear the arteries of plaque. Have a glass of purple grape juice daily.

Potassium and magnesium are heart-protective minerals. Good sources include green vegetables, whole grains, wheat germ, soybeans, garlic, legumes, bok choy, and potatoes. Sea salt, listed previously, is another good choice.

A four-year study published in the *Journal of the American Heart Association* found that people following the Mediterranean diet could reduce their risk of a heart attack by as much as 70 percent.

The Mediterranean diet is associated with a lower incidence of coronary heart disease. It has also been shown to improve the prognosis of those with existing coronary heart disease. One study involved more than twenty-six hundred elderly people who had had a heart attack. Following a Mediterranean diet was associated with an 18 percent lower overall mortality rate than in those who followed a non-Mediterranean diet over a 6.7-year median follow-up.

Follow the Mediterranean diet, which includes the following:
- High consumption of fruits, vegetables, grains, potatoes, beans, nuts, and seeds
- Olive oil
- Low to moderate amounts of dairy, fish, and poultry
- Little red meat
- Eggs zero to four times a week
- Wine in low to moderate amounts

Food to Avoid

If you have heart disease, you must eliminate or drastically reduce your consumption of harmful fats (trans-fatty acids, or hydrogenated fats). Sweet baked goods, for instance, are likely to contain eggs and butter, as well as other fats and oils.

Don't make the mistake of substituting margarine or vegetable shortening for butter. These products are made with oils that have been artificially processed under high heat. This processing creates mutated molecules, called trans-fatty acids, that are most likely even worse for your heart and cholesterol levels than saturated fats are.

People who cut down on fat sometimes end up gorging themselves on non- and low-fat processed foods, especially packaged cookies and other sweets. Avoid this trap. These foods have little or no nutritional content, and they rely on sugar to make up for the elimination of fat. Excess sugar is tied to a number of health problems, and when used as a replacement for starch, it reduces the level of good, heart-protecting cholesterol.

Avoid simple sugars. Simple sugars cause elevated levels of cholesterol, triglycerides, C-reactive protein, insulin, and other markers that contribute to cardiovascular damage.

Radically reduce your consumption of sodium. Packaged and processed foods are by far the highest source of sodium in the Western diet, so stay away from them. A high sodium intake, combined with a low potassium intake, increases your likelihood of having high blood pressure.

℞ Super Seven Prescriptions—Cardiovascular Disease

Super Prescription #1 Magnesium
Take 500 mg daily. The heart uses this mineral to produce energy for contraction and regular rhythm. It also relaxes the blood vessel walls, for improved circulation and reduced blood pressure.

Super Prescription #2 Coenzyme Q10
Take 100 to 300 mg daily. This nutrient is used by the heart cells to pump efficiently and with regular rhythm. Studies show that it lowers blood pressure and helps improve angina, mitral valve prolapse, and congestive heart failure. It also prevents the oxidation of LDL cholesterol.

Super Prescription #3 Fish oil
Take 3,000 to 6,000 mg daily of combined EPA and DHA. Fish oil reduces inflammation in the arteries, lowers triglycerides and cholesterol, lowers blood pressure, and is a natural blood thinner. If you are on blood-thinning medication, consult your doctor about the appropriate dosage for you.

Super Prescription #4 Garlic (*Allium sativum*)

Take 300 to 500 mg of aged garlic twice daily. It reduces cholesterol and homocysteine, has a natural blood-thinning effect, and has antioxidant properties.

Super Prescription #5 Omega-7 fatty acids

Shown in human studies to improve lipid profiles and in animal studies to afford an antiplaque benefit. Take 420 mg of a fatty acid ethyl ester blend.

Super Prescription #6 Hawthorn (*Crataegus oxycantha*)

Take 500 to 900 mg daily. It improves circulation to the heart and reduces blood pressure.

Super Prescription #7 Niacin

Take 500 mg two or three times daily. This redices total, LDL, VLDL, and lipoprotein(a) cholesterol and increases good HDL cholesterol.

General Recommendations

Antioxidant formulas contain a wide spectrum of antioxidants that prevent the oxidative damage of cholesterol. Take as directed on the container.

Ginkgo biloba improves blood flow, has antioxidant benefits, and has blood-thinning properties. Select an extract made with 24 percent ginkgo flavone glycosides and take 80 to 120 mg twice a day.

Vitamin K2 prevents calcification of the arteries. Take 500 mcg to 2,000 mcg daily. If you are on a blood-thinning medication check with your doctor first.

Gooseberry (*Phyllanthus emblica*) has been shown to increase good HDL cholesterol and to lower LDL cholesterol. Take 500 to 1,000 mg daily.

Vitamin E has well-researched cardioprotective properties as an antioxidant and a blood thinner. Take 400 to 800 IU of a vitamin-E complex containing tocotrienols and tocopherols. If you are on blood-thinning medication, take E-complex under the guidance of a doctor at a lower dosage.

Vitamin C prevents cholesterol oxidation and mildly lowers blood pressure. Take up to 3,000 mg daily.

Red yeast rice (*Monascus purpureus*) lowers LDL cholesterol and reduces heart-related deaths. Take 1,200 to 2,400 mg daily.

Cayenne (*Capsicum frutescens*) extract reduces cholesterol levels and improves circulation. Take 500 mg two to three times daily.

Green tea reduces cholesterol oxidation. Take 250 to 500 mg of a standardized extract two to three times daily.

D-ribose is a naturally occurring sugar that fuels the heart for more effective contractions. Take 5 grams twice daily.

L-carnitine is a nutrient that aids normal heart contractions and rhythm. Take 1,500 to 3,000 mg daily.

According to a review of analyses in *Fundamental and Clinical Pharmacology*, consuming dietary fish oil or taking fish oil supplements is associated with a 16 percent reduction in deaths from any cause and a 24 percent reduction in deaths from heart attack in people with or without cardiovascular disease.

Researchers at UCLA Medical Center completed a one-year, double-blind, randomized clinical study with people taking aged garlic extract. Researchers found that people taking aged garlic extract had significantly less coronary plaque formation than did those in the placebo group. Also, the group supplementing the garlic tended to have lower blood homocysteine and cholesterol levels.

New Risk Markers and Their Supplement Solutions

If testing shows that your levels of these markers are elevated, the following supplements can be helpful:

Researchers from Central South University in China studied the effect of red yeast rice extract on the risk of heart disease in 591 Chinese people with a history of diabetes and cardiovascular disease. The group receiving red yeast rice had half as many new coronary events, including nonfatal heart attacks, sudden death from cardiac causes, and other heart-related deaths. Those taking red yeast rice were also 44 percent less likely to die from cancer and stroke than were people in the placebo group.

C-reactive protein
    Vitamin C: 1,000 to 3,000 mg daily
    Vitamin E: 400 to 800 IU daily
    Fish oil: 5,000 mg daily
    Gamma linoleic acid (GLA): 250 to 500 mg daily
    Bromelain: 500 mg three times daily, between meals

Lipoprotein(a)
    Niacin (flush free): 1,500 mg twice daily
    Coenzyme Q10: 100 to 300 mg daily
    N-acetylcysteine: 1,000 mg daily
    Fish oil: 5,000 mg daily

Homocysteine
    Vitamin B12: 800 to 2,000 mcg daily
    Folic acid: 1 to 10 mg daily
    Vitamin B6: 20 to 100 mg daily
    Trimethylglycine (TMG): 500 to 1,000 mg daily
    S-Adenosylmethionine (SAMe): 400 mg daily

Fibrinogen
    Fish oil: 5,000 mg daily
    Vitamin E: 400 to 800 IU daily
    Bromelain: 500 mg three times daily between meals
    Garlic (*Allium sativum*): 350 to 500 mg twice daily

Abnormal LDL density pattern AB or B
    Niacin: 1,000 to 2,000 mg daily
    Phytosterols: 1,000 mg twice daily

Thick Blood

One theory of cardiovascular disease is that *all* the major risk factors for atherosclerosis ultimately do their damage because they increase blood thickness. A commonly cited study is the Edinburgh Artery Study. It involved 4,860 men aged forty-five to fifty-nine years and women aged fifty-five to seventy-four years. The researchers found that the 20 percent of study participants with the thickest and stickiest blood had the majority (55 percent) of the major cardiovascular events over a five-year period. Researchers found that the link between blood viscosity and cardiovascular events was at *least* as strong as that of diastolic blood pressure and LDL cholesterol, and stronger than that of smoking

Homeopathy

If you have cardiovascular disease, see a licensed homeopath for a constitutional remedy. If any of the following remedies seem appropriate for you, try them, but only on a temporary or emergency basis. After that, see a homeopath for further help.

Homeopathy may help you recover from a heart attack. Once you've received emergency help and are under a doctor's care, consult with a naturopathic or homeopathic practitioner.

If you have symptoms of a heart attack, call 911 and follow their instructions. While you are waiting for the ambulance to arrive, you can take a 30C potency every two or three minutes.

Aconitum Napellus is for numbness and pain in the left arm. The person feels very fearful and anxious.

Arnica (*Arnica montana*) is helpful when you have the sensation that your heart is being squeezed or you feel a bruising pain.

Cactus (*Cereus grandiflorus*) can also ease the pain of angina. Take it if you feel as if a band is tightening around your chest.

Acupressure

See pages 787–794 for information about acupressure points and administering treatment.

- If you have a heart attack, first call an ambulance. While you are waiting, you can squeeze the tips of the little fingers. This action may reduce the severity of the attack.
- To stimulate circulation around the heart and the chest, use Heart 3 and 7 (H3 and H7).
- Governing Vessel 24.5 (GV24.5) produces a general sense of calm and wellbeing.
- Conception Vessel 17 (CV17) relaxes chest tension caused by nerves or sadness.
- Pericardium 3 (P3) eases chest pain and anxiety.
- If your anxiety causes heart palpitations, massage Pericardium 6 (P6).

Bodywork

Massage
A full-body massage improves circulation, steadies the body's rhythms, and relieves stress. As such, it is a valuable addition to heart-disease treatment.

If tension causes pressure in your chest, a neck massage may calm you down and regulate your pulse. You can easily give yourself a simple neck rub by learning a few techniques.

Chiropractic or osteopathic treatment can be helpful for improved circulation.

Reflexology
See pages 804–805 for information about reflexology areas and how to work them.

To strengthen a weakened heart, massage the chest and lung area.

Working the sigmoid colon will prevent gas from backing up and causing pain in the chest.

Aromatherapy

Many oils promote relaxation. Try several until you find a few that you like, then alternate them to preserve their effectiveness. Some good oils to start with are lavender and jasmine. A diffuser that releases scent into a room will allow you to benefit from an oil's relaxing qualities all day long.

Add juniper to a massage oil. It will encourage the breakdown of fatty deposits and other toxins.

Stress Reduction

General Stress-Reduction Therapies

Conventional medicine is finally beginning to accept that stress is a primary factor in heart disease. If you have heart disease, you must take several steps to reduce the amount of stress in your life. Dr. Dean Ornish has produced remarkable results by putting his patients on a program of yoga and daily meditation. He's found that even the most resistant of patients have eventually come to enjoy and look forward to these relaxing sessions.

Consider joining a support group for people with heart disease. Again, Dr. Ornish's work shows that when people can talk out their worries and frustrations with others who share some of their experiences, stress levels decline dramatically, along with the risk of a heart attack (or a repeat heart attack).

Other Recommendations

- Quit smoking, and eliminate your exposure to secondhand smoke. Tobacco smoke is known to weaken artery walls and is one of the leading causes of heart disease.
- Exercise is a crucial component of heart fitness, but you don't need to force yourself into a punishing regimen. Just enjoy a brisk thirty-minute walk daily; move quickly enough that you're breathing hard but not so fast that you can't carry on a conversation. If you have heart disease, see a doctor before beginning any exercise program.
- If you're a heart-disease patient and have been told to lose weight, the dietary suggestions given here should help you take off the pounds safely. People who are very heavy will find additional suggestions under the heading Obesity.
- Women who smoke or who are over thirty-five should not take oral contraceptives or synthetic hormone replacements.
- If you suffer from depression, you are at a significantly greater risk of developing heart disease. See the Depression section for more information.
- Chelation therapy from a holistic doctor may improve blood flow through the coronary arteries.
- External counter pulsation involves a device that squeezes the lower limbs to improve blood flow to the heart. This is helpful for those with atherosclerosis or congestive heart failure. It is available from cardiologists or holistic doctors.

REFERENCES

Budoff, M., et al. 2003. Anti-atherosclerotic effect of aged garlic (Kyolic) in the bypass surgery patients analyzed by computed tomography. *FASEB Journal* April 15, San Diego.

De Longeril, M., et al. 1999. Circulation. *Journal of the American Heart Association* 99:733–85.

Gouni-Berthold, I., and H. K. Berthold. 2002. Policosanol: Clinical pharmacology and therapeutic significance of a new lipid-lowering agent. *American Heart Journal* 143(2): 356–65.

Lowe, G. D., A. J. Lee, A. Rumley, et al. Blood viscosity and risk of cardiovascular events: The Edinburgh Artery Study. *Br J Haematol* 1997; 96:168–73.

Sloop, G. D. 1996. A unifying theory of atherogenesis. *Med Hypotheses* 47:321–5. www.ncbi.nlm.nih.gov/pubmed/8910882>.

Taylor, A. J., et al. 2009. Extended-release niacin or ezetimibe and carotid intima–media thickness. *New England Journal of Medicine* 61:2113–22.

Trichopoulou, A., et al. 2007. Modified Mediterranean diet and survival after myocardial infarction: The EPIC-Elderly study. *European Journal of Epidemiology* 22:871–81.

Yzebe, D., et al. 2004. Fish oils in the care of coronary heart disease patients: A meta-analysis of randomized controlled trials. *Fundamentals of Clinical Pharmacology* 18:581–92.

Zhao, S. P., et al. 2007. Xuezhikang, an extract of cholestin, reduces cardiovascular events in type 2 diabetes patients with coronary heart disease: Subgroup analysis of patients with type 2 diabetes from China coronary secondary prevention study (CCSPS). *Journal of Cardiovascular Pharmacology* 49:81–4.

Carpal Tunnel Syndrome (CTS)

The carpal tunnel is a very small opening just below the base of the wrist, between the arm and the hand. It allows the median nerve to pass from the bones and the muscles of the forearm to the palm, the thumb, and the fingers. Because the opening is so small, it is vulnerable to pressure and swelling. Inflammation from overuse, hormonal changes, or arthritis causes the pain and the numbness of carpal tunnel syndrome (CTS). CTS may begin as a mild tingling that's worse in the morning or the evening and can progress to a crippling, excruciating pain.

CTS has always afflicted people who consistently use their hands in a repetitive motion: Knitters, musicians, writers, grocery clerks, and assembly-line workers have traditionally suffered from the effects of CTS. But in the last decade, as work has increasingly centered on the personal computer, CTS has reached near-epidemic proportions. At least 10 percent of people who work at computers have CTS, and that number is projected to rise.

The best way to treat CTS is to prevent it from happening. If you work at a computer, use a wrist rest to relieve pressure on the carpal tunnel, and take a break every hour to rotate your hands. If you think you may already have CTS, see your doctor for a test called an electromyograph. If the test proves that you do have CTS,

In a preliminary trial, people with CTS (some of whom had previously undergone surgery) received either acupuncture or electroacupuncture (acupuncture with electrical stimulation). Researchers found that 83 percent of the participants experienced complete relief that lasted two to eight years after follow-up.

complementary therapies can help relieve your pain. Treatments include removing the source of pain when possible, improving circulation, and reducing swelling. Since a vitamin B6 deficiency has been linked to CTS, complementary treatment also encourages the consumption of that nutrient. Specific treatments from a chiropractor, an acupuncturist, or an osteopath can be very effective in addressing the underlying structural cause of carpal tunnel syndrome. Surgery for this condition should be avoided, if at all possible, because of its high failure rate.

SYMPTOMS

Symptoms can occur in one or both hands.

- Numbness, tingling, or pain in the thumb and the first three fingers
- Pain that is worse at night and/or in the morning
- Weakness of the thumb and the first three fingers
- Inability to make a fist
- Pain that radiates to the forearm or the shoulder

ROOT CAUSES

- Continuous use of the fingers and the hand
- Constant vibration of the fingers and the hand (as in holding a jackhammer for long periods of time)
- Pregnancy or other hormonal changes that cause fluid retention
- Inflammatory arthritis in the wrist
- Bone spurs in the wrist
- Vitamin B6 deficiency

Testing Techniques

The following test helps to assess possible metabolic reasons for carpal tunnel syndrome:

Vitamin B6—blood test

TREATMENT

CTS is often brought on or made worse by pregnancy. If you're pregnant or nursing, check with your doctor before taking any herbs or supplements or making radical changes to your diet.

Diet

Recommended Food

If you're overweight, there's a good chance you will find relief from the pain of CTS by following a wholesome diet based on whole grains, fresh fruits and vegetables, and lean protein (especially beans and soy). This eating plan will help you lose weight safely and will take pressure off the carpal tunnel.

Drink a glass of clean, quality water every two waking hours to combat fluid retention.

A deficiency of vitamin B6 may be a cause of CTS, so consume plenty of beans, brewer's yeast, and wheat germ. Green leafy vegetables are good sources of B6 as well.

Green drinks are also good for reducing inflammation.

Food to Avoid

Fluid retention puts pressure on the carpal tunnel, so eliminate sources of sodium from your diet.

Avoid saturated fat, which slows circulation.

℞ Super Seven Prescriptions—Carpal Tunnel Syndrome

Super Prescription #1 Vitamin B6
Take 100 mg three times daily. Studies show that this vitamin reduces the nerve inflammation that is found with carpal tunnel syndrome. Also, take a B-complex to prevent an imbalance of the other B vitamins.

Super Prescription #2 Bromelain
Take 500 mg three times daily between meals. Look for products standardized to 2,000 MCU (milk-clotting units) per 1,000 mg or 1,200 GDU (gelatin-dissolving units) per 1,000 mg. Bromelain has a natural anti-inflammatory effect. Protease enzyme products also have this benefit.

Super Prescription #3 Boswellia (*Boswellia serrata*)
Take 1,200 to 1,500 mg of a standardized extract containing 60 to 65 percent boswellic acids, two to three times daily. It acts as a natural anti-inflammatory.

Super Prescription #4 Calcium and magnesium
Take a complex containing 500 mg of calcium and 250 mg of magnesium twice daily. This reduces muscle tightness and nerve irritation.

Super Prescription #5 White willow (*Salix alba*)
Take a product standardized to contain 240 mg of salicin daily or 5 ml of the tincture form three times daily. This herbal extract reduces pain and inflammation.

Super Prescription #6 Homeopathy
Pick the remedy that best matches your symptoms in the Homeopathy section. For acute wrist pain, take a 30C potency four times daily. For chronic wrist pain, take twice daily for two weeks to see if there are any positive improvements. After you notice improvement, stop taking the remedy, unless symptoms return. Consultation with a homeopathic practitioner is advised.

Super Prescription #7 *Ginkgo biloba*
Take 120 mg twice daily of a product standardized to 24 percent flavone glycosides. Ginkgo improves circulation.

General Recommendations

Dandelion leaf (*Taraxacum officinale*) is a natural diuretic that is considered to be safe during pregnancy. Take 300 mg or 2 ml three times daily. It should be used under the supervision of a doctor.

DMSO (dimethyl sulfoxide) is a topical pain reliever. Work with a doctor to use this substance. Arnica (*Arnica montana*) and hypericum (Saint-John's-wort) oil can be rubbed over the affected area to reduce pain and swelling.

Homeopathy

Arnica (*Arnica montana*) is for deep pain that feels bruised. It is best used for the first two days after an injury.

Causticum is a remedy for recurring or long-lasting carpal tunnel syndrome. The wrist area feels bruised, with burning or drawing pains. There is often stiffness and contracture of the wrist and the forearm. Symptoms are better with warm applications.

Hypericum (*Hypericum perforatum*) is for shooting nerve pains that extend from the wrist.

Rhus Toxicodendron is for achy pain that improves with movement and dry warmth and is worse with inactivity and windy, rainy weather.

Ruta (*Ruta graveolens*) is for stiff, bruised pain and aching of the wrist. The wrist feels lame and weak from overuse.

Acupressure

See pages 787–794 for information about acupressure points and administering treatment.
- The best points for easing wrist pain are Pericardium 6 and 7 (P6 and P7) and Triple Warmer 5 (TW5). You can easily practice this short acupressure routine while at your desk or when you're taking a break from work.

Work Those Wrists!

Your wrists, like the rest of the body, need exercise to stay strong and supple. Practice the following recommended exercises at the beginning of every workday, and take breaks every few hours to go through the routine again. It's also a good idea to use these exercises as a warm-up for yoga, tennis, rock climbing, and other hand-intensive sports.

- Begin by shaking out your wrists for about ten seconds.

- Gently rotate your wrists clockwise through their full range of motion. Do this five times, and then repeat, this time going counter-clockwise.

- Hold your arm straight out in front of you, palm facing outward, and use the opposite hand to gently pull back your fingertips. Hold for a few seconds and then release. Repeat with the other arm.

Bodywork

Reflexology

See pages 804–805 for information about reflexology areas and how to work them.

Work the areas corresponding to the lymph system, the kidneys, and the adrenals to reduce swelling and inflammation. This gentle therapy is especially good for pregnant women.

Hydrotherapy

Contrast hydrotherapy will improve blood flow and provide pain relief. Submerge your hand and wrist in hot water for a couple of minutes; then immerse them in cold water for about thirty seconds. Repeat the sequence several times.

Other Bodywork Recommendations

An experienced chiropractor or osteopath, especially one who specializes in sports therapy, can perform adjustments of the wrist, the arm, the shoulder, and the neck. Make sure to find a qualified practitioner.

Other Recommendations

- Use a cold compress to reduce swelling.
- Cigar and cigarette smoke disturbs the circulation. If you smoke, quit. If you're exposed to secondhand smoke, remove yourself from the smoky environment as much as possible.
- Pregnant women whose CTS is brought on by edema will find that their symptoms disappear after their babies are born.
- If your CTS has been caused by overuse of the wrist and the fingers, stop all repetitive hand motions for a few days. When you return to your work, you'll need to alternate repetitive tasks with other activities. Take a break every hour to rest and to rotate your wrists, and try to keep your work environment warm and dry, as cool, humid conditions can aggravate CTS.
- If you work on a computer, make sure your screen is two feet away from your body and slightly below your line of vision. Also, use a wrist rest. Most employers are now aware of CTS and will provide ergonomic workspace if you ask for it.
- Laser therapy by a practitioner can be effective for carpal tunnel syndrome.

REFERENCES

Chen, G. S. 1990. The effect of acupuncture treatment on carpal tunnel syndrome. *American Journal of Acupuncture* 18:5–9.

Cataracts

Cataracts are the leading cause of vision loss in the United States and worldwide. Because they develop gradually, and because most of us tend to associate some vision disturbances with "normal" aging, most cases go undetected until it is too late to stop the damage. This is a shame, because when cataracts are caught in their early stages, it is possible to halt or even reverse their progression. If your eyes are healthy, you can also take steps that may help prevent cataracts altogether.

Cataracts are cloudy or opaque spots that develop on the usually translucent lens of the eye. When these spots first appear, you may not notice any difference in your vision.

Over a period of years, however, the cataract spreads across the lens. You may notice that it's harder to make out details or that colors look different. Night driving becomes more challenging. If you've been farsighted for most of your life, a cataract may actually improve your vision—for a short while. As the cataract continues to grow, it will become more difficult to see medium-sized and larger objects. In the worst-case scenario, cataracts can leave a person completely blind. In fact, forty thousand Americans go blind every year as a result of cataracts.

Most cases fall under the category that doctors call "senile cataracts." These are lens spots that commonly accompany old age, although they are by no means an inevitable part of growing older. We now know that senile cataracts are caused by damage from free radicals, the unbalanced, destructive molecules that destroy cells in the body. While the production of free radicals does naturally increase somewhat with aging, most of these dangerous agents are caused by lifestyle choices. Excess sun exposure, poor diet, and smoking are all primary causes of free radicals. Changing these habits can prevent and sometimes stop cataracts, as can taking steps to supply your body with antioxidants, the substances that fight free radicals.

In some instances, cataracts are inherited or caused by a preexisting disorder. Cataracts that begin in youth or middle age are extremely rare and are usually related to an inherited condition. In addition, people with diabetes and Down syndrome have a higher risk of developing cataracts than the rest of the population does.

Poor digestive function can be at the root of cataracts. Low stomach acid can lead to malabsorption of nutrients from foods and can create more free radicals. In addition, toxic metals such as cadmium, mercury, and others accelerate free-radical damage of the lens. Elevated blood sugar levels, as occurs with diabetes, is a major risk factor for developing cataracts.

If at any stage of your life you experience vision changes, it's important to consult a doctor or an optometrist as soon as possible. For many eye disorders, an early diagnosis can mean effective treatment. Nutritional therapy is important in the prevention and the treatment of cataracts.

SYMPTOMS

Symptoms are painless and usually progress in the following order:

- Blurring of details
- Temporary improvement of farsightedness
- Changes in color perception
- Difficulty driving at night
- Blurring of larger objects
- Darkening of vision
- Blindness

ROOT CAUSES

- Exposure to ultraviolet or infrared light
- Poor diet, especially one low in antioxidants
- Obesity
- Poor digestion
- Smoking
- Radiation
- Heavy-metal poisoning
- Mineral deficiencies
- Injury to the eye
- Long-term use of steroids
- Diabetes
- Down syndrome
- Heredity
- Pharmaceutical medications such as statin drugs

Testing Techniques

The following tests help assess possible metabolic reasons for cataracts:
Vitamin and mineral analysis—blood, urine
Intestinal permeability—urine
Digestion—stool analysis
Toxic (heavy) metal toxicity—urine or hair

TREATMENT

Diet

A diet to prevent or reverse cataracts can require some dedication at first. Once you've established healthful eating habits, however, you'll not only improve your eye health, you'll reduce your risk of developing almost every other disease we commonly associate with aging.

Recommended Food

Build your diet around deeply colored fruits and vegetables, which are the best sources of antioxidants, the substances that fight free-radical damage. Of the antioxidants, the carotenoids are most important for eye problems. Good sources of carotenoids are dark-green leafy vegetables, bell peppers, yellow squash, carrots, tomatoes, celery, oranges, red grapes, mangoes, and melons.

Consume spinach and kale, as these foods are high in the carotenoids lutein and zeaxanthin. These carotenoids have been reported to lower the risk of developing cataracts.

Egg yolks are also rich in carotenoids.

Vitamin C and bioflavonoids work in combination to fight free-radical damage. In addition, they improve the tissues and the capillaries of the eye. Good sources of bioflavonoids include berries, cherries, tomatoes, and plums; for vitamin C, eat plenty of citrus fruits.

Food to Avoid

Banish from your diet all fried foods, as well as those that contain saturated, hydrogenated, or partially hydrogenated fats or oils. Refined and processed foods, including white flour, are also out of the question. All of these foods are high in free radicals, the atoms that destroy your body's cells—and your eyesight.

Alcohol puts a heavy burden on the liver and impairs its ability to detoxify your blood, so avoid it.

Some eye doctors have noted a link between cataracts and an inability to digest milk sugars properly. While no one has proven a connection between dairy and eye disorders, it seems prudent for people with cataracts to eliminate milk products from their diet.

Heavy-metal poisoning may cause or contribute to cataracts by preventing antioxidants from doing their job. Consider getting a hair or urine analysis to find out if you have metal poisoning; if you do, be sure to fast regularly, and be sure to look into chelation therapy.

People who consume small amounts of fruits and vegetables and those with low blood levels of antioxidants have been reported to be at high risk for cataracts.

℞ Super Seven Prescriptions—Cataracts

Super Prescription #1 N-acetylcarnosine eyedrops
Apply to affected eyes twice daily. Preliminary research demonstrates benefit. Use under the supervision of a doctor.

Super Prescription #2 Vitamin C
Vitamin C is one of the main antioxidants that protects the eye lens. Take 1,000 mg two to three times daily.

Population studies
show that people
who take multivitamins
or supplements con-
taining vitamin C or E
for more than ten years
have up to a 60 percent
lower risk of forming
cataracts.

Super Prescription #3 Gentian root (*Gentiana lutea*) or betaine HCL

Gentian root and other bitter herbs improve stomach acid and overall digestive function. Take 250 mg or 0.5 to 1.0 ml with meals. Betaine HCL increases stomach-acid levels for improved absorption. Take 1 or 2 capsules with meals.

Super Prescription #4 Bilberry (*Vaccinium myrtillus*)

Take 160 mg two or three times daily of a 25 percent anthocyanosides extract. Phytochemicals in bilberry protect the lens from free-radical damage.

Super Prescription #5 B-complex

Take a 50 mg complex daily. Vitamins B2 and B3 have been shown to have a protective effect against cataracts.

Super Prescription #6 Vitamin E

This potent antioxidant protects against free-radical damage. Take 400 IU of a vitamin-E complex with tocotrienols and tocopherols.

Super Prescription #7 Mixed carotenoid complex

Take 25,000 IU one or two times daily. It provides lutein, zeaxanthin, beta carotene, and other carotenoids that protect the lens.

General Recommendations

Ginkgo biloba has a well-deserved reputation as a free-radical scavenger. It also offers general support and protection to the eyes. Choose an extract standardized to 24 percent flavone glycosides, and take 120 mg twice a day.

Alpha lipoic acid is an important antioxidant. Take 100 mg twice daily.

N-acetylcysteine increases glutathione levels, an important antioxidant for the eyes. Take 500 mg twice daily.

Bioflavonoid complex provides additional protection for the lens. Take with your vitamin C formula or separately at a dose of 500 mg twice daily. *Note*: A separate antioxidant formula can also be used to provide a broad base of antioxidants.

Grapeseed and pine bark extract are both potent antioxidants that improve microcirculation in the eye. Take 50 mg three times daily.

Taking a high-potency multivitamin will provide a base of nutrients that neutralize free radicals.

Homeopathy

Many homeopathic practitioners have reported good success in slowing cataract development. The following suggestions are meant to help you get started, but it is strongly advised that you see a professional for a constitutional treatment. For temporary treatment, choose the appropriate following remedy and take 6C two or three times a day for one month. If you see improvement, take a rest from the remedy for a week, and then keep taking it in a cycle of one month on, one month off.

If a doctor or an optometrist has told you that you have cataracts in the very early stages, take Calcarea. By the time you experience symptoms, you'll need to move on to a different remedy.

Phosphorus is the remedy if you feel that there's a veil over your eyes.
If you have dimmed vision, with hot, red eyes, take Ruta Graveolens.
At the very first sign of impaired vision, take Silica (*Silicea*).

Acupressure

See pages 787–794 for information about pressure points and administering treatment.

- To improve circulation to your head and to deliver oxygen and nutrients to your eyes, work Large Intestine 3 and 4 (LI3 and LI4).

Bodywork

Reflexology

See pages 804–805 for information about reflexology areas and how to work them.
Work the eye/ear region and the neck.
To encourage detoxification, stimulate the liver, the kidneys, and the colon.

Stress Reduction

Although stress is not a direct cause of cataracts, unresolved tension and anxiety inhibit the body's ability to neutralize and eliminate free radicals. Review the stress-reduction techniques in the Exercise and Stress Reduction chapter and find one or two that you'd like to practice on a regular basis

Other Recommendations

- Smoking is a leading cause of free-radical damage and a factor in almost every disease we associate with "natural" aging. If you smoke, stop. And if you don't smoke, you still need to make a conscious effort to avoid secondhand smoke.
- Wear sunglasses that protect against both UVA and UVB rays. Try to avoid excursions that take place in the glare of the full sun.
- Consider the use of intravenous vitamin and mineral therapy. This provides a more aggressive treatment for cataracts.
- For many people with cataracts, surgery is a real option. If the cataract is caught early enough, a doctor can remove the entire lens and replace it with a plastic lens. The operation is not painful, and it has a high rate of success. As always, it's best to try to avoid invasive procedures by employing complementary healing strategies, but if you experience significant loss of vision, surgery may be the only way to restore sight. Talk to your doctor about your options.

REFERENCES

Jacques, P. F., and L. T. Chylack Jr. 1991. Epidemiologic evidence of a role for the antioxidant vitamins and carotenoids in cataract prevention. *American Journal of Clinical Nutrition* 53:352S–55S.

Knekt, P., M. Heliovaara, A. Rissanen, et al. 1992. Serum antioxidant vitamins and risk of cataract. *British Medical Journal* 305:1392–94.

Mares-Perlman, J. A., et al. 2000. Vitamin supplement use and incident cataracts in a population-based study. *Archives of Ophthalmology* 118:1556–63.

Cavities

Cavities, especially in children, are all too common in America. They are the second most common disorder next to the common cold. There are a variety of factors that increase your risk of cavities. The primary one is the foods you consume. The average American drinks more than fifty-six gallons per year of soft drinks. That's an astounding one and one-half twelve-ounce cans per day for every man, woman, and child. Unfortunately, America's children start drinking soda pop at a young age. Twenty-one percent of one- and two-year-olds drink soda pop at an average of seven ounces per day!

Dental cavities are caused by the acidic action of bacteria fermenting on dietary sugars. This leads to minerals such as calcium being leached out of the tooth enamel. Soft drinks, even when carbohydrate free (such as diet sodas sweetened with artificial sweeteners), still cause problems due to their acidic pH. The low or acidic pH erodes the dental enamel. Colas often have a pH of 2.4 or less. To neutralize a glass of cola (pH of 7 is neutral) one would have to consume thirty-two glasses of water!

There are different bacteria that naturally inhabit the mouth. Various forms of sugar feed these bacteria, which form acids and plaque that coat the teeth. Plaque provides a hiding place for the bacteria, which eventually erode the hard, outer tooth enamel. Left untreated, the bacteria erode further layers of the teeth and make their way to the pulp, the inner tooth material that contains blood vessels and nerves. At this point pain and pus formation are symptoms of infection.

Supporters of fluoridation will often point out that there has been a dramatic decline in cavities and tooth decay in the United States during the past half century. But this is misguided since there is also much better dental hygiene being practiced today. And, in addition, many European countries where fluoride water enrichment was stopped in the 1970s show a similar decline in cavities due to better oral hygiene.

In 2011, the U.S. Department of Health and Human Services announced there was too much fluoride in the nation's water supply. They recommended reducing the amount of fluoride added to water to 0.7 parts per million (ppm) everywhere. Previously the limit had ranged from 0.7 ppm in warm climates, where people drink a lot of water, to 1.2 ppm in cooler climates, where people typically consume less water.

When the surfaces of the teeth become damaged, small holes form. If untreated, cavities can lead to toothaches, infection, stained teeth, and tooth loss.

> You should be aware that chewable and powdered vitamin C has been shown to erode tooth enamel. It is likely that buffered vitamin C would not have this detrimental effect.

SYMPTOMS

Cavities may produce no symptoms. Or the following symptoms may present:

- Tooth pain, worse from hot or cold food and drinks, sweets
- Holes or pits in the teeth

ROOT CAUSES

- Poor hygiene (improper flossing and brushing)
- Diet
- Nutritional deficiencies
- Imbalance of mouth flora
- Genetics

- Dry mouth occuring as the result of chemotherapy, radiation, or autoimmune diseases

- Eating disorders
- Acid reflux

Testing Techniques

Dental X-rays
Testing of mouth flora (by holistic dentist)

TREATMENT

Diet

Recommended Food

Hard cheese has been shown to fight cavities in children. It seems to increase the uptake of calcium and phosphate cells by the surface of tooth enamel. Also, components of green tea and oolong tea, both derived from the leaves of *Camellia sinensis,* have been shown to decrease acid production by the common mouth bacterium *Streptococcus mutans.*

Consume fiber-rich fruits and vegetables, which stimulate saliva flow. Pomegranates and pomegranate juice, as well as cranberry, have a unique action of reducing the effects of bacteria that cause cavities.

Chew gum or use lozenges that contain xylitol. This is a natural sugar alcohol derived from corn that reduces acid in the mouth and promotes a strain of *Streptococcus mutans* that is less cavity-causing than typical. This regimen is best started one year before permanent teeth erupt.

Food to Avoid

Soda pop, candy, and other simple sugars including refined carbohydrates like white breads and crackers. Do not keep citrus fruits in your mouth for a long time as the acid can erode enamel.

Rx Super Seven Prescriptions—Cavities

Super Prescription #1 Xylitol
Use a mouthwash containing xylitol. Use as directed. This natural substance prevents cavities.

Super Prescription #2 Probiotics
Specific probiotic species reduce the bacteria that cause cavities. Studied strains include *Lactobacillus GG* and *Bacillus coagulans.* Chewable tablets are available. Use as directed.

Super Prescription #3 Green tea
Drinking green tea or using a tincture form added to water twice daily helps to prevent cavities.

A study was published of 921 children ages three to six years who were randomly assigned to chew one piece of xylitol gum three times daily for five to ten minutes or brush their teeth after lunch. The treatment lasted one to three years with the summers off. At age nine significantly more children in the xylitol group were cavity free compared to the control group. Xylitol gum, mints, and mouthwashes are commonly available over the counter.

Super Prescription #4 Essential oils
Certain blends of essential oils fight the bacteria that contribute to cavities. Look for natural mouthwashes containing a blend of essential oils.

Super Prescription #5 Propolis
Propolis spray and tincture can be used to fight the bacteria that cause cavities. Take as directed on the label.

Super Prescription #6 Vitamin C
Vitamin C improves immunity and strengthens the teeth and gums. Take 500 mg to 2,000 mg daily. Use a nonacidic form if using a powder that mixes in water.

Super Prescription #7 Vitamin D
This vitamin is needed for normal tooth development. Take 2,000 IU to 5,000 IU daily with a meal.

Another exciting natural treatment is the use of the probiotic *Lactobacillus GG*. Research in children has shown that it reduces the incidence of cavities by 49 percent compared to a control group. It is available in chewable tablets from health food stores.

Fluoridated water is not the solution to our epidemic of cavities. Harvard researchers determined that twenty-six of the twenty-seven studies found that a high fluoride level in water negatively affected brain function in children.

Other Recommendations

- Besides cutting down on soft-drink consumption, when you do drink soda pop, make sure to use a straw to keep the acids and sugars away from your teeth. Also, swish your mouth with water afterward to wash out sugar and acid.
- Adequate teeth brushing and flossing are necessary to prevent cavities.
- Consult with a holistic dentist.

REFERENCES

Choi, A. L., G. Sun, Y. Zhang, et al. 2012. Developmental fluoride neurotoxicity: a systematic review and meta-analysis. *Environ Health Perspect* 120(10):1362–68.

Kovari, H., et al. 2003. Use of xylitol chewing gum in daycare centers: a follow-up study in Savonlinna, Finland. *Act Odontol Scand* 61:367–70.

Nase, L., et al. 2001. Effect of long-term consumption of a probiotic bacterium, Lactobacilus rhamnosus GG, in milk on dental caries and caries risk in children. *Caries Res* 35:412–20.

Cervical Dysplasia

The cervix is the lower part of the uterus that connects the body of the uterus to the vagina (birth canal). Cervical dysplasia is a condition characterized by the abnormal growth of cells on the surface of the cervix. These cells can be precancerous or cancerous. Based on testing, dysplasia is classified as low-grade or high-grade, depending on the degree of the abnormal cell growth. Low-grade cervical dysplasia (LSIL, which stands for low-grade squamous intraepithelial lesions) progresses slowly and often resolves without treatment. High-grade cervical dysplasia (HSIL, which stands for high-grade squamous intraepithelial lesions) can lead to cervical cancer. Regular testing is important because 30 to 50 percent of cases of severe cervical dysplasia progress to invasive cancer.

Cervical dysplasia and cancer are almost always caused by the human papillomavirus (HPV), which is sexually transmitted. More than thirty types of HPV can infect the genital area. Fortunately, most women with HPV never develop cervical dysplasia. It has been estimated that up to 70 percent of women have been infected with HPV during their lifetimes. In most people, the immune system has the ability to keep this virus in check.

SYMPTOMS

There are usually no symptoms.

ROOT CAUSES

- Weak immunity that allows the human papillomavirus to replicate
- Hormone imbalance
- Smoking (doubles the risk)
- Poor diet—especially low consumption of fruits and vegetables
- Obesity
- Oral contraceptives (may increase the risk)
- Sexual intercourse with a non-virgin partner (abstinence until marriage with a virgin partner is the most foolproof way to prevent cervical dysplasia)

Other causal factors include the following:

- Youth (the risk of acquiring HPV decreases with age)
- Low socioeconomic status and the resulting poor health care
- Chlamydia infection
- HIV infection
- Multiple male partners

Testing Techniques

Pap smear
Colposcopy (magnified view of the cervix)
Testing that determines the susceptibility to viral infection and inflammation of the cervical tissue:
    Hormone testing—saliva, blood, or urine
    Nutritional deficiencies—vitamins D and B12 and folic acid

---

TREATMENT

Holistic therapy has proven to be very effective in the treatment of cervical dysplasia, particularly the low-grade variety. The authors have also treated some women with high-grade cervical dysplasia solely with natural therapy, and repeat testing shows normalization of the cervical epithelium.

Diet

Recommended Food

Diets rich in fruits and vegetables may help prevent HPV infection. This is particularly true of foods high in carotenoids, which are found in a variety of fruits and

A Brazilian study found that increased dietary intake of dark-green and deep-yellow vegetables and fruit and increased concentrations of blood alpha- and gamma-tocopherols (vitamin E compounds) were associated with a nearly 50 percent decreased risk of aggressive cervical dysplasia. The authors of the study state, "These results support the evidence that a healthy and balanced diet leading to high serum levels of antioxidants may reduce cervical neoplasia risk in low-income women."

Thirty women with cervical dysplasia were randomized to receive a placebo or 200 mg or 400 mg daily of indole-3-carbinol (I3C) for twelve weeks. Four out of eight who were given 200 mg and four out of nine who were given 400 mg had a complete regression of their cervical dysplasia, compared to none of the placebo group.

vegetables as well as in eggs. Foods rich in carotenoids include carrots, cantaloupe, watermelon, yellow squash, peaches, and corn. Green vegetables also have beneficial effects, and some research indicates that lignin-rich foods such as onions, garlic, grapefruit, seeds, and seaweed decrease the risk. Daily consumption of cruciferous vegetables (cabbage, broccoli, brussels sprouts, kale, and cauliflower), which normalize estrogen metabolism and have anticancer properties, is important. Naturally occurring vitamin-E compounds in foods, known as alpha- and gamma-tocopherol, also may help prevent cervical dysplasia.

Women with a high dietary intake of vitamin C have a reduced risk of cervical dysplasia.

A five- to seven-day supervised vegetable-juice fast can help improve immunity and remove harmful estrogen metabolites that can worsen dysplasia.

Food to Avoid

Avoid foods that suppress immunity, such as simple sugars (processed grains, soda, undiluted fruit juice), fried foods, and processed foods.

℞ Super Seven Prescriptions—Cervical Dysplasia

Super Prescription #1 Vitamin B12
Take 1,000 to 5,000 mcg daily, preferably in sublingual form. It is best taken in conjunction with a multivitamin or in a B-complex formula that contains the full spectrum of B vitamins. This is an important nutrient for women with a history of oral contraceptive use. B12 is involved in healthy cell replication.

Super Prescription #2 Folate
Take 2,000 to 10,000 mcg daily. Folate is involved in healthy cell replication. This is an important nutrient for women with a history of oral contraceptive use. Higher doses of folate are available through holistic doctors. L-5 methyltetrahydrofolate is the preferred form.

Super Prescription #3 Indole-3-carbinol (I3C) or Diindolylmethane (DIM)
Take 200 to 400 mg of I3C and/or 200 mg of DIM. These substances are extracts from cruciferous vegetables that support the removal of excess estrogen, which may worsen HPV infection, and that appear to help cervical dysplasia.

Super Prescription #4 Green Tea (*Camellia sinensis*)
Taking 300 mg daily in capsule form (55 percent EGCG, 95 percent polyphenols) has been shown to be effective. Green-tea suppositories are also effective and are available from a holistic doctor.

Super Prescription #5 Carotenes
Take 75,000 IU twice daily of a mixed natural-carotenoid complex. Your skin may turn an orangish hue from the high levels of carotenes, but do not be concerned; the carotenes are nontoxic.

Super Prescription #6 Homeopathic *Conium maculatum* (hemlock)

Take a 6x, 12x, 6C, 12C, or 30C potency twice daily for two weeks. This is best regression of their use under the guidance of a trained homeopathic practitioner.

Super Prescription #7 Vitamin E

Take 400 IU of a mixed vitamin-E complex containing tocopherols and tocotrienols. A low level of vitamin E is associated with an increased risk of cervical dysplasia.

Green tea extract standardized to contain a certain amount of epigallocatechin-3-gallate (EGCG) is used orally and as a vaginal suppository for cervical dysplasia. It is effective since it inhibits epidermal growth factor receptor, a substance needed for cervical cell growth. A study of fifty-one patients with varying degrees of dysplasia were divided into four groups as compared with thirty-nine controls. A green-tea polyphenol vaginal product was applied locally twice a week to twenty-seven patients. Twenty of the twenty-seven patients using the vaginal green-tea product showed a response. As well, an oral 200 mg EGCG capsule was taken every day for eight to twelve weeks in six patients, and three out of the six showed a response. Group three involved eight patients using the vaginal ointment as well as oral capsule. Six of eight showed a response. Group four consisted of ten patients using a higher-dose EGCG capsule (amount not stated). Six out of the ten patients showed a response. Overall, a 69 percent response rate was noted for the green-tea products compared with a 10 percent response rate in the untreated control groups.

General Recommendations

Curcumin has been shown to suppress HPV and reduce inflammation. Take 500 mg twice daily.

Echinacea (*Echinacea purpurea* or *angustifolia*) enhances immunity and has antiviral effects. Take 1 ml of the tincture or 300 mg of the capsule form twice daily.

Lomatium (*Lomatium dissectum*) has antiviral effects and improves immunity. Take 0.5 ml or 500 mg twice daily. Stop using it if you develop a rash.

Astragalus (*Astragalus membranaceus*) enhances immunity and has antiviral effects. Take 1,000 mg or 3 ml twice daily.

Green-tea extract vaginal suppositories have been shown in research to help reverse cervical dysplasia. Discuss with a holistic doctor.

Beta-glucan is a supplement shown to enhance immunity. Take as directed on the label.

Escharotic treatment uses topical agents to remove precancerous cells. A specific protocol developed by Dr. Tori Hudson of the National College of Natural Medicine has been shown to be very effective for cervical dysplasia. For further information, see the book *Women's Encyclopedia of Natural Medicine* or consult a naturopathic doctor.

A double-blind trial looked at the effect of indole-3-carbinol in women with cervical dysplasia. Supplement doses of 200 to 400 mg per day were used and resulted in complete regression of lesions in 50 percent of women with CIN II or CIN III.

Homeopathy

See a practitioner trained in homeopathy for individualized treatment.

Traditional Chinese Medicine

Many Chinese herbal remedies as well as acupuncture can strengthen your immune system against HPV. Consult a practitioner for individual treatment.

Acupressure

See pages 787–794 for information about acupressure points and administering treatment. Rub the points Bladder 23 and 47 (B23 and B47) to fortify the immune system and points Conception Vessel 4 and 6 (CV4 and CV6) to target the reproductive area.

Bodywork

Reflexology

See pages 804–805 for information about reflexology areas and how to work them. Focus on the uterine and cervical area.

Hydrotherapy

Constitutional hydrotherapy can be used to improve immunity. See pages 795–796 for directions.

Aromatherapy

Clove, cistis, and cinnamon are powerful antiviral oils that stimulate the immune system.

Stress Reduction

General Stress-Reduction Therapies

Your immune system and its ability to suppress HPV are greatly affected by stress. Regular exercise, sleep, prayer, biofeedback, meditation, visualization, and other relaxation techniques are important for optimal immunity.

Other Recommendations

It is critical to stop smoking. We also advise forms of birth control other than oral contraceptives because hormone balance seems to play a role for some women with cervical dysplasia. Do not rely on condoms as protection from HPV. The HPV vaccine is still controversial, and safety issues are unclear at the time of the publication of this book .

REFERENCE

Ahn, W., J. Yoo, S. Huh, et al. 2003. Protective effects of green tea extracts (polyphenon E and EGCG) on human cervical lesions. *European Journal of Cancer Prevention* 12(5):383–90.

Bell, M. C., et al. 2000. Placebo controlled trial of indole 3 carbinole in the treatment of CIN. *Gynecol Oncol* 78:123–129.

Tomita, L. Y., et al. 2010. Diet and serum micronutrients in relation to cervical neoplasia and cancer among low-income Brazilian women. *International Journal of Cancer* 126:703–14.

Cholesterol, High

High levels of cholesterol in the blood are one of the many risk factors for serious future health problems (see the Cardiovascular Disease section for information on other risk markers). Too much of certain types of cholesterol can increase the chances of developing heart disease (including possibly fatal heart attacks) and stroke. By inhibiting circulation, too much of this substance can also cause gallstones, impotence, high blood pressure, and loss of mental acuity.

Cholesterol isn't all bad, however. Your body requires it in moderation for the proper function of cells, nerves, brain, immune system, and hormones. It is an essential component of every cell in your body, and life without it would be impossible. To distribute cholesterol throughout the body, substances called lipoproteins transport it in the blood. One class of lipoproteins, called low-density lipoproteins, or LDLs for short, carries cholesterol from the liver, where it is produced, to the cells that need it. Then another kind of lipoprotein, called high-density lipoproteins, or HDLs, picks up the excess cholesterol from the cells and takes it back to the liver, where it is broken down and excreted from the body or reprocessed.

Newer testing allows the analysis of different subtypes of cholesterol. For example, VLDL is a type of LDL cholesterol, and HDL2 is the most protective type of cholesterol.

Under normal conditions, the lipoproteins keep cholesterol levels in balance. But this carefully calibrated system can be overtaxed when the body creates more cholesterol than HDL can sweep away. After the cells take what they need, the existing HDLs remove what they can, and the extra cholesterol simply remains in the blood. Then if cholesterol becomes oxidized (especially LDL cholesterol) and attaches to the artery walls, it sets the stage for inflammation of the arteries. This chronic inflammation contributes to further buildup and deposition of cholesterol and plaque on the interior walls of the arteries. We call this buildup, which narrows the arteries and

limits the amount of blood that can pass through them, arteriosclerosis or hardening of the arteries. Arteriosclerosis is the first stage of heart disease; when left untreated, it will lead to a heart attack or stroke. For more information about arteriosclerosis, see Cardiovascular Disease.

Elevated cholesterol levels are often caused by the standard Western diet, which relies heavily on animal products, processed oils, and refined carbohydrates. It can also be caused by heredity conditions or preexisting diseases like diabetes and insulin resistance, or syndrome X. Although, diet usually plays a role in these cases as well. It stands to reason, then, that high cholesterol can often be treated with dietary changes and exercise. Specific supplements discussed in this section are also excellent nonpharmacological ways to normalize cholesterol levels. Stress reduction has a beneficial effect as well. It is strongly suggested that you employ these natural strategies before trying any of the cholesterol-lowering medications on the market. These drugs, while effective at reducing cholesterol, have a multitude of *potential*

Normal Cholesterol Levels

Total cholesterol:
   165–200 mg/dL.
LDL cholesterol:
   below 130 mg/dL.
HDL cholesterol:
   50 mg/dL or higher.
Total cholesterol/HDL ratio:
   less than 3.7.
LDL/HDL ratio:
   less than 3.0.

Note: The relative amount of total cholesterol to HDL and the ratio of LDL to HDL are considered more important than total cholesterol.

side effects. While they may be necessary in some cases, many doctors prescribe them as a matter of routine—often because they're afraid that their patients won't make the lifestyle changes that can lower cholesterol naturally. If your doctor wants to prescribe a cholesterol-lowering agent for you, explain to him or her that you're willing to embark on a holistic regimen in the hopes of avoiding a lifelong dependency on drugs. Whatever your decision, be sure that it is based on your physician's and your analysis of your individual situation.

The understanding of the role of cholesterol and lipids in the cause of cardiovascular disease has been changing over time. Basing treatment solely on traditional markers such as total cholesterol, LDL cholesterol, HDL cholesterol, and triglycerides is becoming antiquated. While knowing these numbers does provide some value, they are not great predictive markers of one's risk of cardiovascular disease. Instead, leading preventative cardiology now focuses on advanced lipid testing. This includes testing for lipoprotein subfractions and particle sizes. In addition to lipid markers, inflammatory markers are very important in assessing a person's risk. For more information see the Cardiovascular Disease chapter.

The story on cholesterol continues to evolve. Research over the past decade has shown that much of the artery problem caused by cholesterol is the result of oxidation. Oxidation occurs when free radicals (unstable negatively charged molecules) damage cells of the body. Free radicals are the by-product of both energy production by the body's cells and exposure to pollutants and radiation. Oxidized cholesterol (particularly LDL cholesterol) then initiates inflammation and eventual plaque buildup in the blood vessel wall, which inhibits blood flow through the arteries. This oxidation leads to inflammation and damage in the artery walls.

Getting More Specific with Cholesterol

Apolipoprotein B (apoB) is a protein that is believed to promote heart disease by affecting how cholesterol is transported into the arteries and the tissues. ApoB is found in low density lipoprotein (LDL) and other potentially harmful cholesterols, such as very low density lipoproteins (VLDL). Conversely, apolipoprotein A (apoA-1) is found in HDL cholesterol and provides a protective effect against heart disease.

A large study known as the AMORIS (Apolipoprotein-related Mortality Risk) measured the levels of apoA-1 and apoB, as well as other lipids, in more than 175,000 men and women in Sweden. Researchers found that people at greatest risk of dying from a heart attack tended to have the highest ratios of apoB to apoA-1. In this study, these markers were more predictive of a heart attack than were the typically measured total, HDL, and LDL cholesterol and triglycerides. Men with the highest apoB/apoA-1 ratio had almost four times the risk of a fatal heart attack, compared to those with the lowest ratios; and in women the relative risk was threefold. ApoB appears to be an important marker for people with normal to low LDL cholesterol, as well as for those with diabetes and insulin resistance.

ApoB reference range: 55–125 mg/dL
ApoA-1 reference range: 125–215 mg/dL
ApoB/ApoA-1 ratio reference range: 0.30–0.90

SYMPTOMS

Often, there are no symptoms of high cholesterol, so it's important to have your doctor perform a blood analysis regularly. One sign of high cholesterol can be a buildup of cholesterol rings on the skin under the eyes. Make an appointment if cholesterol or heart problems run in your family, or if you experience any of the following:

- Difficulty breathing after minor exertion
- Dizziness
- Mental confusion or dullness
- Circulatory problems

ROOT CAUSES

- Poor diet, especially one high in refined carbohydrates
- Inactivity
- Hereditary tendency to high cholesterol
- Diabetes, insulin resistance
- Hypothyroidism
- Hormone deficiencies such as low testosterone and low estrogen
- Stress

The particle size of LDL cholesterol is very important. The smaller particle size, known as LDL density pattern B, is most likely to cause atherosclerosis, whereas larger LDL particles, known as pattern A, are the least likely to accumulate in arteries and cause atherosclerosis.

There's no doubt about it: Statin drugs are associated with a much higher risk of developing diabetes, and the risk is so strong that even the FDA has issued a warning about it. But that's only the beginning of the risk—because the latest research finds that cholesterol-lowering meds may not only increase your risk of diabetes but also give you more complications from the disease.

If you're healthy before starting statins, the drugs will increase your risk of diabetes by 85 percent and more than double your odds of suffering from diabetes with complications, according to a study in the *Journal of General Internal Medicine*. The higher the dose, the higher your risk— and if you're on high-intensity statin therapy, your risk of diabetes with complications jumps by 368 percent.

Testing Techniques

See the Cardiovascular Disease section for a review of all cardiovascular markers that should be tested.

Lipoprotein particle sizes—blood test

Oxidative damage—blood or urine

Oxidized LDL—blood

TREATMENT

Diet

Recommended Food

One major key to balancing cholesterol levels is to consume a diet that's high in fiber. This means increasing the amount of vegetables, fruits, nuts, seeds, and whole grains in the diet. Soluble fiber is a great choice. This type of fiber does not dissolve in water and binds cholesterol as it passes through the digestive tract. It also decreases your risk of developing many other diseases. Oat bran is a great source of soluble fiber, and more than twenty studies show that it reduces total and LDL cholesterol when consumed on a daily basis. One bowl of oatmeal can lower cholesterol levels between 8 and 23 percent in just three weeks.

Pectin, found in the skin of apples, is also effective, as are ground flaxseeds, beans, apples, peas, and pears.

Consume nuts rich in monounsaturated fatty acids such as almonds and walnuts. A study conducted at the Lipid Clinic in Barcelona, Spain, showed that a walnut-rich diet reduced total cholesterol by as much as 7.4 percent and LDL cholesterol by as much as 10 percent.

Finally, many people with diabetes and insulin resistance find that cutting down on simple carbohydrates and increasing the consumption of protein foods can dramatically reduce cholesterol levels.

The molecules in cholesterol are highly vulnerable to damage by free radicals. Reduce your risk of developing heart disease and other serious degenerative illness by increasing your consumption of deeply colored fruits and vegetables. Eat a wide variety for the broadest protection, and try for at least five raw or lightly cooked servings every day.

Essential fatty acids actually have a heart-protecting effect. Consume two servings a week of heart-healthy omega-3 fatty acids, found in fish such as anchovies, Atlantic herring, sardines, tilapia, and ocean or canned salmon.

Ground flaxseeds are another good source of EFAs; you can sprinkle them over salads or use the oil as a dressing.

Olive oil increases levels of HDL (the "good" cholesterol). The uses for this fruity oil are numerous: it can enrich pasta sauces, or you can add a little to a skillet and sauté your favorite vegetables.

Garlic and onions are savory complements to vegetarian meals—and they help lower LDL cholesterol while raising HDL. Add spices to your meals, such as cayenne, basil, rosemary, and oregano. These spices are rich in antioxidants to prevent cholesterol oxidation.

Food to Avoid

Fats that are hydrogenated or partially hydrogenated (trans fats) tend to raise LDL cholesterol and triglycerides and reduce HDL cholesterol. Fried foods, sweet baked goods, and most crackers are all dangerously full of these bad trans fats. Even margarine and vegetable shortening—items that cholesterol patients often use as substitutes for butter and lard—are high in partially hydrogenated fats.

Sugar and alcohol stimulate the liver to produce more cholesterol. Avoid alcoholic beverages and all sources of refined sugar, including sodas, candy, and low-fat baked goods.

Green tea is rich in the antioxidants that have been shown to prevent cholesterol oxidation.

Hydrogenated and Partially Hydrogenated Fats

Hydrogenation is a process that turns vegetable and seed oils into soft or solid fats that, unlike the oils in their natural state, can be used as table spreads and that hold up when used in cooking or baking. During hydrogenation, the oil's carbon molecules are saturated with hydrogenation and exposed to extremely high heat. The oil is kept in the heat until it reaches the desired consistency. Shortening, for example, remains in the heat until it is completely solid; it is said to be a hydrogenated fat. Margarine, on the other hand, is removed from the heat before the oil completely hardens, just as it reaches a soft, "spreadable" consistency. Products like margarine are called partially hydrogenated oils.

It's ironic and unfortunate that margarine and even vegetable shortening are touted as heart-healthful products. For years, doctors have told us to replace butter with margarine, and most brands of shortening loudly proclaim that they have less saturated fat than butter does. But as you have probably heard, researchers have discovered that the hydrogenating process produces altered molecules called trans-fatty acids. These substances appear to pack a double whammy: not only do they raise LDL, they lower HDL and cause free-radical damage. Instead, eat cold-water fish and sauté your vegetables and dress your salads with oils like olive and flaxseed. These foods fill you up, while raising your "good" cholesterol levels.

℞ Super Seven Prescriptions—High Cholesterol

Super Prescription #1 Niacin
Take 1,500 to 3,000 mg daily. The no-flush form is also available although not as well studied. Niacin reduces total cholesterol and LDL cholesterol and increases the good HDL cholesterol.

Super Prescription #2 Red yeast rice
Take 1,200 mg twice daily. This extract has been shown to reduce total cholesterol levels by 11 to 32 percent and triglyceride levels by 12 to 19 percent. *Note*: Take 25 to 100 mg of CoQ10 when using this product to prevent possible deficiency.

Super Prescription #3 Plant sterols (*beta sitosterol*)
Take 1,000 to 1,500 mg twice daily with meals. Inhibits the absorption of cholesterol from food.

American Journal of Clinical Nutrition published an analysis of twenty-one published studies that tracked almost 350,000 men and women for up to twenty-three years. It showed that people who consumed the largest amounts of saturated fat in their diet did *not* have a higher than average risk of heart disease, stroke, or other types of cardiovascular disease.

The real culprit, according to the author, seemed to be refined carbohydrates—found in candies, desserts, soft drinks, and white bread. These types of carbs increased levels of insulin, cholesterol, and triglycerides. If you cut back on saturated fat but increase your intake of these carbs, you actually boost your risk of a heart attack. However, substituting fruits and vegetables is protective.

Studies have shown that niacin lowers LDL cholesterol up to 25 percent, lowers triglycerides up to 50 percent, and increases HDL cholesterol up to 35 percent.

Fish oil is the primary treatment for high triglycerides in both conventional and alternative medicine. A high dose of fish oil can reduce triglycerides by up to 50 percent.

Super Prescription #4 Fish oil
Take 2,000 to 3,000 mg of combined EPA and DHA to reduce cholesterol and triglyceride levels.

Super Prescription #5 Garlic (*Allium sativum*)
Take 300 to 500 mg of aged garlic twice daily. It reduces cholesterol levels and increases HDL cholesterol.

Super Prescription #6 Guggul (*Commiphora mukul*)
Take a daily total of 1,500 mg standardized to 5 percent guggulsterone (equivalent to 75 mg of guggulsterones). This Ayurvedic herb reduces cholesterol levels and increases HDL.

Super Prescription #7 Artichoke extract
Take 1,000 mg twice daily. Reduces total and LDL cholesterol.

A double-blind, randomized, placebo-controlled study at the UCLA School of Medicine found that red yeast rice extract significantly reduced cholesterol levels compared to a placebo.

General Recommendations

Pantetheine is a metabolite of vitamin B5 that has been shown in studies to reduce total and LDL cholesterol, as well as to increase HDL. It can be particularly effective for people with diabetes. Take 600 to 900 mg daily.

Soy protein has been shown in studies to reduce total and LDL cholesterol and to increase HDL. Take 25 to 50 grams daily.

Reishi (*Ganoderma lucidum*) is a mushroom extract that reduces cholesterol. Take 800 mg two to three times daily.

Gooseberry (*Phyllanthus emblica*) has been shown to increase HDL cholesterol and to lower LDL cholesterol. Take 500 to 1,000 mg daily.

Vitamin E prevents LDL oxidation. Take 400 to 800 IU of a mixed blend daily.

Vitamin C reduces total cholesterol and LDL levels and acts to prevent their oxidation.

Chromium reduces total cholesterol and increases HDL levels. Take 200 to 400 mcg daily.

A twelve-week study demonstrated that 1,500 mg of guggulipid reduced total cholesterol by an average of 22 percent and triglycerides by 25 percent. A different study of 233 people with elevated cholesterol levels showed that guggul worked better than the cholesterol-lowering drug clofibrate. Only people who took guggul had improvements in HDL cholesterol.

Green tea contains potent antioxidants known as polyphenols that reduce cholesterol oxidation. It has also been shown to reduce total cholesterol levels, while increasing good HDL cholesterol.

Sytrinol, a product containing natural citrus and palm fruit extracts, has been shown to significantly lower total and LDL cholesterol and triglycerides.

A tocopherol/tocotrienol complex has been shown to reduce total and LDL cholesterol. Take 100 to 200 mg daily.

Take a complex of antioxidants or a multivitamin as directed on the container. Several antioxidants prevent cholesterol oxidation.

Homeopathy

If you have cardiovascular disease, see a licensed homeopath for a constitutional remedy.

Acupressure

See pages 787–794 for information about acupressure points and administering treatment.

• Keep blood flowing to your heart and chest by working Heart 3 and 7 (H3 and H7).

- If you can feel your chest tense up when you're under pressure, take some time out to work Conception Vessel 17 (CV17).
- Pericardium 3 (P3) is another point for anxiety and chest pain.
- Should tension and anxiety bring on heart palpitations, work Pericardium 6 (P6).

Stress Reduction

General Stress-Reduction Therapies

Persistent, unresolved stress has been linked to high cholesterol problems, as well as to heart disease and stroke. Stress reduction should be part of a comprehensive approach to preventing heart disease.

Other Recommendations

- Know your cholesterol and cardiovascular risk marker levels—all of them. Get regular checkups, and find a doctor who is willing to explain the numbers to you.
- Smoking is the number-one risk factor in heart disease. If you smoke and have high cholesterol, you're in grave danger of having a heart attack. People who smoke must quit immediately; even if you've never picked up the habit but are exposed to secondhand smoke, you must find a cleaner environment in which to live or work.
- Exercise lowers LDL levels, while raising those of HDL. Find an activity you enjoy, and pursue it regularly. A brisk thirty-minute walk every day does wonders for almost everyone.
- If you have diabetes or hypothyroidism, work with a doctor to keep your disease in check and to devise an individual plan for controlling your cholesterol.
- Many cholesterol patients are told to lose weight. The dietary suggestions here will help most people take off excess pounds, but if you're more than twenty pounds overweight, you may need additional help. See Obesity for further suggestions.

Numerous studies have shown that vitamin C reduces the risk of dying from heart disease. One of the mechanisms, in addition to its ability to prevent cholesterol oxidation, is that it is involved in the formation of bile salts. Bile is produced by the liver and released by the gallbladder to digest fats. Cholesterol is converted into bile salts and eliminated through the digestive tract. Vitamin C enhances this process by improving bile-salt formation and thus cholesterol elimination.

REFERENCES

Bargossi, A. M., M. Battino, A. Gaddi, et al. 1994. Exogenous CoQ10 preserves plasma ubiquinone levels in patients treated with 3-hydroxy-3-methylglutaryl coenzyme A reductase inhibitors. *International Journal of Clinical and Laboratory Research* 24:171–76.

Brown, R. 2015. Statins linked to diabetes and complications in healthy adults. Medscape.com. Accessed June 27, 2015 at http://www.medscape.com/view article/845232.

Folkers, K., et al. 1990. Lovastatin decreases coenzyme Q levels in humans. *Proceedings of the National Academy of Sciences of the United States of America* 87(22):8931–34.

Ghirlanda, G., A. Oradei, A. Manto, et al. 1993. Evidence of plasma CoQ10-lowering effect by HMG-CoA reductase inhibitors: A double-blind, placebo-controlled study. *Journal of Clinical Pharmacology* 33(3):226–29.

Heber, D., et al. 1999. Cholesterol-lowering effects of a proprietary Chinese red-yeast-rice dietary supplement. *American Journal of Clinical Nutrition* 69:231–36.

Kishi, T., H. Kishi, and K. Folkers. 1977. Inhibition of cardiac CoQ10 enzymes by clinically used drugs and possible prevention. In *Biomedical and Clinical Aspects of Coenzyme Q*, Vol. I. Ed. K. Folkers and Y.Yamamura. Amsterdam: Elsevier/North Holland Biomedical Press, pp. 47–62.

Mortensen, S. A., et al. 1997. Dose-related decrease of serum coenzyme Q10 during treatment with HMG-CoA reductase inhibitors. *Molecular Aspects of Medicine* 18(Suppl.):S137–S144.

Niyanand, S., et al. 1989. Clinical trials with guggulipid: A new hypolipidemic agent. *Journal of the Association of Physicians of India* 37(5):323–28.

Siri-Tarino, P. W., et al. 2010. Meta-analysis of prospective cohort studies evaluating the association of saturated fat with cardiovascular disease. *American Journal of Clinical Nutrition* 91:535–45.

Srinivasan, S. R., and G. S. Berenson. 2001. Apolipoproteins B and A1 as predictors of risk of coronary artery disease [commentary]. *Lancet* 358:2012–13.

Walldius, G., I. Jungner, I. Holme, et al. 2001. High apolipoprotein B, low apolipoprotein AI, and improvement in the prediction of fatal myocardial infarction (AMORIS study): A prospective study. *Lancet* 358:2026–33.

Chronic Fatigue Syndrome (CFS)

Chronic fatigue syndrome is a disorder that involves severe fatigue that lasts for more than six months. The US Institute of Medicine has proposed that the condition be renamed "systemic exertion intolerance disease" but most clinicians still refer to it as CFS.

Most doctors now acknowledge that CFS is a real disorder. And as its victims well know, it can also be horribly debilitating. Its predominant symptom is persistent, overwhelming fatigue that dramatically reduces its sufferers' ability to participate in the regular activities of life. Along with the fatigue are problems with memory and concentration. It is also usually accompanied by several out of a long list of symptoms, including but not limited to headaches, insomnia, sore throat, and muscle and joint pain. These problems can come and go over a period of years. If you have deep fatigue for more than two weeks, or if for any reason you suspect that you have CFS, do not make a diagnosis on your own. See a doctor so that he or she can rule out other possible disorders. Once other disorders have been ruled out, your best chances of recovery, in our opinion, involve the use of natural therapies.

CFS is probably caused by a combination of factors and often results in a depressed immune system. Of course, the key to treatment is to find out and treat the reason(s) for the immune-system imbalance, which can be related to many factors. For example, chronic infections are thought to play a role for some people, such as the viruses Epstein-Barr (EBV), cytomegalovirus (CMV), and human herpes virus (HHV-6). Other infections, such as mycoplasma, Lyme disease, and chlamydia, are also suspect. The overgrowth of fungi (*Candida albicans*) seems to be a common problem for people with this condition, and health practitioners frequently find parasite infection to be present.

CFS is diagnosed based on patients' symptoms and on ruling out other diseases that have fatigue as a symptom. Besides experiencing severe fatigue for at least six months, one would also have four or more of the following symptoms to qualify for a diagnosis: substantial impairment in concentration or short-term memory, sore throat, tender lymph nodes, muscle pain, multijoint pain without swelling or redness, headaches, unrefreshed sleep, and postexertional fatigue lasting more than twenty-four hours.

One common finding in people with this condition is hormone imbalance. The most common one is adrenal-gland insufficiency, also referred to as "adrenal burnout." (See Adrenal Fatigue.) The adrenal glands, located on top of both kidneys, produce the stress hormones cortisol and DHEA. These hormones are commonly depleted in people with chronic fatigue, and we find that restoring the levels to normal is generally quite helpful. The same can be said of many of the hormones in the body. Low thyroid function can be a core problem and will result in suboptimal energy production within the cells. In addition, deficiencies in testosterone or growth hormone and deficiencies or imbalances of estrogen and progesterone are common. Underlying much of the hormone imbalance can be hypothalamic dysfunction. This refers to an imbalance of the hormonal and the neural messages from the brain to the adrenal and the thyroid glands and other hormonal organs of the body. Low neurotransmitters can also contribute to chronic fatigue.

Poor digestion and impaired detoxification also need to be considered as root causes of chronic fatigue. Malabsorption of foods and nutrients contributes to nutritional deficiencies. Environmental toxins, such as mercury and others, inhibit enzyme functions that are required for energy production.

An unhealthful diet can set the stage for chronic fatigue. A high amount of refined carbohydrates contributes to blood sugar problems, yeast overgrowth, increased demand on the adrenal glands, and chronic inflammation, and immune suppression can set in. In addition, a diet of processed foods is deficient of the nutrients required for energy production and a healthy immune system.

Also of prime importance are the effects of chronic stress on the body. People who do not deal with mental, emotional, and spiritual stresses effectively are more likely to suffer fatigue. In addition, unresolved problems with anxiety and depression contribute to fatigue.

Movement and exercise are fundamental keys to health. Too little exercise contributes to fatigue, while, at the opposite end of the spectrum, overtraining and overexertion lead to breakdown of the organs involved with energy production.

A final area worth mentioning is sleep. This is your body's way of recovering and regenerating. Adequate sleep is essential. If you suffer from a sleep problem, seek medical help and focus on natural ways to alleviate it. See the Insomnia section.

A good complementary-care regimen will address the whole body—and therefore many of the possible causes. If you have CFS, it's important to find the treatments that give you the most relief; what works for one person might not be right for another.

SYMPTOMS

Constant, disabling fatigue is the primary symptom, but CFS usually incorporates several of the following:

- Low-grade fever
- Headache
- Sleep disturbances
- Depression and anxiety
- Difficulty concentrating
- Temporary loss of memory
- Muscle and joint pain
- Weakness
- Exhaustion after even mild exercise
- Loss of appetite
- Upper respiratory tract infections
- Sore throat
- Intestinal problems
- Sore or swollen lymph nodes

In a randomized, double-blind study in the *Journal of Chronic Fatigue*, researchers found that people who received an integrated treatment approach, based on each individual's symptoms and laboratory analysis, experienced significantly greater benefits than did people receiving a placebo. Long-term follow-up found that the active group had increasing improvement.

ROOT CAUSES

- Chronic infection
- Immune-system damage
- Low blood pressure
- Nutritional deficiencies
- Intestinal permeability
- Impaired detoxification
- Parasites and dysbiosis
- Food allergies
- Chemical sensitivities
- Neurological malfunction
- Chronic fungal infection
- Hypoglycemia
- Hypothyroidism
- Poor adrenal function
- Sleep disorders (such as apnea)
- Hormone deficiencies
- Environmental toxins (e.g., toxic metals)
- Unresolved stress
- Side effects of pharmaceutical medications
- Neurotransmitter deficiency

Testing Techniques

The following tests help assess possible metabolic reasons for chronic fatigue syndrome:

Immune system imbalance or disease—blood

Low blood pressure

Hormone testing (thyroid, DHEA, cortisol, testosterone, IGF-1, estrogen, progesterone)—saliva, blood, or urine

Intestinal permeability—urine

Detoxification profile—urine

Vitamin and mineral analysis (especially magnesium, B12, iron, and CoQ10)—blood

Digestive function and microbe/parasite/candida testing—stool analysis

Anemia—blood test (CBC, iron, ferritin, % saturation)

Food and environmental allergies/sensitivities—blood, electrodermal

Blood sugar balance—blood

Sleep disorder—sleep study

Heart function—EKG

Toxic metals—urine or hair analysis

A double-blind, placebo-controlled human clinical trial demonstrated that ashwagandha supplementation boosted energy. The participants who took a standardized form of ashwagandha (8 percent withanolides) experienced a 79 percent increase in energy compared to those who took a placebo.

TREATMENT

Diet

Recommended Food

Your diet should be dense with nutrients and strong in immune-building foods. Sea vegetables and whole grains are high in minerals that your body may lack; cultured foods with probiotics will fight infection, especially candidiasis; cruciferous vegetables are high in nutrients and fiber; and nuts, seeds, and cold-water fish contain lots of essential fatty acids, which support immune function.

Drink a glass of clean, quality water every two waking hours to flush out toxins and encourage good general health.

Intestinal pain is an unpleasant symptom of CFS. Keep your digestive tract working efficiently by eating foods that are high in fiber, especially cruciferous vegetables.

Food to Avoid

People with CFS usually have severely depleted immune systems. Keep as much stress off the body as possible by avoiding caffeine, alcohol, junk and processed food, and refined sugars. In addition to taxing the immune system, some of these items aggravate conditions that may cause CFS. Caffeine depresses the adrenal glands, excess sugar consumption can lead to hypoglycemia, and junk and processed foods contain additives that stimulate chemical sensitivities.

CFS is often accompanied by food allergies; in fact, allergies may cause some cases of CFS. See the Food Allergies section and the accompanying elimination diet to help you determine which foods, if any, trigger an allergic response for you.

Be wary of wheat. Fatigue is a common symptom of wheat or gluten allergy or intolerance. Talk with your nutrition-oriented doctor about testing for a reaction to this food. Or, avoid gluten products for two to four weeks, and see if you notice an improvement.

> **Whiteout**
>
> When eliminating processed foods, a good rule of thumb is to watch out for the "whites." White flour, white sugar, and salt are all hallmarks of artificial or junk-food products.

℞ Super Seven Prescriptions—Chronic Fatigue Syndrome

Super Prescription #1 D-ribose
Take 5 grams two to three times daily. This naturally occurring sugar helps energy production within cells.

Super Prescription #2 CoQ10
Take 200 to 300 mg daily with meals. It is important for energy production in cells.

Super Prescription #3 Ashwagandha
Take 250 mg daily of an 8 percent withanolide extract. It has been shown to increase energy.

Super Prescription #4 Vitamin B12
Take 1,000 to 5,000 mcg of the methylcobalamin sublingual form each morning. The injection form (once weekly) is very effective and is available from a doctor

Super Prescription #5 L-carnitine
Take 2,000 mg daily in divided doses. It has been shown to help chronic fatigue.

Super Prescription #6 NADH
Take 10 mg on an empty stomach each morning.

Super Prescription #7 Rhodiola rosea
Take 300 mg of a 3 percent rosavin extract daily. It has been shown to improve energy production.

A study published in the *Journal of Alternative and Complementary Medicine* found that D-ribose significantly reduced clinical symptoms in patients suffering from fibromyalgia and chronic fatigue syndrome. The dosage in the study was 5 grams taken three times daily.

One double-blind study looked at the effect of using 10 mg of NADH or a placebo each day for four weeks on people with chronic fatigue syndrome. Thirty-one percent of those receiving NADH reported an improvement in fatigue, a decrease in other symptoms, and improved overall quality of life, in contrast to 8 percent of those in the placebo group.

General Recommendations

Vitamin C is used by the adrenal glands to manufacture stress hormones, and it also supports immune function.

A probiotic supplies the good bacteria needed for proper digestion, detoxification, and immunity. Take a product that contains at least four billion organisms daily.

Essential fatty acids are important for healthy cell and brain function. Take 1 or 2 tablespoons of flaxseed oil or 3 to 5 grams of fish oil daily.

L-carnitine is used by the cells for energy production. Take 500 mg three times daily.

Panax ginseng is a strong adrenal-gland tonic. Take 100 mg two or three times daily of a product standardized to between 4 and 7 percent ginsenosides.

Eleutherococcus (Siberian) ginseng is good for energy production. Take 600 to 900 mg of a standardized product daily.

Reishi (*Ganoderma lucidum*) is an adaptogen that can help with energy and mental function. Take 800 mg of a standardized product twice daily.

Ginkgo biloba is a popular herb that improves circulation, which is good for people with low blood pressure, and improves memory. Take 60 to 120 mg twice daily of a standardized product containing 24 percent flavone glycosides and 6 percent terpene lactones.

Saint-John's-wort (*Hypericum perforatum*) can be helpful when depression accompanies fatigue. Take 300 mg three times daily of a 0.3 percent hypericin extract. Do not combine with pharmaceutical antidepressants.

5-HTP is for insomnia and depression related to the fatigue. Take 100 mg two or three times daily. For insomnia, take 100 mg a half hour before bedtime on an empty stomach. Do not combine with pharmaceutical antidepressants.

Olive leaf (*Olea europa*) is for antiviral support. Take 500 mg three times daily.

Phosphatidylserine is a naturally occurring phospholipid that improves memory and increases cortisol levels. Take 300 mg daily.

Ashwagandha, known as "Indian Ginseng," is a revered herb in Ayurvedic medicine and is used as a tonic for fatigue and anxiety. Take 250 mg daily of a 0.8 percent extract.

Enzyme complex can be taken with meals to improve digestion and absorption.

Oregano (*Origanum vulgare*) oil is for chronic infections. Take 500 mg of the capsule form four times daily or as directed on the container.

Malic acid is used by cells for energy production. Take 500 mg two or three times daily.

Vitamin D deficiency can cause fatigue. Take 2,000 to 5,000 IU daily with meals.

Licorice (*Glycyrrhiza glabra*) works to increase the levels of cortisol in the body. Take 1,000 mg two or three times daily. Blood pressure should be monitored, because in some individuals it may elevate blood pressure.

Magnesium is crucial for energy production within the cells. Take 250 mg two or three times daily. Reduce the dosage if diarrhea occurs.

Cordyceps sinensis supports adrenal-gland function. Take 800 mg twice daily.

DHEA is an adrenal hormone that helps with energy production and the effects of stress. Take 5 to 25 mg daily under a doctor's supervision if testing shows that your levels are low.

Note: The use of low doses of cortisol can be effective for people with chronic fatigue syndrome and diagnosed cortisol deficiency. Consult with your local holistic doctor for its proper use.

Homeopathy

Arsenicum Album is helpful for feelings of exhaustion, combined with anxiety and depression. The person is usually chilly, feels worse from cold food or cold environments, and often has trouble sleeping between the hours of midnight and 2 A.M.

Calcarea Carbonica is for a person with fatigue and anxiety who tends to take on too much. He or she also suffers from swollen glands, joint pain, headache, intestinal distress, constipation, and food allergies. The person tends to be chilly, yet sweats easily.

Gelsemium (*Gelsemium sempervirens*) is for fatigue that includes drowsiness, weakness, and a bruising pain in the muscles.

Kali Phosphoricum is for a feeling of fatigue and mental weariness.

Phosphoric Acid is for extreme fatigue, where the person has an unusually strong craving for carbonated drinks. Fatigue may come on after episodes of emotional grief.

Silica (*Silicea*) is for bouts of fatigue and poor stamina. The person gets sick easily and is usually thin and chilly. Constipation is often present.

Acupressure

See pages 787–794 for information about acupressure points and administering treatment.

- Stomach 36 (St36) is an important point for CFS, because it helps your digestive system absorb nutrients.
- Gallbladder 21 (GB21) stimulates circulation. It also alleviates anxiety, irritability, and headaches.
- Pericardium 6 (P6) is good for indigestion, sleeplessness, and nervous tension.
- Bladder 23 and 47 (B23 and B47) support the nervous system and are especially good for fatigue, weakness, and confusion. Do not press on these points if you have severe back pain.
- Lung 3 (Lu3) helps tiredness, head pain, confusion, and lightheadedness.
- Triple Warmer 5 (TW5) soothes joint pain.

Bodywork

Bodywork is a good way to address the many causes and symptoms of CFS. Include at least one bodywork strategy in your treatment program.

Massage

In general, massage improves the systems weakened by CFS: immune, muscular, circulatory, digestive, and limbic. Almost any kind of massage will make you feel better, but if you're seeing a professional, you may want to ask for a lymphatic-drainage massage to stimulate your immune response. Any of the essential oils listed in this section under Aromatherapy will compound the beneficial effects of massage.

You can practice gentle self-massage of your gums, tongue, and lower abdomen to strengthen your digestive system. Chiropractic and osteopathic treatments are also helpful for proper nerve and energy flow. Acupuncture can be very effective for fatigue. Consult with a qualified practitioner.

Reflexology

See pages 804–805 for information about reflexology areas and how to work them. Since CFS is a systemic disorder, it's best to massage the entire foot. If you want to focus on specific symptoms, here are some suggestions. For fatigue, work the adrenals, the diaphragm, the spine, and all the glands. Work the endocrine glands, the solar plexus, the pancreas, and the head in case of depression. If your doctor suspects that hypoglycemia is a cause of your CFS, massaging the pancreas area can help (although it's not a substitute for other treatment). The liver, the gallbladder, and the stomach will ease indigestion.

Hydrotherapy

Constitutional hydrotherapy renews the nervous system. See pages 795–796 for more information.

Aromatherapy

Many oils may reduce your levels of tension and depression. Several suggestions are listed here, but you may want to refer to pages 771–781 and try others that seem best suited to your particular needs. All of the oils mentioned here can be used as inhalants (with steam or without), in baths or diffusers, or as part of a massage.

To stimulate your muscular and nervous systems, use lavender, peppermint, or rosemary.

Geranium, bergamot, and neroli combat fatigue related to depression. Tea tree oil fights bacteria, viruses, and fungi. Because it strengthens the immune system, it's an especially good complement to a lymphatic massage.

For general relaxation and calming benefits, try rose, jasmine, lavender, or bergamot in any preparation you like. If you need all-day stress relief, consider using a diffuser that allows the scent to fill your home or office.

Stress Reduction

General Stress-Reduction Therapies

If you suffer from anxiety, consider EEG biofeedback to teach you to control your brainwaves.

Join a support group for CFS.

If you're ready for a gentle workout, take a yoga class. Yoga relieves joint and muscle pain, and several of the poses help strengthen the digestive muscles.

If you suffer from anxiety, consider EEG biofeedback to teach you to control your brainwaves.

Other Recommendations

- Take a walk every day in the early-morning sunlight. You'll stimulate your immune system, get vitamin D, and ward off the depression and the anxiety that often attend CFS.
- Don't try to do too much. Listen to your body; when it tells you to get rest, do so.
- Don't smoke or expose yourself to secondhand smoke. You'll wreak havoc on your immune system.
- Breathe slowly and deeply to encourage relaxation and to diminish stress.
- Try to keep an optimistic outlook, and focus on a positive outcome.

- Go to bed by 9 P.M. and take a thirty-minute nap after lunch each day.
- Intravenous nutrient therapy and ozone intravenous therapy have been very effective for our patients with CFS.

REFERENCES

Auddy, B., J. Hazra, A. Mitra, et al. 2008. A standardized Withania somnifera extract significantly reduces stress-related parameters in chronically stressed humans: A double-blind, randomized, placebo-controlled study. *Journal of the American Nutraceutical Association* 11(1).

Forsyth, L. M., H. G. Preuss, A. L. MacDowell, et al. 1999. Therapeutic effects of oral NADH on the symptoms of patients with chronic fatigue syndrome. *Annals of Allergy, Asthma and Immunology* 82(2):185–91.

Teitelbaum, J. E., et al. 2006. The use of D-ribose in chronic fatigue syndrome and fibromyalgia: A pilot study. *Journal of Alternative and Complementary Medicine* 12:857–62.

Teitelbaum, J., et al. 2001. Effective treatment of chronic fatigue syndrome and fibromyalgia: A randomized, double-blind, placebo-controlled, intent to treat study. *Journal of Chronic Fatigue Syndrome* 8(2).

Chronic Obstructive Pulmonary Disease (COPD)

Chronic obstructive pulmonary disease, or COPD, is a condition that includes the combination of emphysema and bronchitis (inflammation of the bronchi, the major air-carrying passages between the mouth and lungs). It affects an estimated thirty-two million Americans. It is the third leading cause of death after heart disease and cancer.

With COPD there are detrimental structural changes from tissue damage within the airways and lung tissue. As a result there are symptoms of cough, shortness of breath, exercise intolerance, excess sputum production, and sometimes changes in cognitive function. The inability to breathe properly is the most dominant symptom. COPD is progressive, meaning that it gets worse with time. Most cases are the result of cigarette-smoke exposure.

SYMPTOMS

- Cough with mucus
- Shortness of breath
- Wheezing
- Changes in mental status
- Weight loss

ROOT CAUSES

- Smoking tobacco (most commonly, often even affecting those who stopped smoking decades earlier)
- Long-term exposure to air pollution, chemical fumes, and dust

---

Testing Techniques

Pulmonary function tests (spirometry is the most common)
Chest X-ray
Arterial blood gas analysis
CT scan of chest
Nutrient levels—blood

Treatment

Neither conventional nor alternative medicine has a cure for COPD, and all the drug treatments come with *potential side effects*. However, there are several nutrition-based treatments that can help many COPD sufferers and that are generally used as a complementary treatment to drug therapy.

Diet

Recommended food

A diet that includes fruit, fish, and dairy products and avoids processed foods, red meat, and sweets can improve COPD symptoms and lead to better lung function. Fruits and vegetables are rich in the antioxidants that reduce inflammation. Fish, such as salmon and sardines, contains inflammation-suppressing omega-3 fatty acids. People with COPD are often underweight and malnourished. It is important to maintain adequate protein, which is around 80 to 90 grams daily. Small, frequent meals work best.

Food to Avoid

Dairy products can increase mucus formation for some COPD patients, so eat them with caution. Avoiding foods that trigger food sensitivities can be helpful for some people with COPD. See a holistic doctor for testing, and consult the Food Allergies/Sensitivities chapter.

NAC's ability to reduce COPD symptoms was confirmed in published research. Researchers gave 120 volunteers with stable COPD, mostly older men, either 600 mg of NAC or placebos daily for one year. Tests at the beginning and end of the study measured their lung function. By the end of the study, patients taking NAC had anywhere from a 25 to 75 percent improvement in "forced expiratory flow," a measure of lung function. They also had a 44 percent drop in the average number of COPD symptoms.

℞ **Super Seven Prescriptions—COPD**

Super Prescription #1 N-acetylcysteine (NAC)
Take 600 mg to 2,000 mg daily on an empty stomach. NAC thins mucus, which reduces coughing.

Super Prescription #2 Essential amino acid blend
Take as directed on the label to support muscle and lung health.

Super Prescription #3 Glutathione
Take 250 to 500 mg twice daily on an empty stomach. Glutathione functions as a super antioxidant, protecting the cells of the lungs.

Super Prescription #4 Magnesium
Take 250 mg twice daily. Low magnesium is common in those with COPD. It helps to prevent spasm of the airways.

Super Prescription #5 Fatty acid combo

Take a combination of essential fatty acids to get 1,200 mg of alpha linolenic acid, 700 mg of EPA, 340 mg of DHA, and 760 mg of GLA. This combo improved exercise tolerance in those with COPD.

Super Prescription #6 L-carnitine

Take 2,000 mg twice daily on an empty stomach to improve exercise tolerance.

Super Prescription #7 Proteolytic enzymes

Take as directed on the label on an empty stomach. They help reduce mucus production.

General Recommendations

Garlic (*Allium sativum*) has antimicrobial effects. Take 300 to 600 mg of garlic extract twice daily.

Licorice (*Glycyrrhiza glabra*) reduces coughing, enhances immune function, and soothes the respiratory tract. Use caution when supplementing licorice if you have high blood pressure. It's best used short term under the guidance of a holistic doctor. Take 500 mg of the capsule or 1 ml of the tincture four times daily.

Bromelain has a natural anti-inflammatory effect and enhances the effectiveness of some antibiotics. Take 500 mg three times daily between meals or along with antibiotic therapy. Look for products standardized to 2,000 MCU (milk-clotting units) per 1,000 mg or 1,200 GDU (gelatin-dissolving units) per 1,000 mg.

Vitamin A supports respiratory immunity. Take 5,000 IU daily with a meal.

Other useful herbs that can be found in respiratory formulas include horehound, pleurisy root, plantain, marshmallow, ginger, peppermint, and cherry bark.

Other Recommendations

We have found intravenous nutrients to be helpful for patients with COPD. A team of researchers at the University of Utah treated ten COPD patients, alternating between 2 grams of intravenous vitamin C (IVC) and a placebo. After getting the IVC, patients had less muscle fatigue and were able to breathe better and slower.

Bodywork

Acupuncture can be helpful in improving symptoms. Consult with a licensed acupuncturist.

REFERENCES

Medline Plus. Diet tied to better breathing in COPD patients. Accessed August 3, 2014.

Dal Negro, R. W., R. Aquilani, S. Bertacco, et al. 2010. Comprehensive effects of supplemented essential amino acids in patients with severe chronic obstructive pulmonary disease and sarcopenia. *Monaldi Archives for Chest Disease* 73:25–33.

De Flora, S., C. Grassi, and L. Carati. 1997. Attenuation of influenza-like symptomatology and improvement of cell-mediated immunity with long-term N-acetylcysteine treatment. *European Respiratory Journal* 10:1535–541.

Italian researchers treated thirty-two men and women with severe COPD and sarcopenia (age-related muscle loss). For twelve weeks the volunteers took supplements of all eight essential amino acids (4 grams total daily) or placebos. By the end of the study, people taking the amino acids had gained an average of thirteen pounds, most of which was muscle, not fat. They were also more physically active.

Glutathione is a normal part of the fluid lining the tissue of the lower respiratory tract. It's found in concentrations in the lung fluid that are 140 times that of blood concentrations. In lung disease such as COPD there's an increased demand for antioxidant activity. We have found oral and inhaled glutathione to benefit those with COPD. Consult with your holistic doctor.

Prousky, J. The treatment of Pulmonary Diseases and Respiratory-Related Conditions With Inhaled (Nebulized or Aerosolized) Glutathione. Medscape.com. Accessed August 3, 2014 at http://www.medscape.com/viewarticle/574687.

Rossman, M. J., R. S. Garten, H. J. Groot, et al. 2013. Ascorbate infusion increases skeletal muscle fatigue resistance in patients with chronic obstructive pulmonary disease. *American Journal of Physiology-Regulatory, Integrative and Comparative Physiology* 305:R1163–R1170.

Tse, H. N., L. Raiteri, K. Y. Wong, et al. 2013. High-dose N-acetylcysteine in stable COPD: The 1-year, double-blind, randomized, placebo-controlled HIACE study. *Chest* 144:106–18.

Clostridium Difficile

Clostridium difficile, often referred to as C. difficile, each year causes about thirty thousand deaths and five hundred thousand instances of illness. This infection kills almost as many people in the United States each year as car accidents.

C. difficile bacteria can cause a variety of digestive symptoms, ranging from diarrhea to life-threatening inflammation of the colon, known as colitis. Rates of infection from this nasty bug have been increasing at an alarming rate in the past decade.

Incredibly, about 20 percent of people who are hospitalized acquire C. difficile during hospitalization. More than 30 percent of those infected develop diarrhea. If you have diarrhea within two months of receiving antibiotics, or if you experience diarrhea within seventy-two hours after being hospitalized, you should be tested for C. difficile infection.

Seniors are even more susceptible to the bug than other adults; 25 percent of frail elderly people who get a C. difficile infection die from it. And, frighteningly, the number of kids getting these infections is skyrocketing. A recent study found a twelvefold increase in C. difficile among children, with a stunning three out of four of the infections contracted *outside* of hospital settings!

The *C. difficile* bacterium exists throughout the environment in soil, water, and animal and human feces. It is present in 2 to 3 percent of healthy adults and in as many as 70 percent of healthy infants, who never develop symptoms and do not require treatment. The *balance* of our good bacteria (flora) plays an important role in protecting us against this opportunistic villain.

When levels of good bacteria in our gut get too low, *C. difficile* becomes opportunistic and thrives, producing toxins that inflame the colon. Consuming cultured foods rich in good bacteria known as probiotics (yogurt, miso, tempeh, kefir, sauerkraut) as well as prebiotics that feed your good bacteria (Jerusalem artichoke, onions, leeks, peas, beans, garlic) is important in preventing intestinal infections.

As conventional medicine has learned, the overuse of antibiotics will lead to drug-resistant bacteria. This is one of the biggest challenges we face with *C. difficile*. The bug has become resistant to most of our common antibiotics, making it much more difficult to treat. Antiobiotics also alter gut flora by wiping out the protective good bacteria. This turns the gut into the perfect breeding ground for *C. difficile* to thrive.

Moderate to severe C. difficile is treated with antibiotics. Unfortunately, about one-third of people treated with antibiotics have a relapse within three to twenty-one days after the treatment is discontinued. This means the natural treatments provided in this chapter are very important to help prevent a relapse.

As disturbing as it is to think about, C. difficile is spread through fecal contamination. When someone doesn't wash their hands well enough after using the bathroom, they can quickly contaminate surfaces such as telephones, remote controls, medical equipment, bathroom fixtures, light switches, chairs, tables, door knobs, and other frequently touched items. The spores from the bacteria are hearty and can survive for months on these types of surfaces. If you happen to touch a contaminated surface and then later touch your mouth, the bugs can end up in the intestines, where the damage occurs. This is why frequent hand washing with soap and lots of scrubbing is so important, and why the surfaces inside hospitals, clinics, nursing homes, and other places housing people whose health may be compromised should be cleansed regularly.

Lastly, millions of Americans take acid-suppressing medications known as proton pump inhibitors (PPIs) for acid reflux. Common examples include AciPhex, Dexilant, Nexium, Prevacid, and Prilosec. The FDA issued a statement warning that their use may be linked to an increased risk of C. difficile diarrhea.

The reason for the link between C. difficile and PPIs is not entirely clear. It's possible that stomach acid acts as a natural barrier to bacteria like C. difficile, preventing them from easily entering the digestive tract. Remember, the infection normally makes its way in through the mouth and down through the stomach and intestines. When you suppress your stomach acid you have removed an important barrier to intestinal infections. If you're taking these medications and have diarrhea see your doctor immediately. And, of course, most people can resolve their acid reflux with diet changes and weight loss (see Hiatal Hernia and Acid Reflux Disease).

SYMPTOMS

- Watery diarrhea
- Mild abdominal cramping and tenderness
- Severe abdominial cramping
- Fever
- Blood or pus in stool
- Nausea
- Dehydration
- Loss of appetite
- Weight loss
- Swollen abdomen
- Kidney failure
- Increased white blood cell count

ROOT CAUSES

The fact is *everyone* is susceptible to this infection, but you're even more at risk if you fall into any of the following groups:

- You have cancer or another immune-compromising condition
- You are hospital bound or in a long-term care facility
- You are taking antibiotics (the biggest risk) without simultaneously supplementing with probiotics
- You have recently had abdominal surgery or a gastrointestinal procedure
- You have a colon disease such as inflammatory bowel disease or colorectal cancer
- You have had a previous C. difficile infection

- You are taking any of certain medications, including proton pump inhibitors (PPIs) and the antidepressants mirtazapine and fluoxetine

---

Testing Techniques

Stool culture

White blood cell count—blood

TREATMENT

Diet

Recommended Food

Consuming foods that help to repopulate the colon with friendly bacteria is important to help a current infection and to prevent reinfection. Fermented foods such as sauerkraut, tempeh, and miso are examples. Yogurt with ample amounts of live cultures and that is low in sugar is also a great choice unless one has severe lactose intolerance. Animal research has shown that foods high in soluble (fermentable) fiber such as oatmeal, beans, rice bran, and apple pulp improve recovery. Foods prepared in crockpots and as soups are easier to digest. Prebiotic foods that help to boost gut probiotics include Jerusalem artichoke, onions, leeks, peas, beans, and garlic.

Food to Avoid

To reduce diarrhea avoid foods high in sugar and fructose. This would include juices and soda pop.

℞ Super Seven Prescriptions—Clostridium Difficile

Super Prescription #1 Probiotic *Saccharomyces boulardii* (*S. boulardii*)
Take five to ten billion organisms twice daily. This type of probiotic has been shown to prevent diarrhea associated with C. difficile.

Super Prescription #2 Colloidal silver
Take as directed on the label four times daily. It has antibacterial effects and is well tolerated.

Super Prescription #3 Ginger (*Zingiber officinale*)
Drink a fresh cup of ginger tea, or take 500 mg in capsule form or 2 ml of tincture every two hours. Ginger reduces intestinal inflammation and lessens the effects of food poisoning.

Super Prescription #4 Homeopathic Combination Diarrhea Remedy
For acute diarrhea, take a dose of a combination diarrhea remedy four times daily for twenty-four hours. If you notice improvement, stop taking the remedy unless symptoms return. If your symptoms do not improve within twenty-four hours, then pick the remedy that best matches your symptoms under Homeopathy in this section.

Super Prescription #5 Goldenseal *(Hydrastis canadensis)*

Take 1 ml of the tincture form or 300 mg in capsules four times daily. It helps improve diarrhea that is related to an intestinal infection.

Super Prescription #6 Probiotic

Take a minimum of twenty to one hundred billion organisms daily to support a healthy immune response in the colon to *C. difficile*. Use probiotics containing *Lactobacillus acidophilus* and *bifidus*.

Super Prescription #7 Oregano oil (*Origanum vulgare*)

Take 500 mg of the capsule form four times daily or as directed on the container. Oregano oil has powerful antimicrobial effects.

General Recommendations

Slippery elm (*Ulmus fulva*) is high in mucilage, which has a soothing effect on the intestines. Drink 3 to 4 cups each day. You can also use 5 ml of the tincture or 500 mg in capsules three times daily.

Cranesbill (*Germanium maculatum*) has an astringent effect on the colon for acute diarrhea. Take 3 to 5 ml of the tincture or 500 mg in capsule form three times daily.

Red raspberry (*Rubus idaeus*) tea has historically been used for diarrhea. Drink 4 cups daily to reduce intestinal inflammation. If you prefer to take capsules, spread a dosage of 5 to 10 grams evenly throughout your day. Chamomile and peppermint teas are also good options.

Homeopathy

Aloe Socotrina is helpful when the diarrhea is characterized by rumbling and gurgling in the abdomen, followed by gushing stools. There are often yellow, mucus-filled stools.

Argentum Nitricum is for diarrhea that comes from anticipation anxiety before a stressful situation or event. It is also used for diarrhea that results from sugar ingestion.

Arsenicum Album helps when diarrhea and vomiting occur together. The person is anxious, restless, and chilly. It is good for diarrhea caused by food poisoning. There may be blood in the stool, and the person may feel better from sipping warm drinks.

Chamomilla (*Matricaria chamomilla*) is for green/yellow diarrhea that accompanies teething in infants.

China Officinalis helps when there is extreme exhaustion and weakness from diarrhea.

Ipecacuanha (*Cephaelis ipecacuanha*) is for diarrhea that is accompanied by nausea.

Mercurius Solubilis or Vivus is for burning and bloody diarrhea. The person often has extreme sweating and spasms of the intestines. Phosphorus is for a watery stool. The person feels anxious and craves cold drinks.

Podophyllum is helpful when there is rumbling, gurgling, and cramping in the abdomen, followed by diarrhea. The diarrhea is painless yet explosive, and is often worse in the morning.

Pulsatilla (*Pulsatilla pratensis*) is for diarrhea that results from eating greasy foods or fruits. The person feels better in the open air and worse in a warm room.

Sulfur is for burning, explosive diarrhea that wakes a person up in the morning.

A review of studies published in the highly respected *American Journal of Gastroenterology* found that *Saccharomyces boulardii* was effective in preventing antibiotic-associated diarrhea that occurred with C. difficile infection. The probiotic (which is actually a type of yeast) has been shown to reduce the risk of recurrence of C. difficile when taken in combination with the antibiotics metronidazole or vancomycin. Research even suggests that *S. boulardii* helps decrease the toxicity of *C. difficile* by producing a protein-digesting enzyme that neutralizes the toxins produced by the *C. difficile*.

The stool has a very foul smell, like rotten eggs. The anus is red and excoriated. The person has a great thirst for cold drinks.

Veratrum Album is for painful, profuse diarrhea that resembles rice water. The person is very cold and desires drinks with ice.

Other Recommendations

- One "natural," and perhaps cringe-worthy, solution that's been accepted by conventional medicine is a "stool transplant." A healthy donor's stool (and of course the friendly bacteria it contains) is placed in the recipient's colon by a gastroenterologist with a scope or special tube that goes down the nose. This increasingly popular procedure increases the good bacteria locally within the colon, allowing them to overtake the *C. difficile*.
- Intravenous nutrient replacement helps to maintain energy and immunity while the C. difficile is being treated. Consult with a local holistic doctor.

REFERENCES

Castagliuolo, I., M. F. Riegler, L. Valenick, et al. 1999. *Saccharomyces boulardii* protease inhibits the effects of *Costridium difficile* toxins A and B in human colonic mucosa. *Infection and Immun* 67:302–7.

McFarland, L. V. 2006. Meta-analysis of probiotics for the prevention of antibiotic associated diarrhea and the treatment of *Clostridium difficile* disease. *Am J Gastroenterol* 101:812–22.

McFarland, L. V., C. M. Surawicz, R. N. Greenberg, et al. 1994. A randomized placebo-controlled trial of *Saccharomyces boulardii* in combination with standard antibiotics for *Clostridium difficile* disease. *JAMA* 271:1913–18.

Surawicz, C. M., L. V. McFarland, G. Elmer, et al. 1989. Treatment of recurrent *Clostridium difficile* colitis with vancomycin and *Saccharomyces boulardii*. *Am J Gastroenterol* 84:1285–287.

Ward, P. B. and G. P. Young. 1997. Dynamics of *Clostridium difficile* infection: Control using diet. *Adv Exp Med Biol* 412:63–75.

Colic

Excessive crying, irritability, and apparent abdominal pain are symptoms of colic in babies. This condition is a cause of frustration and concern for many parents. It occurs in approximately 25 percent of babies.

Colic tends to last at least three hours a day, three days a week, and three weeks a month. Pediatricians therefore refer to this condition as the "rule of the threes." The Chinese call it the "hundred days' crying." These crying episodes usually begin in the first three weeks of life and end by three months of age, although they may continue until nine months of age. They frequently begin in the late afternoon and last into the evening.

Colic is not hereditary or affected by birth order. The first baby may be colicky but subsequent siblings may not.

There are different theories about what causes colic. The most likely causes are allergies to milk or formulas, foods that the breast-feeding mother is eating and passing through the breast milk, colon spasms, a hyperactive gastrointestinal tract, tension in the household, or parental anxiety. We find that colic is much less common in children who are breast-fed. This is probably due to the components of breast milk that mature an infant's digestive tract.

Don't dismiss all crying as harmless colic, especially if your newborn exhibits these behaviors:

- A dramatic change in the crying pattern that leads to more painful frequent outbursts
- Crying that is long in duration, inconsolable, and at all times of the day
- Waking up in apparent pain and crying
- Crying that makes you intuitively suspect that your baby has pain somewhere in his or her body

Our experience is that diet changes and natural remedies, especially homeopathy, are highly successful in alleviating this condition.

Conventional treatment involves gas-relieving medications, sedatives, and anti pasmodic medicines.

SYMPTOMS

Crying and fussing are normal behaviors for infants. Signs of colic include the following:

- Episodic crying that occurs the same time each day, often in the afternoon or the evening, with no apparent cause
- Crying that seems nearly impossible to console
- Body-position changes, such as legs drawn up to the abdomen

ROOT CAUSES

- Sensitivity or allergy to infant formula
- Sensitivity or allergy to foods that the breast-feeding mother is consuming and processing through her milk
- Lactose intolerance
- Immature digestive tract
- Fungal overgrowth and/or dysbiosis from antibiotic use
- Gastroesophageal reflux (GERD)
- Feeding too fast, causing gas buildup
- Anxious parents

Testing Techniques

The following tests help assess possible reasons for colic:

Food sensitivity for mother and infant—electrodermal or blood testing

Endoscopy for infant to check for reflux

Elimination diet for mother to see if colic improves

TREATMENT

Diet

Recommended Food

For infant:

- Breast-feeding only is recommended until at least six months of age to prevent colic.
- The formula a bottle-fed infant is using may be the cause of the colic. Switch to a non–cow milk (goat or soy) or a predigested–cow's milk formula. Hypoallergenic predigested protein formulas are readily available. Check with your pediatrician.
- Try feeding your infant more often in lesser amounts.

For the breast-feeding mother:
- Steamed and cooked vegetables are preferable while you're breast-feeding, because they are broken down more efficiently.

Food to Avoid

Foods that the breast-feeding mother is eating can be causing digestive reactions in the infant through the breast milk. Common offenders are dairy products such as cow's milk and cheese, caffeine-containing foods such as coffee and chocolate, spicy foods (such as garlic, onions, or peppers), nuts, and corn. Less common offenders are citrus fruits and juices, soda, wheat, and brewer's yeast. Gas-forming foods such as cauliflower, broccoli, cucumbers, and beans should be avoided as well. Cut out these foods if you are eating a lot of them and see if the infant improves in a week.

A clinical study published in *Phytotherapy Research* reported that breast-fed infants who were given a formula containing fennel, lemon balm, and German chamomile twice daily for a week had a reduction in crying times compared to those given a placebo.

Research has shown that chiropractic spinal manipulation is more effective than the commonly used gas-reducing medication dimethicone for reducing crying in infants with colic.

℞ Super Seven Prescriptions—Colic

Super Prescription #1 Homeopathic Colic Formula
This contains the most common homeopathic remedies for colic. Use as directed.

Super Prescription #2 Homeopathic Chamomilla
This is the most common remedy for colic. Give your baby a 6x, 12x, 6C, 12C, or 30C potency twice daily for two weeks to see if there is any improvement. If you notice improvement, stop giving the remedy unless the symptoms return.

Super Prescription #3 Fennel
Give 3 to 5 drops (room temperature) to your baby of a tea or nonalcohol tincture two to three times daily.

Super Prescription #4 Infant probiotic
Provides good bacteria that help the baby to break down food.

Super Prescription #5 Adult probiotic
Provides good bacteria that help the breast-feeding mother to break down food.

Super Prescription #6 Digestive enzyme (for breast-feeding mother)
Take 1 or 2 capsules with each meal to help you digest food and reduce allergenicity in the breast milk.

> **Super Prescription #7 Chiropractic or craniosacral treatments**
> Improves issues in the baby's nervous system function that may be causing the colic.

General Recommendations

Try different carrying techniques, such as face down, face out, on tummy, or against the bare skin of the parent.

Homeopathy

Pick the remedy below that best matches your baby's symptoms. Give your baby a 6x, 12x, 6C, 12C, or 30C potency twice daily for two weeks to see if there is any improvement. If you notice improvement, stop giving the remedy unless the symptoms return. Consultation with a homeopathic practitioner is advised.

Aethusa is for an infant who is unable to digest milk and is vomiting the milk up. This reaction to milk (breast milk and other kinds) leads to colic.

Calcarea Carbonica is for an infant who fits the Calcarea Carbonica constitutional types (see the Homeopathy section in Part Two). Infant is large and flabby and sweats easily.

Colocynthis is for a child who pulls his or her legs up to the abdomen. Use with warm applications. The child should be lying facedown; it can be irritable.

Dioscorrea is for an infant who arches backward during bouts of colic.

Lycopodium is for an infant who has a lot of gas and bloating after 4 P.M. and does not like tight clothes around the abdomen.

Magnesia Phosphorica is for a child who pulls his or her legs up to the abdomen. It is better with warm applications.

Nux Vomica is for colic that is related to constipation or from a reaction to foods. The child is chilly and irritable.

Pulsatilla is for an infant who feels better being carried and talked to and who cries when left alone.

Acupressure

See pages 787–794 for information about acupressure. This is best done under the direction of a qualified practitioner.

Bodywork

Gentle massage of the abdomen and back can relieve colic for some infants.

Reflexology

See pages 804–805 for information. Use the points that correspond to the stomach, the small intestine, and the large intestine.

Hydrotherapy

Alternating the application of mildly warm and cold cloths to the abdomen may provide colic relief. Wrap a face cloth around the abdomen and cover it with a dry towel.

Craniosacral and Chiropractic

Craniosacral therapy and chiropractic that use gentle adjustments can improve nerve flow and digestive function and may relieve colic.

Aromatherapy

The oils Roman chamomile and lavender are soothing, calming, and relaxing for both mother and child. Rub 2 or 3 drops on the bottom of the baby's feet. Dilute with and equal amount of vegetable oil before applying.

REFERENCES

Savino, F., et al. 2005. A randomized double-blind placebo-controlled trial of a standardized extract of Matricariae recutita, Foeniculum vulgare and Melissa officinalis (ColiMil) in the treatment of breastfed colicky infants. *Phytotherapy Research* 19:335–40.

Wiberg, J. M., et al. 1999. The short-term effect of spinal manipulation in the treatment of infantile colic: A randomized controlled clinical trial with a blinded observer. *Journal of Manipulative Physiological Therapy* 22:517–22.

Common Cold

Colds are caused by any of more than two hundred viruses that infect the upper respiratory tract. Colds are spread through the air, such as by sneezing or coughing, or by contact with a contaminated object. In response to an invasion by a cold virus, the membranes that line the nose and the throat become swollen and start producing additional mucus. The result is congestion, sneezing, coughing, sore throat, and a general feeling of malaise—all of which are your body's way of expelling the virus and getting you to slow down and rest. Although colds can come on at any time of the year, they are most common during late fall and winter. They especially target people whose immune systems are depressed, whether from overwork, preexisting disorders, or a lack of good nutrition and exercise.

The best treatment for a cold is to stimulate your body's natural defenses as soon as the familiar symptoms first appear. Once the virus firmly establishes itself in your system, you can use natural therapies that have direct antiviral activity and that stimulate your immune system to eradicate the virus. Most colds last three to ten days. Do not take over-the-counter medications. The cold symptoms are your immune system's attempts to flush out the virus, so medications that suppress them can actually prolong your cold or cause a recurrence.

Colds can sometimes be difficult to distinguish from allergies The intensity of symptoms usually differentiates a cold from the flu. For adults, the presence of body aches and a fever usually indicates the flu, although a low-grade fever can sometimes exist alongside a cold. Children, on the other hand, may experience fevers as a normal part of a cold. For more information about the flu, see Flu. If your cold symptoms persist, or if they are accompanied by yellow or green mucus, call your doctor. You may have allergies or a different infection, such as sinusitis.

For adults, more than two colds a year may be an indication of underlying toxicity in the body. Some researchers feel that the body uses the cold virus as a way of detoxifying itself through mucus elimination and reduced appetite. In many cases, this could certainly be true. Also, a weakened immune system due to poor lifestyle habits and nutritional deficiencies could be at the root of reoccurring colds.

SYMPTOMS

- Runny nose
- Sneezing
- Congestion
- Cough
- Sore throat

- Swollen lymph glands
- Fatigue
- Loss of appetite
- Mild fever (occasionally, fevers can be higher in children)

ROOT CAUSES

- Toxicity in the body
- A deficient immune system due

to lifestyle factors, nutritional deficiencies, and high stress levels.

TREATMENT

Diet

Recommended Food

Eat lightly. Steamed vegetables, soups and broths, and herbal teas will let your body focus on healing instead of on digestion. If you lose your appetite, don't force yourself to eat.

Stay hydrated. Drink plenty of clean, quality water and other fluids (but see the note in the next section about sugar and juice) to cleanse away toxins and to keep the respiratory tract from drying out.

Increase your consumption of ginger, onions, and garlic. Try adding one or all to chicken soup or miso.

Hot water with lemon, honey, and cinnamon is a traditional cold remedy. Drink a cup every two hours to soothe your throat and chest, prevent mucus buildup, and encourage a cleansing sweat.

Food to Avoid

Sugar decreases the number of white blood cells that your body produces and depresses your immune system, so eliminate refined sugars from your diet for the duration of your illness. Also be wary of fruit juices. Although they are a traditional treatment for colds, fruit juices—especially orange juice—usually contain far more sugar than they do vitamin C. If you want to drink juice, dilute it first.

Avoid milk and other dairy products while you're sick. They encourage the production of mucus and will only make you feel worse.

A randomized, double-blind, placebo-controlled trial was conducted on 323 healthy adults ages eighteen to sixty-five with a history of at least two upper respiratory infections in the previous year. American ginseng (the over-the-counter supplement COLDFX), given at a dose of 200 mg twice daily for four months, was shown to have a statistically significant benefit on immune function in the winter season. It was also shown to be safe and well tolerated.

Rx Super Seven Prescriptions—Common Cold

Super Prescription #1 Homeopathic Combination Cold Remedy

At the first signs of a cold, take a dose of the Combination Cold Remedy four times daily for three days. Then if you notice improvement, stop taking the remedy, unless symptoms return. If your symptoms do not improve within twenty-four hours, pick the remedy that best matches your symptoms under Homeopathy in this section.

Super Prescription #2 *Pelargonium sidoides*

Shown to shorten the duration and reduce the intensity of the common cold.

A randomized, placebo-controlled study of 103 patients with the common cold took a liquid extract of *Pelargonium sidoides* three times a day. After ten days, nearly 79 percent of the *Pelargonium sidoides* group were clinically cured, compared to 31 percent of the placebo group.

A review of twenty-one placebo-controlled studies found that "in each of the twenty-one studies, vitamin C reduced the duration of episodes and the severity of the symptoms of the common cold by an average of 23 percent." A dosage of 1,000 to 8,000 mg was used in these studies.

Super Prescription #3 American ginseng
Take 200 mg of a standardized extract twice daily to reduce the incidence of upper respiratory tract infections.

Super Prescription #4 *Lomatium dissectum*
Take 500 mg or 2 to 4 ml of the tincture four times daily. Lomatium has strong antiviral effects.

Super Prescription #5 Vitamin C
Take 1,000 mg three or four times daily. Reduce the dosage if diarrhea occurs. Vitamin C supports immune-system function through increased white blood cell activity.

Super Prescription #6 Zinc
Take 15 to 25 mg in zinc lozenge form (zinc gluconate or acetate) every two waking hours for four days. Zinc supports immune function and may have antiviral effects. Zinc nasal sprays may be even more effective. Take as directed on the container.

Super Prescription #7 Astragalus (*Astragalus membranaceus*)
Take 500 to 1,000 mg or 3.0 ml of a tincture two or three times daily. Astragalus is an excellent treatment for preventing the common cold. Do not take astragalus if you have a fever.

General Recommendations

Probiotics have been shown to prevent the common cold in children. Take as directed on the label.

Oregano (*Origanum vulgare*) oil has powerful antiviral effects. Take 500 mg of the capsule form four times daily or as directed on the container.

Elderberry (*Sambucus nigra*) is useful for the common cold and the flu. Adults can take 10 ml and children 5 ml three times daily.

Garlic (*Allium sativum*) combats infection and supports the immune system. Take 300 to 500 mg or the liquid form three times daily. It can also be used on a long-term basis for preventing colds.

Thyme extract (*Thymus vulgaris*) optimizes immune activity. Take 1 or 2 capsules twice daily or as directed on the container.

Ginger (*Zingiber officinale*) helps with a sore throat and chills. Take 500 mg in a capsule or drink fresh tea four times daily.

Colloidal silver is used to treat the common cold and to prevent a deeper respiratory infection. Take as directed on the label.

Homeopathy

At the first signs of a cold, take 2 pellets of a 30C potency four times daily for three days of the remedy that best matches your symptoms in this section. Then if you notice improvement, stop taking the remedy, unless symptoms return. If your symptoms do not improve within twenty-four hours, pick another remedy.

Aconitum Napellus is for colds that come on suddenly after exposure to dry, cold weather. There is a scratchy throat and a thin discharge from the nose. You probably feel anxious, restless, and chilly, with a great thirst. This remedy is best taken within four hours of developing cold symptoms.

Allium Cepa is helpful when a person has a clear, burning nasal discharge that irritates the nostrils and the upper lip. The eyes water and have a stinging pain. The nose runs more when indoors and stops when outdoors.

Arsenicum Album is for a cold with a profuse, clear, watery discharge from the nose that makes the upper lip red. The nose may be stuffed but still runs. The person feels chilly, is thirsty for sips of water, and feels anxious and restless.

Ferrum Phosphoricum helps when a person feels feverish but does not act sick. The throat may be sore, and the face is flushed. It's best used at the onset of a cold.

Gelsemium (*Gelsemium sempervirens*) is for a cold accompanied by chills and muscle ache. The person feels drowsy and fatigued and has droopy eyelids. There may be a headache at the back of the neck.

Mercurius Solubilis or Vivus is helpful when the person is sensitive to both hot and cold temperatures. The tongue has a thick coating, and the person has bad breath, has excessive saliva production, and drools on pillow. The throat is often raw and sore.

Natrum Muriaticum is for colds that begin with sneezing and produce a thin clear or white discharge. The person may have a headache that is worse in the sun or the light. The cold may be accompanied by cold sores around the mouth and chapped lips.

Nux Vomica (*Strychnos nux vomica*) is for a person who is very chilly and irritable. Sneezing and coughing, along with a congested nose and sore throat, are common.

Pulsatilla (*Pulsatilla pratensis*) is helpful when there is thick yellow or green nasal mucus. The person has a low thirst and feels warm. The person also feels congested and is better outdoors or with fresh air. There is a desire to be comforted.

Studies on the effectiveness of echinacea for the common cold have been mixed. It appears that the type of standardization and the potency of the product are important for achieving therapeutic effects. One randomized double-blind clinical study looked at the effectiveness of *Echinacea purpurea* for 120 patients with initial symptoms of acute, uncomplicated upper airway infection (in other words, the common cold). Echinacea (20 drops every two hours for the first day and thereafter three times daily) or a placebo was administered for up to ten days, after which patients were questioned about the intensity of their illness, time to improvement, and time until cessation of treatment. The time taken to improve was significantly shorter in the echinacea group, at four days, while people in the placebo group took an average of eight days to recover. No specific adverse events were reported.

Acupressure

See pages 787–794 for information about acupressure points and administering treatment.

- Large Intestine 4 (LI4) is a general tonic for colds and a specific remedy for headaches and congestion.

- If you have a sore throat, a cough, or chest congestion, use Kidney 27 (K27).
- Bladder 2 (Bl2) and Large Intestine 20 (LI20) work on sinus congestion and pain.
- For head pain and congestion, use Gallbladder 20 (GB20) and Governing Vessel 16 and 24.5 (GV16 and GV24.5).

Bodywork

Massage
If you are very congested, try a percussive massage to break up mucus. Percussive motions are best used on people who are relatively strong and healthy. Otherwise, a simple back rub may ease some of the congestion.

Reflexology
See pages 804–805 for information about reflexology areas and how to work them. Work all the toes, as well as the areas corresponding to the lungs, the adrenal glands, the lower spine, the pituitary glands, and the lymph system. If you have a sore throat, also massage the neck area.

Hydrotherapy
Hot baths, showers, and steams all help drain phlegm and detoxify the body. For extra benefits, add any of the essential oils listed in this entry under Aromatherapy.

If you're chilled, take frequent hot foot baths; otherwise, alternating hot and cold foot baths are excellent.

Aromatherapy

Any of the following oils can be added to baths or steam inhalations.

- Lavender has immune-boosting properties and will also help you get to sleep. It's especially soothing if you have a cough.
- Eucalyptus and peppermint relieve congestion and stimulate circulation.
- Tea tree and melissa oils fight viruses and also work against any secondary bacterial infections that may develop.

Stress Reduction

Stress lowers your resistance and makes you much more susceptible to colds. If you get colds frequently, read the chapter on stress reduction in Part Two of this book and incorporate at least one of the techniques discussed there into your daily routine.

Other Recommendations

- Get plenty of sleep and rest.
- Unless you have a fever, take a brisk walk to keep mucus from settling into your body and to chase away the blues. Don't engage in any vigorous exercise, however.
- Keep a humidifier in your room. The moist air will thin secretions.
- If you have a sore throat, gargle with salt water.
- Colds can circulate through an entire family—and even come back to you. Break the cycle by keeping your hands clean and flushing tissues after you

use them. Encourage your family members to eat well, to get rest, and to wash their hands often during your illness.

- Intravenous vitamin C or ozone by a holistic doctor can help one recover more quickly.

REFERENCES

Heisel, O., et al. 1997. Echiniguard treatment shortens the course of the common cold: A double-blind, placebo-controlled clinical trial. *European Journal of Clinical Research* 9:261–68.

Hemilä, H. 1994. Does vitamin C alleviate the symptoms of the common cold? A review of current evidence. *Scandinavian Journal of Infectious Diseases* 26:1–6.

Lizogub, V. G., et al. 2007. Efficacy of a *Pelargonium sidoides* preparation in patients with the common cold: A randomized, double-blind, placebo-controlled clinical trial. *Explore* 3:573–84.

Predy, G., et al. 2005. Efficacy of an extract of North American ginseng containing poly-furanosyl-pyranosyl-saccharides for preventing upper respiratory tract infections: A randomized controlled trial. *Canadian Medical Association Journal* 173:1043–48.

Constipation

In a healthy body, waste travels through the digestive tract in a predictable, regular cycle, usually taking between six and twenty-four hours to pass. Sometimes, however, waste matter passes through the large intestine too slowly, and the result is called constipation. When the bowels are constipated, it may be difficult or impossible to pass stools; in fact, the urge to pass may be absent altogether. Sometimes constipation has no signs other than the lack of bowel movement, but, usually, it is accompanied by a host of uncomfortable symptoms, ranging from a general feeling of malaise to a distended abdomen and painfully hard stools.

A healthy person generally has one to three complete bowel movements daily.

Although constipation is the number-one gastrointestinal disorder in the United States, its unwelcome effects are actually rather easy to avoid. Our Western diet—high in fat and low in fiber and fluids—is the cause of most constipation. When fiber and fluids are lacking, the contracting motions of the large intestine are not stimulated in a regular fashion, and waste is therefore not propelled through the tract. Treatment, then, relies largely on dietary changes. Other factors, such as stress, inactivity, and certain medications, can cause or contribute to constipation as well. Dietary changes are still encouraged in these cases, along with the removal, when possible, of the offending factor. No matter how much or how little discomfort you have, it is always important to address the causes of constipation. When waste matter

Many people think of constipation as an uncomfortable but essentially harmless condition. In reality, recurring long-term bouts can lead to other problems, some merely distressing and others very serious. Constipation has been linked to the following disorders:

Arthritis

Skin disorders

Bad breath

Mood disorders, including depression

Headaches

Irritable bowel syndrome

Fatigue

Hemorrhoids

Hernias

Insomnia

Malabsorption syndrome

Weight gain

Varicose veins

remains in the colon for a long period of time, recent studies show that bacteria and other harmful matter can be reabsorbed into the bloodstream.

Stress or suppressed emotions are often overlooked factors with constipation. There is a direct connection between perceived stress levels and gut motility. In addition, people with hectic lifestyles often do not take the time for regular bowel movements. And sometimes children hold back on stool movements for fear of pain or inconvenience.

A poorly functioning digestive system can also be a major contributor to constipation. This is particularly true with deficient bile flow from the liver and the gallbladder. Herbal therapies in this chapter work to improve bile production and flow.

The use of over-the-counter laxatives is a significant problem for many people with constipation. Although these medications relieve constipation, many of them make the bowels lazier over time.

Occasionally, constipation signals a more serious condition. If you have bloody stools, intense abdominal pain, or a cut near your rectum, see your doctor. And since chronic constipation can cause other illnesses, make an appointment if you have constipation that recurs or a single episode that lasts longer than a week.

SYMPTOMS

- Difficulty passing stools
- Decreased frequency passing stools
- Bloated, tender abdomen
- Loss of appetite
- Flatulence
- Malaise

ROOT CAUSES

- Poor diet (low fiber, low water intake)
- Stress
- Inactivity
- Medications
- Intestinal parasites
- Lack of beneficial intestinal flora
- Colitis
- Laxative or enema abuse
- Underactive thyroid
- Magnesium deficiency
- Liver problems

Testing Techniques

The following tests help assess possible metabolic reasons for constipation:

Stool analysis for good bacteria levels, parasites, fungi, and infection

Thyroid hormones—blood, saliva, or urine

TREATMENT

Diet

Recommended Food

If you're unaccustomed to a high-fiber diet, move into these recommendations slowly. A sudden increase of dietary fiber can be quite a shock to the system and can even cause further digestive problems.

The basic, wholesome diet recommended at the beginning of this book is an excellent source of fiber. Eat lots of whole grains, especially brown rice; raw or lightly cooked fruits and vegetables; and beans, nuts, and seeds. Chew thoroughly, and don't eat too much at one sitting, even of healthful foods.

People with constipation often have a magnesium deficiency. Green leafy vegetables are high in this mineral, as well as in fiber, so now you have another reason to eat kale, broccoli, spinach, brussels sprouts, and the like.

Prunes and figs are time-honored sources of dietary fiber. You may want to plan on making one of these items a regular part of your breakfast.

Flaxseeds are a lesser-known but highly concentrated source of fiber. Don't cook with flaxseeds or subject them to heat; instead, sprinkle them on cereals or salads. Adults should take 1 to 2 tablespoons of ground flaxseeds daily, along with 10 ounces of water. Children can take 1 to 2 teaspoons.

Hot cereals or warm liquids at breakfast can stimulate contractions of the lower intestine. Enjoy some hot oatmeal or herbal tea, or do as our grandmothers did and add lemon juice to a glass of warm water.

Consume fermented products on a regular basis to keep your intestinal flora in balance. Kefir and sauerkraut are good choices, as is live unsweetened yogurt once the acute constipation is relieved.

Drink plenty of water to keep stools soft. A glass of clean, quality water every two waking hours is usually an adequate amount.

Food to Avoid

Do not eat foods that are fried or otherwise high in saturated fat. Fat slows travel time through the intestines.

Avoid mucus-forming foods, which also slow the transit time of waste matter. Foods that encourage mucus production include all dairy products, fried and processed foods, refined flours, and chocolate.

Caffeine and alcohol are hard on the digestive system and are dehydrating as well. During an episode of constipation, avoid them entirely. When you're regular again, consume them only in small quantities. Food sensitivities, such as gluten, may cause constipation.

A *New England Journal of Medicine* study of children with chronic constipation reported that cow's milk was the cause for two-thirds of the children involved in the study.

℞ Super Seven Prescriptions—Constipation

Super Prescription #1 Psyllium
Take 1 teaspoon or 5 grams of psyllium husks twice daily or as directed on the container. Take it with 10 ounces of water. Psyllium acts as a bulk-forming laxative.

Super Prescription #2 Chia seeds or ground flaxseed
Take 1 to 2 tablespoons daily with 8 to 12 ounces of water. This provides fiber to bulk the stool.

Super Prescription #3 *Cascara sagrada*
Take 250 mg or 2.5 ml of tincture two or three times daily for the relief of acute constipation. This herb should not be used as a long-term solution for constipation.

Super Prescription #4 Magnesium

Take 250 mg two to four times daily for the relief of acute constipation. Magnesium improves gut motility and retains water in the colon. Do not use on a long-term basis, as it can lead to malabsorption and electrolyte imbalance.

Super Prescription #5 Probiotic

Take a product containing at least twenty billion active organisms daily. Friendly bacteria (*Lactobacillus acidophilus, bifidus*) help with digestion and elimination.

Super Prescription #6 Triphala

Take as directed on the label. This blend of fruits helps to tonify the digestive tract for those with chronic constipation.

Super Prescription #7 Homeopathic Nux Vomica (*Strychnos nux vomica*)

Take a 30C potency twice daily for relief of acute constipation. See the homeopathic description further on of Nux Vomica, as well as of other indicated remedies.

General Recommendations

Milk thistle (*Silybum marianum*) improves liver function and bile flow. Take 200 to 250 mg of a product standardized to 80 percent silymarin with each meal.

Fenugreek (*Trigonella foenum-graecum*) is an herb that improves bowel contractions. Take 250 mg or 2 ml twice daily with meals.

Aloe vera juice improves bowel movements. Take a quarter cup twice daily or as directed on container.

Gentian root (*Gentiana lutea*) improves overall digestive function. Take 300 mg or 10 to 20 drops five to fifteen minutes before meals.

Enzymes improve digestive function. Take 1 or 2 capsules with each meal.

Senna is helpful for the short-term relief of constipation. Use as directed on the label.

Dandelion root (*Taraxacum officinale*) stimulates bile flow and improves constipation. Take 250 to 500 mg or 2 ml with each meal.

Homeopathy

Pick the remedy that best matches your symptoms in this section. Take a 6x, 12x, 6C, or 30C potency twice daily for two weeks to see if there are any positive results. After you notice improvement, stop taking the remedy, unless symptoms return. Consultation with a homeopathic practitioner is advised.

Alumina is for someone who goes many days without a stool. Stools are hard and dry. The person must strain to pass even a soft stool, and the person may have memory problems.

Bryonia (*Bryonia alba*) is helpful when there is no desire to pass stool. The stool is dry and hard. The person has a great thirst, is irritable, and may have a headache.

Calcarea Carbonica is for the chronically constipated person who feels chilly, with clammy hands and feet. The person feels overwhelmed.

Lycopodium (*Lycopodium clavatum*) is helpful when a person has constipation and problems with gas and bloating. There is a craving for sweets, and symptoms are worse in the late afternoon. The digestive system feels better with warm drinks.

Natrum Muriaticum is for people with constipation who have a strong craving for salt and water. The person may suffer from depression and is often sensitive to the sun or the light.

Nux Vomica (*Strychnos nux vomica*) is helpful when one has an urgent feeling but can't pass stools or stools are never completed. The person feels irritable and over-stressed. Nux Vomica works well for people who work too hard, exercise too little, and eat and drink too much. It also helps those who have become addicted to laxatives.

Sepia is for constipation accompanied by hormonal issues, such as PMS and menopause. The person feels irritable and chilly and has stools that are hard to pass. A heavy sensation in the rectum and the lower abdomen may be present.

Silica (*Silicea*) helps when a person strains for a long time to have a bowel movement. Stool may come a little way out and then recede back in. The person is generally chilly and thin.

Sulfur is helpful if you have constipation alternating with diarrhea. The stool is often dry and hard, and the rectum is inflamed and burning. The person has a strong thirst for ice-cold drinks.

Acupressure

Use these points twice a day until you get relief. For chronic, recurring cases, you may have to work these points for several weeks before the fundamental problem is addressed. For more information about acupressure points and administering treatment, see pages 787–794.

- In acupressure, the most effective point for constipation and abdominal cramps is Conception Vessel 6 (CV6).
- Another point that stimulates intestinal contractions is Large Intestine 4 (LI4).
- Large Intestine 11 (LI11) will strengthen the colon.
- Stomach 36 (St36) is a good general toner that strengthens the digestive system.

Bodywork

Massage

A self-massage of the abdomen feels quite relieving if you're constipated. Better yet, it can induce intestinal contractions. Lie down with your knees bent, and massage your abdomen with the flat of your hand, using pressure that's firm but gentle. Add the stimulating oils listed under Aromatherapy in this section for a more potent effect.

If you prefer, you can get a professional massage of your lower back and pelvis.

Reflexology

See pages 804–805 for information about reflexology areas and how to work them.

Work the areas corresponding to the colon, the liver, the gallbladder, and the adrenal glands.

If stress is a cause or a result of constipation, also work the area that corresponds to the solar plexus.

In cases of chronic constipation, massage the entire foot and hand to address the systemic damage.

Hydrotherapy

Constitutional hydrotherapy is excellent to help with long-term and acute problems with constipation. See pages 795–796 for directions.

Aromatherapy

Black pepper and marjoram stimulate and warm the digestive system. Add them to a carrier oil, and use it in an abdominal massage or a bath.

If you need to relieve stress, you can experiment with many different oils and rotate your favorites so that you don't buildup a tolerance to them. See pages 771–781 for details on oils; you may want to start off with bergamot, jasmine, lavender, rose, sandalwood, or ylang-ylang. Use them in any preparation you like.

Stress Reduction

General Stress-Management Therapies

Yoga and pilates can be a wise choice for people suffering from constipation.

Laugh often. Laughter produces endorphins, the feel-good hormones, and takes you away from your worries, even if just for a few moments. It also stimulates and strengthens your digestive organs.

Other Recommendations

- Exercise helps to stimulate intestinal contractions. You don't need to run a marathon: mild to moderate aerobic exercise should be enough. A brisk walk, taken thirty minutes every morning, is a goal most of us can easily achieve. Crunches done properly are also helpful to strengthen the abdominal muscles.
- Beware of over-the-counter laxatives. They are extremely harsh and can create an unhealthful dependency.
- Never repress the urge to defecate. When you hold back, you are actually training your bowels to misbehave. The result is often chronic—even lifelong— constipation.
- It is possible to retrain your bowels, if necessary. Sit on the toilet at the same time every day, even if you don't have an urge. Early morning or directly after exercise are usually good times. Do not strain—you'll only create hemorrhoids or varicose veins. Instead, breathe deeply, using your abdominal muscles, and try to relax.

REFERENCES

Iacono, G., F. Cavataio, G. Montalto, et al. 1998. Intolerance of cow's milk and chronic constipation in children. *New England Journal of Medicine* 339(16):1100–4.

Congestive Heart Failure

As our population ages, congestive heart failure (CHF) is becoming an increasingly common problem. More than five million people (mostly seniors) in the United States currently have CHF.

CHF occurs when your heart doesn't pump blood efficiently enough to keep up with your body's need for blood and oxygen. This leads to water buildup, decreased kidney function, and circulation problems.

Your heart is a pump, and when you provide it with the nutrients it needs to improve energy and blood flow, you can improve or reverse CHF. In fact, if you catch the condition early enough and receive proper treatment your heart function could even return to normal.

SYMPTOMS

- Shortness of breath during activity
- Trouble breathing when lying down
- Weight gain with swelling in the feet, legs, ankles, or stomach
- Increased urination
- Wheezing
- Generally feeling tired or weak
- Fast heart rate
- Protrusion of eyes
- Distention of neck veins

ROOT CAUSES

- Structural abnormalities of the heart
- Coronary artery disease
- High blood pressure (poorly controlled)
- Arrhythmia
- Infections
- Genetics
- Diabetes
- Hyperthyroidism
- Pregnancy
- Polycythemia vera
- Anemia
- Certain pharmaceuticals (calcium channel blockers, betablockers)
- Obesity
- Nutritional deficiencies (vitamin B1)
- Hormone deficiency (testosterone, thyroid)
- Sleep apnea
- Kidney disease

Testing Techniques

Electrocardiogram—machine

Echocardiogram—sonogram machine

B-type natriuretic peptide and N-terminal pro-B type (increase in heart failure)—blood

Nutrients including CoQ10, magnesium, B1, vitamin D—blood

Hormones (thyroid, testosterone)—blood, urine

TREATMENT

Diet

Recommended Food

A healthy diet and lifestyle are very important to prevent and improve the disease of heart failure. The two diets that have been studied the most for helping heart failure are the DASH (Dietary Approaches to Stop Hypertension) diet and the Mediterranean diet.

Research by the American Heart Association found that women with heart failure who followed a stricter DASH diet had lower mortality rates. The DASH diet is high in fruits and vegetables and low in dairy and salt. Studies have also confirmed the benefits of the traditional Mediterranean diet, which emphasizes lots of healthy fruits and vegetables. In a study published in 2014 in the *European Journal of Heart Failure*, heart-failure biomarkers were slashed in a group of high-risk volunteers who ate a Mediterranean diet, which included extra virgin olive oil or nuts. And in a French study on cardiac patients who were at high risk for death, researchers concluded that the "Mediterranean diet results in a striking effect on survival."

Omega-3 fatty acids are important. Population studies reveal that those who eat more fish have around a 15 percent reduced risk of developing the condition.

Food to Avoid

Limiting sodium will reduce blood pressure and fluid retention, both of which will help reduce workload on the heart. If you have CHF it's recommended that you stick to less than 1,500 mg daily of sodium.

If you're averaging seven or more alcohol drinks a day you could be sending your CHF risk soaring. On the other hand, some studies have found that one to two drinks a day may reduce your risk of heart failure.

Rx Super Seven Prescriptions

CoQ10 is a super nutrient is found in all your cells, and is critical for healthy heart function. There are two different types of CoQ10 on the market: ubiquinone and ubiquinol. Studies show that *both* forms improve heart ejection fraction. A typical daily dose would be 400 to 600 mg of either form of CoQ10 (or a combination of the two). CoQ10 has a mild blood-thinning effect, but those already taking blood-thinning meds can typically tolerate CoQ10 without any problems. Your doctor can monitor your progress.

Magnesium is critical for efficient heart-muscle function. The highest levels of magnesium in the body are found in the left ventricle of the heart, which does most of the heart's work. Magnesium plays an important role in heart contraction. The mineral puts up a roadblock to prevent too much calcium from getting into the heart cells. Excess calcium will cause your heart to work too hard, leading to chest pain and, in some cases, even a heart attack. A 2014 study found that low blood levels of magnesium (and high levels of calcium and phosphorous) are associated with a higher risk of heart failure.

Super Prescription #1 Coenzyme Q10 (CoQ10)

Take 400 to 600 mg daily. This nutrient is needed for heart cells to produce energy and contract with force. Studies consistently show that CoQ10 supplementation improves CHF.

Super Prescription #2 Magnesium

Take 250 to 500 mg twice daily. Magnesium supports heart-cell energy production.

Super Prescription # 3 L-carnitine

Take 1,000 mg of L-carnitine three times a day or 500 mg of propionyl-L-carnitine twice daily. This nutrient helps heart-muscle cells by burning fatty acids for energy.

Super Prescription #4 D-ribose

Take 5 grams three times daily. D-ribose is a naturally occurring sugar that heart cells use to produce energy and improve cardiac function.

Super Prescription #5 Hawthorn

Take 250 to 300 mg three times daily of a hawthorn extract. Some but not all studies show it improves blood flow to the heart as well as ejection fraction.

Super Prescription #6 Taurine

Take 500 mg to 1,000 mg of this amino acid three times daily on an empty stomach. Research has shown it improves heart ejection fraction.

Super Prescription #7 Fish oil

Take 2,000 to 3,000 mg daily of combined EPA and DHA. Omega-3 fats reduce the risk of heart failure. This may be due to their anti-inflammatory benefit or improved circulation.

Research has found that heart failure is associated with low CoQ10 levels. And population studies suggest that low blood levels of CoQ10 may be a predictor of mortality in people with heart failure.

A published study found that CoQ10 supplementation can extend the lifespan of those with CHF. In another two-year, double-blind study, 420 volunteers with CHF were given either a placebo or 300 mg of CoQ10. Those who received the CoQ10 slashed their risk of dying by an astounding 50 percent compared to those who received a placebo. In addition, the CoQ10 takers had about half the number of serious adverse cardiovascular events, and one of the main blood markers doctors use to measure heart function was improved. As the lead author of the study pointed out, CoQ10 was able to do what drugs *don't* do. It improved energy production in heart cells while drugs often do just the opposite. And lastly, in a small study, seven people with congestive heart failure were given an average of 580 mg of CoQ10 per day. Their plasma CoQ10 levels rose dramatically and the heart ejection fraction rose from 22 to 39 percent. The volunteers saw significant improvement in their symptoms as well. And the most impressive was a ten-year study published in the *European Journal of Heart Failure*. CoQ10 supplementation was shown to improve survival for even those with severe heart failure. It also reduced the incidence of hospitalization.

General Recommendations

Creatine has been shown in research to significantly improve breathing difficulties. Take 2,500 mg daily.

L-arginine is an amino acid that increases nitric oxide production in the blood, which in turn improves blood flow. Supplementing L-arginine can have positive benefits on kidney function in those with heart failure. Decreased kidney function or kidney failure due to a lack of blood flow is common with heart failure. L-arginine improves kidney filtration and water elimination. Take 1,000 mg twice a day on an empty stomach.

Vitamin D deficiency is associated with heart failure. In a study of patients rehospitalized for heart failure, 75 percent were found to have vitamin D deficiency. Take 5,000 IU or more depending on your blood level.

Iron deficiency is common in people that have heart failure. It is needed to transport oxygen to your cells. Have your doctor check your levels.

Pycnogenol combined with CoQ10 supplement can help improve ejection

A number of studies have shown that D-ribose supplementation improves quality of life, heart function (based on echocardiography), physical function, and respiratory function in those with heart failure.

Studies have found that carnitine improves exercise capacity and maximum exercise time for those with heart failure. In one study carnitine was shown to improve ejection fraction, and in another—this one focused on a group of advanced heart-failure patients—researchers proved that the nutrient can improve survival rates. It also has an excellent safety record.

Taurine is an underrated amino acid when it comes to helping those with heart failure. Research has shown that taurine helps improves exercise capacity and ejection fraction.

fraction, reduce edema, and improve your ability to walk a longer distance. Take 100 to 200 mg of pycnogenol daily.

Other Recommendations

- It's common for people with heart failure to be prescribed diuretic medications to eliminate the water retention and swelling that overload the hearts and lungs. But ridding your body of all that extra fluid comes at a cost. Nutrients—including thiamine, riboflavin, B12, magnesium, calcium, zinc, and potassium—are in danger of running low.
- Beta-blockers such as atenolol, metropolol, and carvedilol are also commonly prescribed for heart failure. These drugs can deplete your body of CoQ10, an antioxidant that your body needs for basic cell function.
- Enhanced external counterpulsation, also known as EECP, is an effective nondrug therapy for CHF. The patient wears a pair of inflatable pants that cover the legs with sensors that can tell when the heart is beating and when it's at rest. When the heart is at rest (diastole), the pants inflate, increasing pressure in the arteries and blood flow back to the heart arteries. When the heart is about to beat, the pants deflate. This mechanical pumping action improves blood flow to the heart arteries, placing less demand on the heart muscle, reduced artery stiffness, inhibiting inflammatory compounds, reducing plaque formation in the arteries, and improving nitric-oxide production, which also leads to better blood flow. There have been more than 190 papers published on EECP. This outpatient procedure is done at medical centers all around the United States. A general course of treatment typically lasts a total of thirty-five hours, with each session lasting three to four hours.
- Hormone replacement can benefit those with CHF. For example, in both men and women thyroid hormones are very important. Your heart has thyroid receptors and contracts in response to thyroid hormones. And, as is the case with any cell in the body, heart cells use thyroid hormones for energy production. According to a study published in the journal *Circulation*, "A growing body of evidence suggests that thyroid dysfunction may play an important role in the progression to dilated HF (heart failure)." Have your doctor check your free T3 level, and if it's deficient or low, T3 replacement may be beneficial.
- Testosterone is important for all muscles, including heart muscle. It's been estimated that 25 to 30 percent of men with heart failure have low levels of testosterone. Research has shown that exercise capacity can be improved in men with CHF and low testosterone by giving them testosterone supplementation.
- Regular exercise can drastically reduce your risk for heart failure. A study published in the journal *Circulation* found that older adults who got an hour of moderate exercise, or a half hour of vigorous exercise, daily slashed their risk of heart failure by almost half. And remember, exercise doesn't have to include fancy equipment or an expensive gym. Walking, swimming, and biking are all great choices.
- If you smoke, quit. Smoking is a major risk factor for heart failure, and quitting is nearly as effective as the drugs used for CHF.
- If you're carrying around a few extra pounds, consider losing weight. Research shows that gradual weight loss over time will help improve heart function. The simple reason is that your heart has to work harder when you're overweight.

REFERENCES

Azuma, J., A. Sawamura, and N. Awata. 1992. Usefulness of taurine in chronic congestive heart failure and its prospective application. *Jpn Circ J* 56(1):95–9.

Belcaro, G., M. R. Cesarone, M. Dugall, et al. 2010. Investigation of pycnogenol(R) in combination with coenzyme Q10 in heart failure patients (NYHA II/III). *Panminerva Med* 52(2 Suppl 1):21–25.

Beyranvand, M. R., M. K. Khalafi, V. D. Roshan, et al. 2011. Effect of taurine supplementation on exercise capacity of patients with heart failure. *J Cardiol* 57(3):333–7.

Djoussé, L., A. O. Akinkuolie, J. H. Wu, et al. 2012. Fish consumption, omega-3 fatty acids and risk of heart failure: A meta-analysis. *Clin Nutr* 31(6):846–53.

Faculté de Médecine de Grenoble, Université de Grenoble. 2011. Mediterranean diet in secondary prevention of CHD. *Public Health Nutr* 14(12A):2333–337.

Fitó, M. L., R. Estruch, J. Salas-Salvadó, et al. 2014. Effect of the Mediterranean diet on heart failure biomarkers: A randomized sample from the PREDIMED trial. *Eur J Heart Fail* 16(5):543–50.

Gerdes, A. M. 2010. Thyroid replacement therapy and heart failure. *Circulation* 122:385–93.

Levitan, E. 2013. Mediterranean and DASH diet scores and mortality in women with heart failure: The Women's Health Initiative. *Circ Heart Fail* 6(6):1116–23.

Liu, L. C. Y., A. A. Voors, D. J. van Veldhuisen, et al. 2011. Vitamin D status and outcomes in heart failure patients. *Eur J Heart Fail* 13(6):619–25.

Lutsey, P. L. 2014. Serum magnesium, phosphorus, and calcium are associated with risk of incident heart failure: The Atherosclerosis Risk in Communities (ARIC) Study. *Am J Clin Nutr* 100(3):756–64.

Mancini, M., F. Rengo, M. Lingetti, et al. 1992. Controlled study on the therapeutic efficacy of propionyl-L-carnitine in patients with congestive heart failure. *Arzneimittelforschung* 42(9):1101–4.

Molyneux, S. L., C. M. Florkowski, P. M. George, et al. 2008. Coenzyme Q10: an independent predictor of mortality in chronic heart failure. *J Am Coll Cardiol* 52(18):1435–41.

Mortensen, S. A., S. Vadhanavikit, K. Muratsu, et al. 1990. Coenzyme Q10: clinical benefits with biochemical correlates suggesting a scientific breakthrough in the management of chronic heart failure. *Int J Tissue React* 12(3):155–62.

Mortensen, S., A. Kumar, K. Filipiak, et al. 2013. The effect of coenzyme Q10 on morbidity and mortality in chronic heart failure. Results from the Q-SYMBIO study. *European Journal of Heart Failure* 15(S1):S20.

Omran, H., D. McCarter, J. St Cyr, et al. 2004. D-ribose aids congestive heart failure patients. *Exp Clin Cardiol* 9(2):117–8.

Rizos, I. 2000. Three-year survival of patients with heart failure caused by dilated cardiomyopathy and L-carnitine administration. *Am Heart J* 139(2 Pt 3):S120–3.

Soukoulis, V., J. B. Dihu, and M. Sole. 2009. Micronutrient deficiencies an unmet need in heart failure. *J Am Coll Cardiol* 54(18):1660–73.

Stout, M., G. A. Tew, H. Doll, et al. 2012. Testosterone therapy during exercise rehabilitation in male patients with chronic heart failure who have low testosterone status: A double-blind randomized controlled feasibility study. *Am Heart J* 164(6):893–901.

Vijay, N., D. MacCarter, L. M. Shecterle, et al. 2008. D-ribose benefits heart failure patients. *J Med Food* 11(1):199–200.

Watanabe, G., H. Tomiyama, and N. Doba. 2000. Effects of oral administration of L-arginine on renal function in patients with heart failure. *J Hypertens* 18:229–34.

Cough

Coughing is a normal part of the body's immune system and respiratory-defense system. Ejecting quick, sudden bursts of air and fluids from the respiratory tract helps expel microbes, dust, chemicals, and other irritants, as well as foreign objects, from the airway.

Coughing can be a symptom of an underlying infection of the bronchial tubes or lungs, such as bronchitis, pneumonia, or croup. In some cases, it can suggest more serious diseases, such as asthma, lung cancer, or heart problems.

The goal in treating a cough is to address the underlying cause. For example, with infections, the immune system must be stimulated, and for allergy-produced coughs, the allergen must be removed or you must become desensitized to it. In any case, remember not to suppress a cough too much. In cases of infection, this is particularly true. The goal is to allow the body to expel foreign matter and to detoxify, while simultaneously soothing the cough to make a person more comfortable. This will prevent suppression of the disease, so that it doesn't turn into something more serious (such as bronchitis becoming pneumonia).

Be aware that certain drugs, such as some blood pressure medications, are known to cause coughing as a potential side effect.

If a cough lasts more than two weeks or if you have difficulty breathing or blood in the sputum, consult a doctor immediately.

SYMPTOMS

- Dry or wet cough

ROOT CAUSES

- Infection
- Allergens (environmental or food)
- Obstruction in the airway
- Anxiety

Testing Techniques

The following tests help assess possible metabolic reasons for coughing:

Food and environmental allergy testing—blood or electrodermal

Infection—blood work

Obstruction of airway—X-ray

TREATMENT

Diet

Recommended Food

To thin mucus secretions, drink a glass of clean, quality water every two waking hours.

Homemade chicken soup also thins mucus. Add garlic or ginger for flavor and immune support.

To reduce phlegm, have some hot barley soup.

Onions are an old folk remedy and have anti-inflammatory properties, so eat them often.

If you have bacterial bronchitis and are taking antibiotics, consume daily non-dairy sour products, such as kefir or sauerkraut, to replenish disease-fighting bacteria.

Honey has been shown in several studies to reduce cough frequency.

Food to Avoid

Eliminate foods that encourage mucus production: dairy products, chocolate, and bananas, as well as processed, refined, fried, and junk foods. Avoid simple sugars, as they suppress immune function.

℞ Super Seven Prescriptions—Cough

Super Prescription #1 Homeopathy
Use a combination cough remedy, as directed on the container, or pick the remedy that best matches your symptoms under Homeopathy in this section. For acute coughs, take a 30C potency four times daily. For chronic coughs, take twice daily for two weeks to see if there are any positive results. After you notice improvement, stop taking the remedy, unless symptoms return. Consultation with a homeopathic practitioner is advised.

Super Prescription #2 Ivy leaf extract
Take the liquid form as directed on the label. Several clinical studies demonstrate that ivy leaf extract supports bronchial health and alleviates coughing, especially those types which are wet.

Super Prescription #3 Cherry bark
Cherry bark reduces coughing, especially for wet coughs. Take 500 mg of the capsule or 1 ml of the tincture four times daily.

Super Prescription #4 N-acetylcysteine (NAC)
NAC reduces the viscosity of sputum so that it is easier to expectorate. It's useful for acute and chronic wet coughs (especially for smokers or people with asthma or emphysema). Take 300 to 500 mg twice daily.

A 2012 study published in the journal *Pediatrics* found that honey alone was very effective, and even superior to pharmaceutical treatments, for night-time coughs in children.

A different study included ninety-seven adults who had experienced a cough for more than three weeks as the result of an upper respiratory tract infection. Researchers divided participants into three groups, and all were given a tablespoon of a jam-like paste—mixed in warm water—three times a day. The first group received 20.8 grams of honey combined with 2.9 grams of coffee. The second group was given the steroid prednisolone at a dose of 13.3 mg. And the third group—the control group—was given the mucus-thinning medication guaifenesin. At the end of one week, the honey and coffee group had the most significant reduction in cough frequency. The mixture was much more effective than steroids or guaifenesin.

Super Prescription #5 Mullein (*Verbascum thapsus*)

Take 500 mg of the capsule or 2 ml of the tincture four times daily. This herb promotes the discharge of mucus and has soothing and anti-inflammatory effects for the respiratory tract.

Super Prescription #6 Echinacea (*Echinacea purpurea*) and goldenseal (*Hydrastis canadensis*)

For acute bronchitis with a wet cough, take 500 mg or 2 ml of this combination four times daily. Both herbs enhance immune function, and goldenseal works to dry up mucus.

Super Prescription #7 Astragalus (*Astragalus membranaceus*)

Astragalus is an excellent treatment for chronic, as well as acute, bronchitis. It strengthens weak lungs and increases the body's general resistance to infection. Take 500 to 1,000 mg or 3.5 ml of a tincture two or three times daily. Do not take astragalus if you have a fever.

General Recommendations

Vitamin C enhances immune function for acute bronchitis and has anti allergy benefits for chronic bronchitis. Vitamin C is particularly important for smokers. Take 500 to 1,000 mg three times daily.

Garlic (*Allium sativum*) has antimicrobial effects. Take 300 to 600 mg of garlic extract twice daily.

Bromelain has a natural anti-inflammatory effect and enhances the effectiveness of some antibiotics. Look for products standardized to 2,000 MCU (milk-clotting units) per 1,000 mg or 1,200 GDU (gelatin-dissolving units) per 1,000 mg. Take 500 mg three times daily between meals or along with antibiotic therapy.

Colloidal silver has an antimicrobial effect, especially for bacteria. Take ½ to 1 teaspoon, or as directed on the container, three times daily for five days.

Vitamin A enhances immune function. Take 25,000 to 50,000 IU daily for five days.

Ivy leaf (*Hedera helix*) may be helpful for chronic bronchitis for both children and adults. Take as directed on the container.

Licorice (*Glycyrrhiza glabra*) reduces coughing, enhances immune function, and soothes the respiratory tract. Use caution when supplementing licorice root if you have high blood pressure. Take 500 mg of the capsule or 1 ml of the tincture four times daily.

Other herbs that are useful and can be found in respiratory formulas include horehound, pleurisy root, plantain, marshmallow, ginger, peppermint, and cherry bark.

Homeopathy

Antimonium Tartaricum is for a congested, wet cough that produces a rattling noise in the chest. The person has trouble expectorating and may find it hard to breathe at times. The person feels better in a cool room and with the windows open.

Arsenicum Album is for a cough with a burning pain that feels better with sips of warm drinks. The person feels anxious and restless and may be very fatigued. Symptoms are worse from midnight to 2 A.M.

Bryonia (*Bryonia alba*) will treat a dry cough that causes stitching pain in the throat or the chest and that is worse at night. Movement of any type feels worse. The person has a great thirst and prefers to be left alone.

Coccus Cacti is for a cough that produces stringy mucus. The person feels a need to constantly clear the throat. Coughing often leads to vomiting.

Drosera is for a dry, barking cough that may end in gagging. The cough is worse lying down and worse after midnight.

Hepar Sulphuris (*Hepar sulphuris calcareum*) is for a rattling, barking cough that comes on after exposure to dry, cold air. The person coughs when uncovered and feels chilly and irritable. There is often yellowish mucus.

Kali Bichromium is for a hoarse cough that produces thick, stringy, yellow mucus. The cough is worse from eating and drinking.

Phosphorus is for a dry, tickling cough that is worse in the cold air, with talking or laughing, and when lying on the left side. The person may have a burning sensation in the chest and feels better with cold drinks.

Pulsatilla (*Pulsatilla pratensis*) will clear up a cough with yellow or green phlegm that is looser in the morning and drier at night. The person has a low thirst and feels better near an open window. The cough is worse when the person lies down.

Rumex Crispus is for a dry cough that begins as soon as a person lies down. The person feels a tickling sensation in the throat that leads to a cough. The cough is worse in cold air.

Silica (*Silicea*) is for a person who seems to have bronchitis all winter long. The person has weak immunity and low stamina and feels chilly. Coughing up mucus takes a lot of effort.

Spongia Tosta is helpful when someone has a dry, barking cough that is better with warm foods or liquids.

Sulfur is for bronchitis with burning pains that feel better with cold drinks. The person feels warm and desires a cool room. Sulfur is often used after a long bout of bronchitis, for complete recovery.

Acupressure

See pages 787–794 for information about pressure points and administering treatment.

- To relieve chest congestion, massage Kidney 27 (K27), Conception Vessel 22 (CV22), and Lung 1 and 7 (Lu1 and Lu7).
- If you have difficulty breathing and need to calm your emotions, use Bladder 38 (B38).

Bodywork

Massage

A back massage will break up excess phlegm. If you have chronic coughing, you might want to schedule regular sessions with a professional massage therapist. If you're generally a strong and healthy person, ask your therapist to use percussive motions, which are highly effective at releasing phlegm. People who suffer from an occasional bout of acute bronchitis might prefer to rely on a loved one to perform this task each evening.

Hydrotherapy

Sit in a hot, steamy bath or a sauna to thin mucus secretions and sweat out toxins. If you have hypertension, do not use saunas. Constitutional hydrotherapy works well for acute and chronic coughs. Follow the directions for treatment on pages 795–796.

Aromatherapy

Add eucalyptus, peppermint, lemon balm, or tree tea oil to a hot bath or a steam inhalation to drain congestion. You can also add any of these oils to a base oil and rub it directly onto your chest.

Stress Reduction

General Stress-Reduction Therapies

Stress can weaken your immune system and leave your lungs open to infection. If you're vulnerable to frequent bouts of bronchitis or suffer from chronic bronchitis, experiment with the techniques in the Exercise and Stress Reduction chapter until you find one or two that you like. Then practice them on a daily basis, or more often as needed.

Other Recommendations

- Rest, preferably in bed, while the illness is at its worst. When you feel better, move around to keep the infection from settling into your lungs, but continue to rest after periods of activity.
- Don't take a cough suppressant. The lungs must expel phlegm to get healthy; suppressants keep them from doing so. Consistent suppressant use can lead to worse cases of acute bronchitis or even to chronic bronchitis or pneumonia.
- Encourage expectoration by applying warm compresses to your chest.
- Don't smoke or expose yourself to secondhand smoke.
- If you have chronic coughing and live in a damp, cold climate, you may have to move to another location that's dry and warm. You should have your doctor consider mold allergies as a cause of chronic coughing.
- People with chronic bronchitis need to keep their lungs as elastic and strong as possible. Exercise, breath deeply, and, if you enjoy music, take up a wind instrument.

REFERENCES

Cohen, H. A., J. Rozen, H. Kristal, et al. 2012. Effect of honey on nocturnal cough and sleep quality: A double-blind, randomized, placebo-controlled study. *Pediatrics* 130(3):465–471.

Raeessi, M. A., J. Aslani, N. Raeessi, et al. 2013. Honey plus coffee versus systemic steroid in the treatment of persistent post-infectious cough: A randomised controlled trial. *Prim Care Respir J* 22(3):325–330.

Crohn's Disease

Crohn's disease is an inflammatory disorder that leads to severe ulceration of the digestive tract. The disease generally occurs in the last portion of the small intestine (ileum) and the beginning of the large intestine, but it can occur in any part of the digestive tract, from the mouth to the anus. Crohn's disease can affect the small intestine alone (35 percent of cases), the large intestine alone (20 percent), or both—the last portion of the small intestine and the large intestine (45 percent). There may be just one ulceration or several, and they may skip areas of the digestive tract. When these ulcerations heal, they can leave behind scar tissue that narrows a portion of the gastrointestinal passageway.

As its sufferers know, symptoms of Crohn's disease can be exceedingly unpleasant. The most common symptoms include intense abdominal pain and chronic diarrhea, fever, loss of appetite, and weight loss. Other common symptoms include nausea, mouth and anal sores, fatigue, and a general sense of malaise. Crohn's can also lead to other disorders. The chronic diarrhea prevents the absorption of vital nutrients, with malnutrition as a frequent result. Persistent bleeding within the intestines can cause anemia, which only compounds the existing fatigue and the nutritional deficiencies. People with Crohn's may also develop fistulas, abnormal tunnels that connect one part of the intestine to the other, or even to other organs. Sometimes the scar tissue is so thick, it partially or completely obstructs the bowels, a dangerous condition that is always a medical emergency.

The onset of Crohn's disease usually takes place during adolescence or young adulthood, with most cases occurring before age thirty-five, although it can affect the elderly, too. In some cases, the disease strikes once and never returns. For most people, however, Crohn's is a chronic condition that may flare up every few months or every few years. The condition must always be taken very seriously—indeed, the symptoms make it hard to ignore—and sufferers must be under the care of a good doctor, preferably a gastroenterologist with experience in treating the disease. If Crohn's is left untreated, the bowels may eventually stop functioning altogether. Yet natural medicine has a lot to offer for people with this disease, and many find that they can keep the disease under control with a comprehensive natural approach, as described in this chapter.

As with many other intestinal disorders, there can be a variety of causes of Crohn's disease. Crohn's disease is rare in "primitive" societies that follow diets based on whole, unprocessed food. In fact, the disorder was practically unheard of in the United States until the middle of the last century, when consumption of refined and chemically treated products skyrocketed. Food allergies—which tend to afflict societies that rely on unnatural foods—are also thought to play a significant factor in this disorder, as are free radicals, which, again, are best counteracted with good nutrition. Dietary therapy is a crucial component of any treatment plan for Crohn's disease. Good eating habits will prevent many of the secondary disorders, like malnutrition and anemia, that Crohn's can cause; better

Warning Signs of Bowel Obstruction

An obstructed bowel is a medical emergency. Crohn's sufferers are especially vulnerable to this disorder, because the scar tissue from ulcerated areas can partially or completely block the intestine. The classic indicators of bowel obstruction are vomiting and abdominal pain and distention. If you experience these symptoms, get medical help at once.

yet, it will address the underlying problem. Although no one can officially claim a cure for this disease, many sufferers will testify that dietary changes have successfully eliminated their symptoms. Unfortunately, many doctors are unaware of the role that diet plays in this disorder.

It is critical that digestive function be improved with this condition. Increased intestinal permeability is an issue that needs to be addressed. In addition, flora imbalance (dysbiosis), undiagnosed intestinal infection from parasites, harmful bacteria, and fungi need to be tested for and treated. Lifestyle is very important as well. Smokers are more likely to have Crohn's disease, and stress can be a powerful factor in the development of, as well as the recovery from, this disease.

For severe, acute flare-ups, your doctor may prescribe corticosteroids or other medications. The goal, though, is to address the underlying causes with natural therapy so that you can heal the digestive tract and decrease the susceptibility to future attacks. Even if more aggressive measures are needed, the treatments described here can reduce your suffering significantly.

SYMPTOMS

- Abdominal pain
- Chronic diarrhea
- Gas
- Loss of appetite
- Weight loss
- Nausea

- Fatigue
- Malaise
- Mouth and anal sores
- Headaches
- Low-grade fever
- Anemia

ROOT CAUSES

- Diet high in fatty and refined foods and low in fiber
- Food allergies
- Free radicals
- Nutritional deficiencies

- Stress
- Increased intestinal permeability
- Intestinal infection
- Poor lifestyle choices, such as smoking and drinking alcohol

---

Testing Techniques

The following tests help assess possible reasons for Crohn's disease:

Stool analysis—flora balance, possible infection, degree of inflammation

Food-allergy test—blood or electrodermal

Vitamin and mineral analysis—blood or urine for nutritional deficiencies

Stress hormones—DHEA, cortisol

TREATMENT

Diet

Recommended Food
Good nutrition is important for everyone, but people with Crohn's must be especially diligent about eating wholesome meals. It's best to buy fresh ingredients (organic, if possible) and prepare them yourself.

Protein deficiency is common in people with Crohn's. Incorporate quality protein sources into your diet, such as organic chicken, legumes, turkey, and fish, for two meals a day. Soy is also an option unless you are sensitive to it.

Homemade soups and broths are excellent. These meals are liquefied and easy to digest. Use a variety of fresh vegetables and quality protein sources, as described previously. This is particularly helpful during a flare-up.

Juices are ideal for Crohn's sufferers, because they require little work from the digestive system and their nutrients are easily absorbed. Drink vegetable juices every day. Cabbage juice is particularly effective in healing ulcerated areas.

Eat a cultured product like kefir or, if you're not allergic to dairy, live unsweetened yogurt every day. A deficiency of friendly intestinal bacteria is common in Crohn's patients.

Make proper hydration a priority. Drink at least one glass of clean, quality water every two waking hours. You'll replenish the water lost to diarrhea, and you'll also help your bowels regulate themselves.

Many people with Crohn's benefit from the avoidance or restriction of grains. Lactose intolerance is very common, so dairy products should be avoided.

Food to Avoid

Consumption of refined carbohydrates is strongly associated with Crohn's disease. Eliminate white flour, white rice, and both white and brown sugars from your diet. Almost all packaged products are made with at least one of these ingredients, so read labels carefully. A gluten-free diet or a carbohydrate-restricted diet can be very effective for this disease.

Foods that are high in saturated, hydrogenated, or partially hydrogenated fat will irritate your gastrointestinal tract and make diarrhea worse.

Avoid red meat, as well as any fried or greasy foods.

Many people with Crohn's disease have undetected food allergies; when they remove the allergens from their diets, the disease often completely disappears. To determine if a food or foods is causing your problem, read the Food Allergies section and follow the elimination diet that accompanies it. Dairy and wheat are common triggers for people with this disorder.

Be careful with high-fiber foods such as wheat bran, as they are too harsh for some people with this disease. Slowly increase fiber-rich foods in the diet.

Avoid alcohol, caffeine, carbonated drinks, and spicy foods. Although these products don't cause Crohn's disease, they irritate the gastrointestinal system and can make your symptoms worse.

Limit the use of fruit juices, which commonly irritate the digestive tract of people with this condition.

A study that reviewed the diets of people with Crohn's disease and ulcerative colitis found that the risk of Crohn's disease was highest in people who had a high sugar intake. The same study also reported that the consumption of fast foods twice a week tripled the risk of this disease.

℞ Super Seven Prescriptions—Crohn's Disease

Super Prescription #1 Aloe vera
Take ¼ to ½ cup three times daily or as directed on the container. Aloe soothes and heals the lining of the digestive tract.

Super Prescription #2 DGL licorice (*Glycyrrhiza glabra*)
Chew 1 or 2 capsules or take 300 mg of a powdered form twenty minutes before each meal.

Super Prescription #3 Fish oil
Take a total daily dosage of an enteric-coated fish-oil product containing at least 480 mg of EPA and 360 mg of DHA, spread out over three times a day. Fish oil reduces inflammation.

Super Prescription #4 Homeopathy
Use a combination digestive upset or cramping formula for the acute relief of symptoms, as directed on the container. Otherwise, see the description in the Homeopathy section for the most indicated remedy.

Super Prescription #5 Enzymes
Take 1 or 2 capsules with each meal. They aid in the digestion of food and are essential for all the metabolic activity in the body.

Super Prescription #6 Multivitamin and -mineral formula
Take as directed. Most people with this disease will have multiple nutritional deficiencies.

Super Prescription #7 Probiotic
Take a product containing at least twenty billion active organisms daily. It supplies friendly bacteria such as *Lactobacillus acidophilus* and *bifidus*. A product containing *Saccharomyces boulardii* probiotic has proved to be helpful for diarrhea associated with this condition.

In a double-blind trial of people with Crohn's disease, researchers found that people who took an enteric-coated fish-oil supplement had a recurrence rate of 26 percent after one year, while those taking a placebo had a 59 percent recurrence rate.

General Recommendations

Peppermint tea is an excellent tonic for Crohn's sufferers. It reduces nausea, relieves abdominal pain, and has a calming effect. Use with caution if you have reflux problems.

Chamomile (*Matricaria recutita*) will help reduce intestinal inflammation. This herb can be taken as a tincture at 4 to 6 cc three times a day.

Slippery elm (*Ulmus fulva*) is a traditional remedy for bowel disorders. It's high in mucilage, a substance that helps calm the intestines and reduce inflammation. Take 400 to 500 mg three or four times daily, or use 3 to 5 cc three times daily.

Cat's claw (*Uña de gato*) has anti-inflammatory and antimicrobial effects. Take 500 mg three times daily.

Oregano (*Origanum vulgare*) oil can be taken for an infection that accompanies Crohn's disease. Take 500 mg of the capsule form three times daily or as directed on the container.

Take a sublingual form of vitamin B12 and folic acid, to improve energy levels.

Chlorella, spirulina, or a greens formula will provide chlorophyll and other nutrients that promote digestive health. Use with caution, and slowly increase the dose to make sure they are not irritating.

Boswellia (*Boswellia serrata*) has a powerful anti-inflammatory benefit. Take

1,200 to 1,500 mg of standardized extract containing 60 to 65 percent boswellic acids two or three times daily.

Homeopathy

Pick the remedy that best matches your symptoms in this section. Take a 6x, 12x, 6C, or 30C potency twice daily for two weeks to see if there are any positive results. After you notice improvement, stop taking the remedy, unless symptoms return. Consultation with a homeopathic practitioner is advised.

Arsenicum Album is for burning pains in the abdomen that are made better in a warm environment or with warm drinks. The person feels anxious and restless.

Belladonna (*Atropa belladonna*) is the remedy for sudden abdominal pains and a fever that has a throbbing or burning pain. The symptoms are worse with motion.

Colocynthis is for sharp, colicky pains in the abdomen that feel better with pressure.

Ignatia (*Ignatia amara*) is for spasms of the digestive tract that come on after emotional stresses.

Magnesia Phosphorica is for cramping abdominal pain that is better with warm applications and worse from pressure.

Nux Vomica (*Strychnos nux vomica*) is for cramping pain. The person is irritable and chilly.

Pulsatilla (*Pulsatilla pratensis*) can be taken if rich, fatty foods give you diarrhea and if your symptoms are worse at night.

Sulfur can be taken if you are awakened by diarrhea that's urgent and explosive. Burning pain is often present, which feels better with cold drinks. The person may crave spicy foods and alcohol.

Acupressure

See pages 787–794 for information about acupressure points and administering treatment.

- Work Stomach 36 (St36) to increase your body's ability to absorb nutrients into the bloodstream.
- Improve the strength of your colon by working Large Intestine 11 (LI11).
- If you suffer from painful abdominal cramps, use Spleen 16 (Sp16).
- Conception Vessel 6 (CV6) will ease diarrhea and gas.

Bodywork

Massage

To ease pain in the stomach and the intestines, try an abdominal self-massage. Lie down in a comfortable place, bend your knees, and use the flat of your hand to press against the skin of the abdomen gently but firmly. This technique also encourages good digestion. If you like, you can use the antispasmodic oils suggested in the Aromatherapy section.

For stress relief, it's hard to beat a full-body massage. You or your partner can also practice some effective home-care techniques for stress reduction, like a neck or a foot rub.

Reflexology

See pages 804–805 for information about reflexology areas and how to work them. To regulate peristalsis, work the colon. Work the liver area to encourage detoxification. For stress relief, stimulate the solar plexus.

Hydrotherapy

Constitutional hydrotherapy is excellent for improving circulation and enhancing the healing of the digestive tract. It can be used for acute bouts of Crohn's disease and for long-term prevention.

Aromatherapy

Chamomile and lavender are antispasmodic oils that relax abdominal cramps. Dilute some in a carrier oil and use in a massage, or add a few drops to a warm bath. Each oil is also a pleasant stress reducer.

Ginger will soothe an upset stomach. You can use it in a bath, a massage, or a warm compress. If you like, you can combine ginger with chamomile or lavender for a highly potent effect.

Stress Reduction

General Stress-Reduction Therapies

Anxiety and tension play a significant role in every bowel disorder, and Crohn's is no exception. Since the disease itself usually causes further stress, it's important to make time every day to relax. Note that any stress-reduction technique is likely to help.

Other Recommendations

- If you smoke, it is important that you break the habit. And everyone with Crohn's disease must avoid smoky rooms.
- Since intestinal bleeding is a real danger in Crohn's disease, always check your stools for signs of blood, especially if it looks like tar. If you see any, call your doctor at once.
- Exercise promotes bowel health and also helps bring stress under control. Take a thirty-minute walk every day, or find some other aerobic activity you enjoy enough to perform regularly.
- Intravenous nutrient therapy by a holistic doctor is helpful to maintain good levels of amino acids and nutrients in the body. Such therapy is very helpful since multiple nutritional deficiencies are common with this disease. Increasing nutrient levels will not only help symptoms but also help with healing.

Low-dose naltrexone is a drug therapy used by holistic doctors for those with Crohn's disease. It is administered at a dose ten times lower than what is considered a normal dose. It reduces inflammation in the digestive tract. A randomized, double-blind, placebo-controlled study looked at the effect of LDN on adults with active Crohn's disease. The twelve-week study found that LDN improved clinical and inflammatory activity in those with moderate to severe Crohn's disease compared to placebo. Impressively, 78 percent of those treated with LDN showed an improvement in their endoscopy (scope of the lining of the upper digestive tract) compared to 28 percent of those receiving a placebo. The only side effect that was significantly greater than those receiving a placebo was fatigue.

REFERENCES

Belluzzi, A., C. Brignola, M. Campieri, et al. 1996. Effect of an enteric-coated fish-oil preparation on relapses in Crohn's disease. *New England Journal of Medicine* 334:1557–60.

Persson, P. G., A. Ahlbom, and G. Hellers. 1992. Diet and inflammatory bowel disease: A case-control study. *Epidemiology* 3(1):47–52.

Smoth, J. P., et al. 2011. Therapy with the opioid antagonist naltrexone promotes mucosal healing in active Crohn's disease: A randomized placebo-controlled trial. *Digestive Diseases and Sciences* 56(7):2088–97.

Cystitis. See Bladder Infection

Depression

Like many other chronic illnesses, depression can be caused by a wide variety of factors and is characterized by several out of a long list of symptoms. It affects people of all ages, races, and nationalities and, according to the World Health Organization (WHO), is the most costly of all diseases, largely because it disables people who would otherwise be productive. It is estimated that 10 percent of the U.S. population experiences depression severe enough to require medical attention, with women twice as likely as men to develop depression.

A major depressive episode is diagnosed when a patient suffers from a combination of psychological and physical symptoms that are a significant change from the person's prior level of functioning. It requires more than just a sad mood for the diagnosis to be made. A major depressive episode can be devastating and often affects every aspect of a person's life. Beyond a sad mood, there is often great fatigue and apathy, an inability to enjoy once-pleasurable activities, disturbed sleep, increased or decreased appetite, and a low sex drive. Depression generally leaves its sufferers feeling worthless, hopeless, guilty, irritable, or angry. Even a touch of the blues can impair the immune system, and serious cases often go hand-in-hand with other chronic illnesses. People with severe cases have constant thoughts of death and suicide. Depression can be deadly. Approximately one out of eight people will kill themselves during a major depressive episode.

Although it is often normal and healthy to experience sad moods in response to a trauma, such as the loss of a loved one, a major depressive episode is characterized by inappropriate sadness that persists or is out of proportion with its apparent cause. Clinical depression can further be categorized into unipolar depression, marked by recurring episodes of sadness, and bipolar depression, in which the sadness alternates with periods of elation and mania. Unipolar depression is by far the more common of the two. Both kinds of clinical depression can be caused by a number of factors, including constant tension and unresolved stress, genetics, chemical or hormonal imbalances, chronic illness, poor diet, food allergies, nutritional deficiencies, and even inadequate sunlight.

If your depression is clearly reactive to stresses or events in your life, many of the following therapies may ease some of your discomfort and help you work your way through the source of your sadness. Professional counseling is also a good idea. If you suspect that you are clinically depressed, first consult a doctor to rule out any underlying illness (such as a thyroid problem), then see a psychologist or a psychiatrist for a diagnosis and appropriate treatment. Obviously, it is best to work with a doctor who embraces natural therapies and will work with you to find the cause of your depression.

Research has shown that antidepressant medications are overprescribed. The American Psychiatric Association even noted that these drugs are "potentially unnecessary and sometimes harmful." Their recommendations include:

- Don't prescribe antipsychotic medications to patients for any indication without appropriate initial evaluation and appropriate ongoing monitoring.
- Don't routinely prescribe two or more antipsychotic medications concurrently.
- Don't use antipsychotics as the first choice to treat behavioral and psychological symptoms of dementia.
- Don't routinely prescribe antipsychotic medications as a first-line intervention for insomnia in adults.
- Don't routinely prescribe antipsychotic medications as a first-line intervention for children and adolescents for any diagnosis other than psychotic disorders.

Common side effects of antidepressants include:
- Nausea
- Dry mouth
- Loss of appetite
- Diarrhea or constipation
- Sexual problems (loss of desire, erection problems)
- Headaches
- Trouble falling asleep, or waking a lot during the night
- Feeling nervous or on edge
- Feeling drowsy in the daytime
- Weight gain or weight loss

The suggestions here will support your therapy and will also point you toward possible causes or aggravating factors of your disorder.

SYMPTOMS

A depressed person will usually have several of the following symptoms:
- Inability to enjoy things
- Fatigue
- Mood swings, at times characterized by unexplained weeping
- Feelings of apathy, worthlessness, helplessness, hopelessness, irritability, or guilt
- Sleep problems (either insomnia or sleeping too much)
- Appetite disturbances (eating too little or too much)
- Headaches, backaches, and digestive problems
- Difficulty concentrating or making decisions
- Increased anxiety
- Decreased sex drive
- Avoiding social situations
- Recurrent thoughts of death or suicide

ROOT CAUSES

Any of the following can cause depression by itself, but most depressed people are affected by more than one factor:

- Tension and stress
- Unresolved emotional issues
- Chronic illness or pain
- Neurotransmitter imbalance
- Hormonal imbalance, especially after childbirth or as a result of oral contraceptives or other synthetic hormone medications; commonly occurs with PMS and menopause
- Preexisting conditions—most commonly, hypoglycemia, anemia, sleep apnea, low adrenal function, and thyroid gland malfunction
- Alcohol and recreational drug use

- Poor diet
- Food allergies
- Nutritional deficiencies (particularly of B12, folic acid, B6, B1, tyrosine, tryptophan, and omega-3 fatty acids)
- Lack of sunlight
- Medications, including cortico-steroids, antihistamines, blood pressure medications, anti-inflammatory drugs, narcot-ics, and some pharmaceutical antidepressants
- Heavy-metal toxicity
- Fungal overgrowth
- Sleep disturbances

Testing Techniques

The following tests help assess possible reasons for depression:

Fungal overgrowth—stool analysis, blood, or urine

Food allergy test—blood or electrodermal

Hormone testing (thyroid, DHEA, cortisol, testosterone, IGF-1, estrogen, progesterone)—saliva, blood, or urine

Detoxification profile—urine

Vitamin and mineral analysis (especially magnesium, B12, folic acid B6, B1)—blood

Anemia—blood test (CBC, iron, ferritin, % saturation)

Food and environmental allergies/sensitivities—blood, electrodermal

Blood-sugar balance—blood

Toxic metals—urine or hair analysis

Amino acid analysis—blood or urine

Neurotransmitter levels—blood or urine

TREATMENT

Diet

Recommended Food

Depression is often caused by inadequate nutrition. Even if that's not the case with you, a sound diet will help create healthier brain chemistry. Eat a good diet balanced with complex carbohydrates from sources like whole grains, vegetables, and legumes. Complex carbohydrates are high in serotonin, a deficiency of which can cause depression and insomnia.

Soy, beans, lean poultry, eggs, nuts (walnuts are excellent), and seeds are excellent sources of protein, which will boost your energy levels. Have some several times a day.

The brain is primarily composed of fatty acids and requires a constant dietary supply of omega-3 fatty acids. While omega-3 fatty acids are most recognized for their cardiovascular benefit, they are quite important for normal mood. Various studies, including a recent one in *Psychosomatic Medicine*, have demonstrated that a relative imbalance between omega-6 and omega-3 fatty acids is associated with symptoms of depression. Omega-3 fatty acids can be consumed through cold-water fish such as ocean salmon, sardines, and low-mercury-content tuna. Almonds, walnuts, pumpkin seeds, and flaxseeds are also healthy sources.

You need to keep your sugar levels regulated, so instead of eating three large meals a day, try five to six smaller ones.

Consume 1 tablespoon of ground-up flaxseeds daily. This is a good source of fiber and essential fatty acids. Sprinkle on a salad or mix in a shake.

Add 1 tablespoon of flaxseed oil or an oil blend to your salad daily for healthful essential fatty acids.

Food to Avoid

Many depressed people have hidden food allergies. See the Food Allergies section and use the elimination diet on page 316 to determine which foods, if any, may be causing or aggravating your disorder. Any food is a potential allergen, but wheat is the product most often linked to depression.

Dramatically reduce your intake of hydrogenated and saturated fats, which only increase fatigue and sluggishness.

Caffeine and refined sugar may make you feel temporarily better, but your body soon "crashes" from the high, leaving you even more exhausted or irritable. They also deplete vital nutrients from your system. Eliminate these substances from your diet.

Alcohol is a depressant, so avoid wine, beer, and liquor. If you are so unhappy that you feel you need alcohol, talk to a doctor or a therapist. You may have a drinking problem—or you might be headed for one.

If you've been following a diet that's high in saturated fats and refined sugars, or if you've unknowingly been eating foods that have caused allergic reactions, some or even all of your symptoms may be caused by toxic buildup. A detoxification program will help cleanse your body.

If you feel sluggish and dull, and if your doctor has ruled out an underlying disease as the cause, a three-day juice and liquid fast may refresh you. See page 684 for further information.

℞ Super Seven Prescriptions—Depression

Super Prescription #1 S-adenosylmethionine (SAMe)
Take 400 mg of an enteric-coated form two times daily on an empty stomach for two weeks. If you notice improvement, stay on this dosage. If there is little improvement, then increase to 400 mg three times daily. SAMe increases the

Well-designed studies have shown that SAMe is equal to or, in some cases, more effective than pharmaceutical antidepressants. It has also been studied in combination with pharmaceutical antidepressants and was found to quicken the therapeutic effects. A double-blind study at the University of California–Irvine Medical Center found that 62 percent of people taking SAMe and 52 percent of those taking a pharmaceutical antidepressant improved significantly.

concentration of brain neurotransmitters that are responsible for your mood. Take a 50 mg B-complex, as B6, folic acid, and B12 are involved with proper SAMe metabolism. *Note*: People with bipolar disorder should use this supplement only with medical supervision.

Super Prescription #2 5-hydroxytryptophan (5-HTP)

Start with 50 mg taken three times daily on an empty stomach. Dosage can be increased to 100 mg three times daily if necessary. Note that 5-HTP is a precursor to the neurotransmitter serotonin. Take a 50 mg B-complex, as B6 is required for the proper metabolism of 5-HTP. *Note*: Do not take in conjunction with pharmaceutical antidepressants or antianxiety medications.

Super Prescription #3 Saint-John's-wort (*Hypericum perforatum*)

Take 300 mg of a product standardized to 0.3 percent hypericin three times daily (total of 900 mg). Saint-John's-wort has been shown in numerous studies to be effective for mild to moderate depression.

Super Prescription #4 B-complex

Take a 50 mg B-complex one or two times daily. B vitamins such as B12, folate, and B6 are intricately involved in neurotransmitter metabolism. Sublingual B12 and folate supplements are useful for seniors or those with absorption difficulties.

Super Prescription #5 Fish oil

Take a product containing a daily dosage of 1,500 mg of EPA/DHA. Essential fatty acids such as DHA improve neurotransmitter function.

Super Prescription #6 *Ginkgo biloba*

Take 60 to 120 mg twice daily of a standardized product containing 24 percent flavone glycosides and 6 percent terpene lactones. Ginkgo improves blood flow to the brain and enhances neurotransmitter activity.

Super Prescription #7 High-potency multivitamin

This provides a base of the nutrients involved with brain function.

General Recommendations

DL-phenylalanine (DLPA) is an amino acid used by the brain to manufacture neurotransmitters. Take 500 to 1,000 mg on an empty stomach each morning. It should be avoided by people with anxiety, high blood pressure, or insomnia. Do not take in combination with pharmaceutical antidepressants or antianxiety medications.

L-tyrosine is an amino acid that helps depression. Take 100 to 500 mg twice daily on an empty stomach. Do not take in combination with pharmaceutical antidepressants or antianxiety medications.

L-tryptophan has been a historic favorite of nutrition-oriented doctors for the treatment of depression. It acts as a precursor for the neurotransmitter serotonin. Take 500 to 1,000 mg three times daily on an empty stomach. This amino acid requires a prescription from your doctor and is available from compounding pharmacies.

Lithium orotate is a supplement that can be helpful for depression. Take 10 to 20 mg daily as directed by your holistic doctor.

A review of twenty-three randomized clinical studies involving seventeen hundred people found that Saint-John's-wort (*Hypericum perforatum*) was equally as effective as pharmaceutical therapy for mild to moderate depression. One well-publicized study found that Saint-John's-wort was ineffective for major depression. The same study also found the pharmaceutical medication Zoloft ineffective, yet the press focused on the negative aspect of Saint-John's-wort and ignored the fact that health professionals recommend Saint-John's-wort for mild to moderate depression.

Folic acid supplementation has been shown to improve the response to conventional antidepressant therapy.

Ashwagandha (*Withania somniferum*) improves stress-hormone balance and relaxes the nervous system. Take 1,000 mg two or three times daily. This nutrient requires a prescription from a doctor.

If you are low in the hormone DHEA, you should work with a doctor to normalize your levels; 5 to 15 mg is a good starting dosage.

Phosphatidylserine improves memory, and studies show that it's helpful for depression. Take up to 300 mg daily.

Vitamin D has been found in studies to help improve mood. It is particularly important for people who do not get regular sunlight, especially seniors. Take 400 to 800 IU daily.

Methylfolate is the active form of folate. People with the common MTHFR gene mutation may experience benefit for their depression by supplementing methylfolate. Typical dosage is 400 mcg or more.

Acetyl-L-carnitine has been shown to be helpful for seniors with depression. Take 500 mg three times daily.

If you feel tense and on edge, several herbal teas can help you calm down. Peppermint and chamomile have mild relaxing properties, but if you need something a little stronger, try hops (*Humulus lupulus*) or passionflower (*Passiflora incarnata*).

Oatstraw (*Avena sativa*) tea is a good tonic for the nerves. Drink a cup as needed.

For insomnia that accompanies or causes depression, valerian (*Valeriana officinalis*) or kava (*Piper methysticum*) tea, taken before bedtime, can be quite helpful.

Homeopathy

Pick the remedy that best matches your symptoms in this section. Take a 6x, 12x, 6C, or 30C potency twice daily for two weeks to see if there are any positive results. After you notice improvement, stop taking the remedy, unless symptoms return. Consultation with a homeopathic practitioner is advised.

Arsenicum Album is for people susceptible to depression who also suffer from anxiety and insecurity. They are often perfectionists who may have severe phobias. Restlessness and insomnia between midnight and 2 A.M. are common.

Aurum Metallicum is for deep depression, where there are thoughts of suicide. The person feels no joy and is in despair. There is relief from being in the sun. *Note*: Suicidal tendencies should always be discussed with a doctor.

Ignatia (*Ignatia amara*) eases depression brought on by grief or emotional trauma and characterized by rapid mood swings. Frequent sighing and a sensation of a lump in the throat are characteristics of people who benefit from this remedy.

Kali Phosphoricum is for depression as a result of overwork. Mental fatigue is a common symptom that this remedy helps.

Natrum Muriaticum is for depressed people who do not reveal their emotions and who hold their feelings inside. They feel emotionally reserved and withdrawn. Deep inside, they want people to be with them, but then they feel aggravated when others console them. There is often a strong craving for salt and an aversion to sunlight.

Pulsatilla (*Pulsatilla pratensis*) is for people who burst into tears at little or no provocation. They may also be driven to seek constant comfort and reassurance. They are very sensitive and feel better from crying, attention, sweets, and being in the open air. Symptoms are worse in a warm environment. Depression is often worse for women around the menstrual cycle or with menopause.

Sepia is for women who feel indifferent to their families. There are feelings of depression, fatigue, and irritability and a low sex drive. They feel worse when consoled and better from exercise. They are usually chilly and have a strong craving for sweets (chocolate) and salty/sour foods. Depression associated with hormone imbalance, as seen with PMS and menopause, is a strong indication for this remedy.

Staphysagria is for people who have suppressed emotions (such as anger) that contribute to depression. They are usually quiet and do not stand up for themselves, which leads to shame and resentment. Headaches and insomnia are also common.

Acupressure

- Lung 1 (Lu1) is the point of choice to ease anxiety and depression. You can work the point as you would any other.
- Stomach 36 (St36) is a good point for everyone with depression. It restores energy and well-being and soothes digestive troubles.
- For depression accompanied by fear or fatigue, use Bladder 23 (B23).
- Conception Vessel 17 (CV17) will help relieve depression caused by grief or made worse by anxiety.

Bodywork

If you are depressed, you may find that for many reasons—strained relationships, an inhibited sex drive, a decreased desire for stimulation in general—you are touched less than usual. Because touch is necessary for well-being, this situation can lead to further depression. Try one or more of the following techniques and practice them on a regular basis.

Massage

Any massage can help you feel better, but a full-body treatment can be a highly effective way to release stress that has built up in your muscles. You can add any of the oils listed in the Aromatherapy section for added benefit.

People need to touch as much as they need to be touched, so learn some basic techniques and give massages to your loved ones. Hand, neck, shoulder, and foot rubs are easy to give.

Reflexology

See pages 804–805 for information about reflexology areas and how to work them.

For depression in general, work the areas of the foot that correspond to the head, the endocrine glands, the solar plexus, and the pancreas.

If you feel fatigued, working the adrenals, the diaphragm, the glands, and the spine will energize you.

For quick relief of stress or tension, massage the entire foot with rhythmic strokes that are firm but not deep.

Acupuncture

Treatments from a qualified practitioner can help relax the nervous system.

Hydrotherapy

A hot bath or a sauna can relax edgy nerves; the steam will also help detoxify your body. Essential oils can be added to your hot bath as you like. If you have high blood pressure, do not take saunas.

Aromatherapy

Depression can manifest itself in a variety of moods, so you may want to refer to pages 771–781 to find the oils best suited for your particular needs. Following are some suggestions; you can prepare them according to any of the methods described in the Aromatherapy chapter.

To combat fatigue, use geranium, jasmine, neroli, bergamot, or rose.

If you need to calm down, lavender and melissa will have a soothing, quietly uplifting effect.

Ylang-ylang and patchouli are also calming, and they have the additional benefit of stimulating your sex drive.

Stress Reduction

General Stress-Reduction Therapies

If you're depressed, you're experiencing powerful and probably continuous levels of stress. It is vital for your emotional and physical health that you find at least one way to control anxiety, fear, or tension. Prayer, counseling, and positive mental imagery are all helpful.

If you sense that your depression is more than you can handle, don't hesitate to seek help from a psychotherapist, a religious adviser, or a support group. It helps a great deal to talk to people who have worked with others in great emotional pain.

Make an effort to stay in contact with beauty. If you have a garden or live near a nice park, spend as much time there as possible. And try to bring some of that beauty indoors: buy yourself a bouquet of flowers, listen to a favorite CD, or hang a watercolor of a nature scene on the wall in your office.

Regular exercise has been shown to be effective in improving depression. Try to get some physical activity every day for thirty minutes.

It may sound facile, but one quick way to feel better, at least temporarily, is to go dancing. Dancing releases endorphins, powerful hormones that will raise your spirits, and you'll benefit from the touch of other people, not to mention the pleasure of losing yourself in the music.

Helping others with their problems is a great way to relieve depression.

REFERENCES

1994. *Acta Scandinavica Neurologica* 89(154):19–26.

Davidson, J. R. T., et al. 2002. Effect of Hypericum perforatum (St. John's Wort) in major depressive disorder: A randomized controlled trial. *Journal of the American Medical Association* 287:1807–14.

Linde, K., et al. 1996. St. John's Wort for depression—An overview and meta-analysis of randomized clinical trials. *British Medical Journal* 313:253–58.

Medscape.com. "What Not to Prescribe: APA List Aims to Make Patients Safer." Accessed June 26, 2015 at http://www.medscape.com/viewarticle/811389?nlid=33922_1882&src=wnl_edit_dail&uac=130325DZ.

Taylor, M. J., S. M. Carney, G. M. Goodwin, et al. 2004. Folate for depressive disorders: Systematic review and meta-analysis of randomized controlled trials. *Journal of Psychopharmacology* 18(2):251–6.

Diabetes

According to the World Health Organization, 346 million people worldwide now have diabetes! When you count the number of people with prediabetes who are *already* experiencing some organ damage, that number jumps up to about 1.7 billion people with blood sugar problems. Here in the United States, about 10 percent of Americans have diabetes and another 20 percent prediabetes. That means that in this country alone, we're faced with over 70 million people with abnormal blood sugar levels.

Diabetes is a chronic health problem that involves elevated blood sugar levels. The metabolism of carbohydrates, proteins, and fats directly or indirectly leads to the production of the substance glucose, also known as blood sugar. Glucose is needed to supply energy to every cell in the body. If glucose levels become too elevated, then they become toxic to the brain and other body organs. With diabetes, two main problems can occur. One is a deficiency of insulin, a hormone produced by the pancreas that transports glucose into cells. The second is the resistance of the cells to insulin so that blood sugar cannot enter the cells.

Diabetes is categorized into three main types. In type 1 diabetes, also known as juvenile or insulin-dependent diabetes, the production and the secretion of insulin by the pancreas are severely deficient. Type 1 diabetes usually develops during childhood or adolescence. Because insulin levels are absent or dramatically low, people with type 1 need to inject themselves with insulin and monitor their blood sugar daily. This condition is thought to involve an autoimmune reaction, where the immune system attacks and damages its own pancreatic cells that produce insulin. Type 1 diabetes accounts for 5 to 10 percent of US cases of diabetes.

Type 2 diabetes, often called adult-onset or non–insulin dependent diabetes, is by far the more common of the two: about 90 to 95 percent of the diabetes in the United States is type 2. It strikes during adulthood, most often in the elderly or in obese people over forty. It is becoming increasingly common in children, due to lack of exercise, obesity, and poor dietary habits. People with type 2 can produce sufficient insulin, but the insulin and the glucose it transports cannot effectively enter into the cells. This category of diabetes is most often linked to a diet that is high in refined carbohydrates and low in fiber, and it can usually be treated with an effective diet, exercise, and specific nutritional supplements.

The third category is known as gestational diabetes, diabetes that occurs during a woman's pregnancy.

All three types of diabetes are very serious medical conditions. When left unmonitored and untreated, blood sugar levels can swing from dramatically low (hypoglycemia) to dangerously high (hyperglycemia). Hypoglycemia comes on quickly and leaves you feeling dizzy, pale, sweaty, and confused. You may feel uncoordinated or have palpitations. If your glucose levels are not raised, your symptoms could grow worse, and you could lapse into a coma. Hyperglycemia isn't much better. It may take hours or days to develop and can result in diabetic ketoacidosis, a life-threatening condition. Over the long term, both type 1 and type 2 diabetes can lead to heart disease, kidney and nerve disorders, loss of vision, and other problems. The high levels of blood sugar can also leave the body vulnerable to infection.

Researchers from the Indiana University School of Public Health found that higher levels of mercury exposure as younger adults increased the risk of developing type 2 diabetes later in life by a whopping 65 percent! The study involved 3,875 American men and women between the ages of twenty and thirty-two who were followed for eighteen years. Even after controlling for dietary and lifestyle factors such as omega-3 fatty acids and magnesium—both of which help with blood sugar metabolism and reduce the toxic effects of mercury—researchers found that participants who had the highest exposure to mercury as young adults had a tremendously increased risk of developing type 2 diabetes later in life. It appears that one of the many problems with mercury is that it damages the cells of your pancreas that produce insulin, the hormone needed for blood sugar control. Sources of mercury include mercury-laden fish, especially tuna, swordfish, and shark. Other sources include decaying amalgam dental fillings, and a by-product of coal-burning power plants.

Another important aspect of this disease is prediabetes. This is a condition in which the blood glucose level is higher than normal but not high enough to be classified as diabetes. People with prediabetes have an increased risk of developing type 2 diabetes. It is estimated that 57 million American adults have prediabetes.

If you have type 1 diabetes, you must work very closely with a good doctor and follow a lifelong treatment plan that includes medication, diet, and exercise. Complementary therapies, while they may not substitute for conventional medical treatment, can provide helpful support to your taxed endocrine and other systems, help decrease the need for medications, and reduce the long-term complications of the disease. In very rare cases some people are able to get off insulin therapy when a comprehensive natural approach is followed. This, of course, should never be tried without a doctor's supervision.

People with type 2 diabetes must also take their disease very seriously and consult a doctor on a regular basis; however, they will usually find that a comprehensive dietary, exercise, and supplemental program will reduce or eliminate the need for medication.

No matter which kind of diabetes you have, you must always talk to your doctor about any therapies you plan to incorporate into your protocol. And never go off your medication without a doctor's consent.

SYMPTOMS

Because these symptoms may not seem serious, many people with diabetes remain undiagnosed. If they apply to you or to your child, see a doctor as soon as possible.

- Frequent urination (children may be constant bedwetters)
- Strong thirst
- Excessive appetite
- Weight loss
- Fatigue
- Irritability
- Blurred vision

ROOT CAUSES

- Heredity
- A poor diet
- An autoimmune reaction (due to a viral infection, environmental toxin, food allergy)—one proposed theory about the origin of some cases of type 1 diabetes
- Chronic stress and the resulting stress-hormone imbalance
- Nutritional deficiencies, especially of chromium, B vitamins, zinc, vanadium, and vitamin D
- Obesity
- Certain medications such as thiazide diuretics, corticosteroids such as prednisone, antibiotics, cholesterol-lowering drugs such as statin drugs, and possibly some antipsychotic drugs
- Fungal overgrowth

- Chemical toxicity (e.g., pesticides, Agent Orange, mercury)
- Artificial sweeteners

Testing Techniques

The following tests help assess possible reasons for diabetes:

Hormone testing (thyroid, DHEA, cortisol, testosterone,)—saliva, blood, or urine

Intestinal permeability—urine

Vitamin and mineral analysis (especially magnesium, chromium, vanadium, zinc, B vitamins, and potassium)—blood

Digestive function and microbe/parasite/candida testing—stool analysis

Food and environmental allergies/sensitivities—blood, electrodermal

Mercury—urine or blood

Pesticides and other environmental toxins—urine or blood

Your doctor makes a diagnosis of diabetes according to the symptoms you exhibit, in addition to the results of blood and urine tests. Testing will also help your doctor determine whether you have type 1 or type 2 diabetes.

TREATMENT

Diet

The most important therapy for diabetes is a healthful diet. These dietary suggestions will help regulate your levels of blood sugar and also reduce your risk of complications, such as cardiovascular disease.

Recommended Food

Make sure to eat three meals a day at regular times, keeping portions moderate. Never skip breakfast, which leads to blood glucose fluctuations in the morning. Keep your snacks small, choosing nuts, seeds, protein drinks, vegetables, or fruit. Focus on consuming at least two servings of fruits and three or more servings of vegetables per day. Many diabetics notice better glucose control by including small portions of protein at every meal. Examples include nuts such as almonds, walnuts, or cashews, fish, chicken, turkey, or other lean meat. Foods shown to reduce glucose levels include vinegar (use in salad dressings), grapefruit, peanuts and peanut butter, chili, and cinnamon.

It is particularly important to limit refined carbohydrates such as those found in white flours, candy, fruit juice, soda pop, etc. Natural sweeteners such as Luo Han Go, stevia, and xylitol are excellent substitutes for baking or beverage sweeteners and do not adversely affect blood glucose levels. They are commonly available in health food stores.

Follow a diet that's high in fiber (vegetables, nuts, seeds, whole grains). Water-soluble fiber, as found in oat bran, beans, nuts, seeds, and apples, helps to balance blood sugar. Ground flaxseeds should be consumed daily. Consume 1 tablespoon with each meal or ¼ cup daily. Make sure to drink plenty of clean, quality water when you start taking flaxseeds (10 ounces per tablespoon). A daily total of 50 mg of fiber is a great goal.

Consume vegetable protein (legumes, nuts, seeds, peas) or lean animal protein (turkey, chicken, fish) with each meal. Protein drinks that have low sugar levels can be consumed. Protein helps smooth out blood sugar levels. Many people with diabetes benefit from increasing the relative amount of protein in the diet.

Sixty people with type 2 diabetes (thirty men and thirty women) were divided randomly into six groups. Groups 1, 2, and 3 consumed 1, 3, or 6 grams of cinnamon daily, respectively, and groups 4, 5, and 6 were given placebo capsules corresponding to the number of capsules consumed for the three levels of cinnamon. The cinnamon was consumed for forty days, followed by a twenty-day washout period. Researchers found that after forty days, all three levels of cinnamon reduced the mean fasting serum glucose (18–29 percent), triglyceride (23–30 percent), LDL cholesterol (7–27 percent), and total cholesterol (12–26 percent) levels. There were no significant changes found in the placebo groups.

Focus on quality fats. Fish such as salmon is excellent, as are nuts and seeds. Use olive and flaxseed oil with your salads.

Instead of eating three large meals, have several smaller meals throughout the day to keep your insulin and blood sugar levels steady. Or have three main meals with healthy snacks in between.

Chromium deficiency has been linked to diabetes, so eat lots of brewer's yeast, wheat germ, whole grains, cheese, soy products, onions, and garlic. Onions and garlic will also help lower blood sugar levels and protect against heart disease.

Enjoy plenty of berries, plums, and grapes, which contain phytochemicals that protect your vision. Research has shown that consuming three servings of blueberries a week will decrease your risk of diabetes by 25 percent.

Consume turmeric, which has been shown to reduce glucose levels.

Focus on foods with a low glycemic-load value.

Glycemic Index and Glycemic Load

Glycemic index (GI) has become a popular term, as it is more meaningful than the label "simple carbohydrate." GI refers to the rise in blood sugar that occurs after ingesting a specific food. This numerical value is compared to the GI of glucose at a value of 100. Foods with lower glycemic values are recommended for people with obesity, diabetes, and insulin resistance. For example, a Coca-Cola soft drink has a glycemic index of 63, whereas a serving of kidney beans has a value of 23.

Glycemic Index Guidelines:

GI of 70 or more is considered high.

GI of 56 to 69 is considered medium.

GI of less than 55 is considered low.

Glycemic Load

Recently, doctors and researchers have placed more value on the glycemic load (GL) value of foods. The glycemic load takes into account the amount of carbohydrates in a serving of a particular food. The glycemic index tells you how quickly a carbohydrate turns into blood sugar, but it neglects to take into account the amount of carbohydrates in a serving, which is important. The higher the glycemic-load value, the greater the blood sugar level and the resulting stress on insulin levels. This value is attained by multiplying the amount of carbohydrates contained in a specified serving size of food by the glycemic-index value of that food, and then dividing by 100. For example, an apple has a GI of 40, compared to glucose, which is the baseline at 100, but the amount of carbohydrates available in a typical apple is 16 grams. The GL is calculated by multiplying the 16 grams of available carbohydrate times 40 and then dividing by 100 to give a number of approximately 6. Compare this to a serving of Rice Krispies, which has a glycemic index of 82 and available carbohydrates of 26 grams, making a glycemic load of 21. Another example would be macaroni and cheese, which has a glycemic load of 32.

Glycemic Load Guidelines:

GL of 20 or more is considered high.

GL of 11 to 19 is considered medium.

GL of 10 or less is considered low.

Note: Glycemic-index and glycemic-load values for hundreds of different foods are available from the Harvard website at http://www.health.harvard.edu/healthy-eating/glycemic_index_and_glycemic_load_for_100_foods.

Food to Avoid

If you are overweight, it's critical that you implement a diet that promotes healthy weight loss. See Obesity.

Stay away from simple sugars. Obvious no-no's are candy, cookies, sodas, and other sweets.

White, refined bread also spikes blood sugar levels. Whole-grain breads, cereals, and pastas are better choices. Brown rice, barley, oats, spelt, and kamut are complex carbohydrates that are good choices.

Avoid cow's milk. Some studies have found a link between cow's milk ingestion and type 1 diabetes in children. It appears that some children, due to genetic reasons, react to the cow's milk protein (caseins), which causes an autoimmune reaction with the pancreas.

Eliminate alcohol from your diet.

Avoid artificial sweeteners. Instead, use diabetic-safe and more healthful natural sweeteners, such as stevia or xylitol. Diet sodas have been shown to increase the risk for type 2 diabetes.

Avoid high–glycemic load foods.

Diabetics are particularly vulnerable to toxins. Exposure to pesticides, polychlorinated bisphenols (PCBs), and phthalates is increasingly becoming associated with a risk for diabetes. Although fasting is not an option if you have diabetes, other therapies will help flush out toxic buildup and reduce your risk of developing diseases.

Consume detoxifying super green foods, such as chlorella, spirulina, wheatgrass, barley grass, or a mixture of these.

℞ Super Seven Prescriptions—Diabetes

Super Prescription #1 Berberine

Take 500 mg two to three times daily. Research shows berberine is comparable to a common diabetes medication in lowering blood glucose levels. It also reduces lipids, which are commonly elevated in diabetes.

Super Prescription #2 Chromium

Take a daily total of 500 to 1,000 mcg. Chromium improves glucose tolerance and balances blood sugar levels.

Super Prescription #3 *Gymnema sylvestre*

Take 400 mg of an extract daily. Various studies support its use for lowering glucose levels.

Super Prescription #4 Cinnamon extract

Take 500 mg twice daily. Cinnamon improves insulin sensitivity and utilization.

Super Prescription #5 Turmeric

Take 500 mg twice daily or 300 mg of standardized curcuminoids daily. Shown to reduce blood glucose levels.

Super Prescription #6 Alpha lipoic acid

Take 300 to 1,200 mg daily. Alpha lipoic acid improves insulin sensitivity and reduces the symptoms of diabetic neuropathy.

In a study published in *Molecular Nutrition & Food Research*, researchers evaluated one hundred people who were given either 300 mg per day of curcuminoids or placebo for three months. The results were astounding: compared to those in the placebo group those receiving the curcuminoids experienced a significant decline in long-term blood sugar levels, as measured by the marker hemoglobin A1C. It also significantly lowered the levels of free fatty acids. The buildup of these fats is known to contribute to insulin resistance.

> **Super Prescription #7 Resveratrol**
> Take 50 to 250 mg daily for better blood sugar control.

In a study published in *Metabolism,* researchers gave adults with newly diagnosed type 2 diabetes 500 mg of either berberine or the drug metformin three times a day for three months. Researchers found that berberine provided similar results to metformin in terms of the regulation of glucose metabolism and fasting blood glucose. And berberine reduced the amount of insulin needed to turn glucose into energy by 45 percent. In addition, those taking berberine had lower trigylceride and total cholesterol levels than those taking metformin.

In a separate study, researchers compared people with type 2 diabetes who took either 1,000 mg daily of berberine or daily doses of metformin or rosiglitazone. After two months, berberine had lowered subjects' fasting blood glucose levels by an average of about 30 percent, an improvement over the rosiglitazone group and almost as much as the metformin group. Berberine also reduced subjects' hemoglobin A1C by 18 percent—equal to rosiglitazone and, again, almost as good as metformin. In addition, berberine lowered serum insulin levels by 28.2 percent (indicating increased insulin sensitivity), lowered triglycerides by 17.5 percent, and actually *improved* liver enzyme levels.

And in a third study of berberine published in *Journal of Clinical Endocrinology and Metabolism,* researchers found that in type 2 diabetes patients given either berberine or placebo, the berberine group had significant reductions in fasting and postmeal blood glucose, hemoglobin A1C (which measures average blood glucose over time), triglycerides, total cholesterol, and LDL (bad) cholesterol, and also lost an average of five pounds.

General Recommendations

PGX is a type of water-soluble fiber that has been shown in studies to reduce glucose levels in people with type 2 diabetes. Take 2 to 4 capsules before each meal with 8 ounces or more of water.

Biotin is involved with glucose metabolism and is helpful for type 1 and type 2 diabetes. Take 9 to 16 mg daily.

Pycnogenol has been shown to decrease glucose levels. Take 100 mg one or two times daily. It has been shown to decrease glucose levels.

An antioxidant formula supplies additional antioxidants, which are generally required in higher amounts in people with diabetes. Take as directed on the container.

B-complex vitamins are involved in blood sugar metabolism and help treat diabetic symptoms such as neuropathy. Take a 50 mg B-complex daily.

Vitamin B12 is helpful for the symptoms of diabetic neuropathy. Take 1,000 mcg sublingually or by injection from your doctor (1 cc twice weekly).

Vitamin C helps prevent the complications of diabetes. Take 1,000 mg two or three times daily.

Magnesium is involved with insulin production and utilization. Take a daily total of 500 to 750 mg. Reduce dosage if loose stools occur.

CoQ10 tends to be low in people with diabetes. One study found that it has a blood sugar–lowering effect. CoQ10 prevents LDL cholesterol oxidation, which is more prevalent in people with diabetes.

Vitamin E improves glucose regulation and prevents cholesterol oxidation. Take 800 to 1,200 IU daily of a formula containing tocotrienols and tocopherols.

Banaba leaf has been shown in animal and human studies to lower blood sugar levels. Take 16 mg three times daily.

Thyme (*Thymus vulgaris*) extract balances the immune system, which is important for type 1 diabetes. Take 500 mg twice daily on an empty stomach or as directed on the container.

Pancreas extract supports pancreatic function. Take 500 mg twice daily on an empty stomach or as directed on the container.

Adrenal extract supports adrenal gland function, which is also important for blood sugar regulation. Take 500 mg twice daily on an empty stomach or as directed on the container.

DHEA is often low in people with diabetes. If tests show that you have low levels, take 5 to 25 mg daily under a doctor's supervision.

Psyllium has been shown to reduce blood sugar levels. It is a good source of fiber. Take up to 5 grams daily.

Asian ginseng (*Panax ginseng*) has been shown in a study to help improve blood sugar levels in people with type 2 diabetes. Take 200 mg daily.

Bitter melon (*Momordica charantia*) can help balance blood sugar levels. Take 5 ml twice daily of the tincture form or 200 mg in capsule form three times daily of a standardized extract.

Garlic (*Allium sativum*) is an important herb for the diabetic. It stabilizes blood sugar and helps reduce your risk of heart disease and other circulatory disorders by improving blood flow, lowering elevated blood pressure, and reducing levels of "bad" cholesterol. Take 300 to 450 mg twice daily.

Bilberry (*Vaccinium myrtillus*) may help to prevent diabetic retinopathy and cataracts. Take 160 mg twice a day of a product standardized to 25 percent anthocyanosides.

Fenugreek (*Trigonella foenum-graecum*) is another herb that stabilizes blood sugar. Take a product with an equivalent dosage of 15 to 50 grams daily.

Ginkgo biloba stimulates blood flow. Find a brand that's standardized to 24 percent flavone glycosides, and take 60 to 120 mg twice daily.

Evening primrose (*Oenothera biennis*) oil may help prevent and treat diabetic neuropathy. Take a product containing 480 mg daily of GLA (the active essential fatty acid in evening primrose).

Vanadyl sulfate improves glucose tolerance in people with type 2 diabetes. Take 100 to 300 mg daily. Higher dosages should be used under the supervision of a doctor.

Essential fatty acids are needed for proper insulin function, and they support nerve health. Take a fish oil supplement with a combined total of 1,000 mg of DHA and EPA.

Teas made with peppermint, chamomile, and passionflower all have soothing properties and encourage relaxation.

High-potency multivitamin supplies many of the nutrients involved with blood sugar metabolism. Take as directed on the container.

A study published in *Diabetes Care* followed thirty people with type 2 diabetes and found that 50 mg daily of pycnogenol lowered both fasting and post meal blood glucose levels significantly from the baselines. Higher dosages of 100 and 200 mg per day of pycnogenol were more effective.

Homeopathy

Consult with a homeopathic practitioner to individualize your homeopathic treatment.

Acupressure

See pages 787–794 for information about acupressure points and administering treatment.

- Governing Vessel 24.5 (GV24.5) supports the endocrine system.
- To improve circulation, massage Gallbladder 21 (GB21).

Bodywork

Massage

Diabetics often suffer from poor circulation, and a massage is a relaxing way to improve blood flow. Regular massages of the feet may be especially beneficial to help ward off foot ulcers.

Reflexology

See pages 804–805 for information about reflexology areas and how to work them.

Work the points that correspond to the pancreas, the liver, and the thyroid, pituitary, and adrenal glands. You will probably have to massage these points every day for several months to see an effect.

Hydrotherapy

Alternating hot and cold baths will stimulate circulation.

Stress Reduction

General Stress-Reduction Therapies

Diabetes puts additional stress on almost every part of your body and every area of your life. Keep your emotional health in balance by experimenting with the stress-reduction techniques discussed in the Exercise and Stress Reduction chapter. When you find one or two you like, practice them on a regular basis.

Other Recommendations

- Don't smoke or expose yourself to secondhand smoke. If you are diabetic, you are vulnerable to heart and kidney damage, both of which are linked to smoking. You may also have circulation problems, and smoking impairs blood flow.
- Poor circulation and nerve damage can lead to foot ulcers in diabetics. Keep the blood flowing through your feet by wearing comfortable shoes that fit well.
- If you're obese and have type 2 diabetes, you need to lose weight. The previous diet recommendations should help you take off the weight safely, as will the Obesity section in this book, but talk to your doctor about the best weight-loss plan for you.
- Alternating hot and cold compresses, applied to the abdomen, just over the pancreas and the kidneys, will encourage proper insulin production, along with regular elimination of fluids from the kidneys.
- Exercise regularly to maintain optimal blood sugar levels. Walking after meals is effective for some people.

- Have your holistic doctor test you for heavy-metal toxicity. Researchers from the Indiana University School of Public Health found that adults who were exposed to higher mercury levels when they were younger had a 65 percent increased risk of developing type 2 diabetes later in life.

REFERENCES

Anderson, R. A. 2000. Chromium in the prevention and control of diabetes. *Diabetes Metabolism* 26:22–27 [review].

Baskaran, K., B. K. Ahamath, K. R. Shanmugasundaram, et al. 1990. Antidiabetic effect of a leaf extract from Gymnema sylvestre in non-insulin-dependent diabetes mellitus patients. *Journal of Ethnopharmacology* 30:295–305.

Foster-Powell, K., S. H. A. Holt, and J. C. Brand-Miller. 2002. International table of glycemic index and glycemic load values. *American Journal of Clinical Nutrition* 76:5–56.

Hao, Z., et al. 2010. Berberine lowers Blood Glucose In Type 2 Diabetes Mellitus Patients Through Increasing Insulin Receptor Expression. *Metabolism*.

He, K., et al. 2013. Mercury exposure in young adulthood and incidence of diabetes later in life: The CARDIA trace element study. *Diabetes Care*. 36(6):1584–9.

Khan, A., M. Safdar, M. M. A. Khan, et al. 2003. Cinnamon improves glucose and lipids of people with type 2 diabetes. *Diabetes Care* 26:3215–18.

Liu, X., et al. 2004. French maritime pine bark extract pycnogenol dose-dependently lowers glucose in type 2 diabetic patients [letter]. *Diabetes Care* 27:839.

Na, L. X., et al. 2012. Curcuminoids exert glucose-lowering effect in type 2 diabetes by decreasing serum free fatty acids: A double-blind, placebo-controlled trial. *Molecular Nutrition & Food Research* 57(9):1569–77.

Shanmugasundaram, E. R., G. Rajeswari, K. Baskaran, et al. 1990. Use of Gym-nema sylvestre leaf in the control of blood glucose in insulin-dependent diabetes mellitus. *Journal of Ethnopharmacology* 30:281–94.

Yin, J., et al. 2008. Efficacy of berberine in patients with type 2 diabetes mellitus. *Metabolism*.

Zhang, Y., et al. 2008. Treatment of type 2 diabetes and dyslipidemia with the natural plant alkaloid berberine. *Journal of Clinical Endocrinology and Metabolism*.

Diarrhea

Acute diarrhea is a classic symptom of a poisoned, infected, or irritated digestive system. When the body is exposed to a toxic substance, its first priority is to expel that substance, and the digestive system has two basic strategies for performing the task. First, it secretes extra fluid to the intestines; second, it produces an unusual number of very strong intestinal contractions. As a result, loose, watery stools of increased volume and frequency help propel the toxins out of your body.

Most often, the toxin that needs to be expelled is a bacterium or virus, although parasites can be the cause as well. These invaders can enter your body through contaminated food or water or through contact with an infected person. Diarrhea may also result from your body's response to certain foods. An inability to digest milk and dairy products, called lactose intolerance, is a frequent cause of diarrhea, but many other foods can cause problems as well. You may also have diarrhea as a result of dietary overindulgence in general, even when the foods eaten do not usually give you trouble. In addition, anxiety and stress often play a role in all kinds of diarrhea.

While diarrhea is a useful and necessary response to poisoning—you certainly wouldn't want the toxins to remain in your body—it is often very uncomfortable and disruptive. However, for many cases of acute diarrhea (unless directed otherwise by your doctor), you should resist the temptation to take over-the-counter antidiarrhea medications, as they will only suppress the toxins your body is trying to eliminate.

When it comes to most episodes of acute diarrhea, the best thing to do is allow your body to do its work. While no one enjoys the discomfort and the inconvenience, the symptoms usually run their course in a day or two. The main concern is that your intestines may be passing too much fluid, as well as vital nutrients like sodium and potassium, so you'll want to stay hydrated with plenty of fluids and electrolytes. Natural therapies can make you more comfortable and can reduce the intensity and the length of the illness.

Sometimes diarrhea can be a warning sign of a far more serious illness, such as bacterial enteritis, irritable bowel syndrome, colitis, Crohn's disease, celiac disease, hyperthyroidism, parasites, or even cancer. Call a doctor right away if your stools are bloody; if abdominal pain and cramping are not relieved by passing stools; or if the urge is so forceful that you fear incontinence. You should also seek medical help if the episode lasts longer than three days or if it recurs over a period longer than one week. Diarrhea in children under six always requires a doctor's attention.

SYMPTOMS

- Watery, loose stools of increased volume and frequency
- Abdominal pain and cramping
- Gas

ROOT CAUSES

- Viral infection
- Contaminated food or water
- Food allergy or intolerance
- Bacterial, fungal, or parasitic infection
- Drug toxicity
- Anxiety and stress
- Medications (such as antibiotics)
- Electrolyte imbalance and dehydration

Testing Techniques

The following tests help assess possible reasons for diarrhea:

Comprehensive stool analysis—bacterial, fungal, and parasitic infections, flora balance

Food allergy/sensitivity testing—blood or electrodermal

Celiac disease testing for chronic cases—blood testing

TREATMENT

Diet

Although there are several important dietary strategies for diarrhea, the most critical are those to help you stay hydrated.

Recommended Food

While the attack is at its most acute, do not try to take in solid foods. Instead, focus on staying hydrated by drinking two cups of liquid every waking hour. Try water, diluted fruit and vegetable juices, electrolyte drinks, and broths. If you have a dry mouth or suddenly wrinkled skin that does not snap back when gently pulled, you may be on your way to severe dehydration. Drink a large glass of water or fresh vegetable juice immediately.

Food to Avoid

During the most intense stages of diarrhea, you will probably not feel much like eating. Do not force yourself to take in solid food during this time (although you should drink plenty of fluids).

As you feel better and regain your appetite, you should stay away from dairy products, fats, and oils, which will only upset your stomach again. If you do not have an intolerance to any of these foods, reintroduce them to your diet slowly.

Avoid sugar, especially if you have an infection. Bacteria feed on it. Even if a bacterium isn't the cause of your problem, keep sugar out of your diet; it promotes inflammation, which discourages healing.

Avoid caffeine and alcohol, which are too stimulating to the digestive tract.

If the cause of the problem is not clear, determine whether your diarrhea is caused by a food allergy or an intolerance. Once you feel better, use the elimination diet on page 316 to identify troublesome foods. Many cases of diarrhea can be traced to gluten intolerance, so make a special effort to examine the effects of wheat and seeds on your digestive system.

As you feel better, eat basic, simple foods that are easily absorbed. Soups, cooked fruits and vegetables, and brown rice are all good choices. Apples, bananas, carrots, and potatoes tend to taste especially good at this time, and for an excellent reason. They all contain an ingredient, pectin, that has a gentle binding quality.

One study has shown that roasted carob powder reduces the duration of diarrhea. Try a few tablespoons in some water.

Diarrhea is your body's method of self-detoxification. It's generally a good idea to fast on liquids for the first day; most likely, you will not want to eat solid foods anyway. See the dietary recommendations for details.

Tips for Travel

More than 50 percent of travelers to developing nations develop diarrhea from the microorganisms that are present in food and water. You can decrease your risk by taking the following steps:

• Prepare your body before you leave home. Six weeks before you leave, begin to eat lots of fresh garlic for its antibacterial and antiviral properties. You should also consume cultured products—live unsweetened yogurt, kefir, sauerkraut, and so on—to encourage the presence of friendly bacteria in your gut.

- When you arrive, continue eating garlic from your own supply, or take garlic capsules. We also recommend a probiotic supplement.

- This book generally recommends a diet that emphasizes raw plant foods. However, it may be wise to temporarily change your eating habits while traveling. Fried or char-grilled meats are often your best guarantee of thorough cooking. Avoid salads and raw foods, including fruits and vegetables, except those that have a thick outer skin, such as bananas and papayas.

- Use only bottled water, not just for drinking but also for brushing your teeth. Do not add ice to your drinks, unless you've made the ice yourself with bottled water.

- Don't eat at any restaurant or other establishment that is obviously unclean. Street food vendors are best avoided.

- When eating a food that is new to you, try just a little at a time. Even if it is clean and free of microorganisms, your digestive system may not be able to handle large quantities of unusual foods right away.

℞ Super Seven Prescriptions

Super Prescription #1 Homeopathic Combination Diarrhea Remedy
For acute diarrhea, take a dose of a combination diarrhea remedy four times daily for twenty-four hours. If you notice improvement, stop taking the remedy unless symptoms return. If your symptoms do not improve within twenty-four hours, then pick the remedy that best matches your symptoms under Homeopathy in this section.

Super Prescription #2 Ginger (*Zingiber officinale*)
Drink a fresh cup of ginger tea, or take 500 mg in capsule form or 2 ml of tincture every two hours. Ginger reduces intestinal inflammation and lessens the effects of food poisoning.

A study in the *Journal of Gut* reported that live probiotics interact with intestinal cells to protect them from the harmful effect of the bacteria *Escherichia coli.* Researchers found that these good bacteria prevented the *E. coli* from adhering to the cells and invading the body.

Super Prescription #3 Probiotic
Take a product containing at least twenty billion active organisms two or three times daily. It contains friendly bacteria, such as *Lactobacillus acidophilus* and *bifidus*, which aid digestion and fight infection. Studies also show the probiotic *Saccharomyces boulardi* to be effective for diarrhea, especially for diarrhea associated with antibiotic use.

Super Prescription #4 Goldenseal (*Hydrastis canadensis*)
Take 1 ml of the tincture form or 300 mg in capsules four times daily. It helps improve diarrhea that is related to an intestinal infection.

Super Prescription #5 Enzymes
Take 1 or 2 capsules of a full-spectrum enzyme with each meal. Enzymes aid in the breakdown and the absorption of food.

Super Prescription #6 Oregano (*Origanum vulgare*) oil
Take 500 mg of the capsule form four times daily or as directed on the container. Oregano oil has powerful antimicrobial effects.

> **Super Prescription #7 Astragalus (*Astragalus membranaceus*)**
> This is an excellent treatment for chronic diarrhea. It has an astringent effect and improves digestion. Take 500 to 1,000 mg or 3.5 ml of a tincture two or three times daily. Do not take astragalus if you have a fever.

General Recommendations

Activated charcoal binds toxins in the digestive tract. Take 2 tablets three times in one day or as directed on the container for acute diarrhea.

Colostrum has been shown in studies to be effective for diarrhea. It also helps to heal the digestive tract. Take 500 mg three times daily.

Marshmallow (*Althea officinalis*) is soothing to the digestive tract. Take 500 mg in capsule form or 3 ml of the tincture three times daily.

Slippery elm (*Ulmus fulva*) is high in mucilage, which has a soothing effect on the intestines. Drink 3 to 4 cups each day. You can also use 5 ml of the tincture or 500 mg in capsules three times daily.

Cranesbill (*Germanium maculatum*) has an astringent effect on the colon for acute diarrhea. Take 3 to 5 ml of the tincture or 500 mg in capsule form three times daily.

L-glutamine is an amino acid that repairs the digestive tract. It is most useful for conditions associated with chronic diarrhea. Take 1,000 to 2,000 mg three times daily.

Lactase is an enzyme that digests milk sugar (lactose). If you are lactose intolerant and want to eat lactose-containing foods, take 1 or 2 lactase enzymes with each meal.

Vitamin A and zinc have been shown to be helpful for children in third world countries who suffer from infectious diarrhea. Take as directed by a doctor.

Red raspberry (*Rubus idaeus*) tea has historically been used for diarrhea. Drink 4 cups daily to reduce intestinal inflammation. If you prefer to take capsules, spread a dosage of 5 to 10 grams evenly throughout your day. Chamomile and peppermint teas are also good options.

Homeopathy

Aloe Socotrina is helpful when the diarrhea is characterized by rumbling and gurgling in the abdomen, followed by gushing stools. There are often yellow, mucus-filled stools.

Argentum Nitricum is for diarrhea that comes from anticipation anxiety before a stressful situation or event. It is also used for diarrhea that results from sugar ingestion.

Arsenicum Album helps when diarrhea and vomiting occur together. The person is anxious, restless, and chilly. It is good for diarrhea caused by food poisoning. There may be blood in the stool, and the person may feel better from sipping warm drinks.

Chamomilla (*Matricaria chamomilla*) is for green/yellow diarrhea that accompanies teething in infants.

China Officinalis helps when there is extreme exhaustion and weakness from diarrhea.

Ipecacuanha (*Cephaelis ipecacuanha*) is for diarrhea that is accompanied by nausea.

Mercurius Solubilis or Vivus is for burning and bloody diarrhea. The person often has extreme sweating and spasms of the intestines.

Phosphorus is for a watery stool. The person feels anxious and craves cold drinks.

Podophyllum is helpful when there is rumbling, gurgling, and cramping in the

A randomized, placebo-controlled trial looked at the effect of probiotics on acute diarrhea in children from a day-care center. Probiotic supplementation was effective in reducing the duration of the diarrhea. The earlier the probiotics were begun, the more effective the results. In addition, a review of three double-blind clinical trials of diarrhea, which included 242 children ages six months to five years, found "that individualized homeopathic treatment decreases the duration of acute childhood diarrhea."

abdomen, followed by diarrhea. The diarrhea is painless, yet explosive, and is often worse in the morning.

Pulsatilla (*Pulsatilla pratensis*) is for diarrhea that results from eating greasy foods or fruits. The person feels better in the open air and worse in a warm room.

Sulfur is for burning, explosive diarrhea that wakes a person up in the morning. The stool has a very foul smell, like rotten eggs. The anus is red and excoriated. The person has a great thirst for cold drinks.

Veratrum Album is for painful, profuse diarrhea that resembles rice water. The person is very cold and desires drinks with ice.

Acupressure

See pages 787–794 for information about pressure points and administering treatment.
- Spleen 16 (Sp16) will relieve abdominal cramps associated with diarrhea.
- For diarrhea accompanied by gas, use Conception Vessel 6 (CV6).
- Large Intestine 11 (LI11) strengthens the colon.
- Stomach 36 (St36) is an excellent general toner that also strengthens the digestive system and improves the body's ability to absorb nutrients.

Bodywork

Massage
You may want to try a gentle self-massage of your abdomen. Lie down with your knees bent, and stroke the skin gently but firmly. For extra antispasmodic and soothing effects, use the essential oils recommended later in this entry.

Reflexology
See pages 804–805 for information about reflexology areas and how to work them.

Work the areas corresponding to the colon.

If your diarrhea is brought on or made worse by tension, also massage the area connected to the solar plexus.

Aromatherapy

Several oils have antispasmodic properties that will help relieve abdominal cramps.

Chamomile, lavender, peppermint, and lemon balm are some good choices; in addition to soothing cramps, all these herbs will ease stress. Use any of these oils by themselves or in any combination in an abdominal self-massage.

Other Recommendations

Constitutional hydrotherapy can be helpful for acute and chronic diarrhea. See pages 795–796 for directions.

REFERENCES

Jacobs, J., W. B. Jonas, M. Jimenez-Perez, and D. Crothers. 2003. Homeopathy for childhood diarrhea: Combined results and meta-analysis from three randomized, controlled clinical trials. *Pediatric Infectious Disease Journal* 22(3):229–34.

Resta-Lenert, S., and K. E. Barrett. 2003. Live probiotics protect intestinal epithelial cells from the effects of infection with enteroinvasive Escherichia coli (EIEC). *Gut* 52(7):988–97.

Rosenfeldt, V., et al. 2002. Effect of probiotic lactobacillus strains on acute diarrhea in a cohort of nonhospitalized children

Diverticulitis

Approximately 10 percent of American adults over age forty have diverticulosis. This is a condition in which the lining of the colon (and, rarely, the stomach or the small intestine) bulges outward. The bulges, or pouches (called diverticula), can be seen with an X-ray of the colon. As one gets older, the formation of diverticula becomes much more common. About half of Americans older than age sixty have diverticulosis. The most common site for diverticula is the sigmoid colon, the lower part of the large intestine. People with diverticulosis do not usually experience any symptoms and are unaware that they have this condition.

Rarely, diverticula can become infected from bacteria, leading to symptoms such as fever, cramping pain (especially on the lower left side of the abdomen), nausea, and changes in bowel habits. This is known as diverticulitis. In more serious cases, rectal bleeding, abdominal abscess, and perforation may result, requiring antibiotics and emergency surgery. After an initial episode of diverticulitis, the risk of recurrence symptoms ranges from 7 to 45 percent.

The emergence of diverticular disease seems to correlate with the introduction of processed foods in the American diet. Low fiber intake leads to constipation and high pressure in the colon wall, which may explain the formation of diverticula.

SYMPTOMS OF DIVERTICULOSIS

There are usually no symptoms, although some people may experience discomfort in the lower abdomen, constipation, and bloating.

SYMPTOMS OF DIVERTICULITIS

- Sudden pain that can be severe in the lower left side of the abdomen; less commonly, mild abdominal pain that gets worse over time
- Fever

- Change in bowel habits
- Nausea and vomiting
- Constipation
- Diarrhea
- Bloating
- Rectal bleeding

ROOT CAUSES

- Low-fiber diet
- Lack of exercise

- Food sensitivities
- Imbalanced intestinal flora

Testing Techniques

The following tests and procedures help assess possible reasons for diverticulosis and diverticulitis.

To confirm diverticulosis, an X-ray of the colon is performed.

For diverticulitis, a physical exam usually reveals abdominal tenderness (especially in the lower left abdomen) and inflamed diverticula of the colon, and blood work shows an increased white blood cell count.

Preventative tests that help determine the health of the digestive tract:

Stool analysis—flora balance, degree of inflammation, and bacterial, parasitic, or fungal overgrowth

Food sensitivity/allergy testing—blood, electrodermal

TREATMENT

Diverticulosis may be improved through a healthy diet and the treatments outlined in this section. Diverticulitis can also be helped with these treatments, although supervision by a doctor is necessary because of the potential seriousness of this infection. However, natural therapies can be used in conjunction with antibiotic therapy.

Diet

Recommended Food

To treat and prevent diverticulosis, consume a high-fiber, unprocessed diet focused on vegetables, fruits, and whole grains. Eat a cultured product like kefir or natto. If you're not allergic to dairy, eat live, unsweetened yogurt every day. Drink plenty of clean, quality water; 60 ounces daily will prevent constipation.

For those with diverticulitis, consume foods that do not contribute to inflammation. A water, vegetable juice, or broth fast for one to two days under medical supervision can be helpful.

Food to Avoid

Recent studies have not found nuts and popcorn to be associated with an increased incidence of diverticulitis. However, the authors have found them to be a trigger for some people. Food sensitivities, such as those to cow's milk, gluten, and corn, may be triggers for inflammation. Avoid simple sugars, which feed infection and promote inflammation. This includes alcohol.

Laura, a forty-five-year-old housewife, was experiencing moderate abdominal pain and fever for two days. A CT scan of her abdomen showed diverticulitis. A liquid diet of soups and broths, supplementation with aloe vera juice, a high-potency probiotic, colloidal silver, and daily hydrotherapy cleared up her condition in several days.

℞ Super Seven Prescriptions—Diverticulitis

Super Prescription #1 Aloe vera juice or powder
For diverticulitis, take ¼ to ½ cup or 1 teaspoon of powder extract three times daily or as directed on the container. Aloe soothes and heals the lining of the digestive tract.

Super Prescription #2 Colloidal silver
For diverticulitis, take 1 teaspoon four times daily or as directed on the label for up to seven days.

Super Prescription #3 Probiotic
Take twenty to fifty billion active organisms daily for diverticulitis to help fight infection of the colon. For those with diverticulosis, take five billion daily to maintain good healthy flora and prevent inflammation and infection.

Super Prescription #4 DGL licorice (*Glycyrrhiza glabra*)

For those with diverticulitis, chew 1 or 2 capsules or take 300 mg of powdered form twenty minutes before each meal. This herbal extract has anti-inflammatory effects on the lining of the digestive tract.

Super Prescription #5 Digestive enzymes

For those with diverticulosis, take 1 or 2 capsules of a full-spectrum digestive
enzyme with each meal. This aids in the digestion of food.

Super Prescription #6 Boswellia (*Boswellia serrata*)

For those with diverticulitis, take 500 mg three times daily of a standardized
extract. This herbal extract reduces inflammation in the colon.

Super Prescription #7 Psyllium fiber

For those with diverticulosis, take as directed on the label with 8 ounces of
water. This fiber prevents constipation.

General Recommendations

Peppermint (*Mentha piperita*) tea relieves abdominal bloating, pain, nausea, and gas.
Take 2 to 3 cups daily or in supplement form as directed on the label. Use with caution if you have reflux problems.

Chamomile (*Matricaria recutita*) will reduce intestinal inflammation. Take 2 to
3 cups daily or in supplement form as directed on the label.

Slippery elm (*Ulmus fulva*) soothes and reduces inflammation of the colon. Take
400 to 500 mg three or four times daily, or use 3 to 5 cc three times daily.

Cat's claw (*Uña de gato*) has anti-inflammatory and antimicrobial effects. Take
500 mg three times daily.

Oregano (*Origanum vulgare*) reduces infection of the colon. Take 500 mg in
capsule form three times daily or as directed on the container.

Chlorella or spirulina, or a greens formula that provides chlorophyll and other
nutrients, promotes digestive health for those with diverticulosis.

Homeopathy

Pick the remedy that best matches your symptoms in this section. Take a 6x, 12x, 6C,
or 30C potency four times daily for one or two days to see if there is any improvement. If you notice improvement, stop taking the remedy unless the symptoms return.
Consultation with a homeopathic practitioner is advised.

Arsenicum Album is for burning pains in the abdomen that are relieved by a
warm environment or with warm drinks. The person feels anxious and restless.

Bryonia Alba is for sharp left-side abdominal pain that becomes worse with any
movement.

Belladonna (*Atropa belladonna*) is for sudden abdominal pain and fever with
throbbing or burning pain. The symptoms become worse with motion.

Colocynthis is for sharp, colicky pain in the abdomen that is relieved with pressure.

Ignatia Amara is for spasms of the digestive tract that occur after emotional stress.

Magnesia Phosphorica is for cramping abdominal pain that is relieved by warm
applications and that worsens with pressure.

Nux Vomica (*Strychnos nux vomica*) is for cramping pain. The person is irritable and chilly.

Sulfur helps if you are awakened by diarrhea that's urgent and explosive. Burning pain is often present that is relieved by cold drinks. The person may crave spicy foods and alcohol.

Acupressure

See pages 787–794 for information about acupressure points and how to administer treatment.

- Work Stomach 36 (St36) to increase your body's ability to absorb nutrients into the bloodstream.
- Improve the strength of your colon by working Large Intestine 11 (LI11).
- If you suffer from painful abdominal cramps, use Spleen 16 (Sp16).
- Conception Vessel 6 (CV6) will ease diarrhea and gas.

Bodywork

Reflexology

See pages 804–805 for information about reflexology areas and how to work them.

To regulate peristalsis, work the colon.

Work the liver area to encourage detoxification.

For stress relief, stimulate the solar plexus.

Hydrotherapy

Constitutional hydrotherapy is excellent for improving circulation and enhancing healing of the digestive tract. It can be used for acute bouts of diverticulitis and for long-term prevention.

Aromatherapy

Chamomile and lavender are antispasmodic oils that relax abdominal cramps. Dilute some in a carrier oil and use for a massage or add a few drops to a warm bath. Each oil is also a pleasant stress reducer.

Ginger will soothe an upset digestive tract. You can use it in a bath, a massage, or a warm compress. If you like, you can combine ginger with chamomile or lavender for a highly potent effect.

Other Recommendations

- To prevent diverticulosis, exercise daily to maintain bowel regularity.
- Acupuncture and moxibustion can be used to maintain digestive health and treat colon inflammation.

Dizziness

Dizziness is the sensation that you are spinning or that your surroundings are spinning around you. Sometimes the sensation is mild and passes quickly, but it can also be so intense or prolonged that you may lose your balance and fall. Understandably, dizziness frequently produces nausea and vomiting.

Dizziness is not a disease in itself. Like pain, it's a symptom of an underlying problem, and any course of treatment for dizziness must begin with an investigation into the possible causes. Because the body keeps its balance through a complicated interplay of several organs, including the ears, the eyes, the nerves, and the muscles, finding the source of dizziness is not always easy.

Fortunately, dizziness often has its roots in a relatively minor cause. We've all experienced a spinning sensation when standing up too quickly after sitting or lying down for a long period of time; it may happen in airplanes, where there's less oxygen than most of us are used to. Occasional episodes of this kind are nothing to worry about. (If you experience it frequently, however, see a doctor.) Dizziness may also be the result of a fever, motion sickness, hyperventilation, a buildup of a wax in the ear canal, or a reaction to alcohol or drugs—factors that are either easily treated or temporary.

Sometimes, however, the underlying cause takes more effort to address. High blood pressure, anxiety, arteriosclerosis, food allergies, anemia, low blood sugar, hypothyroidism, and diabetes can all lead to dizziness. If nausea, vomiting, and a loss of hearing accompany the dizziness, you may have Ménière's disease, a disorder of the inner ear. In rare cases, dizziness is a warning sign of neurological disease or brain cancer.

If you experience dizziness, first rule out the obvious causes: motion sickness, fever and infection, and drug or alcohol use. In the case of motion sickness or fever, the dizziness will pass when travel or the illness ends. If your problem is related to alcohol or street drugs, stop using them; if you find that you can't, see the Substance Abuse section. For dizziness related to prescription medications, contact your doctor about alternatives.

If you can't immediately determine the cause on your own, see your doctor. He or she will take a thorough medical history to determine the most likely causes and will probably run a battery of tests. As you and your doctor search for the proper diagnosis, you can use the complementary therapies described further on to relieve your symptoms and reduce your chances of triggering an episode. In some cases, these therapies may resolve the problem altogether.

Ménière's disease is an inner-ear disorder characterized by vertigo (feeling as if the room around you is spinning around), tinnitus, and hearing loss.

SYMPTOMS

- Spinning sensation
- Nausea and vomiting
- Loss of hearing

ROOT CAUSES

Dozens of disorders and conditions can cause dizziness. Following are some of the most important:

- Returning to a standing position after a long period of sitting or lying down (orthostatic hypotension)
- Motion sickness
- Anxiety
- Fever
- Medications, street drugs, or alcohol
- Hyperventilation
- Wax buildup in the ear canal
- A disorder of the inner ear (such as Ménière's disease)
- Low blood sugar after a long period of sitting or lying
- Circulatory disorders, such as high blood pressure or arteriosclerosis

- Anemia
- Hypothyroidism
- Diabetes
- Neurological disorders

- Brain tumors
- Allergies (environmental and food)

Testing Techniques

The following tests help assess possible reasons for dizziness:

Anemia—blood

Electrolyte imbalance—blood

Low or high blood sugar—blood, urine

Blood pressure—have your doctor check for orthostatic hypotension

Thyroid disorder—blood or saliva

Inner-ear testing—by an ENT doctor

Food allergies/sensitivities—blood or electrodermal

Food or environmental sensitivities—blood, skin, or electrodermal

---

TREATMENT

Diet

Recommended Food

Nutritional deficiencies can cause dizziness, and they can also cause some conditions that lead to dizziness. Eat meals that are based on a wide variety of basic, whole foods that you have prepared yourself. Keep your blood sugar levels even by planning several small meals throughout the day, rather than three large ones. If you're nauseated, you may find that this strategy helps relieve your discomfort.

Some cases of dizziness have been linked to a deficiency of B vitamins, so add brewer's yeast to your meals. Other good sources of B vitamins are brown rice and leafy green vegetables. These vitamins will also help relieve anxiety.

Dizziness is sometimes caused by impaired circulation to the brain. Improve your blood flow by adding garlic, onions, and cayenne to your meals.

Food to Avoid

A response to a food allergen can cause dizziness. Read the entry on Food Allergies, and follow the elimination diet discussed there, to determine whether a food is the reason for your problem.

Even if your symptoms are not directly related to alcohol, avoid it. Alcohol can upset the inner ear and can aggravate other conditions that cause dizziness.

Excess sodium seems to affect the inner ear. Restrict your intake by avoiding processed, canned, or packaged foods, and don't use table salt to season your meals.

Avoid candy, cakes, cookies, and other sweets. These products will cause your blood sugar levels to spike and then plummet, with dizziness as a possible result.

It's possible that chemicals added to food affect the intricate system that produces our sense of equilibrium. Avoid processed and junk food, along with any food made with additives.

℞ Super Seven Prescriptions—Dizziness

Super Prescription #1 *Ginkgo biloba*

Take 120 mg two or three times daily. Ginkgo improves circulation through the inner ear.

Super Prescription #2 Ginger *(Zingiber officinale)*

Take 300 to 500 mg or 2 to 3 ml three times daily. This ancient remedy is used for nausea and dizziness.

Super Prescription #3 Homeopathic Combination Dizziness and Nausea Formula

Take a 30C potency twice daily to see if there is improvement. If there are no changes within three days, pick another remedy that best matches your symptoms from the Homeopathy section.

Super Prescription #4 Ashwagandha (*Withania somniferum*)

Take 1,000 mg twice daily. If dizzy spells are related to nervous exhaustion or overwork, this tonic herb soothes and strengthens the frazzled mind.

Super Prescription #5 Pycnogenol

Take 100 mg one to two times daily. Improves inner-ear circulation that may be related to dizziness.

Super Prescription #6 B-complex

Take a 50 mg complex twice daily. It combats the effects of stress that may be associated with dizziness.

Super Prescription #7 Vinpocetine

Take 10 mg daily to improve inner-ear circulation, which may help dizziness.

Homeopathy

Pick the remedy that best matches your symptoms in this section. Take a 6x, 12x, 6C, or 30C potency twice daily for two weeks to see if there are any positive results. After you notice improvement, stop taking the remedy, unless symptoms return. Consultation with a homeopathic practitioner is advised.

Aconitum Napellus is for sudden dizziness associated with anxiety, panic, or shock. Your pulse may be rapid, and you may even fear that you're going to die.

Bryonia (*Bryonia alba*) is for dizziness that occurs when you get up from a sitting position, turn your head, or bend over. You are irritable and have a great thirst for cold drinks.

Cocculus is for motion sickness and the dizziness that occurs from looking out the window. Nauseousness and/or vomiting may accompany the dizziness.

Conium is helpful when dizziness is worse from lying down or turning over in bed. Dizziness occurs from moving the head or the eyes.

Gelsemium (*Gelsemium sempervirens*) is for dizziness caused by a viral infection, making a person feel drowsy and droopy. It is also used for dizziness that follows stage fright.

Nux Vomica (*Strychnos nux vomica*) will ease dizziness that's brought on by a hangover or the ill effects of spoiled/contaminated food.

Pulsatilla (*Pulsatilla pratensis*) is for dizziness that comes on when you're in a warm or stuffy room. You feel worse when lying down. There is relief from walking or sitting in the open air.

Acupressure

See pages 787–794 for information about acupressure points and administering treatment.

When you feel dizziness coming on, sit down in a comfortable place, focus on a nonmoving object, and work the following points, all located at the top of your head: Governing Vessel 19, 20, and 21 (GV19, GV20, and GV21). Know these points so that you can use them whenever you need to, without having to look them up.

Bodywork

Massage

A general massage is an excellent way to stimulate circulation throughout the body. You can also practice a simple head and neck rub at home or see a massage therapist.

Reflexology

See pages 804–805 for information about reflexology areas and how to work them.

Work the areas corresponding to the eye/ear and the neck.

Hydrotherapy

Try constitutional hydrotherapy to improve circulation to the brain.

Aromatherapy

Lavender combats the sensation of vertigo. For immediate relief, place a vial of the oil directly under your nose and inhale deeply.

Ginger oil will reduce nausea. You can inhale the aroma directly from the vial or use the oil in an abdominal massage.

Black pepper, eucalyptus, and rosemary increase circulation. You can use these oils separately or in combination; add them to a bath or dilute them with a carrier oil and use in a massage.

Essential oils are perhaps most famous for their stress-relieving properties. If you'd benefit from oils with calming properties, try the following: lavender, berga-mot, ylang-ylang, geranium, or rose. You can use these oils in any preparation you like, but you should avoid using any one for an extended period of time, as you may grow immune to its effects.

Stress Reduction

Anxiety and stress can cause dizziness. Even if your symptoms are caused by an underlying disorder like diabetes or hypothyroidism, stress can aggravate the problem and trigger an attack. That said, you should be wary of any doctor who diagnoses you with stress-related dizziness without first checking for physiological causes. This misdiagnosis frequently happens to women, who are told their dizziness is "just stress," when, in fact, an underlying disorder is at work.

General Stress-Reduction Therapies

Stretching and mild exercise can improve the symptoms of dizziness.

Other Recommendations

- When you feel dizzy, sit down and focus your gaze on a fixed object until the sensation passes. This technique will shorten the duration of the dizziness and reduce nausea. Obviously, it will also prevent you from losing your balance and falling.
- Smoking inhibits circulation and can lead to dizziness. If you smoke, quit. Even if you don't smoke, you must avoid exposure to smoky rooms or bars.
- If you are prone to dizziness, avoid sudden changes in your posture. If you've been lying down or sitting for a long time, don't jump to your feet. Get up slowly.
- Acupuncture, craniosacral therapy, and chiropractic can help correct nerve impingement related to dizziness.

Drug Addiction. See Substance Abuse

Ear Infection

While ear infections can occur at any age, they are most common in early childhood and infancy. In fact, ear infections are the reason for more than half the visits to pediatricians in the United States. Statistics show that acute ear infections affect two-thirds of American children under age two, while chronic ear infections affect two-thirds of children under age six!

There are two main categories of ear infection. The first is an outer ear infection, also known as swimmer's ear or otitis externa. It affects the ear canal, which runs from the ear opening to the eardrum, and happens when a substance (usually water—hence the nickname) enters the ear canal and is trapped there by a buildup of wax. In this stagnant condition, bacteria breed and flourish. The body responds to the infection with inflammation, redness, pain, and sometimes a fever.

The second category, called a middle-ear infection or otitis media, is much more common, especially in very young children and infants. Most ear infections are usually associated with an upper respiratory infection or an allergy. Forty percent of cases involve bacterial infection, with the most common being *Streptococcus pneumoniae*. Many ear infections involve a viral infection that is unresponsive to antibiotics. Chronic middle-ear infections (also known as serous otitis media or glue ear) refer to chronic swelling of the eardrum as a result of fluid accumulation. One of the reasons infants are more susceptible to ear infections is due to the fact that the eustachian tube (which drains fluid from the middle ear) is more horizontal than it is in adults and does not drain as efficiently. This tube becomes more vertical and drains better as children get older. The key is to prevent the buildup of fluid with a proper diet. Food allergens, such as cow's milk and sugar, trigger a cascade of inflammation responses that often result in mucus and fluid. These foods are often

A comprehensive review of studies published in the *British Medical Journal* found that there was no significant difference in children with acute ear infections when antibiotics were given, as compared to a placebo.

The prescribing of antibiotics for otitis media with effusion is controversial. This refers to the presence of fluid in the middle ear, in the absence of signs or symptoms of acute infection. According to the U.S. Agency for Health Care Policy and Research, most cases of otitis media with effusion resolve spontaneously. It must also be recognized that fluid left in the middle ear after antibiotic treatment is normal. Approximately 70 percent of children have fluid in the middle ear at two weeks, 50 percent have fluid at one month, 20 percent have fluid at two months, and 10 percent have fluid at three months after appropriate antibiotic therapy. According to studies, the fluid that remains does not need to be treated with antibiotics, as is typically done.

the root problem. In addition, avoiding environmental allergens is important—particularly secondhand smoke. Addressing food allergies and environmental allergens is crucial so that "germs" do not have an environment to grow in. Of course, a healthy, functioning immune system is also key in preventing infection.

Some infections are the result of a malfunctioning or still-developing eustachian tube, the passage that connects the three bones of the middle ear to the nose and the throat. When the eustachian tube isn't working properly, mucus isn't able to drain from behind the eardrum into the upper respiratory tract; instead, it remains trapped and causes pain and pressure. This situation often leads to infection, especially if there has already been a mucus-producing disease of the upper respiratory system, such as a cold or the flu.

Middle-ear infections can be quite painful. There may be a fever, perhaps a very high one, with some hearing difficulty or nausea and vomiting. If your child pulls or slaps at his or her ear, an infection is a strong possibility. Take all ear infections and ear pain seriously.

The following treatments can be used to relieve pain, but do call a doctor for professional advice in the presence of a sustained fever or if the ear continues to hurt. If you or your child experiences severe ear pain, followed by a sudden relief and/or a discharge of blood or pus, consult a doctor immediately, even if you or the child feels well.

The over-prescribing of antibiotics for childhood ear infections has been a contributing factor to antibiotic-resistant bacteria. In addition, they put your child at risk for candida overgrowth (see Candidiasis).

SYMPTOMS

Not all of the following symptoms need to be present for a diagnosis of ear infection.

- Pain, often throbbing
- Fever
- Pressure or a feeling of fullness in the ear

- Pus from the ear
- Hearing difficulty in the affected ear
- Nausea and vomiting

ROOT CAUSES

- Buildup of wax, often the result of cleaning the ears with cotton swabs
- Upper respiratory infections
- Food allergies/sensitivities (especially overconsumption of dairy products)
- Environmental allergies (molds, dust, animal dander, and hay fever)
- Smoking or secondhand smoke,

which irritates the eustachian tube and causes inflammation behind the ear drum
- Not being breast-fed: Breast-feeding allows for the transport of immune factors from the mother to the child and matures the digestive tract so that the child is less susceptible to food allergies.

- Season: The incidence of earaches is highest in the winter. In northern climates, ear infections increase in frequency beginning in September.
- Fetal alcohol syndrome: More than 90 percent of children with fetal alcohol syndrome (which occurs from the mother drinking alcohol during pregnancy) have problems with ear infections.
- Genetic: Nearly 60 percent of all children with Down syndrome experience problems with otitis media.
- Nutritional deficiencies of vitamins A and C and essential fatty-acid imbalance.
- Injuries: Children who suffered a trauma at birth (e.g., forceps delivery, vacuum extraction) and children with neck and head injuries are more susceptible (an indication for chiropractic, osteopathic, or craniosacral therapy).

Testing Techniques

The following tests help assess possible reasons for chronic ear infections:
Food allergies/sensitivities—blood or electrodermal
Digestive health—stool analysis
Eustachian tube examination by an ENT specialist

TREATMENT

Diet

These dietary suggestions will help alleviate pain. More important, many of them will also prevent recurring infections. Significant changes in your child's diet may be necessary for optimal results. Work with a nutrition-oriented doctor.

Conventional Treatment for Ear Infections

Ear infections have reached nearly epidemic proportions in the United States. In response, frustrated doctors have come up with aggressive treatments, usually in the form of heavy antibiotics and ear tubes. Sometimes these strategies are necessary and effective, but all too often doctors employ them as a first line of defense, rather than as a last resort. Tubes in the ears, which relieve pressure on the eardrum and allow pus to drain, may seem like a good idea, but the tubes themselves often cause a great deal of damage. Interestingly, a study published in the *Journal of the American Medical Association* found that only 42 percent of these surgeries were appropriate. If your doctor recommends ear tubes, question him or her closely. Make sure that any treatment is tailored to your needs or your child's. And as always, try conservative measures—dietary changes, immune enhancement, homeopathy, and gentle herbals—before turning to harsh drugs or invasive procedures.

Recommended Food

A good diet based on whole grains, high-quality protein, and fresh fruits and vegetables will buildup the immune system and discourage infection.

Drink plenty of clean, quality water to thin mucus secretions.

Essential fatty acids, found in cold-water fish, flaxseeds, and flaxseed oil, are useful in reducing the inflammation or the allergies that are often present.

Switch bottle-fed babies to a nondairy formula, with your doctor's supervision.

Breast-feeding mothers should avoid common allergens (e.g., cow's milk), in order to avoid passing the allergenic portion through the breast milk. Food testing can be done with the mother.

Food to Avoid

Investigate the possibility of food allergies, especially to dairy, wheat, sugar, citrus fruits, soy, eggs, or chocolate. See the Food Allergies section, especially the elimination diet on page 316, for further advice. If you discover a trigger food, remove it from your diet.

If ear infections recur or are chronic, suspend the consumption of dairy products indefinitely. For infants and young children who are bottle-fed, replace the regular cow's milk formula with a hypoallergenic/predigested formula.

Simple sugars suppress the immune system, so stay away from refined carbohydrates.

R͓x Super Seven Prescriptions—Ear Infection

Super Prescription #1 Homeopathic Combination Earache Formula
Take a dose of the formula every thirty to sixty minutes for an acute earache. Improvements should be seen within two to four hours. Otherwise, see the remedies listed under Homeopathy in this section for a specific remedy.

Super Prescription #2 Garlic (*Allium sativum*) or garlic/mullein drops
Place 2 warm drops in the affected ear three times daily. Do not use if the eardrum is perforated or if fluid is draining out of the ear. These herbs have antibacterial/antiviral effects and natural pain-relieving qualities.

Super Prescription #3 Echinacea (*Echinacea purpurea*) and goldenseal (*Hydrastis canadensis*)
Adults can take 4 ml and children 2 ml four times daily or as directed on the container. Echinacea and goldenseal enhance immune function.

Super Prescription #4 Vitamin C
Adults should take 1,000 mg three or four times daily and children 500 mg three times daily. Reduce the dosage if diarrhea occurs. Vitamin C enhances immune function and reduces inflammation.

Super Prescription #5 Larix
Dissolve 1 to 2 teaspoons in a formula bottle for bottle-feeding infants or mix in water for older children and give it four times daily. Larix enhances immune function.

Super Prescription #6 Vitamin A
Give 2,000 to 5,000 IU daily (up to five days) for children up to six years of age. It's available in liquid form. Vitamin A supports immune function.

Super Prescription #7 Essential fatty acids

Adults should take 1 to 2 tablespoons of flaxseed oil or 3 grams of fish oil daily, or a formulation that contains a mixture of omega-3, -6, and -9 fatty acids. For children give a children's essential fatty acid formula or ½ to 1 tablespoon of flaxseed oil daily. It can be mixed into the formula for bottle-fed infants. Reduce the dosage if loose stools occur. Essential fatty acids are helpful for the prevention of ear infections, as they reduce inflammation and allergenic tendencies.

General Recommendations

Thyme (*Thymus vulgaris*) extract supports immune function. Take 250 to 500 mg twice daily on an empty stomach or as directed on the container.

Zinc supports immune function. Give 5 mg for children under two and 10 mg for those older than two. Adults should take 30 mg daily.

Chamomile tea is another way to help a child relax and sleep.

Because of its high mucilage content, marshmallow (*Althea officinalis*) is soothing to irritated ear membranes. Adults should take 2 grams three times a day; children six years and under can take 1 ml of the tincture three times daily.

Saint-John's-wort oil (*Hypericum perforatum*) relieves ear pain and fights infection. Place 2 warm drops in the affected ear three times daily. Do not use if the eardrum is perforated or if fluid is draining out of the ear.

Xylitol nasal spray and chewing gums prevent the buildup of bacteria that may cause ear infections. Use preventatively.

Homeopathy

Pick the remedy that best matches your symptoms in this section. For acute earaches, take a 30C potency (or the potency available to you) hourly, up to six doses. After you notice improvement, stop taking the remedy, unless symptoms return. Consultation with a homeopathic practitioner is advised.

Aconitum Napellus is helpful for a painful earache that comes on very quickly. The child experiences violent pain, restlessness, and great thirst. The earache often occurs after being out in the cold, dry wind. The ears are bright red. Aconitum is helpful only if used during the initial six hours of the ear infection.

Belladonna (*Atropa belladonna*) is for a sudden onset of earache, with high fever and a red face and eardrum. The right ear is more affected than the left. The pupils can be dilated, and child looks and feels hot, but the feet are cold.

Chamomilla (*Matricaria chamomilla*) is for a child with an ear infection, who is very irritable, angry, and hard to console. The child appears to be in a lot of pain, screaming and crying. The child wants to be carried, but it helps only for a short period of time. One cheek is often red, the other one pale. This is a great remedy for earaches that occur at the same time as teething.

K. H. Friese, M.D., and his colleagues divided 131 young children (average age five) into two groups. One group of 28 children received conventional treatment, such as decongestants, antibiotics, and fever-reducing medicines (twelve different drugs in all), for ear infections. Another group of 103 children was treated with one or more of twelve homeopathic remedies. Children receiving the homeopathic treatment, on average, experienced two days of ear pain and required three days of therapy. Nearly 71 percent never had another ear infection after one year, and nearly 30 percent had a maximum of three recurrences. By contrast, children treated with conventional medicine, on average, experienced three days of ear pain and required ten days of therapy. Nearly 57 percent did not have a recurrence after one year, while 43 percent experienced a maximum of six recurrences.

Ferrum Phosphoricum is recommended for a child who has a fever and feels warm. The face and the affected ear are red (such as in Belladonna), but the child does not act sick.

Hepar Sulphuris (*Hepar sulphuris calcareum*) is helpful when the ears are very sensitive to the touch and to cold during an infection. The child is irritable and hard to console. There is a sharp pain in the ear that feels better with warm applications. There can be pus or discharge from the ear.

Lachesis is useful when the left ear is affected or when the infection starts in the left ear and moves to the right. The earache is worse with warm applications and at nighttime.

Lycopodium (*Lycopodium clavatum*) is helpful for right-sided ear infections. Ear symptoms are often worse from 4 to 8 P.M. and feel better with warm applications to the ear. The child is irritable and may have more gas and digestive upset than normal.

Mercurius Solubilis or Vivus is a great choice for an earache that has an offensive-smelling pus discharge. The child sweats more than usual. There is a thick coating on the tongue, along with bad breath and increased salivation. The symptoms are worse at night.

Pulsatilla (*Pulsatilla pratensis*) is for a child who has a fever, is weepy, and wants to be held and comforted. Ear pain feels better with cold applications or in the open air, and worse with warmth. The child has a low thirst. The fever and the ear infection often develop at night. There can be a yellow-green discharge from the nose and the ears.

Silica (*Silicea*) is used for children who are thin and frail, with weak immunity, and who suffer from chronic ear infections. It is also used for acute ear infections and for a ruptured eardrum with pus. Cold and wind bother the child.

Acupressure

See pages 787–794 for information about acupressure points and administering treatment.

Triple Warmer 21 (TW21), Small Intestine 19 (SI19), and Gallbladder 2 (GB2) will ease ear pain.

Bodywork

Massage
Massage of the ear, the neck, and the temples is a gentle way to relieve a child's pain (or an adult's).

Reflexology
See pages 804–805 for information about acupressure points and how to administer treatment.

To reduce pain, work the ear/eye area.

Stimulate the lymph area to combat infection.

Hydrotherapy
Alternating hot (two minutes) and cold (thirty seconds) towels over the affected ear helps to relieve pain and inflammation.

Aromatherapy

Chamomile oil makes a gentle wash for the infected ear. First dilute the chamomile in a carrier oil, and place a couple of drops into the ear. After ten minutes, lie down on your side, with the infected ear turned toward the floor. Let the oil drain out (you may want to have a towel handy).

Other Recommendations

- Make sure not to bottle-feed while children are lying on their backs. They should be at a thirty-degree angle or more to prevent fluid accumulation in the eustachian tube.
- Don't smoke or expose yourself or your children to secondhand smoke.
- Follow the old adage that says not to put anything into your ear that's smaller than your elbow. Cotton swabs pack wax into the ear canal.
- During the course of an infection, don't allow moisture into your ears. Put cotton gently in the outside of the ear while taking baths or showers or while washing your face. Don't go swimming until the infection has cleared.
- To reduce pain, apply heat locally. Try a hot-water bottle wrapped in a towel or blow a hairdryer onto the affected ear.
- Chiropractic, osteopathy, and craniosacral treatments can be very helpful for some children with structural and motion abnormalities of the upper neck vertebrae. These abnormalities can cause fluid to buildup and not drain properly, providing a breeding ground for infections. Many parents have reported that these types of treatments helped to prevent further ear infections with their children. Specific treatments by a practitioner can correct these imbalances.

REFERENCES

Friese, K. H., et al. 1997. Acute otitis media in children: A comparison of conventional and homeopathic treatment. *Biomedical Therapy* 15:4, 113–16, 122.

Froom, J., et al. 1997. Antimicrobials for acute otitis media? A review from the international primary care network. *British Medical Journal* 315:98–102.

Kleinman, L. C., et al. 1994. The medical appropriateness of tympanostomy tubes proposed for children younger than 16 years in the United States. *Journal of the American Medical Association* 271:1250–55.

Eating Disorders (Anorexia Nervosa and Bulimia)

Eating disorders are characterized by a distorted body image and an intense fear of being fat. This abnormal mental state leads to extreme and sometimes life-threatening behavior. A person with an eating disorder may binge on large quantities of food and then vomit or use laxatives so that the food exits the body undigested, or the person may refuse to eat at all. Although eating disorders can manifest themselves in many ways, they always result in an unhealthful, obsessive relationship with food. The best-known and most frightening kinds of eating disorders are anorexia nervosa and bulimia.

Anorexia nervosa occurs most frequently in teenage girls and college-age women, and it's estimated that about 1 percent of all young women in this age group suffer from the disease. It is here that eating disorders take their most disturbing form: slow, deliberate starvation. Despite their obviously emaciated bodies, anorexics believe that they are overweight. They refuse food, or they eat just enough to keep their systems minimally functioning. Some may eat occasionally, just to please their families or friends, but they often purge themselves of the food afterward. It's not hard to see that anorexia can lead to grave health problems. Weight loss, weakness, and fatigue are obvious early signs, but as the disease progresses, it can also lead to weak vital signs, irregular menstruation, and cold or tingling extremities. If the dieting continues, the person may go into cardiac arrest.

Bulimia is a more common disorder that affects a slightly older population, usually women in their twenties. Bulimics also have a distorted body image, but instead of dieting down to skin and bones, they use a cycle of bingeing and purging to maintain a relatively normal weight. Bulimics may eat thousands of calories at one sitting and then induce vomiting to expel the food from the body so that they can't gain weight. They may also use laxatives to keep the body from digesting the food. Because many bulimics are quite successful at hiding their purging, the disease may go unnoticed for years. In fact, bulimia is often diagnosed only when a doctor or a loved one notices a pattern of medical conditions associated with bulimia. The stomach acid produced by frequent vomiting often causes tooth decay or a chronically sore throat. Self-induced vomiting produces another telltale sign: sores on the knuckles or the fingers. Not surprisingly, bulimics also tend to suffer from nutritional deficiencies, as well as digestive disorders like constipation or diarrhea. In severe or long-term cases, the complications can be fatal. The stomach or the esophagus may rupture, or a potassium deficiency can lead to kidney failure or heart attack.

We do know that eating disorders are a recent and mostly Western phenomenon, rare before the latter half of the twentieth century and nonexistent in developing nations. Our culture's emphasis on dieting and thinness is one undeniable cause of the disorder; far too many girls—and an increasing number of boys—believe that they are unlovable and even unclean if they can't diet down to the current rail-thin standard. Even if these children don't become anorexic or bulimic right away, it is highly likely that what starts out as "normal" dieting will disrupt the body's metabolism and chemistry and eventually lead to a serious disorder. Family dynamics also play a role: many sufferers come from families that place great pressure on their children to succeed. Although doctors used to believe that anorexia and bulimia were purely psychological in nature, it's now understood that chemical imbalances and the accompanying nutritional deficiencies may lead to eating disorders just as easily as they may lead to depression.

An eating disorder must always be taken seriously. Even if a person does not meet the exact standards for an eating disorder, an obsession with food and dieting can pave the way for more serious problems. If you suspect that you have an eating disorder, find a counselor or a friend you can trust. Talking about the disorder is one of the first and best steps you can take toward healing it. See a doctor for assessment and treatment of any secondary disorders you might have developed; if your eating disorder is severe, you may have to be hospitalized so that your body can regain its strength and balance. Bulimics will need to see a dentist as well. Once you've talked to a doctor, you'll need to follow an eating plan that replenishes the nutrients in your body and helps you reestablish healthful patterns. If you're not already seeing a professional therapist, make an appointment. He or she can help you relearn good habits and thinking patterns.

If you are worried that a friend or a family member has an eating disorder, you may find that confronting the ill person results in the individual's denial or resistance. Sometimes the only way to help a victim of an eating disorder is to ask for professional help. Call a doctor or a psychologist and ask for advice; if you're on a college campus, the school may have an eating-disorder specialist you can talk to. In extreme cases, the person may need to be hospitalized.

SYMPTOMS OF ANOREXIA

- Unexplained and unnecessary weight loss
- Fear of being fat
- Obsession with preparing and serving food
- Obsessive dining rituals
- Fatigue
- Weakness
- Dizziness
- Mood swings
- Menstrual irregularities or delayed onset of menstruation
- Hair loss
- Cold or tingling extremities
- Irregular heartbeat
- Weak vital signs

SYMPTOMS OF BULIMIA

- Sores or calluses on knuckles
- Chronic sore or burning throat
- Erosion of tooth enamel, especially on the back teeth
- "Chipmunk" appearance from swollen salivary glands
- Digestive problems
- Weight fluctuation
- Menstrual irregularities
- Erratic heartbeat

ROOT CAUSES

- Weight-obsessed culture
- Dieting
- Family problems
- Spiritual deficiency
- Chemical imbalance
- Low levels of serotonin
- Nutritional deficiencies (e.g., zinc)

Testing Techniques

The following tests help assess possible reasons for an eating disorder or imbalances that may aid in recovery:

Vitamin and mineral (especially zinc, iron, and B vitamins)—blood test

Blood sugar balance—blood test

Stress-hormone balance—saliva, urine, or blood

Neurotransmitter levels—urine, blood

Amino acid levels—blood, urine

TREATMENT

Diet

The following suggestions will help you get back on track, but it is highly recommended that you work with a nutritional therapist. A professional can help you address the particular deficiencies your disorder has created and can show you how to develop eating habits that work for you.

Recommended Food

Instead of sitting down to a large breakfast, lunch, and dinner, eat small, nourishing meals throughout the day. This strategy will stabilize your blood sugar, and if you're bulimic, it will help you stop bingeing.

A high-fiber diet will restore regularity to your digestive system. Eat plenty of whole grains, oats, and vegetables. Green leafy vegetables are also a good source of potassium, a mineral that bulimics must replenish.

People with eating disorders are often lacking protein. Plan to have fish several times a week, and include servings of soy products or beans at most meals.

Anorexia nervosa has been linked to a zinc deficiency. Pumpkin seeds are an excellent source of this mineral. Eat a quarter to a half cup daily.

Many people with anorexia or bulimia have low levels of the neurotransmitter serotonin. Regulate your serotonin by eating complex carbohydrates like whole grains.

Food to Avoid

Some foods fool your appetite or tastebuds into feeling satisfied, when, in fact, you have received very little nutrition. A goal of your dietary therapy should be to relearn how to listen to your body's needs, so stay away from the following "tricky" products: processed food, junk food, sodas, and diet or "lite" foods.

Keep your blood sugar levels steady by avoiding refined sugar. Do not eat candy, cake, cookies, ice cream, sodas, or other sweets.

Eliminate caffeine and alcohol, substances that upset the digestive system and sometimes produce anxiety.

℞ Super Seven Prescriptions—Eating Disorders

Super Prescription #1 High-potency multivitamin and -mineral
Take as directed on the container. If you have been diagnosed as being iron-deficient anemic, choose a formula that contains iron. It will supply a base of vitamins and minerals for nutritional support.

Super Prescription #2 Homeopathy
Choose the remedy from the list in the Homeopathy section that best matches your situation.

Super Prescription #3 Zinc
Take 45 to 90 mg daily, along with 3 mg of copper. Studies have found that zinc deficiency is common in people with anorexia or bulimia. It is also required for the senses of taste and smell and for appetite.

One clinical trial of twenty women with anorexia looked at the effects of their supplementing 45 to 90 mg of zinc per day. As a result, seventeen out of twenty women experienced weight gain within eight to fifty-six months. Also, a double-blind study of thirty-five women hospitalized with anorexia found that supplementation of 14 mg of zinc per day resulted in a 10 percent increase in weight. This was twice as fast as with the group that received a placebo.

Super Prescription #4 B-complex

Take a 50 mg complex one to two times daily. Many of the B vitamins are depleted because of stress and are required for the formation of brain neurotransmitters that balance mood.

Super Prescription #5 5-hydroxytryptophan (5-HTP)

Take 100 mg two or three times daily. It supports serotonin levels, which reduce anxiety and depression. Do not use in combination with pharmaceutical antidepressant or antianxiety medications.

Super Prescription #6 Gentian root (*Gentiana lutea*)

Take 10 drops in water or 300 mg fifteen minutes before each meal. It improves appetite and digestion.

Super Prescription #7 Saint-John's-wort (*Hypericum perforatum*)

Take 300 mg of a 0.3 hypericin extract two or three times daily. This herb helps with depression and anxiety. Do not use in combination with pharmaceutical antidepressant or anti anxiety medications.

General Recommendations

Take an amino acid complex as directed on the label.

Vitamin B6 is important for the synthesis of neurotransmitters that improve mood and sense of well-being. Take 50 mg daily.

Essential fatty acids are often deficient in people with eating disorders. Take an essential fatty-acid complex, 1 tablespoon of flaxseed oil, or 3 grams of fish oil daily.

Chromium helps to balance blood sugar levels. Take up to 1,000 mcg daily.

Homeopathy

Pick the remedy that best matches your symptoms in this section. Take a 6x, 12x, 6C, or 30C potency twice daily for two weeks to see if there are any positive results. After you notice improvement, stop taking the remedy, unless symptoms return. Consultation with a homeopathic practitioner is advised.

Ferrum Phosphoricum is helpful if you are pale, weak, and anemic.

Ignatia Amara is for people with an eating disorder who have emotional swings. They feel like crying easily, have anxiety and depression, yet are averse to consolation. It is useful for acute emotional upsets, such as grief, which contribute to the eating disorder.

Lycopodium (*Lycopodium clavatum*) is good for an upset stomach and bloating. The person tends to get low blood sugar and suffers from irritability and low self-esteem.

Natrum Muriaticum will help if you are often depressed and have long-standing grief associated with your eating disorder. You often crave salty foods, have a great thirst, and are averse to the sun.

Pulsatilla (*Pulsatilla pratensis*) is helpful if you tend to be sensitive and weepy and feel better with company. You also crave sweets and feel better in cool air.

Acupressure

See pages 787–794 for information about pressure points and administering treatment.

- Bring your appetite back to normal by working Spleen 16 (Sp16).
- Use Stomach 36 (St36) as a general tonic for all body systems and to improve your ability to digest and absorb nutrients.

Bodywork

Massage

A professional massage will help you get back in touch with your body.

Reflexology

See pages 804–805 for information about reflexology areas and how to work them.

Eating disorders wreak havoc on every body system. Work the entire foot for the full benefit. This treatment will also give you a quick mood lift.

To reduce anxiety, work the areas corresponding to the diaphragm, all the glands, the heart, and the solar plexus.

For depression, work the head, the endocrine glands, the solar plexus, and the pancreas.

Aromatherapy

Bergamot and peppermint oils encourage the appetite. Place the vial of oil directly under your nose and inhale deeply.

Stress Reduction

People who are anxious or depressed or exposed to high levels of stress are more vulnerable to eating disorders than others are. Many experts believe that eating disorders are a way of focusing on weight and food instead of on complicated and unpleasant emotions. If you're trying to recover from anorexia or bulimia, you'll find that learning alternative ways to handle stress will reduce your need to exercise control via food.

General Stress-Reduction Therapies

For people who've considered themselves little more than an extension of their appetite, prayer and meditation can work wonders to restore a sense of wholeness.

If you are extremely anxious and nervous, consider EEG biofeedback. It will teach you how to recognize your body's panic signals and show you how to subdue them before they get out of control.

Other Recommendations

- People with eating disorders often become obsessed with burning off calories through physical activity. A far better option is to take a thirty-minute walk at a moderate pace. The mild exercise will boost your spirits, and if you can get out in the fresh air and sunshine, you'll feel even better.
- Girls who are just beginning puberty are particularly vulnerable to losing their self-esteem; they may also fear the upcoming body changes and natural

weight gain. Both of these factors can set the stage for an eating disorder. You can help girls make a healthy transition into adolescence by encouraging them to develop a talent or an ability that improves self-esteem.

- It is imperative that a specialist in eating disorders manage the case of a person with an eating disorder.

REFERENCES

McClain, C. J., M. A. Stuart, B. Vivian, et al. 1992. Zinc status before and after zinc supplementation of eating disorder patients. *Journal of the American College of Nutrition* 11:694–700.

Safai-Kutti, S. 1990. Oral zinc supplementation in anorexia nervosa. *Acta Psychiatrica* Scandinavica 361:14–17.

Eczema

Eczema is a troublesome but common skin disorder that affects up to 15 percent of the population. In its acute form, eczema causes inflamed red, dry, and itchy skin. Some patches may blister and weep, and, eventually, these areas may crust over. If the eczema is a chronic problem, the skin will continue to itch but may thicken and take on a leathery consistency. Usually, dry scales develop, and the skin's color may change.

Most acute cases are brought on by an allergic response. Sufferers may be allergic to a certain food or to other substances; in either case, it's quite possible to have a reaction from ingesting the allergen or just from touching it. If you can identify the irritant and remove it, the eczema will usually disappear. But if the skin continues to be exposed to the irritating factor, the rash may spread and develop into a chronic condition. Stress may aggravate acute eczema and keep it from resolving.

Eczema can appear in infancy or early childhood and most often develops on the face and the head or in the folds of the elbows, the knees, or the groin. In some cases, it will disappear as childhood progresses and either stay away for good or recur in adolescence or adulthood. Chronic eczema is a complex condition that usually involves a family history of eczema, asthma, or hay fever; difficulty handling stress; or food sensitivity. It has also been linked to abnormalities of the immune system, as well as to candidiasis and low levels of essential fatty acids and deficiencies of other nutrients that help keep down inflammation.

Poor digestion and detoxification can also be at the root of eczema. Like most complicated ailments that involve the whole body and lifestyle, holistic treatment is the best approach for both relief and resolution. Conventional therapy for chronic cases is usually quite frustrating for the patient, as it generally just suppresses the skin problem and causes further spreading or intensifies the symptoms. Treating the root cause(s) with natural therapies, as described in this section, is, in our opinion, a superior way to help resolve this aggravating condition.

Dr. Stengler started treating Andrea in May 2010 when she was ten years old. When she came to see Dr. Stengler for the first time her skin was in really bad condition, with blisters all over her body that were full of pus and infected. Andrea was scratching twenty-four hours a day. She was always itching, from her face to the tips of her toes, and she scratched until she bled. Her mother made her wear socks on her hands at night. Sometimes Andrea would ask her mother to tie her hands together to help her sleep at night. Since following Dr. Stengler's treatment Andrea is no longer embarrassed to show her skin, which is clear and beautiful.

SYMPTOMS OF ACUTE ECZEMA

- Red, dry, swollen, and burning skin
- A strong, almost overwhelming desire to scratch
- Skin that blisters, oozes, and crusts over

SYMPTOMS OF CHRONIC ECZEMA

- Recurring cases of acute eczema
- Thick, dry skin with scaly patches
- Continued itching
- Color changes

ROOT CAUSES OF ACUTE ECZEMA

- Food allergies
- Contact with irritants (these can include but are not limited to dyes, perfumes, topical medications, plants, metals, soaps, wool, pollutants, and even sunlight)

ROOT CAUSES OF CHRONIC ECZEMA

- Suppressive treatments of acute eczema (such as long-term topical steroid treatment)
- Heredity
- Stress
- Food allergies or sensitivities
- An imbalanced immune system
- Deficiency of or inability to process essential fatty acids
- Fungal overgrowth
- Low levels of stomach acid and resulting poor digestion
- Poor detoxification
- Low levels of good flora
- Nutritional deficiencies

Testing Techniques

The following tests help assess possible reasons for eczema:

Intestinal permeability—urine

Detoxification profile—urine

Vitamin and mineral analysis (especially magnesium, B6, zinc)—blood

Digestive function and microbe/parasite/candida testing—stool analysis

Food and environmental allergies/sensitivities—blood, electrodermal

Essential fatty acid profile—blood

TREATMENT

Diet

Recommended Food

Eat a diet of basic, whole foods to encourage a healthy internal balance and a balanced immune system.

You should consume essential fatty acids every day. Flaxseeds and flaxseed oil are great sources; use the oil in dressings or sprinkle the seeds on cereal or salads. Flaxseeds and their oil change with heat, so do not bake with them or expose them to high temperatures. Cold-water fish, especially salmon, mackerel, and herring, are also good sources of EFAs.

Eat pumpkin or sunflower seeds daily. They are excellent sources of zinc, a mineral that encourages the proper metabolism of essential fatty acids.

Drink a glass of clean, quality water every two waking hours to flush out toxins and to encourage skin health.

If you're constipated, your body will have to find another way to get rid of wastes—and that usually means that toxins are expelled through the skin. Eat plenty of whole grains, fruits, and vegetables. They're full of fiber and will keep your digestive tract clean.

Vitamin A and beta-carotene are necessary for good skin health, so eat your green leafy and orange-yellow vegetables. Their nutrients are best delivered to your body when the food sources are raw, juiced, or lightly cooked.

Fungal overgrowth is a possible cause of eczema, so eat cultured products every day to stimulate the growth of "good bacteria." For more information, see Candidiasis.

In cases of chronic eczema for adults, undertake a three-day juice fast once a month to sweep away toxic buildup. Green drinks with barley, spirulina, or blue-green algae detoxify the blood and are especially supportive of an eczema fast. Children over the age of five may use these green drinks under the guidance of a nutrition-oriented doctor.

Food to Avoid

Eliminate all additives from your diet. Not only are additives likely to cause a direct reaction, they contribute to a toxic internal environment that can manifest in the skin.

Determine whether you have an allergy or a sensitivity to any foods. See the Food Allergies section for further details. Common food triggers of eczema are dairy, citrus fruits, tomatoes, soy, shellfish, eggs, wheat, and gluten.

Stay away from inflammatory foods, especially sugar, spicy foods, dairy, caffeine, and alcohol. Sugar and caffeine also contribute to anxiety and stress, so you have an extra reason to avoid these substances.

℞ Super Seven Prescriptions—Eczema

Super Prescription #1 Homeopathic Combination Eczema/Rash Formula

Use a combination of the most common remedies indicated for eczema. Take as directed on the container three or four times daily for acute outbreaks and twice daily for chronic cases. If there is no improvement for acute eczema within forty-eight hours, switch to the indicated remedy listed under Homeopathy in this section.

Super Prescription #2 Essential fatty acids

Take a formulation that contains a mixture of omega-3, -6, and -9 fatty acids, as directed on the container. Or adults can take fish oil at a dosage of 1.8 grams of EPA daily or 2 tablespoons of flaxseed oil daily. Children can take fish oil at a daily dosage of 480 mg of EPA or ½ to 1 tablespoon of flaxseed oil. Essential fatty acids reduce inflammation and dryness, and studies show that they heal eczema.

A study in the *Journal of Clinical Allergy and Immunology* reported that when breast-feeding mothers supplemented with a probiotic, their infants with eczema showed improvement after one month. It appears that good bacteria reduce the effect of the infant's food-allergy response.

A double-blind trial researched the effect of fish oil (1.8 grams of EPA) on a group of eczema sufferers. After twelve weeks volunteers who got the fish oil supplement had experienced significant improvement in their eczema.

Super Prescription #3 Probiotic
Adults should take a formula that contains at least five billion organisms per daily dosage and children at least two billion. Friendly flora such as *Lactobacillus* and *bifidobacterium* are involved with proper digestion, detoxification, and immune function.

Super Prescription #4 Burdock root (*Arctium lappa*)
Adults should take 1 ml of the tincture form or 300 mg in capsules with each meal, while children can take 0.5 ml and 150 mg. Burdock root has a cleansing effect on the skin.

Super Prescription #5 Evening primrose oil (*Oenothera biennis*)
Adults can take 3,000 mg daily and children 1,000 mg daily. It contains GLA (gamma linoleic acid), which has anti-inflammatory effects on the skin. Some people with eczema need increased amounts of GLA. It's especially important if other essential fatty acids, such as fish or flaxseed oil, have not been helpful.

Super Prescription #6 Vitamin E
Adults should take 400 IU and children 200 IU daily. It promotes skin healing and prevents the oxidation of essential fatty acids.

Super Prescription #7 Vitamin C with bioflavonoids
Adults take 1,000 mg two or three times daily and children 500 mg two or three times daily. It reduces inflammation and promotes skin healing.

General Recommendations

Zinc is needed for skin healing. Adults should take 30 mg twice daily, along with 3 mg of copper, and children can take 5 to 10 mg twice daily, along with 2 mg of copper.

Vitamin A promotes skin healing. It is particularly helpful for small bumps on the back of the arms. Adults should take 5,000 IU and children 2,000 IU daily.

Quercitin has anti-inflammatory effects. Adults should take 1,000 mg and children 500 mg three times daily.

Dandelion root (*Taraxacum officinale*) assists the liver in its detoxifying functions. Take 500 mg or 3 ml three times a day.

Vitamin D deficiency can be a cause of eczema. Typical dose is 1,000 to 2,000 IU daily for children and 5,000 IU daily for adults.

Many other herbs will reduce itching and swelling when applied topically. You can make a cream, a lotion, a cool compress, or a poultice with any of the following: comfrey, chamomile, calendula, chickweed, and witch hazel.

Red clover (*Trifolium pratense*) is beneficial for many skin disorders, although no one knows exactly how it works. Take 2 to 4 grams or 2 to 4 ml three times daily. If you have oozing skin or weeping blisters, you can also apply a cool infusion of red clover to the affected area.

Calendula (*Calendula officinalis*) heals broken or oozing skin and has an antiseptic quality. It's best used as a succus or cream.

Apply neem oil directly to the skin to heal and soothe patches of inflamed, red, and itchy skin.

Chickweed ointment reduces itching. Use as directed on affected areas for temporary relief.

If you are under stress, drink a cup of peppermint, chamomile, or passionflower tea to help you relax.

Homeopathy

Pick the remedy that best matches your symptoms in this section. Take a 6x, 12x, 6C, or 30C potency twice daily for two weeks to see if there are any positive results. After you notice improvement, stop taking the remedy, unless symptoms return. Consultation with a homeopathic practitioner is advised.

Arsenicum (*Arsenicum Album*) is for a chilly person who has very dry, itchy skin and swollen, tender skin eruptions. The eczema is worse in the winter, and the itching intensifies at night between midnight and 2 A.M. The person feels very restless, and the skin feels worse with warm applications.

Calcarea Carbonica is for people who are flabby and have clammy hands and feet. Their eczema tends to be worse in the winter. They crave eggs and sweets. This is also a good remedy for infants who suffer from cradle cap.

Graphites is for people whose dry skin becomes thick and has a honeylike discharge. The itching is worse in a warm bed.

Medorrhinum is for eczema that has been a problem since birth or a very early age. The person craves oranges and ice, tends to be very warm, and sweats easily.

Mezereum is for eczema that blisters and oozes and then forms a thick crustlike layer. Cold applications and the open air make the skin feel better.

Petroleum is for eczema that is characterized by very dry, cracked skin, especially on the palms of the hands. The itching is worse at night and in the warmth of the bed.

Psorinum is for chronic eczema that causes people to scratch until they bleed. The symptoms are similar to those of people who should take Sulfur, except that in this case, the people are very chilly.

Rhus Toxicodendron is for blistery-looking eczema that is very itchy and feels better from warm applications and movement. The person may crave cold milk.

Sulfur is for dry, red, itchy skin that's made worse with bathing and warmth. The person who will benefit from this remedy feels hot, is restless, and generally has a thirst for cold drinks.

Acupressure

See pages 787–794 for information about pressure points and administering treatment.
- Spleen 10 (Sp10) clears heat from the blood.
- Bladder 23 and 47 (B23 and B47) will relieve eczema.
- Stomach 36 (St36) and Governing Vessel 24.5 (GV24.5) both improve skin all over the body.
- If your eczema causes you stress, use Bladder 10 (B10) to soothe your nerves.
- Large Intestine 4 (LI4) relieves constipation and depression.

Bodywork

Reflexology

See pages 804–805 for information about reflexology areas and how to work them.

Work the areas that correspond to the liver, the kidneys, the intestines, the endocrine glands, the lymph, and the solar plexus.

Hydrotherapy

Constitutional hydrotherapy is helpful for long-standing eczema. See pages 795–796 for directions.

Other Bodywork Recommendations

An oatmeal bath can be very soothing. Tie some oats in a cheesecloth or in a leg from hose, and let water run on the oats under the tap before you soak. This can be purchased as a powder, too. You can also use the wet ball of oats as a compress directly on the affected area.

Aromatherapy

To soothe inflammation and itching and to relieve tension, add chamomile, geranium, or lavender to your bath or to a cream. These oils can be used separately or together.

If you want to relax, there are many oils you can try. See pages 778–780 for information on oils; the following are all excellent: bergamot, jasmine, lavender, rose, sandalwood, or ylang-ylang. Use them in a massage, a bath, lotions, or creams—but make sure you dilute them before applying them directly to the skin.

Stress Reduction

General Stress-Reduction Therapies

Any of the techniques in the Exercise and Stress Reduction chapter will help you control stress-related eczema. To help children, talk with them about how they are feeling and coping with their eczema, and what you are going to do naturally to help them heal.

Other Recommendations

If you have an acute case of eczema, you must avoid the offending irritant. If the source of the irritation is not obvious, review the possible triggers previously listed under "Root Causes of Acute Eczema," and try to avoid or treat each one.

REFERENCES

Bjørnboe A., E. Søyland, G. E. Bjørnboe, et al. 1989. Effect of n-3 fatty acid supplement to patients with atopic dermatitis. *J Intern Med Suppl* 225:233–6.

Majamaa, H., and E. Isolauri. 1997. Probiotics: A novel approach in the management of food allergy. *Journal of Allergy and Clinical Immunology* 99:179–85.

Endometriosis

Endometriosis is a painful condition in which tissue from the uterus attaches itself to other organs. The uterine tissue may appear in the fallopian tubes or the ovaries, or it may implant itself on the outer walls of the uterus itself. In rare cases, the tissue travels outside the pelvic region and appears in organs like the bladder, the lungs, and other areas.

These masses of tissue can be painful in and of themselves, but to make matters worse, they continue to behave as if they're inside the uterus. They continue to fill up with blood over the course of the menstrual cycle, and every month, they shed blood just as the uterus does. Unlike normal menstrual blood, which leaves the body through the vagina, the blood from the abnormal growth has nowhere to go. Instead, it accumulates inside the pelvic cavity, where it often forms cysts. As menstrual cycles repeat themselves and the tissue continues to bleed each month, the cysts may grow so large that they bind organs together. Sometimes a cyst ruptures and leads to agonizing pain. Two out of three women have endometrial growth on the ovaries.

Pain in the pelvis and the lower back is the defining characteristic of endometriosis. The pain usually varies with the menstrual cycle and is at its worst during ovulation, menstruation, or sexual intercourse; sometimes it is so intense as to be incapacitating. A woman with endometriosis may experience heavy or prolonged menstrual bleeding, and this loss of blood can lead to anemia. Digestive problems are common in cases of endometriosis, as are nausea and vomiting. There is a strong connection between endometriosis and infertility, although it is unknown whether the excess tissue actually prevents conception, or if infertility somehow creates conditions hospitable to endometriosis.

No one knows for sure what causes endometrial tissue to leave the uterus and travel to other parts of the body. One prevailing theory is that the disorder is caused by retrograde menstruation, in which menstrual fluid fails to exit the body properly. Instead, some of the endometrial lining that is normally shed during menstruation backs up in the fallopian tubes and enters the pelvic cavity, where the tissue deposits itself and begins to grow. It is also possible that endometrial cells travel to the pelvic cavity via the bloodstream or the lymphatic system. Others believe that endometriosis is caused when the body is still an embryo. In a normal fetus, the cells that are meant to form the uterus differentiate themselves from others and begin to travel to the appropriate site. But according to this theory, the endometrial cells of some fetuses don't make the trip and end up in the wrong places. It is also thought that environmental estrogens may be a causative factor. These xenoestrogens are endocrine disrupters that have estrogenic effects in the body. This category of environmental estrogens includes plastics, detergents, household cleaners, pesticides, herbicides, and hormones found in meat products. In addition, studies have shown immune-system imbalance to be a factor. Specifically, women with endometriosis have higher levels of antibodies that target their own ovaries and endometrial tissue. They also tend to have lower activity of the natural killer cells that usually keep abnormal cells in check. No matter what the cause, it does appear that all cases of endometriosis are linked to hormonal balance and that elevated estrogen levels are a problem.

It is important that liver function be optimized in women with endometriosis. The liver is responsible for breaking down estrogen (and other hormones) and secreting the metabolites into the large intestine for elimination. If the liver does not metabolize estrogen and its metabolites properly, they are recycled throughout the body.

While the liver is the dominant player in estrogen metabolism, the flora or "friendly bacteria" in the large intestine are also important in estrogen metabolism. They prevent the reactivation and the recycling of these unwanted estrogens. Conversely, "unfriendly bacteria" secrete an enzyme called beta-glucuronidase that causes estrogen to be recycled back through the body via the large intestine. A low-fiber and high-fat intake increases the activity of this enzyme.

While endometriosis is not a simple condition to treat, natural therapies often lead to significant improvement. The complementary treatments described here focus on regulating hormones and balancing the immune system and also suggest ways to provide gentle relief of pain and other symptoms.

SYMPTOMS

- Pain in the abdomen and the lower back, associated with menses
- Pain with sexual intercourse
- Prolonged or excessive menstrual bleeding
- Digestive problems
- Nausea and vomiting
- Anemia
- Infertility
- Pain with urination and bowel movements

ROOT CAUSES

- Retrograde menstruation
- Endometrial cells that travel through the bloodstream or the lymphatic system
- Heredity
- Hormonal imbalance (relatively high estrogen and low progesterone) due to poor liver function, diet, xenoestrogens, or ovulatory dysfunction
- Imbalanced immune system
- Flora imbalance (dysbiosis)

TREATMENT

Diet

It is important to eat certified organic foods as much as possible, due to the estrogenic effects of pesticides, herbicides, and hormone-laden meats.

Research has shown that a gluten-free diet can improve pelvic pain in 75 percent of women with endometriosis. Make sure to avoid gluten.

Testing Techniques

The following tests help assess possible reasons for endometriosis:

Immune-system imbalance—blood

Hormone testing (especially for estrogen and progesterone)—saliva, blood, or urine

Detoxification profile—urine

Digestive function (particularly, flora balance and beta-glucuronidase activity)—stool analysis

Food and environmental allergies/sensitivities—blood, electrodermal

---

Recommended Food

Whole grains, beans, and vegetables should form the basis of your diet. All these foods are high in fiber and will help to balance the friendly bacteria involved with estrogen metabolism.

Eat plenty of cold-water fish like salmon, tuna, and mackerel. These fish are good sources of essential fatty acids (EFAs), substances that reduce inflammation and pain.

For additional EFAs, add 2 tablespoons of flaxseeds to your daily protocol, along with 10 ounces of water. Flaxseeds have been shown to help balance estrogen levels.

Eat fruits and vegetables, such as apples, cherries, broccoli, cauliflower, and brussels sprouts. They contain the phytochemical indole-3-carbinol, which supports the liver's detoxification of estrogen.

Regularly consume beets, carrots, artichokes, dandelion greens, onions, and garlic, as these foods stimulate liver detoxification.

Eat organic cultured yogurt to increase the levels of friendly flora in the large intestine.

Once a day, drink 9 to 16 ounces of vegetable juice to support detoxification.

Drink a glass of clean, quality water every two to three waking hours to support detoxification.

Food to Avoid

Avoid red meat and dairy products that are not organic.

To keep pain under control, stay away from inflammatory substances like sugar, caffeine, and alcohol.

Don't eat anything that unbalances your immune system. Processed foods, fried food, refined sugar, and alcohol all limit your body's ability to fight your disorder.

Caffeine consumption appears to be a risk factor for endometriosis. According to researchers at the Harvard School of Public Health, women who consume 5 to 7 grams of caffeine a month had a significantly greater incidence of endometriosis. This is equivalent to about two cups of coffee a day.

℞ Super Seven Prescriptions—Endometriosis

Super Prescription #1 Natural progesterone
This hormone balances estrogen, regulates the menses, and relieves pain. Apply ¼ teaspoon (20 mg) to your skin twice daily from days six to twenty-six of your cycle (stopping during the week of your menstrual flow). It is best used under the care of a health care professional.

Super Prescription #2 Vitex (chasteberry)
Vitex balances the estrogen/progesterone ratio. Take 160 to 240 mg of a 0.6 percent aucubin standardized extract or 80 drops daily. Do not use vitex if you are currently taking a birth-control pill.

Super Prescription #3 Indole-3-carbinol
Take 300 mg daily. It assists the liver in estrogen detoxification.

Super Prescription #4 Dandelion root (*Taraxacum officinale*)
Take 300 to 500 mg in capsule form or 1 ml of tincture with each meal (three times daily). It improves liver detoxification.

Super Prescription #5 Vitamin E
Take 400 IU twice daily. It helps with estrogen metabolism and inflammation.

Super Prescription #6 Essential fatty acids
Take a daily combination of flaxseed (1 to 2 tablespoons) or fish oil (3,000 to 5,000 mg), along with gamma linoleic acid (GLA) from evening primrose oil or borage oil at a dose of 300 mg. These essential fatty acids decrease inflammation.

> **Super Prescription #7 Iodine**
>
> Take 500 mcg or more under a doctor's supervision. Iodine blocks excess estrogen stimulation of cell receptors.

General Recommendations

B-complex vitamins are involved in estrogen metabolism. Take a 50 mg complex twice daily.

Take 500 mg of D-glucarate daily. This phytochemical assists the liver in estrogen breakdown.

Melatonin has been shown to decrease pain scores for women with endometriosis. Take 10 mg at bedtime.

A high-potency multivitamin supplies many of the nutrients required for hormone metabolism. Take as directed on the container.

Vitamin C improves autoimmunity. Work up to 6 grams daily. Reduce the dosage if diarrhea occurs.

Motherwort (*Leonurus cardiaca*) is a good herb to use for acute uterine pain. Take 5 ml three times daily.

Red raspberry (*Rubus idaeus*) is an astringent herb that may help uterine inflammation and pain. Drink it as a tea, three cups daily.

Women with severe endometriosis often find that the pain keeps them up at night. If you need to get to sleep, try tea made with skullcap (*Scutellaria lateriflora*), passionflower (*Passiflora incarnata*), or valerian (*Valeriana officinalis*).

Homeopathy

Many sufferers report long-lasting results from constitutional homeopathic remedies, so it is highly recommended that you see a licensed professional for an individual assessment and remedy. For immediate relief of pain or other symptoms, use one of the following remedies, as appropriate. Take a 6x, 12x, 6C, or 30C potency twice daily for two weeks to see if there are any positive results. After you notice improvement, stop taking the remedy, unless symptoms return.

Arnica (*Arnica montana*) is for a deep, bruising pain.

Colocynthis will reduce cramping pain in the lower abdominal area. The person feels better with pressure on the abdomen and when lying with the knees drawn up.

Dioscorea Villosa is for uterine pain that radiates out from the uterus. The woman arches her back with the pain and feels better standing up and worse lying down.

Cimicifuga Racemosa is for severe menstrual pain that gets worse as the flow increases. There are shooting and cramping pains that radiate across the pelvis or into the thighs.

Lachesis is helpful for menstrual pain and large, purplish clots. The woman feels warm and jealous.

Magnesia Phosphorica is for pelvic pain, cramping, and bloating that feel better when heat is applied. The woman feels worse in the cold air or when the painful area is touched.

Pulsatilla (*Pulsatilla pratensis*) is for menstrual pain when the pain is changeable. The woman feels weepy and better when comforted and has a strong craving for sweets.

Sepia is for hormone imbalance, where the woman feels irritable, has pain with intercourse, and craves sweets, as well as salty and/or sour foods.

Acupressure

See pages 787–794 for information about pressure points and administering treatment.

- Large Intestine 4 (LI4) is a powerful point for relief of pain anywhere in the body.

Bodywork

Massage

Although it can't cure endometriosis, a massage of the belly and the lower back is an effective means of easing an acute attack of pain. Find a massage therapist whom you like and trust; if flare-ups occur at a predictable point in your cycle, you may want to make a standing appointment for treatment.

Reflexology

See pages 804–805 for information about reflexology areas and how to work them. Work the areas corresponding to the uterus, the fallopian tubes, and the ovaries.

Hydrotherapy

A hot bath can help relieve digestive problems as well as pain.

Other Bodywork Recommendations

When you feel an acute episode of pain coming on, lie down and rest, with a hot compress on the affected area.

Acupuncture is highly recommended to help reduce the pain associated with endometriosis. In addition, Chinese herbal therapy from a qualified practitioner can be very helpful.

One study found that auricular (ear) acupuncture was as effective as hormone therapy in treating infertility due to endometriosis.

Stress Reduction

People who suffer from chronic pain live with constant stress—more than their friends and family realize. Stress, too, can contribute to painful flare-ups. If you have endometriosis, it's important that you devote time every day to managing the tension that accompanies a chronic illness.

General Stress-Reduction Therapies

Pilates offers a gentle way to stretch and reduce stress.

Other Recommendations

- Moderate exercise is a natural pain reliever. Try to take a walk every morning, or find some other activity you like well enough to perform regularly.
- Use sanitary napkins instead of tampons. Tampons may encourage retrograde menstruation.
- Human chorionic gonadotropin (HCG) has been shown to relieve pain and other symptoms associated with endometriosis. Consult with a holistic doctor for the use of this bioidentical hormone.

REFERENCES

Gerhard, I., and F. Postneek. 1992. Auricular acupuncture in the treatment of female infertility. *Gynecological Endocrinology* 6:171–81.

Grodstein, F., M. B. Goldman, L. Ryan, and D. W. Cramer. 1993. *American Journal of Epidemiology* 137(12):1353–60.

Fever

A fever is usually regarded as a symptom of an acute infection or an underlying illness. It is the body's way of stimulating the immune system or accelerating detoxification. Anyone with a body temperature elevated at least 1 degree above 98.6 degrees F is said to have a fever. However, in babies, the healthy body temperature can vary from 97 to 100 degrees F because their body temperatures are not yet developed. In healthy children, body temperatures can fluctuate by 2 degrees above or below 98.6 degrees F. The amount of clothing one is wearing, as well as the amount of activity one is engaged in, can influence one's body temperature. Often, a fever is accompanied by a flush to the face and sweat beads on the forehead.

Fevers are often a cause for worry, especially for parents, but they should be regarded as both friend and foe. When a child has a mild fever, it could be a signal that the child's natural defense system is waging a war against an invading microbe. As the army of white blood cells battles, the cells release chemicals called pyrogens. These pyrogens activate the hypothalamus, a part of the brain that serves as the body's thermostat regulator, to turn on the internal heat and raise the body temperature to fight off invaders (many microbes start to die at around 102 degrees F). When this occurs, heat is lost through the skin, and the blood vessels dilate.

The onset of a high fever may lead to a febrile seizure in some children and adults. Their muscles become rigid, and they experience convulsions or even loss of consciousness for up to fifteen minutes. This is an emergency situation that requires immediate medical attention. Upon recovering, a child may sleep for a long time. As horrific as these are to witness, febrile seizures rarely develop into epilepsy or cause permanent harm to the child.

People with temperatures above 102 degrees F may require medical intervention. If your child is younger than three months of age, notify your doctor about the fever.

Be sure to get checked by a doctor if you or someone you are caring for experiences any of these symptoms:

- Acts confused, lethargic, or delirious
- Vomits or has diarrhea
- Complains of a stiff neck or has dilated pupils
- Has had the fever for more than seventy-two hours

And for infants and children, also be aware of these additional signs and symptoms:

- Cries continuously
- Is difficult to awaken
- Has a significant decrease in urine output or appears dehydrated
- Has trouble breathing

Conventional treatment focuses on fever-reducing medications, such as acetaminophen. From a holistic perspective, we look at fever as a generally positive thing since it activates the immune system. We try to work with a fever and not necessarily suppress it, unless it is too high or the patient is very uncomfortable. *Note*: Never give aspirin to a child who has a fever. It can cause an immune reaction, leading to the development of Reye's syndrome, a potentially fatal illness involving vomiting and possible liver damage.

SYMPTOMS

- Flushed face, elevated temperature

ROOT CAUSES

- Infection
- Systemic illness (cancer, etc.)
- Detoxification reaction

TREATMENT

Diet

Recommended Food

Eat lightly. Steamed vegetables, soups, broths, and herbal teas will let your body focus on healing instead of on digestion. If you lose your appetite, don't force yourself to eat.

Stay hydrated. Drink plenty of clean, quality water and other fluids (but see the note about sugar and juice further on) to cleanse away toxins and to keep the respiratory tract from drying out.

Increase your consumption of ginger, onions, and garlic. Try adding one or all to chicken soup or miso.

Regular water intake is important to prevent dehydration. Herbal teas and highly diluted fruit juices can also be given. Fruit-juice popsicles are popular with kids.

Breast-feeding should be maintained for nursing infants.

Food to Avoid

Sugar decreases the number of white blood cells your body produces, and it depresses your immune system, so eliminate refined sugars from your diet for the duration of your illness. Also be wary of fruit juices. Although they are a traditional treatment for colds, fruit juices—especially orange juice—usually contain far more sugar than they do vitamin C. If you want to drink juice, dilute it first.

Avoid milk and other dairy products while you're sick, as they tend to suppress immunity.

℞ Super Seven Prescriptions—Fever

Super Prescription #1 Homeopathic Combination Fever Remedy
To reduce the effects of a fever, take a combination fever remedy four times daily for two days. Then if you notice improvement, stop taking the remedy, unless symptoms return. If your symptoms do not improve within twenty-four hours, pick the remedy that best matches your symptoms under Homeopathy in this section.

Super Prescription #2 Yarrow (*Achillea millefolium*)

Take 300 mg in capsule form, 2 ml of the tincture, or 1 cup of fresh tea four times daily or until the fever breaks. Yarrow induces a sweat to help break high fevers.

Super Prescription #3 Homeopathic Ferrum Phosphoricum

Take a 30C potency four times daily for two days. Then if you notice improvement, stop taking the remedy, unless symptoms return. If your symptoms do not improve within twenty-four hours, pick the remedy that best matches your symptoms under Homeopathy in this section.

Super Prescription #4 Echinacea (*Echinacea purpurea*)

Take 500 mg of the capsule form or 2 to 4 ml of the tincture four times daily. Echinacea stimulates immune function and reduces fever.

Super Prescription #5 Ginger (*Zingiber officinale*)

Take 500 mg of the capsule form or 2 ml of the tincture or drink the fresh tea four times daily. Ginger helps break a fever, especially for people who have a sore throat and chills.

Super Prescription #6 Elderberry (*Sambucus nigra*)

Adults should take 10 ml and children 5 ml three times daily. It's useful for fever related to the flu or other viral infections.

Super Prescription #7 Vitamin C

Take 500 to 1,000 mg three to four times daily. Vitamin C supports immune-system function through increased white blood cell activity. Reduce the dosage if diarrhea occurs.

General Recommendations

Oregano (*Origanum vulgare*) oil has powerful antiviral effects. Take 500 mg of the capsule form four times daily or as directed on the container.

Garlic (*Allium sativum*) combats infection and supports the immune system. Take 300 to 500 mg in capsule or liquid form three times daily.

Thyme extract (*Thymus vulgaris*) optimizes immune activity. Take 1 or 2 capsules twice daily or as directed on the container.

Homeopathy

At the first signs of a fever, take 2 pellets of a 30C potency four times daily for two days of the remedy that best matches your symptoms in this section. Then if you notice improvement, stop taking the remedy, unless symptoms return. If your symptoms do not improve within twenty-four hours, pick another remedy.

Aconitum Napellus is useful at the very beginning of a fever, when there is a sudden onset. This often occurs after a person has been exposed to the cold or the wind. The person is restless and fearful, and children cry with the onset of the fever. This remedy is most useful in the first few hours of a sudden fever. One cheek may be red and the other pale during a fever

Arsenicum Album is for a fever that occurs or increases between midnight and 2

A.M. The person is chilly, along with having a burning fever. Anxiety and restlessness are usually present. The symptoms are better with sips of warm water.

Belladonna (*Atropa belladonna*) is for a sudden, intense fever. The body feels very hot (especially the face), but the feet are cold. The pupils may be dilated, and the cheeks and the face are often bright red. The person is sensitive to light and has a throbbing headache. Some people may become delirious and hallucinate from the fever.

Bryonia (*Bryonia alba*) is for people who have a high fever with a tremendous thirst. They are very irritable and do not want to move.

Chamomilla (*Matricaria chamomilla*) is specific for a fever that accompanies teething. One cheek is red, while the other is pale. The child is very irritable.

Ferrum Phosphoricum is used as a general fever remedy. The person has a fever but does not act sick. The face is red and the body warm.

Gelsemium (*Gelsemium sempervirens*) is for a fever accompanied by chills and muscle aches. The person feels drowsy and fatigued and has droopy eyelids. There is often a headache at the back of the neck.

Mercurius Solubilis or Vivus is helpful when a person has a fever and is sensitive to both hot and cold temperatures. The tongue has a thick coating, and the person has bad breath, has excessive saliva production, and drools on the pillow. The throat is often raw and sore.

Pulsatilla (*Pulsatilla pratensis*) is for someone who has a fever with a low thirst. A feverish child wants to be held and is very clingy. Symptoms are better with the window open or when the person is out in the open air.

Pyrogenium is used when there is a high fever, and the person appears very sick. His or her body aches and feels bruised. The person has a high fever but a slow pulse.

Sulfur is for acute or long-lasting fevers when the whole body is warm. A body rash may accompany the fever. There is a tremendous thirst for cold drinks.

Acupressure

Large Intestine 4 (LI4) is located between the webbing of the thumb and the index finger. Gently push on this spot on both hands to reduce fever.

Bodywork

Hydrotherapy

Constitutional or foot hydrotherapy works very well in helping to control fevers and fight infections. See the Hydrotherapy section for directions.

Fibrocystic Breasts

Though commonly referred to as fibrocystic breast disease, this condition is not really a disease at all; it merely refers to noncancerous lumps or cysts of the breasts that may or may not be painful. It is one of the most common reasons that women consult a gynecologist. Half of all women will experience these lumps in their lifetimes. The most common ages for this condition are the twenties to the fifties. For many women, symptoms of breast tenderness or swelling are noticed prior to menstruation, indicating a hormonal cause. Other women experience these symptoms unrelated to their cycles. It is important for women to regularly monitor their own breast tissue and note changes over time. Although not diagnostic in and of itself, monitoring certainly provides valuable information to their physicians.

SYMPTOMS

- Breast lumps, nodules, or cysts that usually occur in both breasts
- Breast tenderness or pain
- Fluctuating size of breast lumps
- Cyclical increase in breast pain, lumps, or nodules in the two weeks before menstrual flow

ROOT CAUSES

- Hormonal imbalance, particularly estrogen dominance, in which the estrogen level is relatively too high compared to the progesterone level
- Low thyroid hormone
- Poor function of the liver, which metabolizes hormones and plays a role in hormone balance
- Constipation, possibly due to reabsorption of hormones in the colon
- Poor diet, particularly one deficient in fruits and vegetables, and excessive in caffeine and omega-6 fatty acids
- Deficiencies in nutrients such as iodine, omega-3 fatty acids, and vitamin E

Testing Techniques

The following tests help assess possible reasons for fibrocystic breasts:

Hormone testing (thyroid, estrogen, progesterone, prolactin, DHEA, testosterone)—saliva, blood, or urine

Vitamin and mineral analysis (especially calcium, magnesium, vitamin B6, vitamin E, essential fatty acids, iodine)

Liver function—blood

Food sensitivities—blood, electrodermal, stool

Urinary Iodine test

TREATMENT

Diet

Recommended Food

A high-fiber diet is recommended because it promotes the elimination of excess estrogen. This includes the use of ground flaxseed (1 to 2 tablespoons daily with 8 to 12 ounces of clean, quality water per tablespoon). A diet focused on plant foods is most effective, including whole grains, legumes, vegetables, fruits, nuts, seeds, olives, and seaweed. Essential fatty acid balance is important. Cold-water fish, such as salmon or sardines, is recommended twice weekly for inflammation-reducing omega-3 fatty acids. Olive oil is also recommended on salads. Fermented soy foods (tofu, natto, miso, tempeh) have been shown to have a hormone-balancing effect on the breasts. Consume two or more servings weekly.

A one- to two-week detoxification program can be helpful to cleanse the colon and the liver. Also, a three-day vegetable juice fast once a month can be beneficial. You can supplement your fast with plenty of green drinks and cleansing herbal teas.

Food to Avoid

It is important to avoid caffeine (coffee, soda, and chocolate), because some studies, though not all, show such avoidance to be helpful. We find that it makes some difference for most women with this condition.

℞ Super Seven Prescriptions—Fibrocystic Breasts

Super Prescription #1 Natural progesterone cream
Apply ¼ teaspoon (20 mg) to breasts and inner wrists one or two times daily from ovulation until start of menses.

Super Prescription #2 Vitex (chasteberry)
Take 160 to 240 mg or 40 drops of the tincture every day of the month for at least three months. This herb works to balance a woman's progesterone and prolactin levels. Do not use if you are taking birth-control pills.

Super Prescription #3 Vitamin E complex
Some studies show that this vitamin reduces breast tenderness. Part of this benefit may come as a result of its role in estrogen metabolism. Take 800 to 1,200 IU daily for at least two months to see if it is helpful.

Super Prescription #4 Gamma linolenic acid (GLA)
Take 200 to 400 mg daily of GLA. It is available by itself or as part of evening primrose oil, borage oil, or black currant oil.

Super Prescription #5 Iodine
Take 500 mcg daily. Higher dosages and topical application can be effective, too. Consult a holistic doctor.

Super Prescription #6 Indole-3-carbinol (I3C) or Diindolylmethane (DIM)
Take 300 mg of I3C or 200 mg of DIM. These substances are extracts from cruciferous vegetables that support detoxification of excess estrogen in the body.

Super Prescription #7 Dandelion root
Take 300 mg or 30 drops of tincture three times daily with meals for two months. This improves the liver's detoxification of excess estrogen.

A German study of 104 women who suffered from premenstrual breast pain found that vitex extract significantly reduced breast pain.

A review of three studies published in the *Canadian Journal of Surgery* found that iodine supplementation was helpful in allaying the symptoms of fibrocystic breasts in 65 to 74 percent of the participants.

General Recommendations

Probiotics provide friendly flora involved in estrogen metabolism and excretion in the colon. Take as directed on the label.

Phytolacca oil has been used topically by naturopathic physicians and herbalists for breast cysts. Milk thistle promotes liver detoxification. Take 200 mg of an 85 percent silymarin extract three times daily for at least two months.

A multivitamin and multimineral formula provides the nutrients required for hormone detoxification. Take as directed on the label.

Take 200 mg of fish oil daily, combined EPA and DHA, for its natural anti-inflammatory effect on the breasts.

Homeopathy

Calcarea Carbonica is for women with tender breasts associated with menses. These women tend to be overweight, fatigued, and chilly, and they crave dairy products.

Phytolacca Deandra (poke root) is for breast tenderness with obvious glandular swelling, especially of the outer portion of the breast near armpit. Breast tenderness occurs right before and after menses.

Pulsatilla is for aching breasts before menses. These women experience weepiness, irritability, and mood swings with PMS as well as a craving for sweets and a desire for fresh air.

Sepia is for women with fibrocystic breasts that get worse before or with menses. These women become irritable with PMS and have strong cravings for chocolate and sweets.

Acupressure

Rub Stomach 16 (St16) to relieve breast pain.

Bodywork
Reflexology

See pages 804–805 and work the areas that correspond to the lungs, the liver, the ovaries, and the pituitary glands.

Hydrotherapy

Constitutional hydrotherapy can be used short-term and long-term to alleviate symptoms. It also promotes bowel elimination, which is important because constipation is one of the underlying problems in this condition.

Aromatherapy

The essential oil ledum supports liver health and cleansing, which is important for helping this condition. Clary sage oil is important for hormone balancing.

Other Recommendations

Fibrocystic breasts are a symptom of an underlying hormone imbalance. Utilize natural therapies that balance hormone stimulation of the breast tissue. Have your doctor rule out breast conditions other than fibrocystic breasts.

REFERENCES

Ghent, W. R., et al. 1993. Iodine replacement in fibrocystic disease of the breast. *Canadian Journal of Surgery* 36:453–60.

Gayle, a forty-two-year-old nurse, had suffered from severely painful fibrocystic breasts for several days before her menses. Despite diet improvements and supplementation, her symptoms persisted. The use of progesterone cream improved her symptoms by 50 percent in her first cycle. By her third cycle, she noted 90 percent improvement.

Wuttke, W., et al. 1997. Treatment of cyclical mastalgia with a medication containing Agnus castus: Results of a randomized, placebo-controlled, double-blind study. *Geburtshilfe und Frauenheilkunde* 57:569–74.

Fibroids, Uterine

Contrary to their name, fibroids are not fibrous at all. Rather, they are growths of smooth muscle and connective tissue that most often appear on the walls of the uterus. Although it can be frightening to hear that you have a growth of any kind, rest assured that fibroids are noncancerous and usually harmless. They are also quite common: fibroids affect more than 50 percent of women overall and are the most common reason for major surgery. For reasons that we don't yet understand, they appear much more often in women of African or Caribbean descent than in any other group. Most women with the condition tend to have several fibroids at once.

Many women who have fibroids experience no symptoms at all; the growths are usually discovered in the course of a routine exam or an ultrasound. In some cases, however, fibroids inside the uterus wear away the organ's lining, resulting in heavy or prolonged menstrual periods, bleeding between periods, or pain and bleeding during sexual intercourse. Persistent blood loss can cause anemia. A fibroid may also grow so large that it distends the abdomen as it presses on the bladder or the intestines. A woman with a large fibroid may feel pain in her back or lower abdomen; if the growth distorts the bladder, she may feel a frequent urge to urinate. Sometimes the fibroid doesn't cause any pain but simply gives the abdomen a distended appearance. Women may also feel pressure, heaviness, and pain with sexual intercourse, as well as increased urinary frequency. Occasionally, a fibroid will block the fallopian tubes and lead to infertility or compress the ureters (the urinary tract from the kidneys to the bladder), causing impaired kidney function. In some instances the fibroids become calcified.

Fibroids are thought to be dependent upon estrogen; they tend to grow during the reproductive years and pregnancy, and they shrink with menopause, when estrogen levels recede. Fibroids often increase in size during perimenopause, when women do not ovulate regularly and thus have relatively higher estrogen levels (as ovulation increases progesterone). Thus, hormone balance is the key factor with this condition.

Although estrogen is obviously an important factor in the development of fibroids, doctors do not know why the growths appear in some women and not in others. A tendency toward fibroids may run in families; the disorder is also more common in women who are obese or who have an underactive thyroid (which contributes to estrogen excess).

It is important that liver function be optimized in women with fibroids. The liver is responsible for breaking down estrogen (and other hormones) and secreting the metabolites into the large intestine for elimination. If the liver does not metabolize estrogen and its metabolites properly, then they are recycled throughout the body.

While the liver is the dominant player in estrogen metabolism, the flora or "friendly bacteria" in the large intestine are also important in estrogen metabolism. They prevent the reactivation and recycling of these unwanted estrogens. Conversely, "unfriendly bacteria" secrete an enzyme called beta-glucuronidase that causes estrogen to be recycled back through the body via the large intestine. A low-fiber and high-fat intake increases the activity of this enzyme.

Conventional medical treatment for fibroids has long been surgical removal of the uterus, a drastic option that should be considered only in those few cases in which fibroids cause severe pain or bleeding or pose a significant health threat. For mild to moderate cases, it is usually far wiser to follow a treatment program of conservative, noninvasive therapies until menopause is reached and the fibroids abate on their own.

SYMPTOMS

In most women with fibroids, the condition is asymptomatic, especially in the early stages when the fibroids are small. If symptoms do appear, they usually take the following forms:

- Heavy or prolonged menstrual bleeding
- Bleeding or unusual discharge
- Back or abdominal pain
- Pain and bleeding during intercourse
- Anemia
- Swelling in the lower abdomen
- A frequent urge to urinate between periods
- Constipation

ROOT CAUSES

- Relatively high levels of estrogen and low levels of progesterone, due to:
  —Environmental estrogens
  —Obesity
  —Underactive thyroid
  —Ovulatory dysfunction

  —Perimenopause
  —Low-fiber, high-fat diet
  —Iodine deficiency

Caution: If you bleed so much that you need to change tampons or sanitary pads more than once every hour, see your doctor.

Testing Techniques

The following tests help assess possible reasons for fibroids:

Hormone testing (especially for estrogen, thyroid, and progesterone)—saliva, blood, or urine

Detoxification profile—urine

Digestive function (particularly flora balance and beta-glucuronidase activity)—stool analysis

---

TREATMENT

Diet

It is important to eat certified organic foods as much as possible due to the estrogenic effects of pesticides, herbicides, and hormone-laden meats.

Recommended Food

Since diet affects hormone balance, it's wise to give your body good general support with wholesome, freshly prepared meals. Base your diet around whole grains, vegetables, fruits, fish, beans, and soy products. To limit your exposure to pesticides, buy organic food whenever possible, and always wash your produce thoroughly.

Soy products and flaxseeds are good sources of phytoestrogens, substances that regulate the body's estrogen production.

Vitamin K will encourage proper blood clotting and may reduce an excessive flow of menstrual blood. Green vegetables are high in this nutrient.

Include sea vegetables like kelp (*Ascophyllum nodosum*) in your diet. These foods are high in iodine, a mineral that's necessary for a healthy thyroid.

If you have heavy or prolonged periods, you need extra iron to ward off anemia. Take a spoonful of unsulfured blackstrap molasses every day. For more suggestions, see Anemia.

For additional EFAs, add 2 tablespoons of flaxseeds to your daily protocol, along with 10 ounces of clean, quality water. Flaxseeds have been shown to help balance estrogen levels.

Eat fruits and vegetables such as apples, cherries, broccoli, cauliflower, and brussels sprouts. They contain the phytochemical indole-3-carbinol, which supports the liver's detoxification of estrogen.

Regularly consume beets, carrots, artichokes, dandelion greens, onions, and garlic, as these foods stimulate liver detoxification.

Eat organic cultured yogurt to increase the levels of friendly flora in the large intestine.

Once a day, have a green drink to support detoxification.

Drink a glass of clean, quality water every two waking hours. Water will help flush impurities from your body and reduce pain.

Food to Avoid

Avoid red meat and dairy products that are not organic.

To keep pain under control, stay away from inflammatory substances like sugar, caffeine, and alcohol.

℞ Super Seven Prescriptions—Uterine Fibroids

Super Prescription #1 Natural progesterone
This balances estrogen, regulates the menses, and relieves pain. Apply ¼ teaspoon (20 mg) to your skin twice daily from days six to twenty-six of your cycle (stopping during the week of your menstrual flow). It is best used under the guidance of a health care professional.

Super Prescription #2 Vitex (chasteberry)
This balances the estrogen/progesterone ratio. Take 160 to 240 mg of a 0.6 percent aucubin standardized extract or 80 drops daily. Do not use vitex if you are currently taking a birth-control pill.

Super Prescription #3 Indole-3-carbinol
Take 300 mg daily. It assists the liver in estrogen detoxification.

Super Prescription #4 Dandelion root (*Taraxacum officinale*)

Take 300 to 500 mg of the capsule form or 1 ml of the tincture with each meal (three times daily). It improves liver detoxification.

Super Prescription #5 Vitamin E

Take 400 IU twice daily. It helps with estrogen metabolism and inflammation.

Super Prescription #6 Essential fatty acids

Take a daily combination of flaxseed (1 to 2 tablespoons) or fish oil (3,000 to 5,000 mg), along with gamma linoleic acid (GLA) from evening primrose oil or borage oil at a dose of 300 mg. These essential fatty acids decrease inflammation.

Super Prescription #7 D-glucarate

Take 500 mg daily. This phytochemical assists the liver in estrogen breakdown.

General Recommendations

- Iodine blocks excess estrogen stimulation of receptors. Take 500 mcg or more daily.
- B-complex vitamins are involved in estrogen metabolism. Take a 50 mg complex twice daily.
- A high-potency multivitamin supplies many of the nutrients required for hormone metabolism. Take as directed on the container.
- Red raspberry (*Rubus idaeus*) is an astringent herb that may help uterine inflammation and pain. Drink it as a tea, three cups daily.
- If you have heavy menstrual bleeding, take nettle, a blood-building herb, to prevent anemia. Begin using the herb after the last day of your menstrual cycle, and take 500 mg two or three times daily for two weeks.

Homeopathy

Pick the remedy that best matches your symptoms in this section. Take a 6x, 12x, 6C, 12C, or 30C potency twice daily for three weeks to see if there are any positive results. After you notice improvement, stop taking the remedy, unless symptoms return. Consultation with a homeopathic practitioner is advised.

Calcarea Carbonica is for overweight women who get chilly and fatigued easily. They crave sweets and eggs. They have a tendency to get overwhelmed easily and struggle with anxiety. It is used for uterine fibroids that are sometimes characterized by uterine hemorrhage.

Fraxinus Americanus is a specific lesional remedy for uterine fibroids.

Lachesis is for women who experience surges of heat and aggravation from heat. They experience abdominal and uterine pain that improves once menstrual flow begins. They feel anger and suspiciousness.

Phosphorus is for women who have heavy bleeding from fibroids, characterized by bright red blood and clotting. They crave ice-cold drinks.

Pulsatilla is a good choice when there is fibroid pain and menstrual flow that changes. These women feel better having someone around, comforting them. There is a craving for sweets. Symptoms are worse in a warm room and better in the fresh air.

Sabina is for fibroids that cause pain in the lower back and sacrum that extends to the pubic bones. There is heavy uterine bleeding, with clots.

Sepia is for women with fibroids when their uterus feels like it is bearing down and will fall out. They feel irritable and want to be left alone. There is a strong craving for sweets and salty and sour foods.

Sulfur is for fibroids in women who get overheated easily. They desire a cool environment. There is a strong craving for ice-cold drinks.

Acupressure

See pages 787–794 for information about pressure points and administering treatment.
- To stop fibroid pain, work Large Intestine 4 (LI4).

Bodywork

Acupuncture is highly recommended to help reduce the bleeding associated with fibroids. In addition, Chinese herbal therapy from a qualified practitioner can be very helpful.

Reflexology

See pages 804–805 for information about reflexology areas and how to work them.

- Work the areas that correspond to the uterus, the fallopian tubes, and the ovaries.

Hydrotherapy

Regular sitz baths in hot water will improve circulation to the pelvic region and will soothe pain in the abdomen and the lower back. Constitutional hydrotherapy is helpful to reduce congestion in the area containing the fibroid. See pages 795–796 for directions.

Aromatherapy

Warming oils like rosemary, marjoram, and black pepper increase blood flow and relieve pain. If you're constipated, black pepper will also stimulate digestion. You can use these oils separately or in combination. Add a few drops to a sitz bath, or use them in a hot compress.

Stress Reduction

General Stress-Reduction Therapies

For overall hormone balance, utilize techniques such as exercise, yoga, and prayer.

Other Recommendations

- If you have fibroids, you should not take estrogen-replacement therapy.
- Moderate exercise like walking will stimulate blood flow to the pelvic region and will help relieve pain.

Fibromyalgia

Fibromyalgia is the name given to chronic, widespread muscular pain that has no obvious cause. This condition affects over five million Americans. The pain—usually described as aching, stiff, burning, or throbbing—may appear in any location of the body, but for a diagnosis of fibromyalgia to be made, you must have pain in at least eleven of eighteen specific "tender points." The pain from tender points and elsewhere in the body usually feels most severe upon waking and gradually lessens as the day goes on.

Although the pain of fibromyalgia alone can be so severe as to render its victims disabled, the disease can be complicated by any of several other problems. Fibromyalgia is closely linked to chronic fatigue syndrome, and many of its sufferers experience symptoms similar to those of CFS (see the symptom list further on). Irritable bowel syndrome, premenstrual syndrome, palpitations, and temporomandibular joint syndrome (TMJ) may also be present.

As with CFS, there is currently no one agreed-upon cause of this disease. In most cases, many factors combine to produce the varied components of fibromyalgia. Disordered sleep is a very common problem with this condition. The length and the quality of sleep must be improved for long-term success in most cases of fibromyalgia. Also, hormone imbalance is quite common, particularly low thyroid function, imbalances in estrogen/progesterone, and imbalances in the stress hormones DHEA and cortisol. Digestive function and detoxification usually need improvement to help people with fibromyalgia. Along with digestive weakness come leaky gut syndrome and candida overgrowth, as well as general dysbiosis. Chronic infections that include viruses can be a factor. Food allergies are a significant contributor for some people, especially allergies to wheat, sugar, and cow's milk. Nutritional deficiencies, of magnesium, B vitamins, coenzyme Q10, L-carnitine, and several others, are very common. We have also found that many people with fibromyalgia have a brain-chemistry imbalance. Using natural therapies to balance serotonin and other neurotransmitters results not only in a better mood but in less muscular pain. Toxic elements, such as lead, mercury, arsenic, and others, can also be among the root contributors to fibromyalgia. These toxic elements interfere with normal enzyme and cell function in the body. In addition, blood sugar imbalances worsen pain and inflammation. Many people develop symptoms of fibromyalgia after a car accident, and thus structural abnormalities must be addressed through physical therapies. Chiropractic,

The tender points for fibromyalgia exist in pairs (one on the right side of your body and one on the left) at the following locations:

- Base of the skull
- Base of the neck
- Upper chest, a little more than an inch below the collarbone
- Along the top of the shoulder
- Upper back, close to the spine and about an inch below the preceding set of points
- Inside of the elbows
- Lower back, close to the dimples above the buttocks
- Upper outside edge of the thigh
- Inside of the knees

If you are testing yourself for a reaction to these points, you must touch them with enough pressure to whiten your fingernail. A doctor who is knowledgeable in the diagnosis of this condition can test these points for you.

osteopathic, and craniosacral therapy; physiotherapy; and sometimes massage are very helpful in reducing pain.

Fibromyalgia occurs with other rheumatic conditions about 25 to 65 percent of the time, including rheumatoid arthritis (RA), systemic lupus erythematosus (SLE), and ankylosing spondylitis (AS). In essence, all these potential imbalances lead to a defect in how the cells produce energy. Normally, the "energy-producing plant" of the cells, known as the mitochondria, produces energy efficiently. When a defect occurs in mitochondrial metabolism, it can lead to a shortage of energy for the muscle cells and other tissues of the body, resulting in fatigue and pain. Mitochondria require organic acids to act as intermediaries in the energy-creating metabolic pathways in the body. Researchers have found that people with fibromyalgia often have imbalances in these organic acids. To correct this problem, one must address the root causes, listed below. Fortunately, a comprehensive natural approach to fibromyalgia is very effective in eliminating the pain or greatly improving it.

SYMPTOMS

For a diagnosis of fibromyalgia to be made, two factors must be present:

- Unexplained, widespread pain that lasts at least three months
- Pain in at least eleven of the eighteen tender points when gentle pressure is applied

Many other symptoms may exist alongside the pain, including the following:

- Fatigue
- Sleep disturbances
- Irritable bowel syndrome
- Anxiety
- Depression
- Difficulty concentrating
- Memory problems
- Dizziness
- Tingling of the hands or feet
- Premenstrual syndrome (PMS)
- Temporomandibular joint syndrome (TMJ)
- Heart palpitations
- Heightened sensitivity to loud noises, bright lights, and changes in the weather
- Headaches
- Morning stiffness

ROOT CAUSES

- Sleep disorder (including apnea)
- Allergies or sensitivities to certain chemicals, food, or the environment
- Chemical imbalance in the brain, especially of serotonin
- Virus (especially Epstein-Barr, HHV-6, cytomegalovirus)
- Hormone imbalance
- Damage to cells by free radicals (oxidative stress)
- Poor digestion and detoxification
- Toxic metals
- Poor methylation

Testing Techniques

The following tests help assess possible reasons for fibromyalgia:

Chronic infection (human herpes virus type 6 [HHV-6], cytomegalovirus [CMV], Epstein-Barr virus [EBV]—blood

Blood pressure—blood pressure cuff

Hormone testing (thyroid, DHEA, cortisol, testosterone, IGF-1, estrogen, progesterone)—saliva, blood, or urine

Intestinal permeability—urine

Vitamin and mineral analysis (especially for magnesium, B1, B12, iron, and CoQ10)—blood

Digestive function and microbe/parasite/candida testing—stool analysis

Food and environmental allergies/sensitivities—blood, electrodermal

Blood-sugar balance—blood

Toxic elements (such as mercury, arsenic, etc.)—urine, hair

Cellular energy (organic acids)—blood or urine

Amino acids—blood or urine

Detoxification profile—blood or urine

Blood thickness—fibrinogen

MTHFR gene mutation—blood or saliva

TREATMENT

Diet

Recommended Food

Follow a sound diet that is based on whole, unprocessed foods. Emphasize raw or lightly cooked vegetables, especially greens, and other foods that are high in nutrients and fiber.

To keep up a steady supply of energy to your muscles, eat lots of lean protein—beans, raw nuts, soy products, fish, chicken, and turkey are all good sources—and plan on several meals throughout the day, instead of three large ones.

Eat some live, unsweetened yogurt or other cultured food daily to combat candidiasis.

Omega-3 fatty acids help the body create prostaglandin, a hormone that reduces inflammation. Flaxseeds and flaxseed oil, as well as fatty fish, are excellent sources of omega-3 fatty acids.

Fibromyalgia has been linked to a magnesium deficiency, so make sure to consume foods that are high in this mineral, including green leafy vegetables, kelp, soybeans, cashews, and almonds.

Vitamins A, C, and E together help fight free radicals, whose presence may inhibit cells' ability to produce energy. For vitamin A, eat plenty of colored vegetables (especially the green, leafy ones) and skim milk. Good sources of vitamin E are soybeans, broccoli, brussels sprouts, whole grains, and, again, green leafy vegetables.

Drink a glass of clean, quality water every two waking hours. You'll flush out toxins and reduce pain.

Food to Avoid

Determine whether a food allergy is causing or contributing to your pain. Read the Food Allergies section and follow the elimination diet there, or have a nutrition-oriented doctor test your food sensitivities or allergies.

Mineral deficiencies have been linked to fibromyalgia, so avoid caffeine, which interferes with their proper absorption. Caffeine also contributes to sleep disturbances.

Reduce or cut out meat, fried and junk foods, high-fat dairy products, and other foods that are high in saturated fats. They contribute to inflammation and pain, as well as to insomnia; in addition, they slow your circulation and deplete your stores of energy.

Avoid sugar. It increases pain, weakens the immune system, disturbs sleep, saps your energy, and encourages the growth of *Candida albicans*, a fungus that some believe is a cause of fibromyalgia. The most common sources of sugar are sodas and processed food, but you also need to severely restrict your intake of natural sugars, including honey and even fruits.

Dramatically reduce your intake of processed food and carbonated drinks. These items are full of food additives that will only aggravate your condition.

℞ Super Seven Prescriptions—Fibromyalgia

Super Prescription #1 D-ribose
Take 5 grams three times daily. It alleviates the symptoms of fibromyalgia, probably by improving cellular energy.

Super Prescription #2 Magnesium
Take 250 mg two or three times daily. Magnesium glycinate and magnesium aspartate are the preferred forms. Magnesium is important for cellular-energy production and relaxes the nerves and the muscles.

Super Prescription #3 Methylsulfonylmethane (MSM)
Take up to 10,000 mg daily in divided doses. Start with 1,000 mg three times daily, and increase the dosage until pain relief is evident. Reduce the dosage if diarrhea occurs.

Super Prescription #4 S-adenosylmethionine (SAMe)
Take 400 mg twice daily. SAMe is a naturally occurring nutrient that improves the balance of neurotransmitters such as serotonin; improves detoxification; and helps with cartilage formation.

Super Prescription #5 5-hydroxytryptophan (5-HTP)
Take 50 to 100 mg three times daily. This amino acid is a precursor used by the brain to manufacture the neurotransmitter serotonin, which reduces pain, improves sleep, and improves mood.

Super Prescription #6 Coenzyme Q10
Take 200 to 300 mg daily to improve cellular energy and help with fibromyalgia pain and fatigue.

A study of forty-one people with fibromyalgia and/or chronic fatigue syndrome who were given 5 grams of D-ribose three times daily showed a significant improvement in energy, sleep, mental clarity, pain intensity, and well-being.

A double-blind trial involving 800 mg of SAMe (S-adenosylmethionine) per day for six weeks found significant benefit for people with fibromyalgia in regard to pain, fatigue, stiffness, and mood. SAMe has been shown in numerous studies to also be effective for depression and osteoarthritis.

A double-blind, placebo-controlled study of fifty people with fibromyalgia looked at the effect of 100 mg of 5-HTP, taken three times daily for thirty days. In people supplementing with 5-HTP, significant improvement was found in their pain severity, morning stiffness, sleep patterns, anxiety, and fatigue.

> **Super Prescription #7 Malic acid**
> Take 1,000 to 1,200 mg twice daily. Malic acid is important for cellular-energy production.

General Recommendations

A high-potency multivitamin provides a base of nutrients required for cellular energy production. Take as directed on the container.

Nattokinase helps improve circulation, which is often a problem with fibromyalgia. Take 2,000 to 5,000 CFU (fibrinolytic units) daily on an empty stomach. Do not use if you are on a blood-thinning medication.

Acetyl-L-carnitine supports cellular energy production. Take 500 to 1,000 mg daily.

Calcium relaxes the nerves and the muscles. Take 500 mg twice daily, along with 400 IU of vitamin D.

Brown seaweed extract can help with fibromyalgia. Take as directed on the label.

Milk thistle (*Silybum marianum*) supports liver detoxification. Take 250 mg of a 80 to 85 percent silymarin extract three times daily.

Vitamin E has anti-inflammatory benefits. Take 800 IU daily.

Vitamin C has anti-inflammatory and immune-enhancing benefits. Take 1,000 mg two or three times daily.

Grapeseed extract or maritime pine bark improves circulation and has anti-inflammatory effects. Take 100 mg two or three times daily.

Alpha lipoic acid is an antioxidant that supports detoxification. Take 100 to 200 mg daily.

N-acetylcysteine supports detoxification and helps produce glutathione. Take 500 mg daily.

NADH supports cellular energy production. Take 10 to 20 mg on an empty stomach.

Passionflower (*Passiflora incarnata*) relaxes the nerves. Take 300 to 500 mg in capsule form or 1 ml of tincture three times daily. It can also be taken before bedtime to help with sleep.

Valerian (*Valeriana officinalis*) relaxes the nerves. Take 300 to 500 mg in capsule form or 1 ml of tincture three times daily. It can also be taken before bedtime to help with sleep.

Olive leaf extract (*Olea europa*) is good if you have a chronic viral infection. Take 500 mg three times daily.

A probiotic is important for digestive function and immunity. Take a product containing at least four billion active organisms daily.

Thyroid controls cellular energy and mood. If your levels are low, work with a knowledgeable doctor to use natural thyroid hormone (such as Armour or compounded T4/T3 or T3).

DHEA reduces stress and inflammation. If your levels are low, work with a doctor to normalize your levels. The normal starting dosage is 5 to 15 mg daily.

Natural progesterone can be helpful for women with fibromyalgia. Premenopausal women should apply ¼ teaspoon (20 mg equivalent) to the inside of their forearms one or two times daily on days fourteen to twenty-eight of their cycle. Menopausal women should apply ¼ teaspoon (20 mg equivalent) to the inside of their forearms twice daily for three to four weeks of the month. Postmenopausal women should apply ⅛ teaspoon (10 mg equivalent) to the inside of their forearms once daily for three weeks of the month.

Estrogen, cortisol, and testosterone need to be prescribed, based on your levels, by a doctor who is knowledgeable in natural hormone replacement.

Ginkgo biloba improves circulation and memory. Take 60 to 120 mg of a 24 percent flavone glycoside extract three times daily.

Fish oil supplies pain-relieving omega-3 fatty acids. Take a fish oil product containing at least 480 mg of EPA and 360 mg of DHA twice daily.

Flaxseed oil supplies pain-relieving omega-3 fatty acids. Take 1 to 2 tablespoons daily.

Evening primrose (*Oenothera biennis*) oil contains gamma linoleic acid (GLA), which decreases inflammation and pain. Take 2,000 mg daily.

A greens drink containing super green foods, such as chlorella, spirulina, barley grass, and others, supports detoxification and energy production. Take as directed on the container.

Melatonin promotes sleep. Take 0.3 to 0.5 mg a half hour before bedtime.

Black cohosh (*Cimicifuga racemosa*) is a good hormone balancer and relaxes spasms of the muscles. Take 40 mg of a 2.5 percent triterpene glycoside extract twice daily.

Cordyceps sinensis supports adrenal gland function. Take 800 mg twice daily of a standardized product.

Arnica (*Arnica montana*) oil relieves muscle pain and tenderness. Apply the oil to painful areas twice daily.

Homeopathy

Pick the remedy that best matches your symptoms in this section. Take a 6x, 12x, 6C, or 30C potency twice daily for two weeks to see if there are any positive results. After you notice improvement, stop taking the remedy, unless symptoms return. Consultation with a homeopathic practitioner is advised.

Arnica (*Arnica montana*) is the top choice for pain that feels deep and bruised and for allover tenderness. Symptoms are worse after exertion.

Bryonia (*Bryonia alba*) is for pain that is aggravated by the slightest movement. Muscles feel better with cool applications and pressure and feel worse with warmth. The person is irritable and does not want to be touched.

Calcarea Carbonica is for people who get muscle soreness from exertion and cold, damp climates. They are usually chilly, with clammy hands and feet. There is a craving for sweets and eggs. There are often symptoms of anxiety and a feeling of being overwhelmed and easily fatigued.

Causticum is helpful when the muscles and the joints become stiff and sore from overuse and from the cold or dry weather. Symptoms are improved with warm applications. The muscles and the joints feel contracted.

Cimicifuga is for muscles that feel sore and bruised and worse in the cold. The back of the neck is sore and stiff. The person is prone to depression and hormone imbalance.

Ignatia (*Ignatia amara*) is for tight, spasmodic, or cramping muscles and fibromyalgia that comes on from stress or emotional upset.

In one study patients with chronic fatigue syndrome and fibromyalgia had their MTFHR status tested. All of them were found to have some degree of abnormality. In addition, participants who received a naturopathic therapy of intravenous B-complex vitamins (including the active form of folate—methylfolate) had a 55 to 75 percent increase in positive outcomes.

Carol, a fifty-five-year-old nurse, had been unable to work full-time for three years because of her fibromyalgia. Besides having the classic trigger points and fatigue, she also had been struggling with depression for years. After eight weeks of improving her diet and supplementing it with ribose, magnesium, MSM, and 5-HTP, she felt the best she had felt in years. After four months of treatment, she was able to go back to work full-time.

Magnesia Phosphorica is for cramping or spasming muscles that feel better with warm applications.

Nux Vomica (*Strychnos nux vomica*) is for tight muscles that spasm. The person is chilly, and the symptoms are worse in cold weather and better with warm applications. Digestive problems, such as stomachache or heartburn, are often present. The person is irritable and fatigued.

Pulsatilla (*Pulsatilla pratensis*) is helpful if your pain moves from joint to joint, and if you feel tearful and depressed. Fibromyalgia is often connected to the menstrual cycle or hormone imbalance.

Rhus Toxicodendron is for pain and stiffness that's worse in the early morning or after resting and during cold, rainy weather. Symptoms ease with continued movement and warm applications. The person feels restless.

Acupressure

See pages 787–794 for information about pressure points and administering treatment.

- Conception Vessel 17 (CV17) supports the immune system and also eases depression and anxiety.
- Stomach 36 (St36) improves the body's ability to absorb nutrients. It will also lend general support to the digestive system, a helpful quality if you have irritable bowel syndrome.
- To relax cramped muscles and soothe your nerves, use Liver 3 (Lv3).
- Pericardium 6 (P6) relieves anxiety, indigestion, and heart palpitations.
- Bladder 38 (B38) quiets tension and promotes sleep.

Other Recommendations

Acupuncture has a good track record of relieving fibromyalgia pain. See the appendix for agencies that can provide you with lists of qualified acupuncturists in your area.

Bodywork

Many fibromyalgia sufferers have found that bodywork is quite helpful for easing pain and stress. Try several of the following techniques, as everyone responds differently.

Chiropractic or Osteopathic Manipulation
This improves structural alignment and nerve flow, which relieves fibromyalgia pain.

Massage
A gentle allover massage eases pain and brings down stress levels.

Lymphatic drainage massage supports the immune system by detoxifying the tissues. This kind of massage is especially supportive during a fast.

Reflexology
See pages 804–805 for information about reflexology areas and how to work them.

Because fibromyalgia is a systemic, whole-body disease, it is best to work the entire foot, with special attention to the parts corresponding to the areas of your body that hurt.

Hydrotherapy

Hot or warm water can feel wonderful to fibromyalgia sufferers. Try taking a hot shower in the morning, when the pain is likely to be at its worst; at night, when you might have trouble sleeping, try a warm bath. Saunas and heated compresses are other pleasant ways to relax your muscles.

Constitutional hydrotherapy is a good long-term treatment. See pages 795–796 for directions.

Other Recommendations

- A clinical trial published in the journal *Alternative Therapies* demonstrated just how effective intravenous nutrient therapy can be for this condition. Researchers used an intravenous formula containing B vitamins, minerals, and vitamin C to treat a group of female fibromyalgia patients. All the volunteers in the trial suffered with severe symptoms and reported a very poor quality of life as a result. They had all been living with their symptoms for at least five years, and conventional medical treatments had failed. The researchers administered weekly treatments of the cocktail to the volunteers. By week two, when the second cocktail was given, *all* the participants had a decrease in both pain and fatigue. And by the end of the eight-week trial pain levels and fatigue had improved *significantly*.
- Magnet therapy can be helpful to reduce pain. Work with a practitioner who is knowledgeable in this area.
- Moderate, nonjarring exercise is one of the best treatments for fibromyalgia. Daily exercise for half an hour (a brisk walk or a swim are excellent choices) is far preferable to less frequent but more vigorous workouts. Studies show that people with fibromyalgia who exercise regularly have fewer symptoms than those who are inactive.
- Get adequate rest. Most of us need at least eight hours a day; if you need more, however, by all means take it. Overexertion will only aggravate your symptoms.

REFERENCES

Ali, A. 2009. Intravenous micronutrient therapy (Myer's cocktail) for fibromyalgia: A placebo-controlled pilot study. *J Altern Complement Med* 15(3):247–257.

Anderson, P. S. 2012. Active comparator trial of addition of MTHFR specific support versus standard integrative naturopathic therapy for treating patients with diagnosed Fibromyalgia (FMS) and Chronic Fatigue Syndrome (CFS). Poster Presentation, presented at the California Association of Naturopathic Doctors Webinar, February 2014.

Caruso, I., P. Sarzi Puttini, M. Cazzola, and V. Azzolini. 1990. Double-blind study of 5-hydroxytryptophan versus placebo in the treatment of primary fibromyalgia syndrome. *Journal of Internal Medicine Research* 18(3):201–9.

Jacobsen S., B. Danneskiold-Samsoe, and R. B. Andersen. 1991. Oral S-adenosyl methionine in primary fibromyalgia: Double-blind clinical evaluation. *Scandinavian Journal of Rheumatology* 20:294–302.

Teitelbaum, J. E., et al. 2006. The use of D-ribose in chronic fatigue syndrome and fibromyalgia: A pilot study. *Journal of Alternative and Complementary Medicine* 12:857–62.

Flu

The flu, more properly called influenza, is an acute viral infection of the upper respiratory tract. Many people have difficulty distinguishing between the flu and the common cold, and, indeed, many of the symptoms are the same. Colds, however, tend to come on slowly and produce symptoms restricted to the chest, the neck, and the head; in contrast, the flu attacks swiftly and is accompanied by body-wide symptoms, including fever, aches, and general fatigue. While most people recover from colds within a few days, it may take weeks before the lingering fatigue and the cough of a flu completely disappear.

The three classifications of the influenza virus are A, B, and C. The most common virus is influenza A; swine flu is in this group. It often occurs in epidemics during the late fall or the early winter. The highest incidence of the flu is in schoolchildren. It generally takes forty-eight hours after initial exposure for symptoms to begin occurring. Chills, a fever, a headache, and muscular aches and pains are the most common initial symptoms followed by a severe cough. Acute symptoms usually subside in two to three days. People who are most at risk for serious complications include those with chronic pulmonary or heart disease.

The influenza viruses mutate constantly, changing their structure just enough so that it is more difficult to buildup immunity to them. These viruses are also highly contagious. They are communicated via coughs and sneezes, which propel infected droplets into the air and onto surfaces. Most communities see an outbreak of at least one flu virus every winter; every two to three years, the flu reaches epidemic proportions.

As with the common cold, there is no conventional cure for the flu. However, specific natural therapies described in this section have the potential to abort a flu in its early stages. The wisest course of action is to keep your immune system strong and healthy during the winter months, thereby reducing the virus's ability to take hold in your body. Eat well, exercise, rest, and follow the other general recommendations for health outlined in Part Two of this book.

Flu vaccines are highly promoted as the key to preventing the flu yet their effectiveness is controversial. Some flu vaccines have very low rates of effectiveness.

If you have a compromised immune system or a chronic chest condition (such as asthma, emphysema, or cardiovascular disease), see a doctor immediately if you catch the flu. Very young children should also receive medical care right away. No matter what your age or physical condition, if a case of the flu leads to difficulty breathing or tightness in the chest, contact your doctor.

SYMPTOMS

Most people with the flu experience the following symptoms:

- Fever
- Aches in the muscles and joints
- Fatigue and weakness
- Sore throat
- Dry cough

The following symptoms may also accompany the flu:

- Sneezing and runny nose
- Nausea and vomiting
- Swollen glands in the neck
- Insomnia
- Depression

ROOT CAUSES

- If overwork, stress, poor diet, or another illness has run down your immune system, you are much more likely to catch the flu during a community outbreak.

- Similar to the common cold, the flu acts as a means of detoxification for the body.

Testing Techniques

The following tests help assess possible reasons for reoccurring influenza infections:

    Immune system imbalance or disease—blood

    Hormone testing (especially for thyroid, DHEA, cortisol)—saliva, blood, or urine

    Intestinal permeability—urine

    Detoxification profile—urine

    Vitamin and mineral analysis (especially vitamins C and B12, selenium, glutathione, iron, and CoQ10)—blood

    Digestive function and microbe/parasite/fungal testing—stool analysis

    Anemia—blood test (CBC, iron, ferritin, % saturation)

    Food and environmental allergies/sensitivities—blood, electrodermal

    Blood sugar balance—blood

    Flu can be diagnosed by testing in your doctor's office

TREATMENT

Diet

Recommended Food

Eat lightly to allow your body to focus on healing rather than on digestion. During the first two to four days, when you are likely to feel the worst, your diet should consist mainly of liquids—clean, quality water, hot broths, green drinks, herbal teas, and juices—to flush your body of toxins. If you feel like eating, you should have a variety of fruits, especially citrus and berries. These fruits are high in vitamin C and bioflavonoids, which stimulate the production of white blood cells.

After the most acute stage of the illness has passed, continue with the liquids and the fruits but also start eating salads, steamed or lightly cooked vegetables, and whole grains. If you have the stomach for them, nuts are an excellent source of zinc, a mineral that strengthens the immune system. However, if you still don't have an appetite, don't force yourself to eat. Remain on the liquid diet until you're hungry again.

Warmed applesauce or apple juice is soothing and provides high levels of vitamin C. Make sure the sauce or juice isn't overheated or boiled, however, or it will lose some of its potency.

In 1998, the French Society of Homeopathy concluded a ten-year survey of twenty-three homeopathic doctors and their use of Influenzinum for flu prevention in 453 patients. In about 90 percent of the cases, no instances of the flu occurred when Influenzinum was used.

Lomatium (*Lomatium dissectum*) was a lifesaving remedy for Native American Indians living in the Nevada desert during the Spanish flu epidemic that killed over five hundred thousand people in the United States and twenty-two million worldwide. A local medical doctor noted that Native American Indians were recovering from the Spanish flu by ingesting boiled lomatium root. It is believed that phytochemicals found in lomatium root inhibit viruses from replicating and stimulate white blood cell activity.

Stay hydrated. Drink plenty of clean, quality water and other fluids (but see the note about sugar and juice further on) to cleanse away toxins and to keep the respiratory tract from drying out.

Increase your consumption of ginger, onions, and garlic. Try adding one or all to chicken soup or miso.

Hot water with lemon, honey, and cinnamon is a traditional cold remedy. Drink a cup every two hours to soothe your throat and chest, prevent mucus buildup, and encourage a cleansing sweat.

Food to Avoid

Eliminate dairy and refined-sugar products from your diet for the duration of your illness. These foods will only contribute to the formation of mucus and make the virus harder to expel. Sugar also has the extremely undesirable effect of depressing your immune system.

Caffeine depletes the body's stores of zinc, a mineral necessary for healing. Avoid coffee, black teas, and chocolate until the flu passes.

℞ Super Seven Prescriptions—Flu

Super Prescription #1 Homeopathic Combination Flu Remedy
At the first signs of a flu, take a dose of the combination flu remedy four times daily for three days. This contains the most common remedies used for the flu. Another alternative is a flu remedy containing *Anas barbariae*, or Influenzinum. Then if you notice improvement, stop taking the remedy, unless symptoms return. If your symptoms do not improve within twenty-four hours, pick the remedy that best matches your symptoms under Homeopathy in this section.

Super Prescription #2 Elderberry (*Sambucus nigra*)
Adults should take 1 tablespoon four times daily and children 1 tablespoon twice daily. Elderberry inhibits influenza viral replication and reduces coughing.

Super Prescription #3 Vitamin D
Take 5,000 IU daily with meals during flu season to optimize immunity. Children should take 1,000 to 2,000 IU daily during flu season.

Super Prescription #4 *Lomatium dissectum*
Take 500 mg in capsule form or 2 to 4 ml of the tincture four times daily. Lomatium has strong antiviral effects and has traditionally been used by herbalists to treat the flu.

Super Prescription #5 *Pelargonium sidoides*
Take as directed on the label to shorten the duration and intensity of upper respiratory tract infections.

Super Prescription #6 American ginseng
Take 200 mg of a standardized extract (CVT-E002) twice daily to reduce the incidence of upper respiratory tract infections.

Super Prescription #7 N-acetylcysteine

Take 600 mg twice daily for flu prevention and 2,000 to 3,000 mg for flu treatment.

General Recommendations

Garlic (*Allium sativum*) has powerful antiviral and detoxification properties. Add it raw to broths, juices, soups, or vegetable dishes. You can also take 300 to 450 mg of garlic in capsules twice a day.

Astragalus (*Astragalus membranaceus*) is an excellent treatment for preventing the flu. Do not take astragalus if you have a fever. Take 500 to 1,000 mg in capsule form or 3.0 ml of a tincture two or three times daily.

Thyme (*Thymus vulgaris*) extract optimizes immune activity. Take 1 or 2 capsules twice daily or as directed on the container.

Both echinacea (*Echinacea purpurea*) and goldenseal (*Hydrastis canadensis*) enhance immune function, and echinacea has antiviral properties. Take an echinacea and goldenseal combination of 500 mg in capsule form or 2 to 4 ml of tincture four times daily. If you do not have any mucus production, use only echinacea.

Oregano (*Origanum vulgare*) oil has powerful antiviral effects. Take 500 mg of the capsule form four times daily or as directed on the container.

Vitamin C supports immune-system function through increased white blood cell activity. Take 1,000 to 2,000 mg three or four times daily. Reduce the dosage if diarrhea occurs.

Ginger (*Zingiber officinale*) helps with a sore throat and chills. Take 500 mg of the capsule form or drink fresh tea four times daily.

Homeopathy

At the first signs of a flu, take 2 pellets of a 30C potency four times daily for three days, of the remedy that best matches your symptoms in this section. If you notice improvement, stop taking the remedy, unless symptoms return. If your symptoms do not improve within twenty-four hours, pick another remedy.

Aconitum Napellus is for a flu that comes on suddenly after exposure to dry, cold weather. There is a scratchy throat and a thin discharge from the nose. You probably feel anxious, restless, and chilly, with a great thirst. This remedy is best taken within four hours of developing flu symptoms.

Arsenicum Album is for a cold with a flu in which a person feels exhausted, anxious, restless, and chilly and is thirsty for sips of warm water. Diarrhea and vomiting occur with the flu.

Belladonna (*Atropa belladonna*) is for the beginning phase of a flu characterized by a high fever that comes on suddenly. The face is flushed and the skin is hot, but the feet are cold. The pupils are dilated. A throbbing headache is common.

Bryonia (*Bryonia alba*) is for a flu with severe aching of the joints. The person feels worse from the slightest movement and may have a hard, dry cough. There is a great thirst for cold drinks. The person feels very irritable and does not want to move. The joints ache.

Eupatorium Perfolatum is helpful when there is a high fever and tremendous, deep aching of the bones and the muscles. The person has a great thirst for cold drinks.

Italian researchers found that seniors who took N-acetyl-cysteine had virtually no flu symptoms, even though tests showed that they had flu infection, whereas people taking a placebo suffered the brunt of flu symptoms. This powerful antioxidant boosts immunity.

A double-blind, placebo-controlled study in the *Journal of Alternative and Complementary Medicine* reported that people who received elderberry extract (4 tablespoons a day for adults and 2 tablespoons for children) for three days significantly improved their flu symptoms. Ninety percent of people taking this herbal extract were completely well in two to three days, as compared to six days for those taking a placebo.

Ferrum Phosphoricum helps when a person feels feverish but does not act sick. The throat may be sore, and the face is flushed. It's best used at the onset of a flu.

Gelsemium (*Gelsemium sempervirens*) is for a cold accompanied by chills and muscle aches. The person feels drowsy and fatigued and has droopy eyelids. There may be a headache at the base of the head.

Mercurius Solubilis or Vivus is helpful when the person is sensitive to both hot and cold temperatures. The tongue has a thick coating, and the person has bad breath, has excessive saliva production, and drools on the pillow. The throat is often raw and sore. Profuse sweating occurs.

Nux Vomica (*Strychnos nux vomica*) is for a person who has a digestive upset, such as stomach cramping and nausea, with the flu. There is great chilliness and irritability.

Rhus Toxicodendron is for extreme stiffness in the muscles and the joints that feels better with warm applications and when moving around. It is hard to find a comfortable position, so there is a lot of restlessness.

Sulfur is for the end stages of a long flu. Burning in the lungs may occur, as well as fever and sweating. The person has a great thirst for ice-cold drinks.

Acupressure

See pages 787–794 for information about pressure points and administering treatment.

- Large Intestine 4 (LI4), Governing Vessel 24.5 (GV24.5), and Gallbladder 16 and 20 (GB16 and GB20) all ease headache and head congestion.
- To reduce fever and strengthen the immune system, massage Large Intestine 11 (LI11).
- Kidney 27 (K27) relieves a sore throat and chest congestion.

Bodywork

Massage

When most of your symptoms have passed and you're ready to resume a more normal schedule, an all-over massage will help you make the transition more smoothly.

If you have a lingering cough following an episode of the flu, a percussive massage will help break up the mucus. Percussive motions are best used on people who are relatively strong and healthy.

Reflexology

See pages 804–805 for information about reflexology areas and how to work them.

Work the areas corresponding to the chest and the lungs, the intestines, the diaphragm, the lymph system, and all the glands.

Massage the cervicals if your flu is accompanied by a sore throat.

For clogged sinuses, work all the toes.

Hydrotherapy

Constitutional hydrotherapy done each day relieves congestion and stimulates the immune system. See pages 795–796 for directions.

Studies suggest that our wintertime susceptibility to the flu and common cold viruses may be related to less sunlight exposure and lower vitamin D production. Researchers recently discovered that vitamin D controls the production of cathelicidin, a powerful germ-killing immune compound. Other studies show that vitamin D prevents upper respiratory infections, such as those characteristic of the flu.

Aromatherapy

Add any of the following oils to baths or steam inhalations.

Tea tree oil has strong infection-fighting properties. Add to a bath, or mix a few drops of the oil with warm water and gargle with it. (Tea tree oil is quite concentrated, so add no more than 2 or 3 drops to a cup of water for gargling.) To prevent the infection from spreading to the rest of your household, use some in diffusers in the common rooms.

Use lavender in any kind of preparation to strengthen your immune system and help you sleep.

Add eucalyptus and peppermint—either alone or in combination—to a bath, in steam, or in an inhalation to relieve congestion.

Stress Reduction

If chronic stress leaves you constantly vulnerable to the flu and other upper respiratory infections, take some time out every day to detach yourself from any tension you might be experiencing.

Regular stress-management practice can also help you handle future difficult situations with a calm disposition.

General Stress-Reduction Therapies

Regular exercise and a positive attitude and mental imagery improve immune function and may help prevent a flu.

Other Recommendations

- Intravenous vitamin C is very effective as an antiviral treatment for patients with the flu. See a local holistic doctor.
- Rest is absolutely critical to the healing process. As soon as you feel the symptoms strike, get into bed and stay there for several days or even a week, if necessary.
- If you try to exert yourself during a bout of the flu, you may wind up with a secondary infection, such as pneumonia.
- Gargle with warm salt water to reduce sore throat pain.
- Intravenous vitamin C therapy by a holistic doctor is very effective for the treatment of influenza.

REFERENCES

Alstat, E. K. 1987. Lomatium dissectum—An herbal virucide! *Complementary Medicine* 2(5).

Coulamy, A. 1998. Survey of the prescription habits of homeopathic doctors on the subject of a single medication: Influenzinum. French Society of Homeopathy Conference Notes, 1–16.

De Flora, S., et al. 1997. Attenuation of influenza-like symptomatology and improvement of cell-mediated immunity with long-term N-acetylcysteine treatment. *European Respiratory Journal* 10:1535–41.

Grant, W. B., et al. 2009. The possible roles of solar ultraviolet-B radiation and vitamin D in reducing case-fatality rates from the 1918–1919 influenza pandemic in the United States. *Derma-Endocrinology* 1:1–5.

Liu, P. T., et al. 2006. Toll-like receptor triggering of a vitamin D–mediated human antimicrobial response. *Science* 311:1770–73.

Zakay-Rones, Z., N. Varsano, M. Zlotnik, et al. 1995. Inhibition of several strains of influenza virus in vitro and reduction of symptoms by an elderberry extract (*Sambucus nigra L.*) during an outbreak of influenza B in Panama. *Journal of Alternative and Complementary Medicine* 1(4):361–69.

Food Allergies/Sensitivities

Food allergies and food sensitivities (also referred to as intolerances) are terms often used interchangeably. Technically, a food allergy is a measurable immune response to a normally harmless food. Symptoms include itchy hives, lip swelling, nausea, vomiting, diarrhea, wheezing, and difficulty breathing. Common food allergies are to peanuts, wheat, milk, eggs, MSG, and shellfish. Scientists are not sure what exactly causes food allergies. Since many allergies tend to run in families, there apparently is a genetic component. There is also evidence that some allergies are the result of exposure to a certain food or foods too early in life, before the immune system is fully developed. Many infants who are given cow's milk instead of breast milk in the first months develop an allergic reaction; the same goes for children who are fed wheat, eggs, peanut butter, or other products before they are ready. At any age, the overconsumption of a food is thought to lead to allergies. Wheat, for example, is a common allergen in the United States, because most people eat it at every meal and snack.

Food sensitivities are reactions to food where there is not necessarily an immune response, as measured by standard lab tests. These symptoms are not life threatening but are bothersome. These include, but are not limited to, abdominal cramps, bloating, headache, mood swings, reoccurring infections, joint pain, runny nose, skin rashes, dark circles under the eyes, and fatigue. Symptoms may occur up to thirty-six hours after ingesting the offending food. Common food sensitivities that we see with patients are to cow's milk, wheat, corn, soy, chocolate, citrus fruit, and artificial sweeteners and preservatives. Most food sensitivities are acquired throughout life. A lack of variety in the diet, poor digestion and detoxification, and genetics are often the underlying causes. Most people who have multiple food sensitivities have an underlying condition known as leaky gut syndrome. This means that foods are not being broken down effectively (especially proteins), and once absorbed, they cause a heightened immune reaction. The key to these cases is to heal the gut lining and improve food breakdown, something that natural medicine is very effective for. Many cases of food sensitivities can be eliminated or improved with natural therapies.

Food allergies and sensitivities can sometimes be difficult to identify. Immune responses to food may take hours or days to develop, and they may be mistaken for seasonal allergies or for other diseases associated with their symptoms: colds, flu, skin problems, chronic fatigue, and many others. And allergies aren't just triggered by the consumption of large quantities of a problem food: you can have a reaction from a minute quantity or even from simply touching or inhaling an allergen. Use

---

Do be aware that hundreds of conditions can be at least in part caused or worsened by food allergies or sensitivities. Common examples include:

Arthritis

Asthma

Attention-deficit/ hyperactivity disorder

Bedwetting

Canker sores

Colic

Constipation

Depression

Diarrhea

Ear infections

Eczema

Gallbladder disease

Headaches

High blood pressure

Hives

Hypoglycemia

Irritable bowel syndrome

Inflammatory bowel diseases (Crohn's, ulcerative colitis)

Multiple chemical sensitivity

Overweight

Psoriasis

Reflux and ulcers

Sinusitis

Weakened immunity

the elimination diet given here to determine which food or foods, if any, you are allergic to.

In addition, specific testing with blood, electrodermal, or skin-scratch tests, or through applied kinesiology by a holistic practitioner or a doctor, can help you quickly identify your problem foods. They can then be avoided, or you can desensitize yourself to them.

SYMPTOMS

Food allergies can produce a number of symptoms. The most common are listed below:

- Nasal congestion
- Sneezing
- Coughing
- Red, itchy, or watery eyes
- Dark circles or puffiness under the eyes
- Wheezing
- Sore throat
- Difficulty swallowing

- Hives, rashes, eczema, or other skin eruptions
- Nausea or vomiting
- Headache
- Fatigue
- Fluid retention
- Swelling of the throat and the tongue

Common symptoms of food sensitivities:

- Abdominal cramps and bloating
- Headache
- Mood swings
- Reoccurring infections
- Joint pain

- Runny nose
- Skin rashes
- Dark circles under the eyes
- Fatigue

ROOT CAUSES

- Overconsumption of a certain food
- Introduction of a food too early in infancy or childhood

- Stress, which depresses the immune system
- Poor digestion and detoxification
- Heredity

Testing Techniques

The following tests help assess possible reasons for food allergies/sensitivities, as well as determine the offending foods:

Intestinal permeability—urine

Detoxification profile—urine

Digestive function and microbe/parasite/candida testing—stool analysis

Food allergies/sensitivities—blood (IgE and IgG4), electrodermal, skin scratch

Hormone testing (DHEA, cortisol)—saliva, blood, or urine

TREATMENT

If you experience difficulty breathing or develop hives that spread rapidly, *get emergency help at once.* Allergic reactions like these can be quickly fatal. If you know you have severe reactions to certain substances, talk to your doctor about emergency adrenaline kits you can keep on hand.

Diet

Obviously, the most important step in treating allergies is identifying them. Once you've identified the offending substances, adhere to the following suggestions to keep them out of your diet and to reduce your chances of having a bad reaction, should you be accidentally exposed. Food sensitivities can generally be improved or cured by rotating foods in the diet, improving digestion and detoxification, and using the desensitization techniques described in this chapter.

Recommended Food

Fortify your immune system with a healthful, wholesome diet. Eat foods that are high in immune-building nutrients: seafood, beans, and nuts for magnesium; green leafy vegetables and brewer's yeast for B vitamins; and plenty of fresh fruits and vegetables for vitamin C.

A varied diet will discourage the development of allergies, so try to eat different foods every day.

Breast milk is best for infants. If, for some reason, you are unable to provide your baby with mother's milk, use a cow's milk alternative or a predigested, hypoallergenic formula.

Drink a glass of clean, quality water every two waking hours to flush allergens out of your body and to encourage overall health.

Food to Avoid

Of course, you must avoid the foods that trigger a severe allergy response. In general, it is best to buy whole foods and prepare them yourself, so that you are aware of their content, but if you must buy packaged food, learn how to read labels, and scrutinize them carefully. Food preservatives and artificial colorings or flavorings can be at the root of food reactions.

Food sensitivities can generally be rotated in the diet, until you become desensitized to the offending food.

℞ Super Seven Prescriptions—Food Sensitivities

Super Prescription #1 Diamine oxidase
Take 1 or 2 capsules within fifteen minutes of ingesting a food that you are intolerant of but not allergic to. This helps to regulate histamine levels in the body.

Super Prescription #2 Digestive enzyme complex
Take a full-spectrum digestive complex with each meal.

Super Prescription #3 Homeopathic Desensitization Drops
Take a homeopathic dilution of the food(s) you are sensitive to, up to three times daily or as directed on the container. This approach of like curing like helps desensitize the immune response to sensitivity reactions.

Super Prescription #4 Probiotics
Take a product that contains at least five billion active organisms daily, thirty minutes after a meal. These good bacteria favorably alter the way the immune system perceives foods and also helps with their metabolism and digestion.

Super Prescription #5 Gentian root (*Gentiana lutea*)
This improves stomach-acid levels and overall digestive function. Take 300 mg in capsule form or 10 to 20 drops five to fifteen minutes before meals. It can also be used as part of a digestive bitters formula.

Super Prescription #6 Thyme (*Thymus vulgaris*) extract
Take 1 or 2 capsules or as directed on the container three times daily on an empty stomach. Thyme extract balances an overactive immune system.

Super Prescription #7 Methylsulfonylmethane (MSM)
Take 1,000 mg twice daily. MSM has a natural antiallergy benefit that includes aiding with food sensitivities.

General Recommendations

L-glutamine repairs the lining of the small intestine for improved absorption. Take 500 mg three times daily.

An adrenal-glandular supplement supports adrenal-gland function and allergy control. Take 1 capsule three times daily between meals.

Pantothenic acid (vitamin B5) supports adrenal-gland function and allergy control. Take 500 mg three times daily.

Milk thistle (*Silybum marianum*) supports liver function and detoxification. Take 250 mg of a 85 percent silymarin extract with each meal.

Betaine hydrochloric acid improves stomach-acid levels. Take 1 or 2 capsules with each meal.

Quercitin has antiallergy benefits. Take 500 mg three times daily.

Vitamin C with bioflavonoids reduces allergy reactions. Take 1,000 mg two or three times daily.

Take 1 or 2 protease enzyme capsules two or three times daily on an empty stomach, unless you have an ulcer or gastritis.

Studies done with infants and nursing mothers have found that probiotics help improve food allergies. It appears that probiotics directly reduce the immune response to food allergens and indirectly improve symptoms, due to improved food digestion.

Homeopathy

Pick the remedy that best matches your symptoms in this section. For acute food reactions, take a 30C potency four times daily. For chronic food sensitivities, take 6x, 12x, 6C, 12C, or 30C potency twice daily for two weeks to see if there are any positive results. After you notice improvement, stop taking the remedy, unless symptoms return. Consultation with a homeopathic practitioner is advised. *Note*: Homeopathy is not a replacement for medical treatment for serious acute food-allergy reactions.

Lycopodium (*Lycopodium clavatum*) is for people who have problems with food reactions and also suffer tremendous bloating and gas. They crave sweets. Symptoms are usually worse in the early evening.

Nux Vomica (*Strychnos nux vomica*) is for people with multiple food sensitivities and digestive problems, such as heartburn, reflux, constipation, or stomach cramps. They tend to be chilly and irritable.

Urtica Urens is helpful if you have welts or hives with itchy, burning skin, especially after eating shellfish. If your hives or welts are rapidly spreading, get emergency help at once.

Elimination Diet to Detect Food Allergies

Although it takes some time and dedication, an elimination diet is the best way to uncover any hidden food allergies. The first step is to come up with a list of possible trigger foods. Do this by keeping a food diary, writing down everything you eat each day for a week (or longer, if you sense that one week can't adequately represent your eating habits). At the end of the week, note the foods you've consumed most often during the week. This is your list of possible triggers.

Next, you should eliminate all the suspect foods on your list from your diet for a total of two weeks. For most people, this stage is difficult, as you're asked to give up the foods you love and rely upon the most; try to keep in mind that you'll be able to return to your usual diet, perhaps with a few modifications, soon.

If, after two weeks, your symptoms have disappeared, you know that you are allergic to at least one of the foods on your list. To identify which food or foods are the culprit, reintroduce the suspect foods to your diet one at a time. When reintroducing foods that have been eliminated, be sure to use the purest form of the food. For example, if milk is on your list of suspects, add whole milk back to your diet, not skim. If you've eliminated wheat, reintroduce it by eating cream of wheat or shredded wheat. Allow two full days to pass between reintroducing foods, as it may take a while for symptoms to manifest themselves. Should your symptoms reappear, you can assume that the food most recently reintroduced is an allergen, and you should banish it from your diet or work to have your immune system desensitized to it. Continue to make your way through the list, however, as you may be allergic to more than one food. Wait at least forty-eight hours after the onset of symptoms before reintroducing the next eliminated food.

At the end of the elimination diet, you will know which, if any, foods produce an allergic response in your body. Depending on your reaction, you can avoid or reduce your intake of this food.

Acupressure

See pages 787–794 for information about pressure points and administering treatment.

- Large Intestine 4 (LI4) relieves headaches and sneezing.
- If you have fatigue, swollen eyes, or head pain, use Bladder 10 (B10).
- Triple Warmer 5 (TW5) fortifies the immune system.
- Stomach 36 (St36) strengthens the entire body and promotes a healthful balance.

Bodywork

Massage

If food allergies have left you chronically or severely congested, consider a percussive massage to help break up mucus. Percussive motions are best used on people who are relatively strong and healthy. If you are frail, thin, or elderly, check with your massage therapist about the suitability of this treatment for you.

To reduce stress, get a relaxing massage that incorporates any of the soothing essential oils listed in the Aromatherapy recommendations.

Reflexology

See pages 804–805 for information about reflexology areas and how to work them.

To ease allergic reactions in the upper respiratory tract, work the big toes and the inside of the heels.

If you have been exposed to an allergenic food, work the liver and the colon to speed the processing and the release of toxins.

Hydrotherapy

Hydrotherapy enhances gut healing. See pages 795–796.

Aromatherapy

Use melissa in a bath, an inhalation, or a massage oil to reduce the intensity of an allergic attack.

Lavender and chamomile will relax and soothe the body after the stress of an allergic reaction. Use either oil according to your particular symptoms. If you have acne, mix into a lotion and apply directly to the skin. For other reactions, you can use a compress to apply the oil to a specific body part, add to a bath, or use in a massage for allover relief.

If you're congested, try any of the following oils in a steam inhalation, a bath, a diffuser, or a massage: eucalyptus, peppermint, melissa, and tea tree.

Stress Reduction

General Stress-Reduction Techniques

Stress can impact your immune and digestive systems and can contribute to food sensitivities.

Read the Exercise and Stress Reduction chapter in Part Two, and choose a couple of stress-reduction techniques you'd like to try. Once you've found one or two that you like, incorporate them into your daily routine. Regular practice will help you handle daily tension with detachment and equanimity.

REFERENCES

Laiho, K., A. Ouwehand, S. Salminen, et al. 2002. Inventing probiotic functional foods for patients with allergic disease. *Annals of Allergy, Asthma, and Immunology* 89(6 Suppl 1):75–82.

Majamaa, H., and E. Isolauri. 1997. Probiotics: A novel approach in the management of food allergy. *Journal of Allergy and Clinical Immunology* 99:179–85.

Food Poisoning

One of the most unpleasant and certainly potentially dangerous conditions is food poisoning. A person's body reacts to toxins produced by bacteria that contaminate food. The most common types of food poisoning result from the bacteria of salmonella, campylobacter, and staphylococcus.

Symptoms range from nausea, overall body weakness, fever, and abdominal cramps to violent episodes of vomiting and diarrhea as the body tries to rid itself of the contaminated food.

Most cases of food poisoning can be avoided. Food poisoning occurs as a result of improper handling, storing, or cooking of food. That is why it is important for people to always wash their hands thoroughly with soap before eating and especially before preparing a meal.

It is important to refrigerate foods like mayonnaise, egg salad, potato salads, rice puddings, and fried rice. These foods can be easily contaminated. Another common mistake is not to cook foods thoroughly and at high-enough temperatures. This is especially true with meats.

Follow the old adage in deciding whether or not to eat leftovers: "When in doubt, throw it out."

Food poisoning can also occur from eating plants that contain toxic chemicals (certain types of mushrooms) or foods contaminated with chemicals (e.g., heavy metals like lead). If you suspect that your child has eaten a poisonous plant, seek medical attention immediately.

Fortunately, most cases of food poisoning are short-lived, and your appetite will return within one to two days. However, head to the emergency room if you or your child has a medical condition that impairs the immune system (e.g., HIV, hepatitis) or displays any of these severe symptoms:

- Violent vomiting
- A fever exceeding 102 degrees F
- Vision problems
- Severe diarrhea that lasts more than one day or contains blood
- Trouble breathing or talking
- Headache and dizziness
- Dehydration

EXAMPLES OF FOOD POISONING

Staphylococcus

Foods that have been handled by people with skin infections can be contaminated when left at room temperature. The classic example is a potato salad left out for a long time at a picnic. Symptoms usually come on very quickly, within two to eight hours, and usually begin to resolve within twelve hours. Symptoms may include:

- Severe nausea and vomiting
- Abdominal cramps
- Diarrhea
- Headache and fever

Campylobacter

This infection usually results from poultry that has been infected and not cooked properly. It can also occur from unpasteurized milk and contaminated drinking water. Symptoms usually begin two to five days after exposure. Symptoms may include:

- Diarrhea
- Nausea and vomiting
- Fever
- Abdominal pain and cramping

Salmonella

Infection is by one of the many types of *Salmonella* bacteria. The most common contaminated foods include unpasteurized milk and undercooked poultry and eggs. This infection causes acute intestinal distress, with a sudden onset of headache, fever, abdominal pain, diarrhea, nausea, and sometimes vomiting. Dehydration in infants can be severe. Symptoms start sixteen to forty-eight hours after eating and can last up to seven days.

Botulism

Home-canned foods are the most common source of the spores that cause toxicity to the nervous system. Commercially prepared foods can also be at fault. The botulinum spores are very resistant to heat. It is recommended that canned foods be exposed to moist heat at 212 degrees F (120 degrees C) for thirty minutes to kill the spores. The toxins that are produced by the spores can be killed through heat by cooking the food at 176 degrees F (80 degrees C) for thirty minutes. Symptoms usually come on eighteen to thirty-six hours after ingestion of the botulinum toxin. This can be a very severe and potentially fatal poisoning. Symptoms can include:

- Nausea, vomiting, and abdominal cramps, followed by neurological symptoms such as
  - Vision changes
  - Muscle weakness
  - Difficulty breathing
  - Constipation

Note: Infant botulism occurs most often in children who are less than six months old. Botulinum spores may be present in honey, so it is recommended that children under one year of age not be given honey (as their immune systems may not be able to handle it).

E. Coli

This infection usually occurs as a result of undercooked beef or unpasteurized milk or through fecal-oral contamination. The bacterium infects the digestive tract and typically leads to bloody diarrhea and possibly kidney failure. Young children (younger than five years old) and the elderly are most susceptible to the damaging effects of this infection. Symptoms usually include:

- Severe abdominal cramps
- Watery diarrhea, followed by bloody diarrhea (usually lasts one to eight days)
- Fever is usually absent or low grade

Clostridium Perfingens

This bacterium is found in feces, water, soil, air, and water. Contaminated meat left at room temperature is the main source of infection. Symptoms usually begin six to twenty-four hours after ingestion and resolve within twenty-four hours. Common symptoms include:

- Watery diarrhea
- Abdominal cramps

Traveler's Diarrhea

Bacteria endemic to the local water cause this infection. Viruses can also cause it. It occurs in areas that lack adequate water purification. Common symptoms include:

- Nausea and vomiting
- Loud gurgling noises in the abdomen
- Abdominal cramps
- Diarrhea beginning twelve to seventy-two hours after ingesting the contaminated water or food

Parasitic Infections

Giardia is the most common example. This parasite is transmitted through the feca–loral route, mainly through water contamination. In most cases there are no symptoms, and symptoms usually take one to three weeks after exposure to appear. In cases where symptoms occur, the most common are:

- Watery, malodorous diarrhea
- Abdominal cramps and distention
- Flatulence and burping
- Nausea
- Low-grade fever
- Fatigue

Chemical Food Poisoning

Plants or animals that contain a naturally occurring poison fall under the heading of chemical food poisoning. Common examples include:

- Wild mushrooms (e.g., *Amanita phalloides*)
- Wild and domestic plants (yew, nightshade, castor bean, morning glory, and many others)
- Fish
- Shellfish

In addition, fruits and vegetables sprayed with insecticides or other chemicals can cause chemical poisoning if the foods are not washed.

Obviously, severe cases require conventional treatment that focuses on identifying the type of infectious organism and then prescribing an antimicrobial medicine (e.g., antibiotics for bacterial infections). However, natural therapies are often effective for mild cases and can be used adjunctively for more severe cases.

Testing Techniques

The following test helps assess possible reasons for food poisoning:
Comprehensive stool analysis—bacterial and parasitic infection, flora balance

---

TREATMENT

Diet

Recommended Food

The most important thing is to keep hydrated by drinking two cups of liquid every waking hour. Try clean, quality water, diluted fruit and vegetable juices, electrolyte drinks, and broths. If you have a dry mouth or suddenly wrinkled skin that does not snap back when gently pulled, you may be on your way to severe dehydration. Foods that are easy to digest, such as soup, broths, and steamed vegetables, are recommended.

Food to Avoid

During the most intense stages of diarrhea, you will probably not feel much like eating. Do not force yourself to take in solid food during this time (although you should drink plenty of fluids).

As you feel better and regain your appetite, you should stay away from dairy products, fats, and oils, which will only upset your stomach again. If you do not have intolerance to any of these foods, reintroduce them to your diet slowly.

Avoid sugar, especially if you have a bacterial infection. Bacteria feed on it. Even if bacteria aren't the cause of your problem, keep sugar out of your diet; it promotes inflammation, which discourages healing.

Avoid caffeine and alcohol, which are too stimulating to the digestive tract.

If the cause of the problem is not clear, determine whether a food allergy or intolerance caused your diarrhea. Once you feel better, use the elimination diet on page 316 to identify troublesome foods. Many cases of diarrhea can be traced to gluten intolerance, so make a special effort to examine the effects of wheat and seeds on your digestive system.

As you feel better, eat basic, simple foods that are easily absorbed. Soups, cooked fruits and vegetables, and brown rice are all good choices. Apples, bananas, carrots, and potatoes tend to taste especially good at this time, and for an excellent reason. They all contain pectin, which has a gentle binding quality.

One study has shown that roasted carob powder reduces the duration of diarrhea. Try a few tablespoons in some water.

℞ Super Seven Prescriptions—Food Poisoning

Super Prescription #1 Homeopathic Combination Diarrhea Remedy and Homeopathic Combination Nausea/Vomiting Remedy
For acute diarrhea and nausea/vomiting, alternate doses of a combination diarrhea and combination nausea/vomiting remedy four times daily for

twenty-four hours. Then if you notice improvement, stop taking the remedy, unless symptoms return. If your symptoms do not improve within twenty-four hours, pick the remedy that best matches your symptoms under Homeopathy in this section.

Super Prescription #2 Ginger (*Zingiber officinale*)

Drink a cup of fresh-ginger tea, or take 500 mg in capsules or 2 ml of a tincture every two hours. Ginger reduces intestinal inflammation and lessens the effect of food poisoning.

Super Prescription #3 Probiotic

Take a product containing at least four billion active organisms two or three times daily. It contains friendly bacteria, such as *Lactobacillus acidophilus* and *bifidus*, which fight intestinal infection.

Super Prescription #4 Goldenseal (*Hydrastis canadensis*)

Take 1 ml of the tincture or 300 mg in capsule form four times daily. It helps improve diarrhea that is related to an intestinal infection.

Super Prescription #5 Oregano (*Origanum vulgare*) oil

Take 500 mg of the capsule form four times daily or as directed on the container. Oregano oil has powerful antimicrobial effects.

Super Prescription #6 Peppermint (*Mentha piperita*)

Take 1 ml of a tincture or 250 mg in capsule form or drink 1 cup of fresh tea every two hours. Peppermint reduces nausea and cramping.

Super Prescription #7 Activated charcoal

Take 3 capsules every two hours for three doses. Activated charcoal capsules taken internally can help to absorb toxins from food poisoning. Charcoal works best when taken in the first stages of food poisoning (when you first realize you have food poisoning).

General Recommendations

Parasite Blend

If your doctor suspects that you have a parasite infection, take an herbal parasite blend with herbs such as garlic, black walnut (*Juglans nigra*), wormwood (*Artemisia absinthium*), and grapefruit extract. Take as directed on the container.

Homeopathy

Pick the remedy that best matches your symptoms in this section. For acute symptoms, take a 30C potency four times daily. After you notice improvement, stop taking the remedy, unless symptoms return. Consultation with a homeopathic practitioner is advised.

Arsenicum Album is the most common remedy for food poisoning. Symptoms include diarrhea (especially burning diarrhea), vomiting, chilliness, anxiety, and restlessness. Symptoms tend to be worse between midnight and 2 A.M. The person experiences burning pains in the abdomen. Symptoms are better from warm drinks.

China (*Chinchona*) is a good remedy for diarrhea and bloating that has led to exhaustion and weakness. It is useful to take after an acute bout of food poisoning, to regain strength.

Ipecacuanha (*Cephaelis ipecacuanha*) is for extreme nauseousness and vomiting. The person experiences a sinking sensation in the stomach. Vomiting does not relieve the symptoms.

Mercurius Corrosivus is for food poisoning that causes bloody, burning diarrhea. The person may alternate between feeling chilly and sweaty.

Nux Vomica (*Strychnos nux vomica*) is for food poisoning that causes heartburn, cramping, and painful diarrhea that feels better temporarily from passing stool or from warm applications. The person is chilly and irritable. This is also a good general remedy to use for the ill effects from food, such as spicy or rich foods.

Phosphorus is a remedy for burning diarrhea, abdominal pain, and vomiting that feel better with cold drinks or cold food.

Podophyllum is for profuse, watery, explosive diarrhea with gas. Stool may contain yellow mucus.

Veratrum Album is indicated when there are profuse, rice-water stools that occur simultaneously with forceful vomiting. The person experiences violent cramping and feels very cold.

Acupressure

Work Stomach 36 (St36)—four finger widths below the kneecap and one finger width toward the outside of the leg (outside of the shin bone on the muscle).

Bodywork

Hydrotherapy

Constitutional hydrotherapy helps relieve abdominal pain and bring good immune cells into the digestive tract to fight the infection.

Aromatherapy

Add 2 drops of German chamomile and 1 drop of black pepper into a carrier oil, and rub over the person's abdomen.

Other Recommendations

Intravenous nutrients will help a person prevent and recover from dehydration related to diarrhea.

REFERENCES

Resta-Lenert, S., and K. E. Barrett. 2003. Live probiotics protect intestinal epithelial cells from the effects of infection with enteroinvasive Escherichia coli (EIEC). *Gut* 52(7):988–97.

Gallbladder Problems

The gallbladder is a digestive organ located in the upper right portion of the abdomen, directly underneath the liver. It is responsible for storing and concentrating the bile that is produced by the liver. Bile is a greenish-yellow color and is composed of bile acids, water, electrolytes, bilirubin, cholesterol, and phospholipids. As food enters the small intestine, hormonal and nervous system activity cause the gallbladder to contract, sending bile through the common bile duct into the beginning portion of the small intestine, known as the duodenum. Bile has several different functions, including the digestion and absorption of fats, the absorption of fat-soluble nutrients, the retention of water in the colon to promote bowel movements, the excretion of bilirubin (degraded red blood cells), the elimination of drugs and other compounds from the body, and the secretion of various proteins involved in gastrointestinal function. As you can see, dysfunction in bile production and secretion can result in many different health problems.

The most common problem associated with the gallbladder is gallstones. It is estimated that 20 percent of people over the age of sixty-five have gallstones. Every year, more than five hundred thousand people have surgery to remove their gallbladders. The symptoms of gallstones can greatly vary from person to person. Most people with gallstones often have no symptoms throughout their lives, as the stones pass without problems. Symptoms may include right-sided abdominal pain (or pain anywhere in the abdomen) and radiating pain that goes to the right shoulder blade. Abdominal bloating, gas, belching, and recurrent pain are common, too. Most often, gallstones are found with a routine exam, and if they are causing no symptoms, they are left alone. Gallstones that cause pain and other symptoms are treated conventionally, with surgery (often using laparoscopy), bile acids taken orally (for stones that are noncalcified), or, more commonly, lithotripsy, the use of shock waves to fragment the stones so that they will pass.

Gallstones are formed as a result of the bile's becoming saturated with cholesterol. This can be due to an increase in cholesterol secretion or decreased bile and lecithin secretion. Other particulate matter then attracts cholesterol and sets the stage for stone formation. As you will read in this chapter's treatment section, there are natural ways to decrease the saturation of cholesterol in the bile via diet and nutritional supplementation.

Risk factors for gallstones include:
- Sex: Women are two to four times more likely than men to have gallstones. This, in part, may be due to the use of oral contraceptives and synthetic hormone replacement.
- Race: Gallstones are more common in women of North American Indian ethnicity.
- Obesity causes an increased secretion of cholesterol into bile. Also, it should be noted that rapid weight loss (during the initial phases) can contribute to gallstone formation.
- Age: The frequency increases with age.
- A Western diet is a contributing factor.
- A positive family history predisposes one to this problem.
- Digestive-tract diseases, such as Crohn's disease, increase one's risk.

A persistent obstruction of the bile duct can also result in fever, nausea, and vomiting. At this point, the condition is termed acute cholecystitis. This is an acute inflammation of the gallbladder wall as a response to the gallstone obstruction. In rare cases, infection and pus may fill the gallbladder or cause perforation of the gall-bladder wall. These situations are dangerous and require immediate surgery. While most cases of acute cholecystitis are surgically treated, people who improve greatly within one to two days may not require surgery if the gallstones are small enough to pass into the intestinal tract. Ultrasound and X-rays are used to diagnose gallstones and acute cholecystitis.

The natural approaches in this chapter are highly successful in preventing further gallstone formation and gallbladder inflammation/attacks, as long as the present stones are not too large. People with asymptomatic or "silent" gallstones should not require surgery if the proper diet and supplemental measures are followed.

SYMPTOMS (GALLSTONES AND ACUTE CHOLECYSTITIS)

- Right-sided abdomen pain (or pain anywhere in the abdomen) and radiating pain that goes to the right shoulder blade
- Fever
- Nausea
- Vomiting

ROOT CAUSES

- Drugs, such as oral contraceptives and synthetic hormone replacement and some cholesterol-lowering drugs
- Race (more common in women of North American Indian ethnicity)
- Obesity
- Rapid weight loss
- Constipation
- Western diet (high in saturated fat, low in fiber, alcohol)
- Food allergies/sensitivities (root cause for gallbladder attacks)
- Positive family history
- Increased risk from digestive tract diseases, such as Crohn's

---

Testing Techniques

The following tests help assess possible reasons for gallstone attacks:

    Food allergy/sensitivities—blood or electrodermal

    Stool analysis—analyze fat digestion

    Essential fatty-acid balance—blood test

TREATMENT

Diet

Recommended Food

Fiber-rich foods are important in reducing the likelihood of gallstones. A variety of fruits, vegetables, whole grains, and oat bran is recommended. Include five to seven servings of fruits and vegetables a day.

Regularly eat beets, globe artichokes, and organic dandelion greens, as they improve bile flow.

Olive oil has historically been used by nutritionists and naturopathic doctors to improve bile flow. Use it on salads regularly.

Flaxseeds are a highly concentrated source of essential fatty acids, the "good" fats that reduce inflammation. Add flaxseeds to juices, salads, or fruit plates, or use the oil as a salad dressing.

Studies have shown that vegetarians are at a lower risk for gallstones. This does not mean you need to be a strict vegetarian if you have gallstones, but you should greatly increase the amount of plant foods in your diet.

Food to Avoid

Avoid consumption of fried foods and foods with a high percentage of saturated fat (dairy products and red meat).

It is important to limit your intake of simple carbohydrates and sugars. Researchers have found that gallstones are rare in countries like Africa, where the diet is low in refined sugars and high in fiber. In one study, thirteen people with gallstones ate a diet containing refined carbohydrates for six weeks, then consumed a diet of only unrefined carbohydrates for an additional six weeks. The cholesterol-saturation index of bile (indicating a tendency to form gallstones) was higher in twelve of the thirteen people during the period of time they ate refined carbohydrates.

Food allergies or sensitivities can be a root cause of gallbladder attacks. Since the 1940s, James Breneman, M.D., the former chairman of the Food Allergy Committee of the American College of Allergists, reported that food allergies can initiate gallbladder attacks and gallbladder disease. One study found that 100 percent of a group of patients were symptom free after following an elimination diet that included beef, rye, soy, rice, cherries, peaches, apricots, beets, and spinach for one week. Foods that were most likely to cause gallbladder symptoms in this study included eggs, pork, and onions. Other common triggers included fowl, citrus fruits, milk, coffee, corn, beans, and nuts. Dr. Breneman believes that food allergies cause inflammation and swelling of the bile duct, which restricts bile flow from the gallbladder.

One study found that men who drank coffee had a lower risk of gallstones than men who did not drink coffee. However, coffee initiates gallbladder contractions, so people with known gallstones should avoid its use.

℞ Super Seven Prescriptions—Gallbladder Problems

Super Prescription #1 Wild yam root (*Dioscorea villosa*)
Take 2 to 3 ml or 500 mg of the capsule form every hour for the relief of gallbladder spasms and pain. Wild yam root has an antispasmodic effect on the bile duct.

Super Prescription #2 Bile salts
Take 1 or 2 tablets of bile salts with each meal to improve digestion and the absorption of fats.

Super Prescription #3 Lipase enzymes
Take 1 or 2 capsules of lipase enzymes with each meal to improve fat digestion.

Super Prescription #4 Homeopathic China

Take a 30C potency twice daily for two weeks and then stop using it, unless symptoms return. This remedy is helpful for people with gallstones and gall-bladder disease that causes bloating, nausea, flatulence, and diarrhea, as well as gallbladder pain.

Super Prescription #5 Dandelion root (*Taraxacum officinale*)

Take 2 ml of tincture or 500 mg of the capsule form with every meal. Dandelion root improves bile flow.

Super Prescription #6 Turmeric (*Curcuma longa*)

Take a product standardized to contain 150 mg of curcumin with each meal. Turmeric has anti-inflammatory properties, improves bile flow, and relaxes the bile duct.

Super Prescription #7 Globe artichoke (*Cynara scolymus*)

Take 1 to 2 ml of the tincture or 500 mg of the capsule form with each meal. Globe artichoke improves bile flow.

General Recommendations

Take milk thistle extract standardized to contain a daily total of 420 mg. Milk thistle increases bile flow and decreases bile cholesterol saturation.

Vitamin C is required to convert cholesterol into bile. Take 500 to 1,000 mg three times per day with meals.

Phosphatidylcholine is a component of lecithin that helps increase the solubility of cholesterol. Take 1,000 mg twice daily.

Fish oil reduces inflammation, and animal studies show that a deficiency of essential fatty acids predisposes you to gallstones. Take a daily dosage of an enteric-coated fish oil product containing at least 480 mg of EPA and 360 mg of DHA twice daily.

Full-spectrum digestive enzymes aid in the digestion of food and make food sensitivities less likely. Take 1 or 2 capsules with each meal.

A probiotic supplies friendly bacteria, such as *Lactobacillus acidophilus* and *bifidus*. These good bacteria are involved with cholesterol and bile acid metabolism. Take a product containing at least four billion active organisms daily.

Homeopathy

Pick the remedy that best matches your symptoms in this section. For acute gallstone pain, take a 30C potency four times daily. For chronic gallstone pain, take a 6x, 12x, 6C, 12C, or 30C twice daily for two weeks to see if there are any positive results. After you notice improvement, stop taking the remedy, unless symptoms return. Consultation with a homeopathic practitioner is advised.

Berberis Vulgaris is for sharp, stitching, or colicky pains that radiate from the gallbladder to the stomach or the shoulder. Abdominal pain makes you double over in pain.

Calcarea Carbonica is a good remedy for people with a predisposition to gallbladder problems. The abdomen feels swollen on the right and is sensitive to pressure. The person feels worse from standing, worse from exertion, and better from lying on the painful side. People requiring this remedy are usually overweight and chilly and tire easily. They also tend to feel anxious and overwhelmed. There is a craving for sweets, eggs, and dairy products.

Chelidonium Majus is used when there is pain in the right upper abdomen that radiates to the right shoulder blade. Symptoms are worse from eating fatty foods and better from warm drinks.

China Officinalis is a remedy that is helpful for people with gallstones and gallbladder disease who experience bloating, nausea, flatulence, and diarrhea, as well as gallbladder pain.

Colocynthis is for cramping pains that make a person double over or lie down and apply pressure on the abdomen. Symptoms may come on after anger or suppressed emotions.

Dioscorea is a specific remedy for when people bend backward to relieve the gallbladder pain. Their symptoms are worse from lying down or bending forward.

Lycopodium is a remedy for gallbladder pain accompanied by bloating and a distended abdomen that feel better from warm drinks or warm applications and from rubbing the abdomen. Gas often occurs in the evening (4 to 8 P.M.). People requiring this remedy are often chilly and crave sweets.

Magnesia Phosphoric is helpful for right-sided abdomen pain and gas pains that feel better with warm drinks or warm applications. It is also used for gallbladder spasms.

Nux Vomica is for stitching pains and cramps accompanied by nausea or heartburn. Symptoms may come on after the consumption of spicy foods, coffee, alcohol, or other stimulants. The person feels chilly, impatient, and irritable.

Pulsatilla is specific for gallbladder pains that come on after eating rich or fatty foods like ice cream. The person feels better in the fresh air and desires consolation when not feeling well.

Acupressure

See pages 787–794 for information about acupressure points and administering treatment.
- Work Stomach 36 (St36) to improve digestion.
- Liver 21 (LV21) improves gallbladder function.

Bodywork

Reflexology

See pages 804–805 for information about reflexology areas and how to work them.
Work the gallbladder and the liver area to reduce pain and spasm.

Hydrotherapy

Constitutional hydrotherapy is excellent for improving and reducing gallbladder pain and spasms. It can be used for acute bouts and for long-term prevention.

Aromatherapy

Chamomile and lavender are antispasmodic oils that relax abdominal cramps. Dilute some in a carrier oil and use in a massage, or add a few drops to a warm bath. Each oil is also a pleasant stress-reducer.

Stress Reduction

General Stress-Reduction Therapies

For some people, anger and anxiety worsen existing gallbladder problems. Take time to meditate and relax.

Other Recommendations

Exercise should be part of a program to prevent gallstones. In a study of over sixty thousand women, an average of two to three hours per week of exercise reduced the risk of gallbladder surgery by approximately 20 percent. Choose an exercise system you like and be consistent with it.

REFERENCES

Breneman, J. C. 1968. Allergy elimination diet as the most effective gallbladder diet. *Annals of Allergy* 26:83–87.

Leitzmann, M. F., E. B. Rimm, W. C. Willett, et al. 1999. Recreational physical activity and the risk of cholecystectomy in women. *New England Journal of Medicine* 341:777–84.

Leitzmann, M. F., W. C. Willett, E. B. Rimm, et al. 1999. A prospective study of coffee consumption and the risk of symptomatic gallstone disease in men. *Journal of the American Medical Association* 281:2106–12.

Thornton, J. R., et al. 1983. Diet and gallstones: Effects of refined carbohydrate diets on bile cholesterol saturation and bile acid metabolism. *Gut* 24:2–6.

Gastritis. See Ulcers

Gingivitis

Gingivitis, a type of periodontal disease, is very common in the United States. According to the Centers for Disease Control and Prevention, approximately 34 percent of Americans over thirty years of age have periodontal disease, and 13 percent have a severe case of the disease.

Periodontal disease is an infection of the tissues of the mouth that support the teeth, such as the gums, or gingiva. In periodontal disease, these tissues become inflamed and degenerate. When the gums are involved, the condition is called gingivitis. When the bone and connecting tissues are involved, it is called periodontitis. This chapter focuses on gingivitis.

Those who have this condition often notice swollen gums and bleeding when they brush their teeth. This is a sign of infection and inflammation of the gum tissue.

SYMPTOMS

- Swollen, tender, and/or soft gums
- Gums that bleed easily when brushing or flossing
- Bad taste in mouth
- Bad breath
- Gums reddish rather than pink

ROOT CAUSES

- Poor dental hygiene
- Bacteria buildup in the gums and teeth that forms plaque
- Viral and fungal infections
- Smoking
- Decreased immunity, such as that seen with cancer, diabetes, HIV/AIDS
- Stress
- Pregnancy
- Medications: birth-control pills, steroids, antiseizure, cancer, blood pressure, and those that reduce saliva flow
- Poor-fitting dental restorations
- Substance abuse, such as alcohol and recreational drugs
- Poor nutrition and nutritional deficiencies (such as zinc, vitamin C, folic acid, essential fatty acids, flora imbalance, and coenzyme Q10)
- Food sensitivities

Testing Techniques

The following tests help assess possible reasons for gingivitis:
    Dental exam
    Flora balance—culture of tongue and gum flora
    Vitamin and mineral analysis—blood or urine
    Food sensitivities—blood or electrodermal
    Blood sugar—blood
    Immunity—blood

TREATMENT

Diet

The modern Western diet, which is plentiful in sugar, appears to be a big factor in the prevalence of this disease. Along with proper dental hygiene and nutritional supplements, improved nutrition that reduces inflammation of the gums produces the best results.

Recommended Food

A diet that focuses on whole foods is important in the treatment of this condition. Fish such as sardines, salmon, and trout contain anti-inflammatory essential fatty acids. Consume 2 or 3 servings weekly. Increase your intake of vegetables, nuts, seeds, and whole grains. Fresh vegetable juice daily will help to reduce inflammation. Use chewing gum that contains xylitol, which prevents the buildup of bad bacteria.

Food to Avoid

Sugar feeds the bacteria that accumulate on the gums and teeth. Limit processed foods, candy, undiluted fruit juices, refined grains, and other simple sugars.

R̥ **Super Seven Prescriptions—Gingivitis**

Super Prescription #1 Coenzyme Q10
Take 100 mg daily with a meal. Studies show that this nutrient has a healing effect on periodontal disease.

Super Prescription #2 Folic acid mouthwash
Use 5 ml twice per day of a 0.1 percent solution. This has been shown to reduce the symptoms of gingivitis.

Super Prescription #3 Vitamin C
Take 1,000 mg twice daily. Vitamin C is required for good immunity and healthy tissue formation. It also reduces inflammation.

Super Prescription #4 Green tea
Drink 1 to 3 cups daily. The polyphenols have been shown to fight the bacteria that cause gum disease.

Super Prescription #5 Calcium
Calcium deficiency has been shown to increase the risk of periodontal disease. Take 500 mg twice daily along with vitamin D (1,000 IU).

Super Prescription #6 Bioflavonoids
Take 500 mg twice daily to strengthen gum tissue so that it is more resistant to bleeding.

Super Prescription #7 Tea tree oil mouth rinse
Take as directed on the label to destroy the bacteria linked to gum disease.

Chronic periodontal disease is a risk factor for various systemic diseases that go far beyond the mouth. For example, people with periodontal disease are almost twice as likely to have coronary artery disease than those without periodontal disease. This condition can also worsen existing heart conditions. Those with this disease also seem to be more susceptible to a stroke. Although the mechanism isn't totally clear, it is thought that the bacteria of the mouth travel to the arteries and create inflammation, or else they just create a systemic inflammatory response. Recent studies also suggest a relationship between periodontal disease and rheumatoid arthritis.

A study published in *Molecular Aspects of Medicine* found that the topical application of coenzyme Q10 resulted in a significant alleviation of gingivitis. Other studies have shown it to be helpful when taken internally as a supplement.

General Recommendations

Essential fatty acids reduce inflammation of the gums. Take a fish oil product containing 1,000 mg of EPA and DHA or 1 tablespoon of flaxseed or hempseed oil daily.

Betaine hydrochloride improves the absorption of the nutrients required for good gum health. Take 1 or 2 capsules with each meal. Xylitol-containing mouth rinses fight the bacteria associated with gum disease. Probiotics contain species specific for gum health. Take as directed on the label.

Homeopathy

Pick the remedy that best matches your symptoms in this section. Take a 6x, 12x, 6C, 12C, or 30C potency twice daily for two weeks to see if there is any improvement. If you notice improvement, stop taking the remedy unless your symptoms return. Consultation with a homeopathic practitioner is advised.

Kreosotum is for gums that are inflamed, along with infected teeth or jaw.

Mercurius solubilis or vivus is for spongy gums that have a bad odor and/or pus formation.

Phosphorus is for gums that bleed very easily and feel better from cold applications.

Silica is for swollen, painful gums that have a tendency to form boils and pus.

Acupressure

- Stomach 36 (St36) improves digestion and absorption related to gum health.
- Large Intestine 4 (LI4) is used for inflamed gums.

Bodywork

Reflexology

Work on the areas of the foot that correspond to the mouth. See pages 804–805 for more information about reflexology areas and how to work them.

Hydrotherapy

If poor digestion is present, follow the constitutional hydrotherapy treatment on pages 795–796.

Other Recommendations

Work with a holistic dentist and a holistic doctor to address the root causes of your gum disease. Laser therapies and essential-oil mouth rinses can be helpful.

REFERENCES

Hanioka, T., et al. 1994. Effect of topical application of coenzyme Q10 on adult periodontitis. *Molecular Aspects of Medicine* 15(Suppl):S241–48.

Glaucoma

Glaucoma affects more than two million Americans and is the second leading cause of blindness in this country. This can be a very serious disease that must be given medical care as soon as possible if permanent vision loss is to be avoided. In the healthy eye, fluid is produced and drained at equal rates. If the fluid cannot drain properly, it builds up and puts pressure on the optic nerve, the retina, and the lens. This pressure can partially damage or even completely destroy the retina and the optic nerve.

If the outflow channels are open and become blocked with debris, the disorder is called open-angle glaucoma. Chronic open-angle glaucoma is the most common form and usually occurs over years. Fluid drains too slowly from the anterior chamber of the eye and pressure builds up. At first, increased pressure in the eyes produces no symptoms. As the disease progresses, symptoms may include narrowing peripheral vision, mild headaches, and vague visual disturbances, such as seeing halos around electric lights or having difficulty adapting to darkness. At some point, tunnel vision—where the visual field narrows and makes it hard to see anything on either side when looking forward—may develop.

If the channels are blocked by the iris, the disorder is called closed-angle glaucoma. Fluid pressure increases quickly and causes intense pain in one eye, along with headaches and vision problems, including blurring or a "halo effect" around lights. The eyeball feels hard to the touch, and the pain may be so severe that it causes nausea and even vomiting. The eyelid swells, and the eye becomes red and watery. These symptoms are warning signs that you must receive medical care immediately. Permanent vision loss and even total blindness can settle in after just a few days. Fortunately, acute glaucoma is rather rare and accounts for only 10 percent of all glaucoma cases. Certain medications, long periods spent in darkness, and stress are all potential triggers for an attack.

Since the disease targets older people most frequently, anyone over sixty-five should make glaucoma tests part of their annual eye exam. African Americans, who have a much higher incidence of glaucoma than the rest of the population, should start getting annual tests after the age of forty, as should anyone with diabetes. If at any age you experience a loss of peripheral vision, constant low-level headaches, eye pain, or blurred vision that is not corrected with one new lens prescription, see a doctor at once. If you test positive for glaucoma, you may not be able to recover the damage that's already been done, but there's a good chance that you can significantly slow the progress of the disease.

There does not seem to be one single cause of glaucoma. Most likely, a variety of factors come into play. A good strategy for prevention, as well as treatment in conjunction with a doctor's care, incorporates reducing the general number of toxins in the body, eating foods that support the eye, correcting nutritional deficiencies associated with glaucoma, enhancing digestion, avoiding medications that predispose one to glaucoma, and reducing stress.

SYMPTOMS OF OPEN-ANGLE GLAUCOMA

- Narrowing peripheral vision
- Mild headaches
- Vague visual disturbances
- Tunnel vision

SYMPTOMS OF CLOSED-ANGLE GLAUCOMA

Chronic glaucoma is usually asymptomatic until irreversible damage has already been done. Signs that chronic glaucoma has already progressed include the following:

- Intense pain in one eye, with vision problems
- Nausea and vomiting
- Swollen eyelid
- Red, watery eye
- Vision loss

ROOT CAUSES

- Accumulation of wastes and metabolic slowdown related to aging
- High blood pressure
- Some prescription drugs, including corticosteroids, antidepressants, and blood pressure medication
- Certain illnesses, such as other eye disorders (especially macular degeneration) and diabetes
- Nutritional deficiency
- Heredity

Testing Techniques

The following tests help assess possible reasons for glaucoma:

    Blood pressure

    Hormone testing (thyroid)—saliva, blood, or urine

    Intestinal permeability—urine

    Detoxification profile—urine

    Vitamin and mineral analysis (especially magnesium, vitamin C)—blood

    Food and environmental allergies/sensitivities—blood, electrodermal

    Blood sugar balance—blood

TREATMENT

If you have glaucoma of either kind, you must be under a doctor's care. The therapies listed here will complement and support your conventional treatment. Natural therapies work very well for chronic and open-angle glaucoma.

Diet

Recommended Food

Eat a basic, wholesome diet based on whole grains and fresh fruits and vegetables.

Carotenoids are essential for optimum eye health. Consume plenty of orange, yellow, and green leafy vegetables. It is also highly recommended that you drink live juice made from these and other fruits and vegetables several times a day.

The bioflavonoid anthocyanidin fights free radicals and helps keep the collagen around the eye healthy and flexible. Blueberries and cherries are excellent sources.

Drink a glass of clean, quality water every two waking hours to flush out toxins and to keep the eye tissues supple. Spread your consumption of water and other liquids out across the day, so that you do not buildup pressure in your eye.

Some studies have shown fish oils to lower eye pressure. Incorporate fatty fish such as salmon, mackerel, and cod into your meals two or three times a week.

Chromium and magnesium both have beneficial effects on glaucoma. Brewer's yeast is the best source of chromium; kelp, leafy greens, apples, and safflower and sesame oils will provide you with magnesium.

Food to Avoid

If you have glaucoma, do not take the herb ephedra (*Ma huang*), which dilates the pupils and may increase eye pressure.

Fluid retention in the eye may be a response to food allergies. See the Food Allergies section to determine whether a food is contributing to your problem. If you find that consumption of a certain food makes your eyes red, irritated, painful, or tender, you must avoid that product from now on.

Caffeine has been shown to reduce blood flow to the eye, so avoid coffee, chocolate, and caffeinated teas and sodas.

A toxic liver may be related to eye problems. Avoid alcohol, which puts a terrible burden on this essential organ.

℞ Super Seven Prescriptions—Glaucoma

Super Prescription #1 Magnesium

Take 250 mg twice daily. Magnesium relaxes the blood vessel walls and improves blood flow to the eye.

Super Prescription #2 Curcumin

Take 500 mg twice daily. Research shows curcumin can reduce intraocular eye pressure and slow the progression of glaucoma.

Super Prescription #3 Fish oil

Take a formula containing a daily dose of 600 mg of EPA and 400 mg of DHA. Animal studies using this supplement show a significant drop in intraocular pressure.

Super Prescription #4 Vitamin C

Take 1,000 mg two to four times daily. Studies show that vitamin C supplementation reduces eye pressure.

Super Prescription #5 Bilberry (*Vaccinium myrtillus*)

Take 160 mg twice daily of a 25 percent anthocyanosides extract. Bilberry improves blood flow and contains flavonoids that support eye structure and function.

Super Prescription #6 *Ginkgo biloba*

Take 60 mg three times daily of a 24 percent flavone glycoside extract. Ginkgo has been shown to be helpful for glaucoma. It improves blood flow and contains flavonoids that support eye structure and function.

Super Prescription #7 Chromium

Take 250 to 500 mcg twice daily. It is particularly important for people with diabetes to supplement for blood sugar balance and the prevention of glaucoma.

Studies using 2,000 mg or more a day of vitamin C demonstrate that this nutrient lowers intraocular pressure in people with glaucoma. One study found that vitamin C reduced intraocular pressure by a whopping 16mm Hg. An even more aggressive approach is to consult with a physician who uses intravenous vitamin C. The benefits of vitamin C are only present as long as one is supplementing this nutrient.

General Recommendations

Grapeseed extract or maritime pine bark improves circulation. Take 100 to 200 mg daily.

Rutin is a bioflavonoid that has been shown in older studies to help glaucoma. Take 20 mg three times daily.

Homeopathy

Chronic glaucoma is a constitutional disorder, so see a homeopathic practitioner for a specific remedy that suits your individual tendencies and needs.

Acupressure

The following points are especially helpful for people who use their eyes a great deal and suffer from eyestrain. For information about pressure points and administering treatment, see pages 787–794.

A proprietary formula containing 80 mg of pycnogenol and 160 mg of bilberry extract was found to significantly improve intraocular pressure (IOP) and maintain a healthier IOP over the six-month investigational period. No side effects were observed.

- Stomach 3 (St3) relieves pressure on the eyes.
- Bladder 10 (B10) soothes eyes that are tired and red from eyestrain.
- Improve blood flow to your head and eyes by working Large Intestine 3 and 4 (LI3 and LI4).

Bodywork

Massage can't relieve glaucoma directly, but neck and head massage will ease stress and improve circulation to the eye area.

Chiropractic, craniosacral, or osteopathic treatments may also be helpful.

Reflexology

See pages 804–805 for information about reflexology areas and how to work them. Work the areas corresponding to the eyes, the neck, and the kidneys.

Aromatherapy

Stress is a trigger for acute glaucoma and may be a contributing factor in the chronic version. Many oils can help you handle tension and anxiety, but here are some good ones to start: bergamot, jasmine, lavender, rose, sandalwood, or ylang-ylang. You can use them in any preparation you like, but do be sure not to rely on just one oil, as it might lose some of its effects from overuse.

Stress Reduction

General Stress-Reduction Therapies

Stress may contribute to glaucoma, and it's definitely caused by glaucoma. For many people, vision problems mark a significant change of life. Consider learning to meditate. You'll reduce daily tension, and you can practice the technique for the rest of your life, no matter what the condition of your eyes.

Other Recommendations

- Avoid eyestrain from reading or working at computer terminals for long periods. Take frequent breaks and look away from the screen or your reading material often.
- Don't watch television in the dark. Prolonged periods in the darkness with the pupils dilated can bring on acute glaucoma.
- Tobacco smoke reduces blood flow to the retina, so don't smoke. You must also avoid smoky rooms, bars, and restaurants.
- Mild to moderate aerobic exercise can reduce eye pressure, so find an activity you enjoy and make it a daily habit.
- Wear sunglasses that block UVA and UVB rays; both kinds of light create free radicals that have been linked to glaucoma.

REFERENCES

Filina, A. A., N. G. Davydova, S. N. Endrikhovskii, et al. 1995. Lipoic acid as a means of metabolic therapy of open-angle glaucoma. *Vestnik Oftalmologii* 111:6–8.

Ringsdorf, W. M., Jr., and E. Cheraskin. 1981. Ascorbic acid and glaucoma: A review. *Journal of Holistic Medicine* 3:167–72.

Steigerwalt, R. D., et al. 2008. Effects of Mirtogenol on ocular blood flow and intraocular hypertension in asymptomatic subjects. *Molecular Vision* 14:1288–92.

Virno, M., et al. 1967. Oral treatment of glaucoma with vitamin C. *Eye Ear Nose Throat Monthly* 46:1502–8.

Gluten Sensitivity

Gluten sensitivity (GS) is a very common condition that affects the health of millions of Americans. While it is slowly being recognized by conventional medicine, holistic doctors have been helping people with a variety of health problems by identifying this intolerance to gluten-containing grains such as wheat, rye, barley, and possibly oats.

A class of proteins known as prolamins, which are found in several grains, is what people with celiac disease or GS react to. Gluten is made up of the proteins (prolamins) glutenin and gliadin, found in wheat. The reactive prolamin in rye is secalin, and in barley it is hordein. Gluten has become the general term for the prolamins that those with celiac disease and GS react to.

Celiac disease (CD) is similar to but different from gluten sensitivity. It, too, is underdiagnosed in the United States. About three million Americans, or 1 out of every 133 people, have CD. Many people with CD have not been diagnosed. This is an autoimmune disease in which the immune system attacks the gluten particles and then cross-reacts with the tissues of the digestive tract. This reaction to gluten damages the fingerlike projections (villi) of the small intestine that are responsible for the absorption of food and nutrients. This leads to the malabsorption of foods and nutrients. The result is nutritional deficiencies.

CD also contributes to leaky gut syndrome, in which toxins and larger-than-normal food particles, including gluten particles, are absorbed into the bloodstream and further worsen autoimmunity.

There are two key genes that have been identified in CD, and they can be identified with testing. These are HLA DQ2 and HLA DQ8. If you don't have either gene, there is a 99 percent chance that you won't develop CD. However, this does not rule out gluten sensitivity, which often does not show up in conventional blood, stool, or small intestine biopsy testing.

CD is diagnosed by blood tests and, in some cases, with a biopsy of the small intestine. Many people who have a normal blood test or biopsy may still have GS.

People with CD must strictly avoid all foods, medications, supplements, and other substances that contain gluten, because it can make them very ill. Those with GS may be able to tolerate various amounts of gluten, depending on their overall sensitivity and intestinal health.

"After three days of following a gluten-free diet, the diarrhea I have experienced for twenty-five years is gone!" These are the words of Arthur, a fifty-six-year-old engineer who, despite being under the care of gastroenterologists, had never gotten relief for his chronic diarrhea. His previous doctors had done various diagnostic images and a biopsy of his small intestine. This had included testing for CD, which was negative. Yet alternative testing that included a stool test found severe GS, which was the key to his recovery.

SYMPTOMS

- Fatigue
- Digestive upset (gas, bloating, diarrhea, constipation, reflux, abdominal pain, nausea)
- Headaches (including migraine, tension, and sinus headaches)
- Hormone imbalance, infertility, irregular periods
- Hair loss
- Bone and muscle pain
- Skin problems, including eczema, psoriasis, and vitiligo

- Poor memory
- Weight loss
- Weight gain
- Mood problems (anxiety, depression)
- Stunted growth

- Canker sores
- Anemia
- Autoimmune conditions, especially Hashimoto's thyroiditis
- Seizures

ROOT CAUSES

- Genetics
- Excessive consumption of gluten-containing products
- Leaky gut syndrome and malabsorption (including acid-suppressing medications that result in poor digestion and

  absorption)
- Fungal infection (often caused by overuse of antibiotics)
- Hybridization of wheat and other grains that create foreign proteins

---

Testing Techniques

The following test can help determine GS:

Can be diagnosed by the strict avoidance of gluten for several weeks to see if the symptoms abate.

Lab tests to diagnose GS—stool, saliva, blood, or urine. This type of testing is available through specialized laboratories used by holistic doctors.

TREATMENT

Diet

Recommended Food

Alternative foods to gluten that can be consumed include the following:

- Amaranth
- Arrowroot
- Buckwheat
- Corn
- Millet

- Potatoes
- Quinoa
- Rice
- Soy
- Teff

One can also consume fruits, vegetables, dairy products, eggs, fish, legumes, red meat, seafood, nuts, and poultry (all are gluten free).

Yogurt with live cultures and with friendly flora aid digestion. *Note*: Many people with a gluten allergy or sensitivity also have problems with the cow's milk protein known as casein.

Food to Avoid

- Wheat (including wheat flour, wheat germ, wheat bran, cracked wheat, einkorn wheat, emmer

  wheat)
- Couscous
- Kamut

- Spelt
- Semolina
- Rye
- Triticale
- Barley

- Oats (most oats are often contaminated with wheat, but certified gluten-free varieties are available)

℞ Super Seven Prescriptions—Gluten Sensitivity

Super Prescription #1 Digestive enzyme complex
Choose a formula that contains DPP-IV, which reduces the reaction to gluten. Take as directed on the label.

Super Prescription #2 Probiotic
Take five to ten billion colony-forming organisms daily. Studies show that people on a gluten-restricted diet tend to have lower levels of good bacteria.

Super Prescription #3 Multivitamin and -mineral formula
Take as directed on the label to supply nutrients that may be deficient on a gluten-free diet.

Super Prescription #4 Vitamin D
Take 2,000 to 5,000 IU daily with meals.

Super Prescription #5 Fish oil
Take 1,500 mg of EPA and DHA combined to reduce inflammation of the digestive tract.

Super Prescription #6 Betaine hydrochloride
Take 1 or 2 capsules with each meal to improve digestion.

Super Prescription #7 Calcium
Take 500 mg daily along with 250 mg of magnesium to supply extra nutrients that may be needed by those with GS.

Homeopathy

See a practitioner for the remedy that best meets your body's imbalances.

Acupressure

See pages 787–794 for information about pressure points and administering treatment.
- Stomach 36 (St36) is an overall toner and strengthens the digestive system.
- Large Intestine 4 and 13 (LI4 and LI13) and Triple Warmer 5 (TW5) relieve the reactions that accompany GS.

Bodywork

Reflexology

See pages 804–805 for information about reflexology areas and how to work them. Focus on the stomach and the small intestine areas.

Hydrotherapy

Constitutional hydrotherapy is healing to the intestinal walls. See pages 795–796 on how to use these treatments at home.

Aromatherapy

The essential oil black pepper has anti-inflammatory properties. Peppermint oil supports the digestive system and is a pain reliever.

Gout

Gout is an intensely painful disorder caused by the buildup of uric acid. Although it affects both sexes, men are much more likely—by a factor of ten—to suffer from gout. The condition was once known as the "rich man's disease," and, in fact, it often strikes people who eat heavy, fatty foods and who overindulge in alcohol. Although this kind of diet was once solely the province of the wealthy, one no longer has to be rich to eat poorly. Today, the disease affects people across the entire spectrum of economic classes.

Uric acid is a metabolic by-product of protein breakdown. Purines raise uric acid levels in the body. Most purines are created by the body, but a few are taken in through food and drink. Since purines can't be absorbed, they are normally broken down by a digestive enzyme that allows them to be dissolved and passed out of the body in urine. If there is more uric acid than the enzymes can break down, the acid accumulates in the tissues and the bloodstream. Eventually, it crystallizes into needle-shaped deposits. These sharp crystals of uric acid poke their way into the tissue that surrounds a joint and ultimately penetrate the joint itself. The resulting pain is extreme and is usually followed by redness and swelling of the joint, which may be highly sensitive to the touch. The pain may go on for days or even weeks, and unless the cause of gout is addressed, the attack is likely to recur. A person with gout is also more likely to suffer from uric acid kidney stones. Gout most often occurs in the joint at the base of the big toe, but it may also appear in other locations like the ankle, the thumb, the wrist, the elbow, and even the earlobe.

Newer research is demonstrating that people with insulin resistance are more susceptible to gout. It is estimated that 76 percent of people with gout have insulin resistance. With this condition, the cells become resistant to the hormone insulin, and blood glucose levels remain high. This in turn leads to increased insulin levels and a resulting uric acid increase. If you follow a syndrome X–type diet (one rich in plant foods, moderate protein consumption—especially fish—and low in saturated fat and refined carbohydrates), uric acid decreases and the resultant gout flare-ups can be prevented. This, along with a calorie-restricted diet and exercise, should be the primary plan for people with gout. Also, fungal overgrowth in the body may increase uric acid levels.

Conventional medicines that lower the levels of uric acid are available, but you should consider them a last resort. For hundreds of years, the best way to treat gout has been with diet and detoxification therapies. Sometimes doctors automatically prescribe medication for gout because they don't believe their patients will commit to changing their diets. If your doctor suggests medication for you, explain to him or her that you're willing to try a new eating plan. You may find that you can forgo harsh medicines entirely.

SYMPTOMS

- Sharp pain, usually in a single joint and most often in the big toe
- Fever
- Inflamed, red joints that feel hot and are tender to the touch

ROOT CAUSES

- A diet high in saturated fats, refined carbohydrates, and alcohol
- Insulin resistance
- Dehydration (in people susceptible to gout)
- Obesity
- Kidney disease
- Surgery
- Joint injury
- Stress
- Pharmaceutical medications that increase uric acid (e.g., aspirin, diuretics, and high-dose niacin therapy)
- Lead toxicity
- High blood pressure
- Acidic system

A study of twelve people with gout found that eating one-half pound of fresh or canned cherries or drinking a full quart of cherry juice prevented gout attacks. In all twelve people, uric acid levels returned to normal, and the gout attacks ceased. Black, sweet yellow, and red sour cherries were all effective.

Testing Techniques

The following tests help assess possible reasons for gout:

Urinary pH—urine

Detoxification profile—urine

Vitamin and mineral analysis (especially magnesium, folic acid, B6, B12)—blood

Food and environmental allergies/sensitivities—blood, electrodermal

Blood-sugar balance—blood

Uric acid—blood

Fungi—stool

TREATMENT

Diet

Recommended Food

For the first stages of an attack, see the detoxification suggestions further on.

After the pain has subsided, introduce whole grains, nuts, seeds, and soy products into your meals. These foods are high in fiber, which encourages the elimination of uric acid, and soy products are excellent vegetarian sources of protein. Continue to eat several helpings of raw fruits and vegetables daily.

Berries, especially cherries, strawberries, and blueberries, neutralize uric acid. Eat fresh berries as snacks or for dessert, and drink a glass of cherry juice every day.

Flaxseeds are a highly concentrated source of essential fatty acids, the "good" fats that reduce inflammation. Add flaxseeds to juices, salads, or fruit plates, or use the oil as a salad dressing.

One of the most important foods you can eat to prevent gout is fish. Eat fish such as salmon, cod, halibut, and sardines, as they reduce inflammation.

Drink as much clean, quality water as you can. One glass every two waking hours should be your minimum consumption.

Food to Avoid

The traditional approach for treating gout has been to eliminate from your diet foods that are high in purines: red meat, meat broths and gravies, bouillon, consommé, sweetbreads, shellfish, anchovies, sardines, herring, mushrooms, asparagus, brewer's yeast, fish, poultry, eggs, dried beans, peas, lentils, cooked spinach and rhubarb. However, for people with insulin resistance (the majority of gout sufferers), this can make your gout problem worse. Instead, focus on eating the foods in the recommended food list.

Rich foods aggravate gout pain. Stay away from saturated, hydrogenated, and partially hydrogenated fats and oils, and do not eat products made with refined flour or sugar.

Alcohol increases uric acid levels. If you suffer from gout, you must not drink alcohol in any form.

A study published in *Archives of Internal Medicine* found that higher vitamin C intake is associated with a significantly decreased risk of gout in men. Ingesting 500 to 1,500 mg of vitamin C daily from the diet and/or supplements is associated with a 17 to 34 percent reduced risk of gout compared to consuming less than 250 mg daily.

℞ Super Seven Prescription—Gout

Super Prescription #1 Homeopathic Colchicum
Take a 30C potency every waking two hours for two days. This homeopathic remedy is specific for gout pains that are worse with any motion.

Super Prescription #2 Celery seed extract
Take 450 mg two to three times daily to treat and prevent gout. Celery seed extract has anti-inflammatory effects and may reduce uric acid levels.

Super Prescription #3 Nettle root (*Urtica dioica*)
Nettle root encourages the elimination of uric acid from the kidneys. Select a product made with the concentrated root extract, and take 250 mg three times a day.

Super Prescription #4 Cherry extract
This reduces the uric acid level and inflammation. Take as directed on the label.

Super Prescription #5 Vitamin C
Take 500 mg two to three times daily to reduce the risk of gout.

Super Prescription #6 Fish oil
Take a daily dosage of a fish oil product containing at least 480 mg of EPA and 360 mg of DHA. Fish oil reduces inflammation in the joints.

Super Prescription #7 Folic acid
Take 10 to 40 mg daily, under the supervision of a doctor. High doses of folic acid may help reduce uric acid levels.

General Recommendations

Quercitin has natural anti-inflammatory effects. Take 500 to 1,000 mg three times daily.

Devil's claw (*Harpagophytum procumbens*) should not be taken if you have a history of gallstones, heartburn, or ulcers. Take 1,500 to 2,500 mg of the standardized powdered herb in capsule or tablet form daily, or use 1 to 2 ml of a tincture three times a day.

Dandelion root (*Taraxacum officinalis*) cleanses the kidneys. Take 500 mg or 1 to 2 ml three times daily. Be sure the preparation you use is made from the dried root.

A cream made with capsicum (cayenne pepper) has a remarkable and documented ability to relieve pain. You can find capsicum cream at most health food stores. Apply the cream to the affected area two to four times daily for symptomatic relief. Choose a cream standardized to 0.025 to 0.075 percent capsaicin. Capsaicin depletes the nerves of substance P, a neurotransmitter that transmits pain messages.

Chlorella is rich in chlorophyll and works to alkalinize the body. Take 500 mg four times daily.

Bromelain has a natural anti-inflammatory effect. Take 500 mg three times daily between meals. Look for products standardized to 2,000 MCU (milk-clotting units) per 1,000 mg or 1,200 GDU (gelatin-dissolving units) per 1,000 mg.

Protease enzyme products also have a natural anti-inflammatory benefit.

Homeopathy

Pick the remedy that best matches your symptoms in this section. For acute gout pain, take a 30C potency four times daily. For low-grade gout pain, take a lower potency, such as 6x, 12x, or 12C, twice daily for two weeks to see if there are any positive results. After you notice improvement, stop taking the remedy, unless symptoms return. Consultation with a homeopathic practitioner is advised.

Arnica (*Arnica montana*) is for deep, bruising pain.

Belladonna (*Atropa belladonna*) is for intense, throbbing, and burning pain that comes on quickly. The joint looks red and is worse from jarring.

Bryonia (*Bryonia alba*) is for pain that intensifies with the slightest touch or movement. The person becomes very irritable.

Ledum (*Ledum palustre*) is the remedy for throbbing pain that is better from ice and cold-water applications. The knees and the feet are affected.

Pulsatilla (*Pulsatilla pratensis*) will ease pain that moves around within the joint and that improves with gentle motion and the application of a cold compress.

Rhododendron is for gout of the big toe that flares up before a storm. Warm applications feel better.

Sulfur is for gout where there is a burning sensation and itching of the skin. Symptoms are better with cold applications and worse from any heat.

Acupressure

No matter where gout surfaces in your body, you can use Large Intestine 4 (LI4) to significantly reduce the pain.

People with gout should avoid high doses of niacin (more than 1,000 mg), as it can increase uric acid in some individuals.

South African researchers placed men with a history of gout on a nonconventional diet more suited for people with insulin resistance. The diet was higher in protein, complex carbohydrates (instead of refined carbs), and polyunsaturated and monounsaturated fats (instead of saturated fats). High-purine foods, such as poultry and fish, were not restricted. After four months on this diet, the average number of gout attacks fell by two-thirds. The average decrease in uric acid was 18 percent. In addition, there were an average loss of seventeen pounds and improvements in lipid markers (e.g., lowered LDL cholesterol and triglycerides, and improved HDL cholesterol.)

Bodywork

Massage

Do not rub the painful joint, as a local massage will only aggravate the pain. (During an acute attack, you probably won't even want to touch the area.) However, a lymphatic massage for the rest of the body will help break down toxins, and it will help distract you, albeit temporarily, from the gout. Add juniper oil to the massage for added detoxification benefits.

Reflexology

See pages 804–805 for information about reflexology areas and how to work them. Work the areas corresponding to the kidneys and to the body part affected by gout.

Hydrotherapy

Some people find that cold water is welcome relief for a "hot" joint; others find that warm or hot hydrotherapy is more soothing. You will probably know instinctively which is best for you, so choose between the following suggestions accordingly.

During an acute attack, hold the joint under cold running water. Follow up with a cool bath.

Constitutional hydrotherapy can be used to help with acute gout and prevent further problems, due to its detoxifying qualities.

Other Bodywork Recommendations

Apply a hot or cold compress to the affected joint. To speed up the expulsion of uric acid, you can add juniper oil to the compress.

Acupuncture can be very helpful for acute gout.

Aromatherapy

Juniper oil helps break down toxic deposits and carry them away from the body. Add it to a hot sitz bath or a compress, or dilute it in a carrier oil and use in a massage (but don't rub the affected joint directly).

Other Recommendations

- Exercise will stimulate blood flow and decrease pain. Try a nonimpact sport like swimming.
- Magnet therapy can be effective in alleviating the pain of gout. Use as directed by a knowledgeable practitioner.
- People who are overweight are more vulnerable to gout than others are. If you need to lose weight, the dietary suggestions here can help. For further suggestions, see Obesity.

REFERENCES

Blau, L. W. 1950. Cherry diet control for gout and arthritis. Texas Reports on Biology and Medicine 8:309–11.

Choi, H. K., et al. 2009. Vitamin C intake and the risk of gout in men. *Archives of Internal Medicine* 169:502–7.

Dessein, P. H., E. A. Shipton, A. E. Stanwix, et al. 2000. Beneficial effects of weight loss associated with moderate calorie/carbohydrate restriction, and increased proportional intake of protein and unsaturated fat on serum urate and lipoprotein levels in gout: A pilot study. *Annals of the Rheumatic Diseases* 59(7):539–43.

Hair Loss

In the body's renewal process, most of us lose fifty to one hundred hairs every day. The average rate of growth is approximately ½ inch per month. Interestingly, hair grows fastest in the summer, as heat and friction speed up growth. Conversely, it grows more slowly in the cold and the winter months. More rapid hair loss begins in both sexes by age forty and tends to accelerate once people reach their fifties. A human adult body has an average of five million hairs, with 100,000 to 150,000 of those located on the scalp.

Since most of us grow new strands to replace the ones that have been shed, there's usually no reason to worry about a few stray hairs that come out with a good brushing or that swirl down the drain after a shower. Hair loss poses a potential problem only if it leads to noticeable thinning or balding, and even then it is often a normal part of life.

Genetics and hormones determine the most common reasons for hair loss. Male-pattern baldness is characterized by a receding hairline and loss of hair, especially on the crown of the head. By age forty, two-thirds of Caucasian men are noticeably bald. Female-pattern baldness is characterized by a general thinning of the hair all over the head and a moderate loss of hair on the crown or the hairline. It also occurs between the ages of thirty and forty and often becomes more apparent during and after menopause. About 50 percent of children with a balding parent of either sex will inherit the dominant baldness gene. Besides age and genetics, the main culprit in balding appears to be an overabundance or overactivity of the male hormone dihydrotestosterone (DHT) within the hair follicle. DHT is a derivative of testosterone and is driven by an enzyme called 5-alpha reductase, which is produced in the prostate, the adrenal glands, and the scalp. The activity of this enzyme tends to increase as people, especially men, age. It also causes the hair follicle to degrade, and it shortens the growth phase. Some follicles die, but most shrink and produce weaker hairs that become thinner, many to the point where they fall out from daily activities. Another important hormone is progesterone. Menopausal women commonly find improvement with the use of natural progesterone and estrogen for excessive hair loss.

Other physiological factors might cause hair loss. Recently, a group of Japanese researchers reported a correlation between excessive sebum in the scalp and hair loss. Excessive sebum, often accompanying thinning hair, is attributed to an enlargement of the sebaceous gland. The researchers believe that excessive sebum causes a high level of 5-alpha reductase and pore clogging, leading to malnutrition of the hair root. Animal fat in the diet is believed to increase sebum production. Medical researchers in Asia also believe that hair loss is caused mainly by an insufficient blood supply to the scalp.

The effects of stress can cause hair loss and thinning in both men and women. Generally, this type of hair loss or thinning is reversible once the levels of stress have come down or the person has dealt with the stress sufficiently.

In addition, various autoimmune and other systemic diseases can lead to hair loss. The list includes many conditions, ranging from psoriasis to thyroid disease to cancer.

Other reasons for hair loss and thinning may include strict dieting (the loss is

It is common for women who are going through menopause to experience hair loss and thinning. This is due to the fluctuating changes in many of their hormones. Natural hormone-balancing protocols, administered by a knowledgeable doctor, can reverse this hair loss. Also, low levels of thyroid hormone can result in hair loss in women and men of all ages. This can include thinning of the eyebrows. Hypothyroidism often develops around menopause or during pregnancy. On the other hand, hyperthyroidism can be the cause of hair loss as well.

due to malnutrition), heavy-metal toxicity (e.g., arsenic), chemotherapy, and severe illness. Several different nutrient deficiencies can contribute to hair loss, brittleness, or thinning. In women, the most common deficiency contributing to hair loss is iron deficiency. You will need a blood test by your doctor to see if this is occurring.

No matter whether you have a temporary or permanent condition, many complementary therapies exist that can help you improve your hair and scalp health. While they can't completely reverse permanent baldness, many treatments can encourage small but significant regrowth.

Genetic Baldness . . . or Medication?

If you experience thinning or receding hair, chances are that you're seeing the first signs of genetic-pattern baldness. Before you come to a conclusion, however, you should run a check of any medications you might be taking. Many pharmaceutical medications cause hair loss, such as the following:

Cholesterol-lowering drugs:
clofibrate (Atromid-S) and gemfibrozil (Lopid)

Parkinson medications:
levodopa (Dopar, Larodopa)

Ulcer drugs:
cimetidine (Tagamet), ranitidine (Zantac), and famotidine (Pepcid)

Anticoagulants:
Coumarin and heparin

Agents for gout:
allopurinol (Loporin, Zyloprim)

Antiarthritics:
penicillamine, auranofin (Ridaura), indomethacin (Indocin), naproxen

(Naprosyn), sulindac (Clinoril), and methotrexate (Folex)

Drugs derived from vitamin A:
isotretinoin (Accutane) and etretinate (Tegison)

Anticonvulsants for epilepsy:
trimethadione (Tridione)

Antidepressants:
tricyclics, amphetamines

Beta-blocker drugs for high blood pressure:
atenolol (Tenormin), metoprolol (Lopressor), nadolol (Corgard), propranolol (Inderal), and timolol (Blocadren)

Antithyroid agents:
carbimazole, iodine, thiocyanate, thiouracil

Others:
Blood thinners, male hormones (anabolic steroids), and chemotherapeutic agents

---

SYMPTOMS

- Receding hairline
- Thinning hair
- Hair that falls out in patches

ROOT CAUSES

- Heredity
- Hormone imbalance (particularly, thyroid)
- Serious illness, especially with a high fever
- Pregnancy

- Menopause
- Stress
- Chemotherapy
- Hypothyroidism
- Autoimmune disorders
- Crash or fad diets

- Syphilis
- Extremely high doses of vitamin A
- Nutritional deficiencies
- Heavy-metal toxicity
- Poor scalp circulation
- Malabsorption, parasites

Testing Techniques

The following tests help assess possible reasons for hair loss:

Hormone testing (thyroid, cortisol, DHEA, testosterone, dihydrotestosterone, estradiol, progesterone)—saliva, blood, or urine

Intestinal permeability—urine

Vitamin and mineral analysis (especially iron)—blood

Heavy-metal toxicity—hair or urine

Stool analysis—parasites, fungal overgrowth

TREATMENT

Diet

Recommended Food

Hair loss can be caused or aggravated by poor diet. Make sure to eat varied, well-rounded meals made from basic foods. Include plenty of whole grains, vegetables, and quality protein (such as beans, nuts, fish, and lean poultry).

Biotin promotes hair and scalp health and, in some cases, can even prevent hair loss. The best sources of biotin are nuts, brown rice, brewer's yeast, and oats. Many of these foods are also high in B vitamins, which promote hair growth.

Iron is essential for hair growth. Take a spoonful of unsulfured blackstrap molasses every day, and include several of the following foods in your meals: green leafy vegetables (except spinach), leeks, cashews, berries, dried fruits, and figs.

Your body needs vitamin C to absorb iron; eat citrus fruit after an iron-rich meal.

Eat nuts, seeds, and avocados for vitamin E, a nutrient that keeps the scalp in good condition. Olive oil is another excellent source.

Foods containing essential fatty acids, as found in nuts (walnuts), flaxseeds, and fish, are important.

Food to Avoid

Avoid foods that deplete your system of nutrients and impair circulation, such as saturated and hydrogenated fats, refined flour and sugar, and processed food.

℞ Super Seven Prescriptions—Hair Loss

Super Prescription #1 Saw palmetto (_Serenoa repens_)
Take 320 to 400 mg daily of an 85 percent liposterolic extract.

A study in the Journal of _Alternative and Complementary Medicine_ reported that a product containing saw palmetto (_Serenoa repens_) and a plant compound called beta-sitosterol (also found in saw palmetto and other plants) may increase hair growth in men. This study included nineteen men between the ages of twenty-three and sixty-four years who had mild to moderate hair loss. They were given either a placebo or a supplement containing 400 mg of a standardized extract of saw palmetto and 100 mg of beta-sitosterol per day. After about five months, hair growth in 60 percent of the men taking the herbal combination had improved, compared with their initial evaluation. Only 11 percent of those receiving the placebo had any improvement.

Super Prescription #2 Silicon (*Orthosilicic acid*)
Take 10 mg daily to support healthy hair growth.

Super Prescription #3 Biotin
Take 2,000 to 3,000 mcg daily.

Super Prescription #4 Essential fatty acids
Take a combination formula containing a blend of omega-3 and omega-6 fatty acids. Take 4,000 mg of fish or flaxseed oil and evening primrose or borage oil containing 200 mg of GLA daily.

Super Prescription #5 Methylsulfonylmethane (MSM)
Take 3,000 mg daily. It contains the mineral sulfur, which helps promote hair development.

Super Prescription #6 Fo ti (*Polygonum multiflorum* or *He shou-wu*)
Take 500 mg three times daily. This Chinese herb is used by practitioners of Oriental medicine to slow or stop hair loss, although it is mainly used in formulas with other herbs.

Super Prescription #7 Rosemary essential oil
Apply 3 to 5 drops per 1 ounce of shampoo daily to improve scalp circulation.

General Recommendations

Zinc is a mineral required for hair development. Take 30 mg daily, along with 3 mg of copper.

Natural progesterone cream can be helpful for women with low levels, particularly women in menopause. See the Menopause section for proper use.

Enzymes improve the absorption of foods and nutrients. Take a full-spectrum complex with each meal.

Take a high-potency multivitamin daily to provide a base of the nutrients required for healthy hair.

A B-complex supplement combats the effects of stress and contains vitamins in the B family that contribute to healthy hair. Take a 50 mg complex twice daily.

A greens formula that includes super green foods, such as chlorella, spirulina, barley, and wheatgrass, provides a host of hair-healthy nutrients. Take as directed on the container.

A vitamin B12 deficiency may be at the root of hair loss. Take as part of a B-complex or take 200 to 400 mcg of the sublingual form daily.

Homeopathy

Pick the remedy that best matches your symptoms in this section. Take a 6x, 12x, 6C, 12C, or 30C potency twice daily for two weeks to see if there are any positive results. After you notice improvement, stop taking the remedy, unless symptoms return. Consultation with a homeopathic practitioner is advised.

Arsenicum Album is helpful when hair loss is the result of stress. The person is very fearful and restless.

Ignatia (*Ignatia amara*) is for hair loss that comes on with acute grief or an emotional trauma.

Lycopodium (*Lycopodium clavatum*) is for premature balding and graying of the hair. People who require this remedy often have digestive problems and crave sweets.

Natrum Muriaticum is for hair loss accompanied by depression, a strong salt craving, and an aversion to being in the sun.

Phosphoric Acidum is for hair loss that is accompanied by fatigue and mental debility. Hair loss may come after grief or sorrow. There is often a craving for carbonated beverages.

Sepia is helpful when there is a hormone imbalance–related hair loss, as seen during menopause or after using the birth-control pill.

Silica (*Silicea*) is helpful when there has been a chronic illness accompanied by hair loss. The hair is brittle, and the person tends to be thin, chilly, and easily fatigued.

Acupressure

See pages 787–794 for information about pressure points and administering treatment.

- If you have been eating poorly or have suffered from an illness, work Stomach 36 (St36) to encourage maximum absorption of nutrients into your bloodstream.

Bodywork

Massage

A scalp massage will increase circulation to the head and will help hair follicles receive nutrients from the blood.

Aromatherapy

Rosemary oil will stimulate hair growth. Take a few minutes before a shampoo to rub some into your hair and scalp.

If you need to reduce stress, essential oils can help. Lavender, chamomile, jasmine, rose, and geranium all have relaxing properties, as do many others. See pages 771–781 for more suggestions. Find a few that you enjoy and use them in baths, massages, or diffusers, or just hold the bottle under your nose and inhale deeply.

Stress Reduction

If you experience so much stress that your hair is falling out, you may need a therapist to help you cope. Hair loss is often related to shock or grief; look for a professional who has experience with your particular problem.

Any of the strategies in the Exercise and Stress Reduction chapter can help you with long-term stress management. Find the therapy you like best and practice it regularly.

Other Recommendations

- Exercise increases circulation everywhere, including the scalp. Talk a walk daily.
- Be gentle to your hair. When it's wet, use a wide-toothed comb to separate the strands, or, if possible, let your hair dry completely before combing it into

place. Do not use a blow dryer, and don't dye your hair or use bleach on it. If you want to pull your hair back, do so loosely, and use a special coated elastic that won't grip the individual strands and pull them out.

- Sleep is essential for hair renewal and growth. Try to get eight hours a night, or more, if that's what your body needs.

REFERENCES

Barel, A., et al. 2005. Effect of oral intake of choline-stabilized orthosilicic acid on skin, nails, and hair in women with photo-damaged skin. *Research* 297:147–53.

2002. *Journal of Alternative and Complementary Medicine* 8:143–52.

Prendiville, J. S., and L. N. Manfredi. 1992. Skin signs of nutritional disorders. *Seminars in Dermatology* 11(1):88–97.

Halitosis. See Bad Breath

Headache

Headaches are one of the most frequently occurring disorders; they're more prevalent than even the common cold. Most of us have experienced headaches of varying intensity and kind, and most of us will continue to have them now and then. More than forty-five million Americans suffer from chronic recurring headaches. This includes 20 percent of children and adolescents who suffer from significant headaches. The vast majority of headaches are caused by tension in the muscles of the head, the shoulders, and the neck. If you have a tension headache, you may feel tightness, pressure, or throbbing anywhere in your head or neck. Often the pain is worse as the day goes on but disappears upon waking the next day.

Migraine headaches are another matter. They account for only 6 percent of headaches, but what they lack in numbers they make up for in severity. They are intensely painful and are often accompanied by vision disturbances, extreme sensitivity to light, nausea, and vomiting. A migraine episode, which is usually incapacitating, may last a few hours, or it can go on for several days. Unlike tension headaches, migraines are not caused by muscular tension but by disturbances in blood flow to the head. In addition, it is rare to have just one migraine; most migraine sufferers get them at least once a month. The disorder can run in families and affects far more women and girls than it does men or boys.

Cluster headaches are a different type of headache, characterized by painful one-sided headaches that usually occur in clusters of several headaches in a short period of time. There may be no headaches for weeks or months.

Headaches can be triggered by a variety of factors, most often stress and anxiety but also allergies, hormone imbalance, poor digestion and detoxification, low blood sugar, fatigue, and drugs (including caffeine and alcohol). Most headaches are best addressed by identifying and removing the trigger or triggers, along with implementing strategies for natural pain relief.

If you have recurring or extremely severe headaches, however, you should consult a doctor to rule out any serious underlying causes, which can range from glaucoma to high blood pressure to brain tumors. Check with your doctor before combining herbs with prescription headache medications.

SYMPTOMS OF A CLUSTER HEADACHE

- One-sided headaches that are intense for a number of days or weeks and then disappear and reappear later

SYMPTOMS OF A TENSION HEADACHE

- Sensation of a tight band around the head
- Tension in the neck or the shoulders
- Pressure or throbbing anywhere in the head or the neck

SYMPTOMS OF A MIGRAINE HEADACHE

- Severe pain, usually on one side of the head
- Vision disturbances that precede or accompany head pain
- Sensitivity to light
- Nausea and vomiting
- May last for several days

ROOT CAUSES

- Emotional stress
- Fatigue
- Allergies (food or environmental)
- Sinusitis
- Eyestrain
- Poor posture and spinal misalignment, especially of the neck and the jaw (TMJ)
- Excessive intake of or withdrawal from drugs like alcohol, caffeine, nicotine, or illegal substances
- Low blood sugar
- Hormonal imbalance
- Constipation and poor digestion/ detoxification
- Nutritional deficiencies (especially of magnesium, B6, essential fatty acids)

Testing Techniques

The following tests help assess possible reasons for headaches:

Blood pressure

Hormone testing (thyroid, cortisol, estrogen, progesterone)—saliva, blood, or urine

Intestinal permeability—urine

Detoxification profile—urine

Vitamin and mineral analysis (especially magnesium, B6, iron)—blood

Digestive function and microbe/parasite/candida testing—stool analysis

Food and environmental allergies/sensitivities—blood, electrodermal

Blood sugar balance—blood

Toxic metals—hair, urine

TREATMENT

Diet

Recommended Food

To avoid headaches caused by food additives, eat meals that you've prepared from whole foods. To keep your blood sugar steady, try to have five small portions throughout the day, instead of three large meals.

Make sure you get enough fiber to reduce the chance of headaches induced by constipation or toxic buildup. One to two tablespoons of ground flaxseeds, along with 10 ounces of water, is a good way to start the day.

Drink a glass of clean, quality water every two waking hours. The fluid will keep the muscles in your head and neck supple and will also flush out toxins.

If you want to prevent headaches, include sources of both calcium and magnesium in your diet. Soy products, green leafy vegetables, and beans are all rich in calcium. Green leafy vegetables and beans are good sources of magnesium, as are nuts, bananas, and wheat germ. If food allergies keep you from eating these foods, take a good calcium/magnesium supplement every day to ensure adequate intake.

Fish such as salmon and mackerel are rich in the omega-3 fatty acids that may help prevent migraine headaches. Consume a serving three to five times weekly.

Food to Avoid

If you suffer from migraines or recurring headaches, see the Food Allergies section and the accompanying elimination diet to determine whether your problem may be caused by an allergic reaction or a sensitivity. Common triggers of both tension and migraine headaches include foods that contain either tyramine or phenylalanine. Tyramine can be found in cheese, chocolate, citrus fruits, coffee, cold cuts, herring, smoked fish, wine, alcohol, sausage, sour cream, and vinegar.

Sources of phenylalanine include monosodium glutamate (MSG), the artificial sweetener aspartame, and nitrates, which can be found in processed meats, especially hot dogs. If you have an allergy or a sensitivity, eliminate the troublesome food or foods from your diet.

Avoid caffeine, alcohol, and sugar products (including artificial sweeteners).

Do not consume sugary foods. They cause your blood sugar level to rise sharply and then crash; often, the result is a headache.

Very cold foods can also cause headaches. Ice cream and cold drinks are frequent culprits, so avoid them.

If you suffer from chronic headaches, a detoxification program can be effective. Try a two- to three-day vegetable juice fast, unless low blood sugar levels bring on your headaches.

Constitutional hydrotherapy can aid detoxification. See pages 795–796 for directions.

A study published in *Neurology* found that butterbur extract, at a dose of 75 mg twice daily for four months, reduced migraine attack frequency an average of 48 percent, compared to 26 percent for a placebo.

By Any Other Name, It's Still MSG

Monosodium glutamate is notorious for triggering headaches, and for that reason, food companies try not to list it on their product labels. Here are some common additives that are really hidden sources of MSG:

Calcium caseinate

Sodium caseinate

Autolyzed yeast

Hydrolyzed protein

℞ Super Seven Prescriptions—Headache

Super Prescription #1 Homeopathic combination headache formula

This contains the most common homeopathic remedies for headaches. Take as directed on the container for the treatment of all three types of acute headaches. For an individualized remedy, see the Homeopathy section further on.

Super Prescription #2 Butterbur

Take a standardized extract of 75 mg twice daily. Children can take 50 to 75 mg twice daily. Studies have demonstrated that this herbal extract prevents headaches in both adults and children.

Super Prescription #3 Magnesium

Take 200 mg two or three times daily. Reduce the dosage if diarrhea occurs. Magnesium has been shown in several studies to be effective in alleviating migraine headaches, and we also find it very helpful in preventing tension headaches. Intravenous magnesium can be very effective for acute headaches. Consult with a nutrition-oriented doctor for intravenous treatments.

Super Prescription #4 Riboflavin (vitamin B2)

Take 400 mg daily for at least three months. Studies have shown it to be effective in preventing migraine headaches.

Super Prescription #5 Feverfew (*Tanacetum parthenium*)

Take a product standardized to contain 250 to 500 mcg of parthenolides daily. Several studies have shown it to be effective in reducing the severity, the duration, and the frequency of migraines.

Super Prescription #6 Coenzyme Q10

Take 100 mg three times daily to decrease migraine frequency by about 50 percent.

Super Prescription #7 5-hydroxytryptophan (5-HTP)

Take 50 to 100 mg three times daily. Several studies have shown 5-HTP to be effective in preventing migraine and tension headaches. It has a direct effect on serotonin levels, which affect circulation in the blood vessels of the brain, and increases the body's endorphin levels (natural painkillers). Do not use if you are currently on a pharmaceutical antidepressant or antianxiety medication.

General Recommendations

Calcium relaxes the nervous system, the muscles, and the blood vessels, making it helpful for all types but especially for tension headaches. Take 500 mg twice daily.

Ginkgo biloba improves circulation to the brain and has anti-platelet activity. Take 60 mg two or three times daily of a 24 percent flavone glycoside extract.

Melatonin has been shown in preliminary research to help migraine headaches. This is a hormone supplement to consider, especially if you have insomnia. Take 0.3 to 0.5 mg before bedtime.

In a double-blind trial of eighty-one people with migraines, ages eighteen to sixty-five, a dose of 600 mg of magnesium per day was significantly more effective than a placebo at reducing the frequency of migraines. In weeks nine through twelve, the attack frequency was reduced by 41.6 percent in the magnesium group and by 15.8 percent in the placebo group.

In one study, forty-nine people with reoccurring migraines were given 400 mg of riboflavin daily for at least three months. The average number of acute migraine attacks decreased by 67 percent, and migraine severity was reduced by 68 percent. In a separate double-blind trial, 59 percent of patients assigned to receive vitamin B2 had at least a 50 percent reduction in the number of headache days, whereas only 15 percent of those taking a placebo experienced that degree of improvement.

Peppermint or menthol cream applied to the temple area has been shown in studies to be helpful for tension headaches.

White willow bark (*Salix alba*) contains salicin, the ingredient from which aspirin is derived. White willow bark is a highly effective pain reliever that's much easier on the stomach and the entire body than its pharmaceutical counterpart is. Take 60 to 120 mg daily.

Take a few quiet moments with a relaxing cup of tea to reduce tension/stress headaches. Peppermint, chamomile, and passionflower are all good choices.

Enzymes taken with meals improve digestion and absorption. Take a full-spectrum enzyme with each meal or as directed on the container.

Essential fatty acids improve circulation and reduce inflammatory prostaglandins that may contribute to migraine headaches. Take 5,000 mg of fish oil or 1 tablespoon of flaxseed oil daily.

Vitamin B6 is involved in the synthesis of neurotransmitters, such as serotonin, which may be deficient in migraine sufferers. Take 50 mg of vitamin B6 daily.

Homeopathy

Pick the remedy that best matches your symptoms as described in this section. For acute headaches, take a 30C potency four times daily. For chronic headaches, take a 6x, 12x, 6C, 12C, or 30C twice daily for two weeks to see if there are any positive results. After you notice improvement, stop taking the remedy, unless symptoms return. Consultation with a homeopathic practitioner is advised.

Belladonna (*Atropa belladonna*) helps when it is a right-sided headache that starts on the back of the head (right side) and extends to the right eye or the forehead. There is throbbing pain, as if the head would burst. The face is flushed and the skin feels hot, but the feet are cold. The person feels better lying down in a dark, quiet room.

Bryonia (*Bryonia alba*) is for pain in the left eye or the forehead that extends to the whole head. Symptoms are worse with any movement and feel better with pressure and stillness. Constipation may be associated with the headache. There can be nausea and a great thirst. The person is irritable and wants to be alone.

Calcarea Phosphorica is for schoolchildren who get chronic headaches and stomachaches. The pain is intense at the back of the head. The child craves smoked meats, may be homesick, and is often irritable.

Cimicifuga is helpful when there is severe neck stiffness and pain with the headache, which often occurs with the menstrual cycle or with hormonal changes during menopause.

Gelsemium (*Gelsemium sempervirens*) is for a dull, heavy pain at the back of the neck, which then spreads like a tight band around the head. The person feels tired and dizzy and may have blurred vision. The headache improves after urinating.

Glonoinum is for a congestive headache with intense pounding. Symptoms are worse from the sun and from heat and better from cold applications.

Ignatia (*Ignatia amara*) is for headaches associated with neck or back spasms. It feels as if a nail were driven into the head. It's also good for headaches that begin after emotional grief or a trauma.

Iris (*Iris versicolor*) is for right-sided migraine headaches that feel as if the head is constricted. Nausea and vomiting occur with the headache. There is often blurry vision. The person feels better with movement.

Lachesis is for left-sided headaches, with a burning, congestive, pulsating feeling. The face can be flushed. The person wakes up with a headache. Heat and touch worsen the headache, and the open air improves it.

Lycopodium (*Lycopodium clavatum*) is for a right-sided headache in the temple or the forehead area. Symptoms are worse from 4 P.M. to 8 P.M. and from being overheated or going too long without eating.

Magnesia Phosphorica is for tension headaches. This remedy helps to relax tight muscles.

Natrum Muriaticum is a great remedy for migraine headaches caused by being in the sun or headaches that come on from stress or grief. The person feels better lying down in a dark, cool room.

Natrum Sulphuricum is for headaches that come on after a head injury.

Nux Vomica is for headaches caused by stress, overwork, and bad reactions to food. The headache feels better with cold applications. There is often a stomachache and nausea. This remedy is used for headaches caused by alcohol or food allergies. The person is irritable from the headache and feels worse from noise, light, and opening the eyes. Nux Vomica is also useful for headaches caused by constipation.

Pulsatilla (*Pulsatilla pratensis*) is helpful when headaches occur around the menstrual cycle. The location of the headache changes rapidly. Symptoms are worse from the heat or from stuffy rooms and better in the open air.

Sanguinaria is for a headache that begins in the right side of the neck or the shoulder and radiates to the right eye. There is relief from vomiting.

Spigelia is for a stitching, sharp headache around the left eye. Symptoms are worse with movement or any jarring and better with heat or hot bathing.

Acupressure

See pages 787–794 for information about pressure points and administering treatment.

- Large Intestine 4 (LI4) is good for all kinds of aches, but it is especially successful at treating pain in the front of the head.
- For headaches accompanied by tired, painful eyes or sinus congestion, use Bladder 2 (B2).
- Gallbladder 20 (GB20) will ease headaches of any sort, including migraines.

Bodywork

Massage

For almost immediate relief, have someone rub the back of your neck and your upper back with ice.

If your headache is caused by sinus pain, you can practice an effective self massage. Lean forward over a sink or a towel to allow the sinuses to drain, and gently rub the areas over and below your eye sockets. You can also extend out from beneath your eye socket in a straight line across your cheeks.

An allover massage can help relieve stress before it turns into a headache. If you're prone to anxiety and tension, you may want to schedule regular sessions with a massage therapist.

Reflexology

See pages 804–805 for information about reflexology areas and how to work them. Work the areas corresponding to the head, the neck, the spine, and the solar plexus.

Other Bodywork Recommendations

Postural problems are at the root of many recurring headaches. See a chiropractor or an osteopath for a diagnosis and, if necessary, an adjustment of your vertebrae.

Acupuncture can be very helpful for all three types of headaches.

Aromatherapy

Lavender and peppermint will soothe both head pain and stress. Add a few drops of either to a carrier oil, and massage the temples. You can also add these oils to a cold compress.

If your headache is brought on by sinusitis, use eucalyptus in a steam inhalation. The oil will open up your sinus cavities quickly.

Stress Reduction

General Stress-Reduction Therapies

Many headache sufferers experience excellent results with biofeedback. People with tension headaches tend to clench their head and neck muscles unconsciously throughout the day, but they can use EMG muscle biofeedback to learn how to spot this clenching reflex and how to stop it, thus avoiding headaches. People with migraines can learn to increase blood flow to their head via thermal biofeedback. If biofeedback is too expensive or too complicated for you, find another stress-management technique and practice it daily. Read the Exercise and Stress Reduction chapter and experiment with the therapies there until you find one or two you enjoy.

Other Recommendations

- Breathe deeply. Some headaches are caused or made worse by an inadequate supply of oxygen.
- To reduce muscular spasms, lie down in a darkened room and apply a cold compress to the painful area. Some people may find that a warm compress is more effective.
- A heating pad, a warm compress, or a hot towel on the neck or the shoulders is a relaxing way to ease muscular tension.
- Place an ice pack (wrapped in a thin towel) on the back of the neck and put the feet in a bucket of warm water for ten minutes.
- Poor posture and the resulting misalignment of the vertebrae can lead to headaches. Wear flat or low-heeled shoes that fit well, and if you work long hours at a telephone, ask your company to invest in a headset for you. Ergonomic chairs are also recommended for people who sit a long time during the day.
- Women on the birth-control pill should consider discontinuing it to see if

their migraine headaches improve. Also, women using synthetic hormone replacement should switch to natural HRT or nutritional supplements to see if their headaches go away. See the Menopause section for more information.

• Get checked for temporomandibular joint problems, which can be a cause of tension or migraine headaches.

REFERENCES

Lipton, R. B., et al. 2004. Petasites hybridus root (butterbur) is an effective preventive treatment for migraine. *Neurology* 63:2240–44.

Peikert, A., C. Wilimzig, and R. Kohne-Volland. 1996. Prophylaxis of migraine with oral magnesium: Results from a prospective, multi-center, placebo-controlled and double-blind randomized study. *Cephalalgia* 16:257–63.

Schoenen, J., J. Jacquy, and M. Lenaerts. 1998. Effectiveness of high-dose riboflavin in migraine prophylaxis. A randomized controlled trial. *Neurology* 50:466–70.

Schoenen, J., M. Lenaerts, and E. Bastings. 1994. High-dose riboflavin as a prophylactic treatment of migraine: Results of an open pilot study. *Cephalalgia* 14:328–29.

Hearing Loss

Hearing loss is always a disturbing problem, but it's one that too often goes untreated. Many people who experience diminished hearing simply accept it as an unfortunate but normal part of life. While it's true that for some people, age-related hearing loss is unavoidable, the progression of many cases can be halted, significantly slowed, or even reversed with proper diagnosis and treatment. And with good nutrition and ear care, it's often quite possible to prevent hearing loss in the first place.

Hearing is a complex combination of many processes in the ear, the nerves, and the brain, and any disruption of these functions can lead to partial or complete deafness. Nevertheless, hearing problems can generally be categorized according to one of two types: conductive and sensorineural. Conductive hearing loss, which is caused by mechanical problems in the ear's structures, is by far the more common of the two. Although its tendency to come on suddenly can be frightening, it can often be resolved.

The most frequent cause of conductive hearing impairment is a buildup of wax in the ear canal. Normally, wax (or cerumen, to use its medical name) lines the ear canal and serves as a lubricant. When too much wax accumulates, it can block the canal and can lead to hearing loss, as well as to pain and ringing in the ears. A middle-ear infection can also cause a blockage, especially if the infected fluid remains in the ear for a long time and coagulates around the small bones (ossicles) that are responsible for transmitting sound waves. Ear infections and excessive earwax are both readily treatable, often with home care, and several highly effective nutritional strategies can prevent the problem from recurring.

In some instances, conductive hearing damage is more serious. If you suffer hearing loss after a fall or a blow to the ear or the head, or if you experience a sudden, intense pain in your ear, see your doctor at once. You may have a ruptured ear drum or damage to the hearing sensor, called the organ of Corti. Even innocuous-looking cotton swabs can cause grave damage, including ruptures, when inserted deep into the ear canal. Some drugs can affect the organ of Corti, so talk to your doctor if you experience hearing loss after starting a new prescription drug. Finally, some conductive hearing damage may simply be a part of aging. As the body gets older, the eardrum can thicken and other ear structures may grow weak, leading to partial loss of hearing. More than 40 percent of people seventy-five and older experience some degree of hearing problems. Sensorineural hearing damage affects the nerves that receive sound waves and transmit their impulses through the ear and to the brain, where the impulses are registered as the sensory perception of sound. Almost all sensorineural hearing damage is due to high levels of noise. Loud concerts and stereos turned up to full volume may be the most obvious source of excessive noise, but sirens, airplanes, trains, jackhammers, and construction sounds are common culprits as well. Every time you're exposed to a loud noise, your auditory nerves are damaged; a lifetime of noises can add up to permanent hearing loss. In some cases, sensorineural hearing problems are caused by other disorders, including diabetes, arteriosclerosis, lupus, and hypothyroidism. And again, sometimes nerves simply weaken with age and lose their ability to conduct sound effectively. However, recent research has shown that loud noises form free radicals that damage the inner ear. Antioxidants such as vitamin E, zinc, NAC, magnesium, and vitamin A appear to protect against this cause of damage, although they have not been shown to reverse hearing loss.

In some cases, tumor growths on the nerves involved with hearing are responsible for the hearing loss. One must also consider other structural possibilities, such as vertebral and soft tissue misalignment in the neck and the jaw (TMJ), as well as in cranial bones.

No matter what you suspect the source of your hearing problems to be, it's important that you consult a doctor about any sudden hearing loss or any gradual hearing damage that does not resolve itself within a few weeks. For one, the problem may be treatable. Even if you're older and believe that the hearing problem is due to age-related deterioration of ear structures or nerves, you may be surprised to find that the cause is actually wax buildup (something to which people over sixty-five are prone) or a side effect of medication. If the cause is not obvious to your doctor, he or she should run tests to rule out an underlying disorder. Finally, even hearing problems that are not reversible by natural means can often be significantly improved with hearing aids, electronic implants, or even surgery.

SYMPTOMS

- Gradual or sudden loss of hearing ability
- Partial or total inability to hear

ROOT CAUSES

- Accumulation of earwax
- Middle-ear infection
- Poor diet and nutritional deficiencies
- Food allergies
- Trauma to the ear
- Medication
- Loud noise
- Age-related weakening of the ear structures and the nerves

- Structural abnormalities (especially cervical spine, TMJ, and cranial bones)
- High cholesterol
- Other disorders that cause hearing loss

Testing Techniques

The following tests help assess possible reasons for hearing loss:

Specialized hearing tests by an otologist

Blood pressure

Vitamin and mineral analysis (especially magnesium, folate, B12, zinc, and iron)—blood

Food and environmental allergies/sensitivities—blood, electrodermal

---

TREATMENT
For further information about treating infections of the middle ear, see Ear Infection.

Diet

Recommended Food
Although no one has proven (yet) that antioxidants can reduce or prevent hearing loss, we do know that they slow many aspects of the aging process. Increasing your antioxidant intake by consuming more deeply colored fruits and vegetables certainly can't hurt you, and it may prevent or slow hearing damage (along with many other disorders we tend to associate with old age).

Eat plenty of fiber at every meal. Good sources include whole grains, especially oats and brown rice; beans; nuts and seeds; and raw or lightly cooked fruits and vegetables. Fiber will improve circulation to your entire body, including your ears. Fibrous foods also tend to require chewing, an activity that discourages wax from accumulating in your ear canals.

Since hypothyroidism can lead to hearing loss, include sea vegetables such as kelp, in your diet. These foods are high in iodine, a mineral that's necessary for good thyroid health. You can easily incorporate sea vegetables into soups, especially miso broth, or add them to a stir-fry with brown rice and tofu.

Food to Avoid
If you experience frequent ear infections or a buildup of earwax, you may have a food allergy. Read the Food Allergies section, and follow the elimination diet there; if a certain food provokes ear problems or excess mucus (which can lead to infection), avoid it.

Even if you are not allergic to milk or dairy products, stay away from them for the duration of an infection or a wax problem. Dairy encourages mucus to accumulate, which can encourage infection or excess wax.

If you have a chronic hearing problem, eliminate saturated fat, especially red meat and fried foods, from your diet. Saturated fat contributes to earwax and slows circulation to the ear structures. Removing saturated fat from your meals and snacks will also help reverse arteriosclerosis, a disorder that may cause hearing loss.

Bacteria feed on sugar, so people who are prone to ear infections should radically reduce their consumption of it. The best course of action is to cut out all refined sugars and have fruit or naturally sweetened products for dessert.

If you have recurring ear infections or wax problems, a short juice fast will help clear your body of excess mucus. Fasting is also helpful for people whose hearing loss is connected to food allergens, as a three-day respite from solid food will rid your system of the toxic substance.

℞ Super Seven Prescriptions—Hearing Loss

Super Prescription #1 *Ginkgo biloba*
Take 60 to 120 mg twice a day of a 24 percent flavone glycosides standardized extract. This herb increases blood flow, which helps ear tissues receive the oxygen and the nutrients they need for good health.

Super Prescription #2 Magnesium
Take 200 mg daily to prevent hearing loss induced by noise exposure.

Super Prescription #3 Vitamin B12
Take 200 to 400 mcg of sublingual B12 daily. This B vitamin is important for nerve health.

Super Prescription #4 Folate
Take 800 mcg daily.

Super Prescription #5 Vitamin E
Take 400 to 800 IU daily. It acts as an antioxidant and improves circulation.

Super Prescription #6 Cayenne (*Capsicum annuum*)
Take 300 mg twice daily. Cayenne improves circulation.

Super Prescription #7 Garlic (*Allium sativum*)
Take 300 to 600 mg of aged garlic twice daily. Garlic decreases cholesterol levels and improves blood flow.

A placebo-controlled double-blind study in Israel involving three hundred healthy young adults found that 167 mg of magnesium aspartate reduced the likelihood of permanent hearing loss.

General Recommendations

If you have an ear infection, an herbal solution made from 3 or 4 drops of warm olive oil combined with oil of Kyolic garlic, mullein, or lobelia can work wonders. Either lie down on your side until the oil works its way into the ear, or place a cotton ball loosely in the outer ear to the keep the oil from running out.

Marshmallow will help drain excess mucus. Take 2.5 to 3.0 grams twice a day, or take 5 to 15 cc of a tincture three times a day.

Bromelain has a natural anti-inflammatory effect. Take 500 mg three times daily between meals. Look for products standardized to 2,000 MCU (milk-clotting units) per 1,000 mg or 1,200 GDU (gelatin-dissolving units) per 1,000 mg.

Protease enzyme products also have a natural anti-inflammatory benefit.

Homeopathy

For prolonged hearing loss, it's best to see a homeopathic practitioner for a constitutional remedy.

Acupressure

See pages 787–794 for information about pressure points and administering treatment.

- To stimulate better hearing, work these two ear points: Gallbladder 2 (GB2, also known as Reunion of Hearing) and Small Intestine 19 (SI19, Listening Place).

Bodywork

Massage

A head rub will improve circulation; a gentle head massage will also help ease the pain caused by an ear infection.

Reflexology

See pages 804–805 for information about reflexology areas and how to work them.

To release pain and stimulate circulation, work the eye/ear area and the neck.

Other Bodywork Recommendations

Spinal and cranial treatments from a chiropractor, an osteopath, a craniosacral practitioner, or a naturopath can be helpful in improving nerve flow and circulation.

Aromatherapy

Several oils benefit circulation, including marjoram, ginger, rosemary, and black pepper. You can combine any of these with a carrier oil to use in a head massage. If you prefer not to get oil in your hair, you can add the oils to a steam inhalation.

Other Recommendations

- Protect your ears from loud noises. If you are outdoors and hear a loud sound such a siren or a train whistle, cover your ears; if you're in a car, roll up the windows.
- Play music at a low to moderate level, and wear earplugs if you must attend a loud concert.
- For those of you who cannot avoid exposure to noises because of your job, invest in earphones that cover your ears, and rest in a quiet place as often as you can.
- Excessive earwax can often be treated successfully at home. Buy an over-the-counter preparation containing carbamide peroxide and gently squeeze a few drops in your ear canal. This solution will help soften the wax so that it comes out easily. (You can also use hydrogen peroxide, if you prefer.) Allow the liquid to remain in your ear for a few minutes; for very hard wax, you may want to wait a day or two. Then use a bulb syringe filled with warm water to gently flush out the ear. If the plug of wax does not come out immediately, keep trying. It may take some time, but most people find that the wax does come out eventually.

REFERENCES

Attias, J., et al. 1994. Oral magnesium intake reduces permanent hearing loss induced by noise exposure. *American Journal of Otolaryngology* 15:26–32.

Hemorrhoids

It is estimated that 50 to 75 percent of Americans suffer from hemorrhoids at least once, and nearly one-third of the population has an ongoing problem with this often painful condition. Hemorrhoids are usually caused by increased pressure on the veins of the anus and the rectum. This pressure inflames and swells the veins, much in the same way that pressure on the veins of the legs creates varicose veins. Increased pressure on the anal veins can occur for many reasons but is most commonly the result of constipation, especially straining to pass stools, and pregnancy and childbirth. There may also be a genetic component to this disorder.

Hemorrhoids can be divided into three categories. Internal hemorrhoids develop inside the rectum, where they cannot be seen. Because they are usually painless, you may not even be aware of them unless they bleed. External hemorrhoids are located at the lower end of the anal canal, at the opening of the anus and under the skin. They are likely to become inflamed; when they do, they turn blue or purple and feel tender to the touch. Because of the high number of nerves in the anus, these hemorrhoids can be quite painful.

If an internal hemorrhoid becomes enlarged, it may collapse and descend so that it partially protrudes outside of the anus. These lumpy-looking masses of tissue are called prolapsed hemorrhoids. They usually appear after a bowel movement and produce both mucus and heavy bleeding. Prolapsed hemorrhoids can be excruciatingly painful.

Most cases of hemorrhoids are linked in some way to a lack of dietary fiber. They are best treated at home with increased fiber intake, detoxification, and soothing treatments for the pain and the itching. If your hemorrhoids don't improve with these conservative strategies, see a doctor about more aggressive treatments. In rare cases, surgery is required to remove large and very painful hemorrhoids. If you have any rectal bleeding at all, consult with a doctor so that he or she can rule out a more serious underlying condition.

SYMPTOMS

- Pain, itching, burning, or bleeding in the anal area
- Lumpy tissue protruding from the anus
- Blue or purple patches of hard skin near the anus

ROOT CAUSES

- Constipation and straining
- Pregnancy and childbirth
- Lifting heavy objects
- Obesity
- Inactivity, especially standing or sitting for extended periods
- Food allergies
- Portal hypertension and poor liver function
- Poor anal hygiene
- Hypothyroidism

Testing Techniques

The following tests help assess possible reasons for hemorrhoids:

Hormone testing (hypothyroid can contribute to sluggish bowel and liver function)—saliva, blood, or urine

Digestive function and microbe/parasite/candida testing—stool analysis

Food and environmental allergies/sensitivities—blood, electrodermal

---

TREATMENT

If sluggish digestion is a cause of your hemorrhoids, you will find additional suggestions for relief in the Constipation section.

Diet

Almost everyone who suffers from hemorrhoids—even people who aren't constipated—will benefit from dietary changes.

Recommended Food

If you're unaccustomed to a high-fiber diet, incorporate these suggestions incrementally. If you try to introduce too much fiber at once, you'll only place more pressure on your digestive tract.

The best way to relieve hemorrhoids is to consume more fiber. Eat lots of whole grains, raw or lightly cooked fruits and vegetables, and beans, nuts, and seeds. Rather than sitting down to three large meals every day, plan on several smaller meals.

To allow stools to pass more easily, drink a glass of clean, quality water every two waking hours.

Add prunes or figs to your breakfast to speed up a sluggish intestine.

Have a tablespoon of flaxseed oil every day to encourage elimination, or sprinkle 1 to 2 tablespoons of ground flaxseeds onto cereal or salads.

Vitamin K will help stop or prevent bleeding. Green leafy vegetables, especially kale, are a good source of this nutrient, as are kelp and alfalfa sprouts.

An overgrowth of candidiasis is an often-overlooked aggravator of hemorrhoids. Consume soured food like unsweetened live yogurt, kefir, and sauerkraut to increase the numbers of friendly bacteria that inhibit this fungal growth. These products will also help you absorb vitamin K.

Eat wheat germ for its high level of vitamin E. You'll promote circulation and prevent blood clots in your already-stressed circulatory system.

Bioflavonoids have been shown to significantly reduce inflammation and to strengthen capillaries, so enjoy some berries a few times daily.

If you're pregnant, you have another reason to eat your leafy greens. These vegetables are high in B6, a vitamin that many pregnant women lack; a deficiency may contribute to hemorrhoids. Brewer's yeast and wheat germ are also good sources.

Food to Avoid

Fats and oils slow down the digestive system. Stay away from foods that are fried or otherwise high in saturated fat.

Caffeine and alcohol are dehydrating and worsen hemorrhoids.

Avoid sugars and spicy foods, as they tend to worsen this condition.

Some cases of hemorrhoids are caused by food allergies. Read the Food Allergies section, and try the elimination diet to determine whether you need to remove certain foods from your diet. The most common ones that lead to hemorrhoids are cow's milk, wheat, citrus fruit, tomatoes, and peanuts.

If hemorrhoids result from constipation or straining on the toilet, go on a three-day juice fast to cleanse accumulated waste matter from your digestive tract. If you are constipated when you begin taking the fast, add psyllium husks or flaxseeds to your juices for fiber.

℞ Super Seven Prescriptions—Hemorrhoids

Super Prescription #1 Butcher's broom (*Ruscus aculeatus*)
Take a standardized extract that gives you 200 to 300 mg of ruscogenins daily. Ruscogenins are believed to constrict and reduce inflammation of hemorrhoidal tissue.

Super Prescription #2 Pycnogenol
Take 100 mg twice daily to heal acute hemorrhoids.

Super Prescription #3 Horse chestnut (*Aesculus hippocastanum*)
Take a standardized extract that contains 100 mg of aescin daily. This herb improves circulation and reduces swelling.

Super Prescription #4 Collinsonia (stone root)
Take 500 mg three times daily. Collinsonia reduces hemorrhoid swelling.

Super Prescription #5 Witch hazel (*Hamamelis virginiana*)
Apply as a gel or a cream to external hemorrhoids, or add 1 ounce to a sitz bath daily.

Super Prescription #6 Bioflavonoid complex
Take 1,000 mg two or three times daily. Various flavonoids, such as rutin and hesperidin, have been shown to be effective in treating hemorrhoids. They reduce swelling and prevent bleeding.

Super Prescription #7 Bilberry (*Vaccinium myrtillus*)
Take a standardized extract containing 25 percent anthocyanosides at 160 mg twice daily. Bilberry improves circulation and strengthens capillary walls.

General Recommendations

A greens drink that contains a blend of super green foods, such as chlorella, spirulina, and so on, provides fiber and improves liver function. Take as directed on the container.

Aloe vera juice is healing and soothing to the entire digestive tract. Drink 4 ounces daily or as directed on the container.

Vitamin C strengthens the rectal tissue. Take 500 mg two or three times daily.

A probiotic contains friendly bacteria, such as *lactobacillus* and *bifidobacterium*, which improve digestion and constipation. Take a product that contains at least four billion active organisms daily.

Dandelion root (*Taraxacum officinalis*) promotes bile flow and improved regularity. Take 300 mg in capsule form or 2 ml of tincture three times daily.

Psyllium is a good fiber supplement and has been shown to reduce the pain and the bleeding associated with hemorrhoids. Take 5 to 7 grams daily, along with 10 ounces of water.

Flaxseed oil improves regularity and reduces straining. It also contains essential fatty acids that promote tissue healing. Take 1 to 2 tablespoons daily.

A study of fifty-one pregnant women found that supplementation of bilberry significantly improved the pain, the burning, and the itching associated with their hemorrhoids.

Homeopathy

Pick the remedy that best matches your symptoms in this section. Take a 6x, 12x, 6C, 12C, or 30C potency twice daily for two weeks to see if there are any positive results. After you notice improvement, stop taking the remedy, unless symptoms return. Consultation with a homeopathic practitioner is advised.

Aesculus (*Aesculus hippocastanum*) is for pain that feels as if the rectum is being poked with sticks. The pain extends to the back.

Aloe vera is for large, painful hemorrhoids. The doctor states that the hemorrhoids look like a "bunch of grapes." They feel better with cold compresses. The person may be prone to having diarrhea.

Calcarea Fluorica is helpful when bleeding and itching occur with the hemorrhoids. Often, lower back pain is present. The person may have problems with flatulence and constipation.

Ignatia (*Ignatia amara*) is for hemorrhoids that cause a stabbing or sticking pain, along with rectal spasms. The symptoms feel worse from emotional upset.

Nux Vomica is for painful hemorrhoids that come on as a result of chronic constipation and straining with bowel movements. The person is irritable and has a tendency to overuse alcohol, drugs, or medications.

Ratanhia is helpful when a person experiences a lot of pain after a bowel movement. There is a cutting pain that feels like one is sitting on broken glass.

Sulfur is for large, itching, burning hemorrhoids that tend to be worse at night. The anal area is red and inflamed, and there is often flatulence with a foul odor.

Consider the Keesey Technique

A procedure known as the Keesey Technique (also referred to as hemorrhoidolysis) is available from alternative doctors. This procedure, which takes about ten minutes per treatment, utilizes a galvanic current to shrink hemorrhoidal tissue. During this painless procedure the practitioner touches the protruding hemorrhoid(s) with an electrode probe that conducts an electrical current. The result is shrinkage of tissue over the following ten days. Severe cases may require a series of treatments.

Acupressure

See pages 787–794 for information about pressure points and administering treatment.

- To relieve constipation, work Conception Vessel 6 (CV6) and Large Intestine 4 (LI4).

- Keep the colon strong and healthy by working Large Intestine 11 (LI11) on a regular basis.
- Use Stomach 36 (St36) to improve the assimilation of nutrients into the body.

Bodywork

Massage

If you're constipated, a self-massage of the abdominal area can induce intestinal movement. Lie down with your knees bent, and massage your abdomen with the flat of your hand, using firm but gentle pressure.

A professional massage of your lower back and pelvis may also relieve constipation.

Reflexology

See pages 804–805 for information about reflexology areas and how to work them.

Work the areas corresponding to the sigmoid colon, the rectum, and the lower back.

If you are constipated, also work the areas related to the liver, the gallbladder, and the adrenal glands.

Hydrotherapy

Constitutional hydrotherapy is a good long-term treatment for hemorrhoids. See pages 795–796 for directions.

An alternating warm (one minute) and cold (thirty seconds) sitz bath offers relief and improves circulation.

Aromatherapy

Geranium relaxes your system by easing anxiety and depression, which often lead to constipation. Add it to your bath water or use a few drops in a compress.

Tea tree oil reduces the chances of infection. You can also add this to a bath or a compress. This is a potent oil, so start off with just 2 or 3 drops. If you don't have a reaction, you can increase the amount by a few more drops the next time you make a preparation.

If you need to stimulate your digestive system, marjoram and black pepper will help. Add either or both to a bath, or combine with a carrier oil and use it in a massage.

Stress Reduction

General Stress-Reduction Therapies

Regular exercise is very important to reduce the effects of stress and improve circulation.

Other Recommendations

- If you're constipated, do not strain when sitting on the toilet. Try to relax and breathe deeply.
- Do not use laxatives. They only address the surface of the problem and can cause your bowels to become dependent on them. If you need temporary relief, see the Constipation section.
- Get regular exercise. Any kind will do, but a daily walk is always a good idea.

- For temporary relief of pain and itching, use any of the following as a topical lotion: cocoa butter, zinc oxide, olive oil, or calendula gel.
- If you must stand or sit for long periods of time, take frequent breaks to stretch and move around.
- Special foam-rubber pillows known as a "doughnuts" are helpful when you need to sit. They have a hole in the middle so there is less pressure on the hemorrhoids.
- If you're obese, losing weight will reduce or even eliminate your hemorrhoids. The dietary suggestions in this section should help you take the weight off safely, but if you'd like additional recommendations, see Obesity.

REFERENCES

Teglio, L., et al. 1987. Vaccinium myrtillus anthocyanosides (Tegens) in the treatment of venous insufficiency of lower limbs and acute piles in pregnancy. *Quaderni di Clinica Obstetrica e Ginecologica* 42(3):221–31.

Heart Attack and Heart Disease. See Cardiovascular Disease

Hepatitis

Hepatitis is the general term for the inflammation of the liver, which is the body's largest internal organ and is located beneath the breastbone, extending under the bottom of the right side of the rib cage. Hepatitis can result from the use of alcohol, drugs, and chemicals but is most commonly caused by one of several specific hepatitis viruses.

One of the liver's functions is to produce and metabolize bile, which is necessary to break down fats and expel toxins out of the body. With hepatitis, bilirubin, a pigment normally excreted in bile, builds up in the bloodstream and accumulates in the skin. This causes the characteristic yellowish color of the skin and the eyes, as well as dark urine. Classic symptoms of hepatitis include nausea, fatigue, loss of appetite, weight loss, clay-colored stools, fever, and diarrhea. Blood tests show an elevation of one or more liver enzymes.

At least six different viruses cause acute viral hepatitis. The main three are hepatitis A, B, and C. Other hepatitis viruses include D, E, and G.

Hepatitis A, which has a 15- to 45-day incubation period, is highly contagious and is spread mainly by fecal-tainted food or water. Epidemics are common in underdeveloped countries. Contaminated raw shellfish can be a causative factor. It can also be transmitted through blood or saliva secretions. Hepatitis A is an acute infection, and people do not become chronic carriers of the virus. It does not play a role in the development of chronic hepatitis or cirrhosis. A vaccine for hepatitis A is available.

Hepatitis B has an incubation period of 30 to 180 days. It is contracted by contaminated blood or blood products, as happens with drug users who share needles. It can also occur from sexual contact and, less commonly, from transfusions tainted with infected blood. People can become chronic carriers of this virus. A wide spectrum of liver diseases is associated with hepatitis B, including cirrhosis and liver cancer. A vaccine for hepatitis B is available.

Hepatitis C has an incubation period of 15 to 150 days. This is the most common form of viral hepatitis. In the past, it was more commonly contracted through contaminated blood. The main causes of hepatitis C infection worldwide include unscreened blood transfusions and the reuse of needles and syringes that have not been adequately sterilized. In developed countries, it is estimated that 90 percent of people with chronic HCV infection are current and/or former injecting drug users or those with a history of transfusion of unscreened blood or blood products. Hepatitis C can also be transmitted by sexual activity and from mother to infant. It is estimated that 3 percent of the world's population (170 million people) are chronically infected with hepatitis C virus. Most people with hepatitis C have no symptoms. According to the World Health Organization, about 80 percent of newly infected patients progress to develop the chronic infection. Cirrhosis develops in about 10 to 20 percent of people with chronic infection, and liver cancer develops in 1 to 5 percent of those with chronic infection over a period of twenty to thirty years. Currently, there is no vaccine to prevent hepatitis C. Antiviral drugs are the standard conventional treatment. Effectiveness of these drugs varies, but side effects prevent many people from continuing treatment.

Hepatitis D virus occurs only in the presence of acute or chronic hepatitis B virus infection. Drug addicts who share needles are at high risk for this infection. It is characterized by an unusually severe acute hepatitis B infection.

Hepatitis E virus is most commonly transmitted via contaminated water in developing countries. The infection can be severe but is not chronic.

Hepatitis G virus can be transmitted by blood. Currently, not a lot is known about this virus, although it can become chronic.

The early symptoms of acute hepatitis may include a loss of appetite, fatigue, nausea, vomiting, and fever. Hivelike eruptions and joint pains occasionally occur. After a period of three to ten days, the urine darkens and is followed by jaundice (yellowing of the skin). The liver is usually enlarged and tender, and the spleen may enlarge as well. Blood tests will show elevated liver enzymes from the beginning stage of the illness.

Hepatitis usually resolves within four to eight weeks, especially hepatitis A. However, 5 to 10 percent of hepatitis B infections become chronic, and up to 80 percent of hepatitis C infections become chronic. Hepatitis lasting for six months or longer is generally termed chronic.

Natural therapies can be very helpful in preventing liver damage and decreasing the viral load or the infectiousness of the hepatitis viruses. Holistic therapies are becoming very popular for people with hepatitis C—an emerging world epidemic. The effectiveness of conventional antiviral drug therapy has greatly improved in recent years for chronic hepatitis. Natural treatment is used to augment the immune system to fight the viral infection and to improve and protect liver function. Our experience is that most cases can be helped with natural treatment, and sometimes the improvements are dramatic.

Many natural therapies in this chapter can be combined with conventional therapy.

SYMPTOMS

- Nausea
- Fever
- Fatigue
- Diarrhea
- Loss of appetite

- Dark urine
- Weight loss
- Jaundice
- Clay-colored stools

ROOT CAUSES

- Viral infection
- Alcohol
- Adverse reaction to drugs and

other toxins
- Weakened immune system

Testing Techniques

The following tests go beyond regular conventional testing and identify reasons for weakened immunity:

Blood work (conventional testing)—immune function, liver enzymes, viral load

Stool analysis—digestive health

Hormone analysis by saliva, urine, or blood (testosterone, DHEA, cortisol, melatonin, IGF-1, thyroid panel)

Toxic metal—hair or urine

Oxidative stress analysis—urine or blood testing

TREATMENT

Diet

Recommended Food

During the acute phase, it is recommended that you consume soups, broths, diluted vegetable juices, herbal teas, steamed vegetables, brown rice, and nonred-meat protein sources, such as free-range turkey or chicken, legumes, and fish.

To promote healing of the liver and to provide a diet that is supportive to the immune system, consume lots of vegetables and moderate amount of fruits, whole grains, and legumes. Reduce or eliminate foods that are taxing to the liver, such as fried foods; refined sugar products; foods containing trans-fatty acids, such as margarine and vegetable shortening; and saturated fats, found in meat and dairy products. Make fresh juices out of foods such as apples, beets, and carrots. Start with small amounts to see how you tolerate them. Steamed artichokes are healing to the liver. Eating smaller and more frequent meals is recommended. Soups and stews are good, as they are easy to digest. Purified water should be consumed, an 8-ounce glass every two to three waking hours.

Food to Avoid

Cut out junk food, sugar, and alcohol, all of which suppress your immune system and tax your entire body.

Avoid saturated fats and hydrogenated oils, which stress the immune system and the liver. Stay away from fried foods and solid fats, such as margarine, lard, and vegetable shortening.

Find out now if you have any food allergies or sensitivities, because they weaken the immune system. See the elimination diet on page 316 for further details.

℞ Super Seven Prescriptions—Hepatitis

Super Prescription #1 Milk thistle (*Silybum marianum*)
Take a daily dosage of a product standardized with regard to silymarin, so that you supplement a daily total of 600 to 1,000 mg of the active constituent silymarin daily. This herb protects the liver, promotes liver-cell regeneration, and helps reduce liver-enzyme count. Products standardized to silybin are very effective, too.

Super Prescription #2 Vitamin C
Take 1,000 mg three or four times daily of a buffered (nonacidic) vitamin C. A more therapeutic technique is to keep gradually increasing the dosage until loose stools occur, and then cut back on the dosage. Intravenous vitamin C treatments from a holistic doctor are even more effective. Vitamin C improves immune function and has antiviral properties.

Super Prescription #3 Catechin
Take 750 mg three times daily. Catechin is a type of flavonoid that was shown in studies to be helpful for acute and chronic hepatitis. It is best used under the supervision of a doctor.

Super Prescription #4 Thyme extract
Take as directed on the container. Look for a high-quality purified thyme extract. A typical dose is 200 to 300 mg three times daily. Thyme extract has been shown to improve immune function and be helpful for people with hepatitis C.

Super Prescription #5 Licorice root (*Glycyrrhiza glabra*)
Take 500 mg three times daily. One of the active phytonutrients in licorice root, known as glycyrrhizin, has been used as part of injectable formulas to treat chronic hepatitis B and C, with favorable outcomes. Licorice root has been shown to have immune-enhancing and antiviral properties. Holistic doctors also administer glycyrrhizin intravenously for a strong therapeutic effect. *Note*: High doses of licorice root may cause high blood pressure. High doses, as recommended in this section, are best used under the supervision of a physician.

Super Prescription #6 Reishi extract
Take 3,000 to 6,000 mg daily of a standardized extract. Preliminary studies have shown reishi extract to be effective for hepatitis B and elevated liver enzymes. Reishi is commonly used by health practitioners for liver support.

Super Prescription #7 Schisandra extract (*Schisandra chinensis*)
Take 500 mg three times daily. Studies have found that this Chinese herb is effective in treating chronic hepatitis.

Milk thistle (*Silymarin*) was studied in a group of twenty-one people who had active liver disease (cirrhosis). People who took 420 mg of silymarin had a 15 percent reduction in the liver enzyme AST and a 23 percent decrease in the enzyme ALT.

A preliminary trial involving five thousand people with various types of hepatitis found liver enzymes normalized in 75 percent of people supplementing schisandra.

General Recommendations

Turmeric (*Curcuma longa*; 90 to 95 percent curcumin) has anti-inflammatory benefits for liver infection. Take 500 mg three times daily.

Alpha lipoic acid supports immune function and has anti-inflammatory properties. Take 300 mg twice daily.

Phosphatidylcholine helps the liver to process fats and protects the liver cells. One study demonstrated benefits for people who had chronic hepatitis B. Take 3,000 mg daily.

Astragalus is an excellent herb for long-term immune support and is used for chronic viral hepatitis. Take 2 ml of the tincture or 1,000 mg of the capsule form three times daily.

A high-potency multivitamin and mineral formula should be supplemented, for general immune system support.

Selenium is important, because a deficiency can make it easier for viruses to replicate. Make sure you are getting a total of 400 mcg daily.

Zinc supports immune function. Take a daily total of 30 to 50 mg.

Vitamin E complex is important for protection against liver damage and to support immune function. Take 800 mg of a blended formula containing tocopherols and tocotrienols.

Phyllanthus (*Phyllanthus amarus*) was shown in one study to be effective for people who were chronic carriers of hepatitis B. Take 200 mg three times daily.

Dandelion root improves liver function. Take 3 ml of the tincture or 500 mg in capsule form three times daily with meals.

Liver glandular extract supports liver function. Take as directed on the container.

A greens drink that contains super green foods, such as chlorella, spirulina, and others, supports liver detoxification and immunity. Take as directed on the container.

Homeopathy

Pick the remedy that best matches your symptoms in this section. Take a 6x, 12x, 6C, 12C, or 30C potency twice daily for two weeks to see if there are any positive results. After you notice improvement, stop taking the remedy, unless symptoms return. Consultation with a homeopathic practitioner is advised.

Cardus Marianus is a specific remedy for inflammation of the left lobe of the liver. The person's symptoms are worse when lying on the left side. There is abdominal or liver pain that is worse from breathing in or from movement.

Chelidonium is used when there is pain under the right rib cage, radiating to the right shoulder blade. Abdominal pain is ameliorated after eating or by lying on the left side with the legs drawn up. The person feels better from warm drinks. Jaundice is usually present.

China is used when the liver is very sensitive to the touch. There is tremendous bloating of the abdomen, which is not relieved from passing gas.

Lycopodium is used for hepatitis in which bloating, indigestion, and flatulence are prominent symptoms. There is discomfort in the upper right area of the abdomen. The symptoms feel better from warm drinks. The person feels irritable and craves sweets.

Natrum Sulphuricum is used to treat jaundice that is accompanied by diarrhea. The tongue has a greenish coating. It is used for hepatitis that causes headaches, accompanied by nausea and vomiting. The person feels better from firm pressure or rubbing of the abdomen.

Nux Vomica is helpful when constipation, cramping, or reflux accompanies hepatitis. Common symptoms also include fatigue and irritability. The person is chilly and feels better from heat.

Phosphorus is indicated for hepatitis that occurs from solvent and toxin exposure. The person feels a thirst for ice-cold drinks but tends to vomit after drinking them.

Sulfur is a remedy for chronic hepatitis with jaundice and diarrhea. The person feels very warm and desires a cool environment.

Acupressure

Acupressure and acupuncture can be very effective in treating hepatitis. See a practitioner of Asian medicine for a specific treatment.

- Pericardium 6 (P6) is used to relieve nausea.
- Stomach 36 (St36) is used for fatigue.

Bodywork

Massage
Lymphatic massage detoxifies the body while improving circulation. Consult with an experienced practitioner.

Reflexology
See pages 804–805 for information about reflexology areas and how to work them.

Massage the liver points to relieve liver congestion.

To detoxify cells and tissues, work the area corresponding to the lymph system.

Other Bodywork Recommendations
Constitutional hydrotherapy helps to improve liver detoxification and stimulate the immune system for viral hepatitis. See pages 795–796 for directions.

Stress Reduction

General Stress-Reduction Therapies
A diagnosis of chronic hepatitis can be very stressful. Although family and friends are always a welcome source of strength, you may also want to recruit the help of a professional who has experience working with people suffering from chronic illness. A religious adviser, a psychotherapist, or a support-group leader can offer you invaluable advice and help.

In a world of expensive and invasive medical treatments, meditation and positive mental imagery can come as a relief.

Exercise is a healthful way to relieve stress and improve immune function.

Other Recommendations

- Avoid the use of acetaminophen and over-the-counter painkillers and other pharmaceuticals, if possible, as they stress the liver.
- Chinese herbal therapy from a practitioner of Asian medicine can be highly effective.

- Intravenous vitamin C, ozone, glutathione, and other nutrients can be very effective for various forms of hepatitis.

REFERENCES

Chang, H. M., and P. But (eds.). 1986. *Pharmacology and Applications of Chinese Materia Medica*, Vol. 1. Singapore: World Scientific.

Lirussi, F., and L. Okolicsanyi. 1992. Cytoprotection in the nineties: Experience with ursodeoxycholic acid and silymarin in chronic liver disease. *Acta Physiologica Hungarica* 801(1–4):363–67.

Herpes

The herpes family of viruses includes more than seventy known members. The most common ones that humans encounter include herpes simplex 1 and 2, Epstein-Barr virus, varicella zoster, and cytomegalovirus. This section contains information on herpes simplex 1 (HSV-1) and herpes simplex 2 (HSV-2).

Both of the herpes simplex viruses cause small, irritating, fluid-filled blisters or eruptions on the skin and the mucus membranes. Herpes simplex virus 1 is often at the root of cold sores, also known as fever blisters, since sun exposure can bring on an outbreak.

The initial symptoms of a cold sore include burning and tingling sensations around the edges of the lips and the nose, where itchy, painful blisters and/or small, red pimples will form within a few hours and last a few days. They usually dry up and crust over in eight to twelve days after onset, although natural and conventional therapy can often greatly reduce the healing time. A person may complain of localized pain, as well as have a mild fever and swollen lymph nodes in the neck.

Herpes simplex virus 2 causes blisters on the genitals and is typically spread through sexual contact (although herpes simplex virus 1 can also cause genital herpes and vice versa). The burning and tingling sensations surrounding the genital areas are its initial symptoms. The moist linings surrounding the sex organs will soon become the sites of blisters that later turn into sores or lesions that can easily become infected and irritating. It should be noted that a pregnant woman carrying the herpes simplex virus 2 may pass it along to her baby during birth, allowing the baby to form lesions from contact, as well as problems with its nervous systems, such as seizures and mental retardation. Women are screened for this infection during their pregnancy, and cesarean section birthing can prevent the transfer of herpes simplex 2.

Herpes simplex virus 1 and 2 are extremely common. Once they enter the body, herpes viruses can remain dormant in the nervous system for several years or life. Their outbreak is more likely when the immune system is under stress, such as during infectious illness (common cold), when the patient is under physical or emotional stress, from excessive exposure to sunlight, and from nutritional deficiencies and allergies to food or drugs.

Conventional treatment for a cold sore is to let it run its course, apply antiviral topical solutions, or use pain-relieving medications. The antiviral drug acyclovir (Zovirax) is used to suppress outbreaks of oral and genital herpes. Antibiotics may be given for secondary skin infections.

Natural therapy focuses on enhancing the immune system so that one is not as susceptible to a herpes outbreak. In addition, this section discusses some natural remedies that have direct antiviral effects. It has been estimated that 90 percent of the population has one or both herpes viruses. The key is to have a resilient immune system that can fight off and contain the herpes virus. In the case of genital herpes, the best approach is prevention through avoidance of casual sexual contact. However, natural therapies can make a dramatic impact in reducing outbreak recurrence and severity for people with genital herpes.

SYMPTOMS

- A burning, tingling sensation on reddened skin, accompanied by one or more clusters of fluid-filled vesicles

ROOT CAUSES

- Sexual contact
- Nutritional deficiencies
- Immune-system suppression

Testing Techniques

The following tests help assess possible reasons for repeated herpes outbreaks:

Immune-system imbalance or disease—blood

Hormone testing (thyroid, DHEA, cortisol, testosterone, IGF-1, estrogen, progesterone)—saliva, blood, or urine

Intestinal permeability—urine

Detoxification profile—urine

Vitamin and mineral analysis (especially iron)—blood

Digestive function and microbe/parasite/candida testing—stool analysis

Food and environmental allergies/sensitivities—blood, electrodermal

Amino acid imbalance—blood or urine

TREATMENT

Diet

Recommended Food

Consume foods that are rich in the amino acid L-lysine, as they may inhibit herpes virus replication. These includes legumes, fish, turkey, chicken, and most vegetables.

Bell peppers, brussels sprouts, broccoli, potatoes, and other brightly colored vegetables and fruits provide vitamin C and bioflavonoids that help heal the skin.

Fish such as salmon, nuts like walnuts, and seeds such as flaxseeds provide essential fatty acids that are necessary for tissue repair.

Food to Avoid

Avoid foods that are high in the amino acid L-arginine, as it may stimulate HSV replication. These foods include peanuts, almonds, and other nuts, as well as whole wheat and chocolate.

Reduce or eliminate sugars, as they interrupt the healing of tissue and suppress immune function.

Acidic foods, such as grapefruit, tomatoes, oranges, and other citrus fruits, may aggravate cold sores and should be avoided during an outbreak.

℞ Super Seven Prescriptions—Herpes

Super Prescription #1 L-lysine
Take 1,000 mg three times daily between meals for an acute outbreak. For preventative purposes, take 500 mg two or three times daily between meals. This supplement has been shown in some studies to help treat acute outbreaks and may reduce recurrence.

Super Prescription #2 Lemon balm extract (*Melissa officinalis*)
Apply a lemon balm topical cream four times daily to the affected area. It has mainly been studied for healing cold sores.

Super Prescription #3 Homeopathic Herpes Nosode
Take a 30C potency three times daily for three days. This remedy stimulates an immune response to the herpes virus. It can be used for both oral and genital herpes and is also used to prevent recurrences.

Super Prescription #4 Lomatium root (*Lomatium dissectum*)
Take 1 ml or 500 mg four times daily for acute outbreaks. Lomatium root has immune-enhancing and antiviral properties.

Super Prescription #5 Propolis
Apply propolis tincture or ointment four times daily to the affected area. Propolis has been shown to heal genital herpes and most likely helps cold sores.

Super Prescription #6 Vitamin C
Take 1,000 mg, along with 500 mg of bioflavonoids, three times daily. Vitamin C improves immune function and reduces the duration of the infection.

Super Prescription #7 Zinc
Take 30 mg twice daily, along with 3 mg of copper. Zinc supports immune function and has been shown in studies to reduce the frequency, the severity, and the duration of a herpes outbreak. Topical application of zinc sulfate has been shown to reduce the recurrence of herpes outbreaks.

In one double-blind trial, topical application of an extract of lemon-balm cream, applied four times daily for five days, led to significantly fewer symptoms and fewer cold sore blisters than experienced by people using a placebo cream. Lemon balm has also been shown to help prevent recurrence of cold sores.

General Recommendations

Licorice root extract (*glycyrrhetinic acid*) cream has been shown to be effective for herpes outbreaks. Apply to lesions four times daily.

Research on the herpes virus shows that in a culture dish, the amino acid arginine stimulated growth of the virus, while the addition of lysine inhibited growth. In a study, forty-five patients who experienced frequent herpes outbreaks received 312 to 500 mg of L-lysine for two months to three years. The dosage was increased to 800 to 1,000 mg for acute outbreaks, and foods that are high in the amino acid arginine were restricted (chocolate, seeds, nuts). This therapy reduced the frequency of outbreaks and greatly accelerated the recovery from acute outbreaks. Another double-blind study found that 1,200 mg of L-lysine significantly reduced the recurrence of herpes simplex outbreaks.

B-complex is important for people who are prone to cold sore outbreaks. Take a 50 mg complex one or two times daily.

Take a probiotic product containing at least four billion active organisms twice daily, thirty minutes after meals. It supplies friendly bacteria, such as *Lactobacillus acidophilus* and *bifidus*, that are important for immune function.

Echinacea (*Echinacea purpurea*) supports immune function and has antiviral properties. Take 500 mg or 2 to 4 ml of a tincture three times daily.

A high-potency multivitamin provides a base of nutrients required for a healthy immune system. Take as directed on the container.

A super-green-food supplement, such as chlorella or spirulina, or a mixture of super green foods, supports immune function. Take as directed on the container.

Thyme (*Thymus vulgaris*) extract supports the activity of the thymus gland, an important component of the immune system. The dosage is 1 or 2 tablets/capsules twice daily between meals or as directed on the container.

Homeopathy

Pick the remedy that best matches your symptoms in this section. For acute herpes outbreaks, take a 30C potency four times daily. For chronic herpes infections, take a 6x, 12x, 6C, 12C, or 30C twice daily for two weeks to see if there are any positive results. After you notice improvement, stop taking the remedy, unless symptoms return. Consultation with a homeopathic practitioner is advised.

Arsenicum Album is for people with cold sores who have symptoms of burning herpetic lesions that feel better with warm applications and warm drinks. They tend to feel anxious and restless.

Hepar Sulphuris is for very painful and sensitive mouth sores. The lesions feel very sensitive and are aggravated from cold drinks and cold air. The person feels chilly and irritable.

Mercurius Solubilis or Vivus is helpful when bleeding gums, a thickly coated tongue, heavy salivation and drooling, and offensive breath accompany the cold sores. The lesions burn and are worse at night.

Natrum Muriaticum is a specific remedy for cold sores that break out from sun exposure, fever, or emotional stress. The lesions are often near the lips. The corners of the mouth are often cracked as well. There is often a strong craving for salty foods. This remedy is also used for cases of chronic genital herpes. The person has a tendency toward depression and avoids the sun.

Rhus Toxicodendron is helpful for painful, swollen, itchy vesicles that burn and break out quickly. The person feels restless. Symptoms are worse from the cold or the damp.

Sulfur is a useful remedy for red, inflamed, itchy, and burning herpetic lesions. Symptoms are better from cold applications or ice-cold drinks. People requiring this remedy are very warm, with a great thirst for cold drinks.

Aromatherapy

Mix 1 drop of lemon and 1 drop of myrrh in a carrier oil, and with a Q-tip, dab the oil onto the herpes lesion.

Other Recommendations

- Acupuncture is helpful for some people with recurrent herpes. See a qualified practitioner for treatment.
- Intravenous vitamin C and ozone are effective in reducing the viral load associated with acute and chronic herpes.
- Magnet therapy can be effective in reducing pain and stimulating skin healing. maceutical acyclovir. Use under the guidance of a knowledgeable practitioner.
- Applying ice to a cold sore at the first sign of symptoms can help prevent a full-blown outbreak. Apply for ten minutes and then stop. Repeat every hour. An adult should apply it to the lesion of a young child to prevent damaging the skin.

REFERENCES

Griffith, R. S., et al. 1978. A multicentered study of lysine therapy in herpes simplex infection. *Dermatologica* 156:257–67.

Koytchev, R., R. G. Alken, and S. Dundarov. 1999. Balm mint extract (Lo-701) for topical treatment of recurring herpes labialis. *Phytomedicine* 6:225–30.

McCune, M. A., et al. 1984. Treatment of recurrent herpes simplex infections with L-lysine hydrochloride. *Cutis* 34:366–73.

Vynograd, N., I. Vynograd, and Z. Sosnowski. 2000. A comparative multi-centre study of the efficacy of propolis, Acyclovir and a placebo in the treatment of genital herpes. *Phytomedicine* 7(1):1–6.

In one study involving ninety men and women with genital herpes, investigators compared propolis ointment to the pharmaceutical acyclovir. The participants were examined during their course of treatment. The authors of the study concluded that propolis ointment appeared to be more effective than acyclovir and a placebo in healing genital herpes lesions.

Herpes Zoster. See Shingles

Hiatal Hernia and Acid Reflux Disease

A person is said to have a hiatal hernia when part of the stomach protrudes, or herniates, through the opening of the diaphragm and into the chest cavity. While almost half of all Americans over the age of forty have this disorder, many of these people experience few, if any, symptoms. Hiatal hernias are generally not considered dangerous unless they produce persistent or severe symptoms.

The food you eat starts its digestive journey in the mouth and then slides down the esophagus, a long tube that leads to the stomach. Because food is meant to travel through the digestive system in one direction only, the base of the esophagus is outfitted with a ring of muscles that acts as a sentry. At the stomach entrance, the muscles relax and allow the food to pass into the stomach, where acids start to break it down into a digestible stew. Once you're finished eating and the esophagus is empty, the muscular rings and valves tighten. This action keeps the food and the acids from backing up out of the stomach and refluxing into the esophageal tube.

Hiatal hernias can keep this system from working properly. When part of the stomach slides out of place (herniates), the ability of the muscular rings to keep food and acid in the stomach may be inhibited. In a phenomenon known as acid reflux, food and acid splash up into the esophagus, causing heartburn, chest pains, and belching. A person with severe symptoms may regurgitate stomach acid into the throat and the mouth. Sometimes the acid reflux leads to angina-like chest pains and spasms; the symptoms may be so intense that they are mistaken for a heart attack. Over long periods of time, the constant irritation of the esophagus can lead to inflammation, scarring, ulceration, hemorrhaging, and even esophageal cancer.

As with almost all digestive disorders, poor diet plays a large role in the unpleasant symptoms of hiatal hernias. Anything that contributes to an overly full stomach— eating too much, or eating foods that are not easily digested—encourages the stomach's contents to back up. In many cases, food allergies make the condition worse. Stress can trigger severe gastric upset as well. Anything that traumatizes the stomach muscles, such as injury, surgery, or pregnancy, can lead to hiatal hernias, as can the general weakening of muscles most people associate with aging. Finally, some people inherit a genetic tendency to this condition.

Bodywork therapies can be utilized to improve the structural problem that occurs with this condition. This involves manipulating the soft tissue, as well as the stomach itself, in a downward direction. This is described further in this chapter.

Acid reflux can also be caused by being overweight, from stomach infections, and from the effects of stress.

No matter what the cause, hiatal hernias respond well to dietary, herbal, and stress-reduction therapies. If you have this disorder, you'll also want to get regular checkups to monitor the health of your esophagus.

SYMPTOMS

- Symptoms that are usually worse after eating
- Heartburn that's worse when bending over or lying down
- Belching
- Pains and muscle spasms in the chest
- Acid reflux

ROOT CAUSES

- Poor diet
- Trauma to the stomach area
- Food allergies
- Stress
- Weakness of stomach muscles
- Inherited tendency
- Pregnancy

Testing Techniques

The following tests help assess possible reasons for hiatal hernia and acid reflux:

Hormone testing (progesterone for women)—saliva, blood, or urine

Digestive function and microbe/parasite/candida testing—stool analysis

Food and environmental allergies/sensitivities—blood, electrodermal

TREATMENT

Diet

Recommended Food

Eat basic, unrefined foods that have not been stripped of their natural fiber. Whole grains, raw vegetables, and raw nuts and seeds are all good choices.

Avoid overeating by planning several light meals throughout the day.

Drink plenty of water. To maintain good digestive health, you need to drink a glass of clean, quality water every two waking hours. In addition, have a large glass or two whenever you feel symptoms coming on. The water will dilute and neutralize the rising stomach acids.

The powers of cabbage juice to soothe the digestive tract are extraordinary. Drink a glass every day.

Add flaxseeds or flaxseed oil to your meals every day.

Food to Avoid

Avoid overeating. Don't eat on the run; take time to enjoy your meals and to savor each bite. Stop eating before you feel full.

Do not eat just before bedtime. Allow two to three hours for your stomach to empty.

Stay away from foods that are hard to digest. Saturated, hydrogenated, and partially hydrogenated fats linger in the stomach and often lead to acid reflux. The most frequent culprits are fried and greasy foods, red meat, and heavy sauces.

Food allergies are linked to hiatal hernias, so see the Food Allergies section and follow the elimination diet given there. If a food causes you trouble, eliminate it from your diet. You may find that your symptoms improve significantly or even disappear.

Avoid caffeine, alcohol, chocolate, and spicy or minty foods. They irritate the stomach and can aggravate your symptoms.

℞ Super Seven Prescriptions—Hiatal Hernia and Acid Reflux

Super Prescription #1 Licorice root (DGL)
Chew one or two 400 mg tablets (or take in powder form) twenty minutes before each meal. DGL is a special type of licorice extract that soothes and heals the stomach and the esophagus. It does not cause high blood pressure.

Super Prescription #2 Aloe vera juice
Take 1 to 2 tablespoons three times daily or as directed on the container. Aloe vera promotes healing and soothes the digestive tract.

Super Prescription #3 Homeopathic Nux Vomica
Take a 30C potency two or three times daily. This homeopathic is specific for heartburn and reflux.

Super Prescription #4 Orange peel extract
Take 1 capsule that contains D-limonene 98.5 percent extract every other day for twenty days, then as needed, to reduce heartburn.

DGL is a special type of licorice-root (*Glycyrrhiza glabra*) extract used by holistic doctors to relieve acid reflux and ulcer pain. DGL stimulates cell growth of the mucus layer that lines the stomach and the intestines. It also improves blood flow and reduces muscle spasms. A study involving one hundred people compared the effects of DGL to those of the pharmaceutical antacid drug Tagamet and found that both were equally effective for healing ulcers.

Super Prescription #5 Slippery elm (*Ulmus fulva*)

Take 1 teaspoon, 300 mg of the capsules, or 3 ml of the tincture three times daily. This herb is used to soothe and reduce inflammation of the lining of the esophagus and the stomach.

Super Prescription #6 Digestive enzymes

Take 1 or 2 capsules of a full-spectrum blend with each meal. Enzymes help you to digest foods more effectively so they are less likely to cause irritation. *Note*: Some people may need to use a formula that contains no protease, as this protein-digestive enzyme may irritate the stomach.

Super Prescription #7 Probiotic

Take a product containing at least five billion active organisms daily. It contains friendly bacteria, such as *Lactobacillus acidophilus* and *bifidus*, which improve digestive function.

General Recommendations

Gentian Root (*Gentiana lutea*) improves overall digestive function. Take 300 mg or 10 to 20 drops five to fifteen minutes before meals.

A super-green-food supplement, such as chlorella, spirulina, or a mixture of super green foods in a drink, helps to neutralize acidity. Take as directed on the container.

Chamomile tea is soothing to the digestive tract. Drink one to two cups daily.

Liquid calcium is soothing to the stomach. Take a formula containing 500 mg of calcium and 250 mg of magnesium twice daily. Magnesium helps to relax tightened muscles of the esophagus and the stomach.

Take 300 mg of marshmallow root three times daily.

Homeopathy

Pick the remedy that best matches your symptoms in this section. For relief of acute acid reflux, take a 30C potency every fifteen minutes up to four doses. For chronic acid reflux, take a 6x, 12x, 6C, 12C, or 30C dose twice daily for two weeks to see if there are any positive results. After you notice improvement, stop taking the remedy, unless symptoms return. Consultation with a homeopathic practitioner is advised.

Arsenicum Album is for a burning sensation in the esophagus or the stomach that is alleviated by drinking milk or frequently sipping on warm water and sitting up. The person feels anxious and restless.

Carbo Vegetabilis will help people whose sluggish digestion leads to flatulence, belching, and bloating in the upper abdomen. People who benefit from this remedy are often pale and cold. Despite their chilliness, they feel better with cool air and drinks.

Lycopodium (*Lycopodium clavatum*) is also for gas and bloating, but in this case the symptoms are usually brought on by anxiety and lack of confidence. The person feels worse when wearing tight clothes and better when sipping warm drinks. There may be a sour taste in the mouth. Symptoms are often worse in the late afternoon and the evening.

Natrum Carbonicum is for people who have trouble digesting most foods, especially milk.

Nux Vomica is for people with heartburn and reflux that occurs from stress, spicy foods, and alcohol. They are generally chilly, irritable, and oversensitive to stimuli (noise, light). Constipation is often a problem as well.

Pulsatilla (*Pulsatilla pratensis*) is helpful if you feel worse after eating rich and fatty foods. Symptoms are worse in a warm room and better with fresh air. You also tend to feel tearful when ill, and you greatly desire comfort.

Phosphorus helps when you have a burning pain in the stomach that feels better from cold drinks. However, soon after drinking, you feel nauseous and may vomit.

Sulfur is for burning pain and belching, accompanied by diarrhea. The person tends to be very warm and gets relief from ice-cold drinks.

Acupressure

See pages 787–794 for information about pressure points and administering treatment.

- Strengthen your upper digestive tract and reduce tension by working Pericardium 6 (P6).
- Stomach 36 (St36) gives general support to the entire body while improving your ability to absorb nutrients.
- Lung 1 (Lu1) reduces stress.
- Conception Vessel 12 (CV12) reduces heartburn.

Bodywork

Reflexology

See pages 804–805 for information about reflexology areas and how to work them.

Work the areas corresponding to the stomach, the diaphragm, and the adrenal glands. To reduce stress, also work the solar plexus.

Other Bodywork Recommendations

A chiropractor, an osteopath, or a naturopath can perform a gentle manipulation of your stomach with a downward pull. This helps reduce the stomach protrusion and soft tissues that have gone too far up through the diaphragm. Noticeable improvements can be noted within a few treatments.

Also, acupuncture can be quite effective in managing the symptoms. See a qualified practitioner.

Aromatherapy

Add any of the following oils to a warm bath, or dilute them in a carrier oil and use them in a gentle massage of your abdomen or lower back.

If your digestive system is slow to break down the food in your stomach, black pepper will stimulate the process.

Chamomile and ginger oils will help soothe stomach pain.

Stress Reduction

General Stress-Reduction Therapies

Any stress-reduction technique will help calm your stomach, so feel free to use any of the strategies listed in the Exercise and Stress Reduction chapter. You may find that yoga is especially helpful, as it not only reduces stress but also builds up the abdominal muscles. Regular exercise and Pilates are excellent as well.

Other Recommendations

- If you are obese, your symptoms will greatly improve if you lose weight. The dietary suggestions here may help, but see the Obesity entry if you need further advice.
- Do not wear clothes that fit tightly around your midsection. Constrictive clothing can push the stomach even farther out of place.
- Smoking aggravates heartburn, so if you smoke, quit. If you don't, you must still avoid exposure to secondhand smoke.
- Do not bend over, lie down, or put any great strain on your body within a few hours after eating. Organize your activities so that you can perform them when your stomach is empty.

REFERENCES

Morgan, A. G., et al. 1982. Comparison between Cimetidine and Caved-S in the treatment of gastric ulceration, and subsequent maintenance therapy. *Gut* 23:545–51.

High Blood Pressure. See Blood Pressure, High

High Cholesterol. See Cholesterol, High

HIV. See AIDS and HIV

Hives

Hives, medically known as urticaria, are raised white or yellow bumps surrounded by red, inflamed patches of skin. Hives usually cause a burning sensation at first, which soon gives way to intense itching. Aside from these symptoms, the course of hives is unpredictable. The rash may erupt suddenly and then disappear almost as quickly, or it may linger for weeks or even longer. It most often appears on the arms, the legs, or the trunk, but it can develop on any part of the body; sometimes it erupts in one place and then vanishes, only to appear somewhere else.

Although we don't tend to think of skin as an excretory organ, it actually plays a significant role in allowing toxins to pass out of the body. During the flu, for example, the body's temperature rises so that the virus can be expelled through a cleansing sweat. Just as poisons leave the body through sweat, they can also be excreted via skin eruptions like hives. Hives, like the symptoms of the flu, are an indicator that your body has detected a toxin and is trying to eliminate it.

An episode of hives is most frequently a response to an allergen or an irritant, which in either case is a normally harmless substance that produces a toxic response in your body. Possible allergens and irritants include insect bites, cosmetics, perfumes, detergents, and household cleaners. Certain foods may also trigger an allergic response. Shellfish are notorious for causing hives, but dairy, meat, and poultry are frequent instigators as well. Any food made with additives, preservatives, or pesticides may also produce a reaction. Some people with chronic or recurring cases of hives find that their triggers are frustratingly ubiquitous: heat, cold, sunlight, and stress have all been known to bring on a rash.

Drugs and viruses can also cause hives. Antibiotics, especially penicillin, cause hives in some unfortunate people; during a bacterial infection, they will need to work closely with their doctors to determine the best course of medical action. Lately, doctors have linked viruses like hepatitis B and Epstein-Barr to hives, and the fungus *Candida albicans* has also been known to trigger the disorder.

Some people suffer from reoccurring hives due to the effects of stress. In these cases, it is important for them to incorporate stress-reduction techniques into their lifestyle. Also, hives can be symptoms of more serious conditions, such as parasitic infections, hepatitis, cancer, hyperthyroidism, and rare blood disorders.

Anyone who sufferers from chronic or recurring hives should consider that his or her digestive system may not be functioning properly, thereby forcing the skin to throw off toxins that would normally be excreted by the intestines. A close review of dietary and lifestyle habits is in order.

The good news is that hives, although irritating and itchy, rarely pose a significant health threat. In almost all cases, they disappear from the skin without leaving a scar or other marks, and they do not damage any other organs. The best treatment is to identify the irritant or the toxin and then avoid it; you'll also want to employ methods that help you speed up the detoxification process. Sometimes, however, hives can cause the tongue and the throat to swell up; breathing becomes difficult, if not impossible. If you have hives and experience any trouble breathing or swallowing, you have a medical emergency. Call for medical help immediately. If you know that you are prone to severe hives, keep an emergency adrenaline kit on hand.

SYMPTOMS

- Burning or itchy white bumps, surrounded by areas of redness and inflammation
- May appear anywhere on the body, and may come and go without warning

ROOT CAUSES

- Response to an allergen or an irritant
- Certain drugs, especially antibiotics and aspirin
- Infectious agent
- Poor digestion
- Vitamin D deficiency

Testing Techniques

The following tests help assess possible reasons for hives:

    Immune-system imbalance or disease—blood

    Hormone testing (thyroid, DHEA, cortisol)—saliva, blood, or urine

    Intestinal permeability—urine

    Detoxification profile—urine

    Digestive function and microbe/parasite/candida testing—stool analysis

    Food and environmental allergies/sensitivities—blood, electrodermal

    Vitamin D—blood

TREATMENT

Diet

Recommended Food

If you have a chronic case of hives and cannot identify the cause, it is highly recommended that you buy food in its natural state whenever possible and prepare it yourself. This eating plan will drastically reduce your chances of encountering a food allergen.

Everyone with hives should make it a priority to follow a high-fiber diet that includes oats, brown rice, beans, and raw fruits and vegetables. You'll improve your digestion and reduce the necessity of expelling toxins through your skin.

If your hives are triggered by sunlight, eat lots of deeply colored vegetables. They're high in carotenoids and will improve your skin's resistance to the sun.

Essential fatty acids reduce inflammation. Eat cold-water fish several times a week; if you're following a vegan diet, add flaxseeds to your salads, or use flaxseed oil as a dressing.

Candidiasis may be a factor in persistent hives. Although live active yogurt is generally recommended for people with candidiasis, you should stay away from it if you are allergic to dairy. Instead, try kefir or sauerkraut. Many people with dairy allergies choose to drink sauerkraut juice daily—an acquired taste, to be sure, but one that goes a long way toward replacing the friendly bacteria that fight *Candida albicans*.

Drink a glass of clean, quality water every two waking hours. You'll flush out impurities and encourage the health of nearly every body system, including the skin.

Food to Avoid

Hives are often caused by a response to a food allergen or an irritant. Read the Food Allergies section and follow the elimination diet to find out if a certain food triggers hives for you; if so, it goes without saying that you must banish that food from your diet. Some people can't even come into contact with allergenic foods, let alone ingest them, so stay as far away from these as you can. Any food can conceivably cause hives, but shellfish, dairy, eggs, cured meats, citrus fruit, and peanuts are the most common triggers.

Avoid foods that prevent your body from functioning optimally. Processed, junk, and refined foods all unbalance your immune and digestive systems, even if you're not allergic to them.

Alcohol and caffeine are diuretics that pull nutrients out of your body. Since your poisoned system needs all the support it can get, stay away from these substances.

Digestive problems are linked to all skin disorders. Do not eat meat, fried foods, or foods high in saturated fat; they take too long to travel through the intestines and lead to constipation. Avoid dairy products, as they slow food down on its way through the digestive system.

 Super Seven Prescriptions—Hives

Super Prescription #1 Homeopathic Apis (*Apis mellifica*)
Take a 30C potency every fifteen minutes, up to four doses. This remedy is specific for hive outbreaks where there is itching and swelling.

Super Prescription #2 Vitamin D3
Take 4,000 to 5,000 IU daily with a meal. Research has shown it to reduce the severity of symptoms.

Super Prescription #3 Quercitin
This nutrient reduces the effects of histamine, a chemical that is released by the body during an allergic reaction. Take 1,000 mg three times daily.

Super Prescription #4 Vitamin B12
Taking 1,000 mcg of the injected form (given by your doctor) one to three times weekly can help reduce the severity of acute hives. The oral form is not as effective, but you can take 400 mcg of sublingual B12 daily.

Super Prescription #5 Greens drink
Take daily, as directed on the container, a blend containing super green foods such as chlorella or spirulina. You can also take these supplements individually. They support detoxification and neutralize acidity.

Super Prescription #6 Burdock root (*Articum lappa*)
Take 300 mg or 3 ml three times daily to support detoxification of the skin.

Super Prescription #7 Nettle leaf (*Urtica dioica*)
Take 300 mg three times daily of a freeze-dried nettle product. Nettle leaf has an antihistamine effect.

A study by researchers at the University of Nebraska Medical Center and published in the *Annals of Allergy, Asthma, and Immunology* found that supplementation of 4,000 IU daily of vitamin D3 caused a 40 percent decrease in the severity of subjects' hives over three months' duration.

General Recommendations

Aloe vera reduces inflammation and is soothing to the skin. You may smooth a cream or a lotion directly onto the hives for temporary relief; to address the body's imbalances more directly, drink aloe vera juice.

Chamomile (*Matricaria recutita*) is a good all-around tonic for hives. Used in a cream, it relieves itching. Drunk as a tea, it eases stress.

If you need more potent relief from stress or anxiety, drink valerian (*Valeriana officinalis*) tea once during the day and again just before bedtime.

People with skin disorders often have stressed livers. Milk thistle (*Carduus marianus*) will help cleanse this crucial organ. Find a product standardized for 70 to 80 percent silymarin, and take 200 to 250 mg twice daily.

Homeopathy

Pick the remedy that best matches your symptoms in this section. For relief of acute hive outbreaks, take a 30C potency every fifteen minutes, up to four doses. For chronic hives, take a 6x, 12x, 6C, 12C, or 30C twice daily for two weeks to see if there are any positive results. After you notice improvement, stop taking the remedy, unless symptoms return. Consultation with a homeopathic practitioner is advised.

Apis (*Apis mellifica*) is for red, swollen, burning hives that feel better with cold applications and in the fresh air.

Histaminum is a remedy used for general allergy reactions. It calms down the release of the chemical called histamine that leads to allergy reactions.

Rhus Toxicodendron is for hives that are caused by getting chilled in the rain or in dampness and that itch violently. They feel better when heat is applied.

Urtica Urens is for hives that feel like prickly heat and are caused by insect bites or from eating shellfish.

Acupressure

See pages 787–794 for information about pressure points and administering treatment.
- To remove heat from the blood, work Spleen 10 (Sp10).
- Other points that ease heat-related skin conditions are Bladder 23 and 47 (B23 and B47) and Stomach 2 and 3 (St2 and St3).
- If stress is a trigger for you, work Bladder 10 (B10) whenever you feel tense and likely to break out.
- Spleen 10 (Sp10) clears heat from the blood.
- If you are constipated, work Conception Vessel 6 (CV6) and Large Intestine 4 (LI4) to stimulate intestinal contractions.

Bodywork

Reflexology
See pages 804–805 for information about reflexology areas and how to work them.
Work the liver and the colon to encourage detoxification.
If you need to reduce tension, stimulate the solar plexus.

Hydrotherapy
A cool bath will not cure hives, but it can temporarily relieve the itching.

Aromatherapy
Chamomile, lavender, and melissa will reduce inflammation, itching, and stress. Use any one of the oils or all of them together in a bath, a compress, or a lotion. As it's

possible that you'll have a reaction to one of these oils, start off by using them in small quantities, and test them on a small area of skin before plunging into a bath.

Stress Reduction

General Stress-Reduction Therapies

Folk wisdom has always noted the link between anxiety and hives, and now at least one scientific study seems to confirm this traditional knowledge. If you get hives frequently—even if they're caused by an identifiable trigger—you should seek out a relaxation therapy and practice it regularly.

Other Recommendations

An oatmeal bath can reduce itching. Add a cup of oatmeal powder, such as Aveeno, to a warm bath. The other alternative is to put oatmeal into a cheesecloth bag and tie it with a string, hang it under the faucet or float it in the tub. Soak in the warm bath for five to fifteen minutes. When you're done, pat your skin dry so that a film of oatmeal is left on your skin. This film contains the anti-itch properties of the oatmeal.

REFERENCES

Rorie, A., et al. 2014. Beneficial role for supplemental vitamin D3 treatment in chronic urticaria: A randomized study. *Ann Allergy Asthma Immunol* 112(4):376–82.

Hyperthyroidism (Overactive Thyroid)

This condition occurs when the thyroid gland produces too much of the thyroid hormones known as thyroxine (T4) and triiodothyronine (T3). Since thyroid hormones increase the metabolism of cells, one can experience many symptoms related to high metabolism. These include irregular heartbeat, nervousness, sudden weight loss, insomnia, and rapid heartbeat.

The most common cause is an autoimmune condition known as Graves' disease. This condition is more common in women over the age of twenty. As the immune system attacks the thyroid gland, it stimulates the release of an antibody known as thyrotropin receptor antibody (TRAb), which causes the thyroid to make excessive amounts of thyroid hormones.

Conventional therapy offers three main treatment options: antithyroid medications that suppress the production of thyroid hormones, radioactive iodine (which destroys the thyroid gland), and surgical removal of the thyroid. Those who receive radioactive iodine or surgery will develop hypothyroidism (low thyroid), which then requires thyroid-hormone supplementation for the rest of their lives.

Hyperthyroidism can sometimes be reversed solely with natural therapy when it's treated in the early stages. The root causes of the autoimmune response, such as stress, hormone imbalance, chronic infections, or gluten allergy, must be identified and treated. Otherwise, natural therapies can be integrated with antithyroid medications such as methimazole to maintain a better thyroid balance.

SYMPTOMS

- Anxiety and nervousness
- Increased sweating
- Breast enlargement in men
- Insomnia (possible)
- Menstrual irregularities
- Diarrhea
- Muscle weakness
- Difficulty concentrating
- Rapid or irregular heartbeat
- Double vision
- Restlessness
- Eyeballs that protrude (exophthalmos)
- Shortness of breath with exertion
- Thyroid enlargement (goiter)
- Eye irritation and tearing
- Tremor
- Fatigue
- Weight gain (rare)
- Heat intolerance
- Weight loss
- Increased appetite

ROOT CAUSES

The following are the causes accepted in conventional medicine:

- Genetics—a family history of the disease
- Sex—women are seven times more likely to develop Graves' disease than men are
- Age—Graves' disease usually develops after age twenty
- Smoking
- Pregnancy
- Stress

Holistic doctors also look at:

- Food allergies such as gluten (which can trigger autoimmunity)
- Toxic metals
- Poor digestive function
- Overall hormone balance, particularly stress hormones such as DHEA and cortisol, which modulate the immune system
- Environmental toxins (such as pesticides)

Testing Techniques

The following tests help assess possible reasons for hyperthyroidism:

Thyroid-hormone levels and antibodies—blood

Food allergies and sensitivities—blood, stool, electrodermal

Toxic metals—urine, blood, hair

Digestive function and absorption—stool analysis, urine

Environmental toxins—blood, urine

TREATMENT

Diet

A healthy diet can reduce the autoimmune response involved in hyperthyroidism.

Recommended Food

Consume a diet that is focused on whole foods in their natural state as much as possible. This should include vegetables, fruits, fish, legumes, nuts and seeds, and nongluten grains. Shakes made with protein, anti-inflammatory herbs, and nutrients can be helpful.

Food to Avoid

Many of those affected with this condition benefit from a gluten-free (no rye, barley, wheat, and most oats) and casein-free (cow's milk) diet. Avoid artificial dyes, colorings, sweeteners, and simple sugars.

℞ Super Seven Prescriptions—Hyperthyroidism

Super Prescription #1 Homeopathic Iodum
Take 2 pellets of a 30C potency three times daily for five days or 2 pellets of a 200C one time only. See if there is any improvement. Do not repeat the remedy if improvement continues. This treatment is best done under the supervision of a homeopathic practitioner and works best in the first week or two of the symptoms.

Super Prescription #2 Bugleweed
Take 2 ml three times daily. Bugleweed contains organic acids that are believed to inhibit antibody binding to the thyroid gland.

Super Prescription #3 L-carnitine
Take 1,000 mg two to four times daily. One study found that it reduced hyperthyroid symptoms.

Super Prescription #4 Lemon balm (*Melissa officinalis*)
Take 2 ml three times daily. It contains substances that inhibit antibody binding to the thyroid gland.

Super Prescription #5 Lithium
Lithium supplementation can suppress thyroid-hormone production. Use under the direction of a holistic doctor.

Super Prescription #6 Iodine
Higher doses of iodine can suppress thyroid-hormone production. Use under the direction of a holistic doctor.

Super Prescription #7 B-complex
Take 50 mg twice daily to help with symptoms of hyperthyroidism.

A study in the *Journal of Endocrinology and Metabolism* found that L-carnitine supplementation significantly alleviated the symptoms associated with hyperthyroidism. The randomized, double-blind, placebo-controlled six-month trial involved fifty women. The researchers found that 2,000 to 4,000 mg daily of oral L-carnitine was able to relieve many symptoms associated with hyperthyroidism without any toxicity or medication interaction. It also helped to reduce elevated liver enzymes.

General Recommendations

B12 injections from a holistic doctor may alleviate some symptoms of hyperthyroidism.

Plant-sterol supplementation can be used to balance and modulate the immune system. Use as directed on the label.

Thyme extract helps to balance the immune system. Use as directed on the label.

Bodywork

Reflexology
Work the areas of the thyroid gland.

Hydrotherapy
Constitutional hydrotherapy can be used to balance the immune system. See pages 795–796.

Other Recommendations
Acupuncture and Chinese herbal therapy can be helpful in managing symptoms. See a qualified practitioner.

Hypoglycemia

Hypoglycemia is a condition of low blood sugar (glucose). Since glucose is your body's primary fuel source, a variety of symptoms can occur when the level drops too low. Symptoms include fatigue, irritability, weakness, and poor concentration. Diet, exercise, and supplements work very well for this condition.

Dietary changes should be the first line of therapy to stabilize the blood sugar level. At a deeper level, stress-hormone balance can help many with this condition because stress hormones such as cortisol affect blood sugar balance.

Many doctors such as ourselves find that hypoglycemia can be a precursor to the opposite problem in the future: high glucose level and diabetes.

SYMPTOMS

- Fatigue
- Anxiety
- Weakness
- Sweating
- Irritability
- Hunger
- Poor concentration
- Heart palpitations
- Headache
- Seizures (not common)
- Visual changes
- Loss of consciousness (not common)

ROOT CAUSES

- Dietary, including:
  Not eating enough or frequently enough
  Eating too many simple sugars
  Not eating enough protein or complex carbohydrates
  Excessive alcohol consumption
- Hormonal imbalance among the pituitary, adrenal, and pancreatic hormones
- Nutritional deficiencies such as of chromium
- Tumors
- Chronic illnesses
- Medications such as diabetes drugs

Testing Techniques

The following test can help determine underlying reasons for hypoglycemia:
  Oral glucose-tolerance test—blood
  Stress-hormone balance—blood, urine, or saliva
  Food sensitivities—blood or electrodermal

TREATMENT

Diet

A balanced diet will go a long way in helping those with hypoglycemia. Many people find that eating four or five smaller meals daily prevents their blood sugar from dropping so easily.

Recommended Food

Follow a diet high in fiber (vegetables, nuts, seeds, whole grains). Water-soluble fiber, found in oat bran, beans, nuts, seeds, and apples, helps to balance blood sugar. Ground flaxseed or chia seeds should be consumed daily. Consume 1 teaspoon with each meal or ¼ cup daily. Make sure to drink plenty of clean, quality water when you start taking flaxseed (10 ounces per tablespoon). A daily total of 50 mg of fiber is a great goal.

Consume vegetable protein (legumes, nuts, seeds, peas) or lean animal protein (turkey, chicken, fish) with each meal. Protein drinks that have low sugar levels may be consumed. Protein helps to stabilize blood sugar levels. Many people with hypoglycemia benefit by increasing the relative amount of protein in the diet.

Focus on quality fats. Fish such as salmon is excellent, and so are nuts and seeds. Use olive and flaxseed oil on your salads.

Instead of eating three large meals, have several smaller meals throughout the day to keep your insulin and blood sugar level steady, or have three main meals with healthy snacks in between. Do not go longer than three hours without eating.

Chromium deficiency has been linked to hypoglycemia, so eat lots of brewer's yeast, wheat germ, whole grains, cheese, soy products, onions, and garlic.

Food to Avoid

Stay away from simple sugars such as candy, cookies, soda, and other sweets.

Refined white bread spikes the blood sugar level and then leads to a rapid drop. Whole-grain breads, cereals, and pastas are better choices. Brown rice, barley, oats, spelt, and kamut are complex carbohydrates that are good choices.

Eliminate alcohol and caffeine from your diet; they cause blood sugar fluctuations. Avoid artificial sweeteners. Instead use diabetic-safe and healthier natural sweeteners such as Stevia, lo han, or xylitol. Avoid high-glycemic foods.

℞ Super Seven Prescriptions—Hypoglycemia

Super Prescription #1 Chromium
Take 200 to 500 mcg daily for better blood sugar balance. Chromium is involved in the transport of glucose into the cells.

Super Prescription #2 Whey protein
Take 20 grams once daily between meals for better glucose balance.

Super Prescription #3 PGX
This is a type of water-soluble fiber that has been shown to balance glucose levels. Take 2 to 4 capsules before each meal with 8 ounces or more of water.

Super Prescription #4 Ashwagandha
Take 125 to 250 mg of an ashwagandha extract for adrenal support and better glucose balance.

Super Prescription #5 Multivitamin/ -mineral
Take a high-potency multivitamin and multimineral formula to provide a base of nutrients for glucose balance.

Super Prescription #6 Fish oil
Take 1,000 mg of EPA and DHA daily for better glucose balance.

Super Prescription #7 Resveratrol
Take 100 to 250 mg daily for glucose balance.

A three-month double-blind crossover study published in *Metabolism* found that chromium supplementation at 200 mcg daily for three months reduced symptoms and improved glucose levels in patients with reactive hypoglycemia.

General Recommendations

Adrenal glandular helps with stress-gland function and glucose balance. Take 1 tablet twice daily.

Alpha lipoic acid helps with glucose control. Take 300 mg twice daily.

Chia seeds contain fiber and protein that help glucose balance. Take as directed on the label.

Take a 50 mg B-complex supplement daily. Many of the B vitamins are involved in blood sugar metabolism.

Homeopathy

Consult a homeopathic practitioner to individualize treatment.

Bodywork

Reflexology

See pages 804–805 for information about reflexology areas and how to work them. Work the points that correspond to the pancreas, the liver, and the thyroid, pituitary, and adrenal glands.

Other Recommendations

Exercise regularly to maintain good blood sugar balance. Make sure to have a snack thirty minutes before exercise to prevent a low glucose level.

REFERENCES

Anderson, R. A., M. M. Polansky, N. A. Bryden, et al. 1987. Effects of supplemental chromium on patients with symptoms of reactive hypoglycemia. *Metabolism* 36:351–55.

Hypothyroidism (Underactive Thyroid)

Hypothyroidism, also referred to as low thyroid or underactive thyroid, is a very common condition that affects millions of North Americans. The most widely prescribed drug in the United States is Synthroid, a synthetic thyroid-hormone replacement used by more than twenty-two million Americans every month.

The thyroid gland, situated at the base of the neck, below the Adam's apple, secretes hormones that control metabolic activity in every cell of the body. This means the thyroid has an impact on processes as varied as temperature control, weight regulation, heart rate, and energy production. It also affects the balance of other hormones in the body, including the neurotransmitters, which influence mood. In hypothyroidism, the thyroid fails to produce sufficient quantities of its hormones. There are many possible symptoms of hypothyroidism. Common ones include fatigue, weight gain, dry skin, hair loss, constipation, intolerance to cold, and poor memory. See the symptom section below for a complete listing.

The most common cause of hypothyroidism in the United States is Hashimoto's thyroiditis, an autoimmune disease in which the immune system attacks and destroys thyroid cells. It makes the affected person less able to produce thyroid hormone. In addition, they have an increased risk of thyroid cancer. Hashimoto's is diagnosed by blood tests that detect elevated thyroid antibodies. The exact cause is unknown, although there seems to be a genetic predisposition. Vitamin D deficiency and gluten sensitivity/allergy increase one's risk as well. Other possible risk factors include increased intestinal permeability, other hormone imbalances, environmental toxins, other infections, and the effects of stress.

Worldwide, the most common cause of hypothyroidism is iodine deficiency. Iodine is required for the thyroid gland to produce thyroid hormones. Iodine deficiency has become more common in North America in recent years as people avoid iodized salt due to concerns about high blood pressure. Other than in certain seafood and algae products, iodine is not readily available in the diet. In addition, certain chemicals present in the environment and the food supply block iodine from being received by the thyroid gland. These include bromine, fluoride, chloride, and perchlorate. Some research suggests that iodine overload can suppress thyroid function, although this is much less common than iodine deficiency.

Hypothyroidism can also be caused by hormonal changes that accompany pregnancy, certain medications, infectious/inflammatory reactions, and problems with the hypothalamic and pituitary areas of the brain.

Hypothyroidism is more common in women. The balance of estrogen and progesterone can have an indirect influence on the thyroid glands. Most common is estrogen dominance, wherein relatively higher estrogen levels suppress thyroid function. This predisposition can occur throughout a woman's life. Women on synthetic estrogen therapy are particularly susceptible to decreased thyroid function.

The effects of stress and the balance of stress hormones are also important in thyroid function. Chronic elevation of the stress hormone cortisol suppresses thyroid function, while low levels of DHEA appear to make one more susceptible to hypothyroidism. Toxic metals, such as mercury, lead, arsenic, and others, can also interfere with thyroid activity.

Although hypothyroidism can wreak havoc upon a patient's entire body, it is easy to treat, especially if caught in its early stages. If you suspect that you have an underactive thyroid, measure your basal body temperature by taking your temperature at the same time every morning, before you get out of bed, for several days in a row. If your body temperature is consistently low, you should see a doctor for an evaluation. For mild cases, nutritional supplements can set you back on track quickly. For people with more severe cases, the use of thyroid-hormone replacement may be required. Even if you require a thyroid-hormone supplement, you should complement this regime of supplementation with dietary changes, stress-reducing activities, exercise, and general hormone balancing.

A word of caution: Many doctors rely on a blood test known as TSH to diagnose hypothyroidism. Unfortunately, this test by itself is extremely unreliable and often fails to catch mild to moderate cases of the disorder. If your basal body temperature is consistently low and if you experience the symptoms described here, but your blood test does not reveal hypothyroidism, consider working with a more holistic doctor for preventative care.

SYMPTOMS

- Fatigue
- Anxiety and panic attacks
- Apathy
- Poor memory and concentration
- Depression and irritability
- Low libido
- Weight gain
- Headaches
- Aches and pains
- Premenstrual syndrome
- Sensitivity to cold and heat
- Lowered immunity
- Constipation
- Carpal tunnel syndrome
- Menstrual problems (irregular periods and heavy periods)
- Raynaud's phenomenon
- Water retention
- Recurring infections
- Dry eyes/blurred vision
- High cholesterol
- Eyebrow loss (outer one-third)
- Hair loss
- Anemia and easy bruising
- Dry skin and hair
- Slow healing
- Brittle, peeling nails
- Hoarse voice
- Infertility
- Tingling hands and feet
- Insomnia
- Decreased perspiration
- Decreased hearing
- Full sensation in throat, hoarseness
- Swelling of the face
- Slow pulse
- Swelling of the ankles
- Slow reflexes
- Chilliness
- Low body temperature
- Muscle aches
- Muscle weakness

ROOT CAUSES

- Hashimoto's disease and other inflammatory disorders of the thyroid
- Hormone imbalance (especially estrogen/progesterone, cortisol/ DHEA)
- Iodine and other nutrient deficiencies
- Stress
- Surgery on or radiation of the thyroid
- Poor diet

- Inactivity
- Certain medications, most notably lithium, arrhythmia medications, and synthetic estrogen
- Pregnancy
- Failure of the pituitary gland
- Pituitary gland imbalance
- Genetics
- Head or thyroid injury

Testing Techniques

The following tests help assess possible reasons for hypothyroidism:

Thyroid-hormone testing (thyroid: TSH, Free T4, Free T3, Reverse T3, anti-thyroglobulin antibodies, anti-thyroid peroxidase)—blood, urine

General hormone testing (DHEA, cortisol, testosterone, IGF-1, estrogen, progesterone, insulin)—saliva, blood, or urine

Intestinal permeability—urine

Toxic metals (e.g., mercury, lead)—hair or urine

Vitamin and mineral analysis (especially vitamin A, selenium, zinc, iodine, copper, magnesium, vitamin D)—blood, urine

Amino acid analysis (especially L-tyrosine)—blood or urine

Digestive function and microbe/parasite/fungal testing—stool analysis

Food and environmental allergies/sensitivities—blood, electrodermal

TREATMENT

Diet

Recommended Food

It stands to reason that hypothyroidism is most frequently found in landlocked regions, where iodine-rich foods from the sea are less available. If you have an underactive thyroid, it may be helpful to consume plenty of organic sea vegetables, such as kelp, nori, dulse, kombu, and wakame. Fish and sea salt are also good sources of iodine.

Hypothyroidism can be worsened by deficiencies in several other minerals, including zinc, selenium, and copper. A deficiency of the amino acid tyrosine is often present in those with hypothyroidism. To make sure you're getting enough of these nutrients, incorporate pumpkin seeds, beans, almonds, and fish into your diet.

Essential fatty acids found in flaxseeds, walnuts, and fish are important for thyroid function. Brazil nuts are also recommended since they are a rich source of selenium, a mineral required for thyroid hormone production.

Consume organic, hormone-free meats and poultry since environmental hormones disrupt thyroid function.

A slow metabolism often means a slow digestive process. Encourage faster elimination by eating more fiber in the form of whole grains, beans, fruits, and vegetables.

Medications that can cause hypothyroidism:

Amiodarone
Interferon alfa
Thalidomide
Lithium
Stavudine
Oral tyrosine kinase inhibitors
– Sunitinib, imatinib
Bexarotene
Perchlorate
Interleukin (IL)-2
Ethionamide
Rifampin
Phenytoin
Carbamazepine
Phenobarbital
Aminoglutethimide
Sulfisoxazole
p-Aminosalicylic acid
Ipilimumab

You must stay adequately hydrated. Drink a glass of clean, quality water every two waking hours.

Food to Avoid

Certain vegetables known as goitrogens may suppress thyroid function. Most of the research has been on animals and overall results are conflicting. Goitrogenic foods include kale, broccoli, cauliflower, cabbage, millet, and brussels sprouts. Cooking the vegetables inactivates the goitrogens. However, for most people consuming these foods raw in moderate amounts is fine. Excess soy consumption, especially of non-fermented soy, may be problematic.

It's never advisable to drink tap water, but people with hypothyroidism must be especially wary of it. Most tap water is full of fluorine and chlorine, two chemicals that inhibit your ability to absorb iodine.

℞ Super Seven Prescriptions—Hypothyroidism

Super Prescription #1 Iodine
Take 150 to 500 mcg daily or more under a holistic doctor's supervision. Iodine provides the building block of thyroid hormones.

Super Prescription #2 Selenium
Take 200 mcg daily. Selenium is necessary for the production of free T3, the most active thyroid hormone. Also, selenium has been shown in research to reduce the levels of thyroid antibodies.

Super Prescription #3 Thyroid glandular
Take 350 to 500 mg daily or as directed on the container to stimulate thyroid function.

Super Prescription #4 L-tyrosine
Take 500 mg twice daily on an empty stomach. This amino acid is used in the synthesis of the thyroid hormone.

Super Prescription #5 Ashwagandha
Take 125 to 250 mg of an extract daily. This supports T3 production.

Super Prescription #6 Guggul (*Commiphora mukul*)
Take a product containing 25 mg of guggulsterones three times daily to support thyroid function.

Super Prescription #7 Bladderwrack (*Fucus vesiculosus*)
Take 250 mg or 1 ml twice daily to support thyroid function.

General Recommendations

A high-potency multivitamin provides a base of nutrients required for thyroid-hormone synthesis. Take as directed on the container.

Essential fatty acids are important for thyroid function. Take 3,000 mg of fish oil or 1 tablespoon of flaxseed oil and 150 mg of GLA from evening primrose or borage oil.

TSH (thyroid stimulating hormone) is the hormone released by the pituitary gland, located in the brain. Its job is to stimulate thyroid-hormone secretion when the brain senses that thyroid levels are getting low. Perhaps you've seen TSH listed on the results of your blood test. A normal lab range is referenced as 0.5 to 5.5 uU/ml. We feel that 0.2 to 2.0 is an optimal TSH range. Furthermore, it is important to have your free thyroxine (T4) and free triiodothyronine (T3) levels tested, as these are the two most metabolically active thyroid hormones, especially the free T3. Finally, since Hashimoto's thyroiditis is the most common cause of low thyroid, you should have your thyroid antibody levels tested.

Take DHEA if tests show that your levels are low. Take 5 to 15 mg each morning, under the supervision of a doctor.

Pituitary glandular stimulates thyroid function. Take 1 tablet or capsule three times daily on an empty stomach or as directed on the container.

Natural progesterone helps women who have low thyroid hormones and low progesterone levels. See the Menopause and Premenstrual Syndrome sections for the proper dosage.

Homeopathic Thyroidinum 3x or 6x is used to gently stimulate thyroid activity. Take 5 pellets three times daily.

Iron deficiency contributes to hypothyroidism. If your doctor finds that you are iron deficient then increasing dietary amounts and taking supplements can be helpful.

Vitamin D deficiency may increase the risk of Hashimoto's thyroiditis. Supplement vitamin D3 if your levels are low.

Homeopathy

Although homeopathic remedies are not a substitute for thyroid supplementation, they are quite useful for easing the symptoms of an underactive thyroid. In mild cases, these remedies may stimulate the thyroid enough to avoid having to supplement thyroid hormone.

Pick the remedy that best matches your symptoms in this section. Take a 6x, 12x, 6C, 12C, or 30C potency twice daily for two weeks to see if there are any positive results. After you notice improvement, stop taking the remedy, unless symptoms return. Consultation with a homeopathic practitioner is advised.

Calcarea Carbonica is helpful when there is low thyroid function, accompanied by chilliness, fatigue, and a sense of being overwhelmed. The person tends to be flabby and may have excessive sweat on the head at nighttime. There is a craving for eggs and milk products.

Lycopodium (*Lycopodium clavatum*) is helpful if you have a right-sided enlargement of the thyroid. You also experience a tremendous amount of gas and bloating. There is a strong craving for sweets. You tend to be chilly and irritable.

Pulsatilla (*Pulsatilla pratensis*) is for women who are warm and who desire cool, fresh air. There is a craving for sweets, a low thirst, and symptoms of hormone imbalance, possibly due to PMS or menopause, that are characterized by weeping and sadness.

Sepia is for women with low thyroid hormone who are irritable and chilly. They crave salty, sweet, and sour foods.

Nux Vomica is helpful if you suffer from fatigue and also feel chilly, achy, irritable, and constipated. It is good for thyroid burnout from overworking.

Acupressure

See pages 787–794 for information about pressure points and administering treatment.

- Triple Warmer 17 (TW17) has a balancing effect on the thyroid.
- For depression, work Lung 1 (Lu1). You'll find yourself taking air more deeply into your lungs and relieving stress with each breath.

- If you feel weak and fatigued, work Bladder 23 and 47 (B23 and B47). Do not press on these points if you have severe back pain.
- Work Conception Vessel 6 (CV6) to ease constipation.

Bodywork

Massage
A full-body massage will reduce stress, improve circulation, and lift your energy level. If you like, you can add any of the essential oils listed in the Aromatherapy section to further enhance the treatment.

Reflexology
See pages 804–805 for information about reflexology areas and how to work them. Work the area corresponding to the thyroid.

Aromatherapy

Geranium oil will regulate the thyroid hormone. Use it in a bath, or better yet, add to a carrier oil and incorporate into a massage. Geranium can also help lift fatigue and depression. So can jasmine, neroli, bergamot, and rose.

If your skin is dry, add chamomile (*Matricaria chamomilla*) to a lotion, a cream, or a carrier oil and apply the mixture to the affected area.

Oil of black pepper or marjoram will stimulate a sluggish digestive system and improve overall circulation.

Stress Reduction

General Stress-Reduction Therapies
High levels of stress inhibit the thyroid's ability to properly manufacture its hormone. Exercise has been shown to improve thyroid function and should be done on a daily basis.

Other Recommendations

For those that require medication, bioidentical thyroid replacement is available. The first type is desiccated thyroid extracts (DTE). This is a group of bioidentical thyroid medications derived from purified porcine (pig) thyroid tissue. The levels of T3 and T4, the two most active thyroid hormones, are standardized in DTEs. They also contain two other thyroid hormones, T2 and T1, which have activity in the human body but about which less is known. The second type of bioidentical thyroid hormone is called compounded hormones. A compounding pharmacy manufactures a preparation containing the exact dose and type of hormone prescribed by a doctor based on the patient's blood work and symptoms. Both types require a prescription. Consult with a holistic doctor.

REFERENCES

Gartner, R. 2003. Selenium in the treatmetnt of autoimmune thyroiditis. *Biofactors* 19(3–4):165–70.

Medscape. Accessed June 26, 2015 at http://emedicine.medscape.com/article /122393-overview#a4.

Impotence

Impotence, also referred to as erectile dysfunction, is a man's inability to attain or sustain an erection sufficient for normal, satisfying sexual intercourse. It was once thought that almost all impotence was caused by psychological factors, but we now know that as many as 85 percent of cases are brought on by physiological disturbances. No matter what the cause, it helps most men to realize that they are not alone. Nearly every man experiences impotence at some point, and almost thirty million have chronic or recurring problems.

Many physiological factors may contribute to impotence, but the most common are hormonal changes, medications, diet, and chronic illness. Low levels of testosterone, the male sex hormone, are a critical link to male impotence. The most common cause of impotence is atherosclerosis, which is hardening of the arteries with plaque buildup. This causes a problem with blood flow to the penis. See the Cardiovascular Disease section for a comprehensive program to reverse this vascular problem. Also, dilation of the arteries and blood flow to the genital area are dependent on a chemical produced in the body known as nitric oxide.

The following classes of drugs can cause impotence: antihypertensives (drugs to treat high blood pressure), antidepressants, antipsychotics, antiulcer agents, 5-alpha reductase inhibitors, and cholesterol-lowering durgs.

Diet is another common cause. Just as a high-fat, low-fiber routine can inhibit blood flow to the heart, it can also block the arteries that lead to the penis. Men with high blood pressure or arteriosclerosis may have difficulty maintaining erections. Other chronic illnesses, especially diabetes, can take a toll as well.

It is important to note here that aging is not a cause of impotence. While it's true that impotence affects older people more frequently than it does the rest of the population, this situation can be attributed to the increased incidence of disease and medication in the elderly. And disease itself is not an inevitable part of aging; see Aging for information about staying healthy throughout the full span of your life. If you are healthy and content, you can be sexually vigorous well into your eighties and beyond.

If you are not chronically impotent—that is, if you are impotent only in certain situations or can achieve an erection on your own or in your sleep—then it's likely that psychological factors are causing or contributing to your problem. Overwork and fatigue have reached epidemic levels in our society, and many men—especially those who have children—simply feel too tired to enjoy sex. Depression, anxiety, stress, fear of failure, and fear of pregnancy are other frequent causes.

Many cases of impotence can be successfully treated with an improvement in lifestyle and dietary habits, as well as with nutritional supplements, but anyone with a chronic problem should see a doctor first to rule out underlying disorders.

SYMPTOMS

- Inability to achieve or maintain an erection

ROOT CAUSES

- Low levels of DHEA and testosterone
- Prescription medications
- Street drugs
- A diet that's high in fat and low in fiber

- Underlying illness (most often, arteriosclerosis, high blood pressure, and diabetes)
- Depression
- Other psychological factors (fear of pregnancy, fear of failure, lack of desire)
- Hormonal imbalance (low testosterone, thyroid imbalance)

- Fatigue
- Heavy-metal poisoning
- Stress or anxiety
- Injury from radiation (such as radiation therapy for prostate cancer)
- Surgery for prostate cancer
- Overweight

Testing Techniques

The following tests help assess possible reasons for impotence:

Immune system imbalance or disease (such as leukemia, anemia)—blood

Blood pressure—blood pressure machine

Hormone testing (thyroid, DHEA, cortisol, testosterone, IGF-1, estrogen, progesterone)—saliva, blood, or urine

Intestinal permeability—urine

Detoxification profile—urine

Vitamin and mineral analysis (especially magnesium, B12, iron, zinc, and CoQ10)—blood

Anemia—blood test (CBC, iron, ferritin, % saturation)

Blood sugar balance—blood (hemoglobin A1C)

Lipids—blood

Ultrasound of penis vasculature

TREATMENT

If an underlying condition or a medication is causing impotence, check with a doctor before undertaking any changes in your diet, medication, or habits. If you have cardiovascular disease or diabetes, see the appropriate section in this book for further recommendations.

Diet

Recommended Food

Eat a healthful diet that's high in fiber and nutrients. Good sources of fiber include fresh raw vegetables, apples, oats, and whole grains.

Vitamin E dilates blood vessels and improves blood flow. Foods that are high in this nutrient include wheat germ, soy products, leafy green vegetables, and whole grain cereals.

Enjoy soybeans, pumpkin seeds, and sunflower seeds as snacks or in salads. They're excellent sources of zinc, which aids the prostate and improves testosterone levels.

Watercress leaves, sesame seeds, and bee pollen are libido enhancers. Add some to your meals every day.

Food to Avoid

Avoid foods that are high in saturated, hydrogenated, or partially hydrogenated fats, including red meat, butter, margarine, shortening, and refined vegetable oils. A high-fat diet causes circulatory problems and blocks the flow of blood to the genitals.

Eliminate junk and processed foods from your diet. Not only are they generally fatty and lacking in nutrition, they contain chemicals that might affect sexual performance.

Moderate your intake of caffeine and alcohol. While a cup of coffee or a glass of wine should not pose a problem for most people, overindulgence can lead to temporary or chronic impotence.

℞ Super Seven Prescriptions—Impotence

Super Prescription #1 L-arginine
Take 1,000 mg three times daily on an empty stomach. This amino acid leads to blood vessel dilation and improved blood flow, which are required for an erection.

Super Prescription #2 L-citrulline
Take 500 mg three times daily. This natural substance has been shown in studies to improve erectile function by boosting L-arginine levels. It is often used in combination with the supplement L-arginine.

Super Prescription #3 Pycnogenol
Take 100 mg to 200 mg daily. Research has shown that in combination with L-arginine it can improve sexual function in middle-aged men.

Super Prescription #4 *Panax ginseng*
Take 100 mg two or three times daily of a product standardized to between 4 and 7 percent ginsenosides. This herb is revered in China for its ability to improve libido and sexual function for men.

Super Prescription #5 DHEA
If lab testing shows that your levels are low, take 25 to 50 mg daily under the supervision of a doctor. Studies show that some men who are low in this hormone improve their erectile function with supplementation. DHEA is also a precursor hormone to testosterone.

Super Prescription #6 Maca
Take 500 mg three times daily to improve sexual desire and performance.

Super Prescription #7 *Ginkgo biloba*
Take 120 mg twice daily of a standardized product containing 24 percent flavone glycosides and 6 percent terpene lactones. Ginkgo improves blood flow, and studies show it to be effective for erectile dysfunction.

Several studies have shown that *Ginkgo biloba* extract improves erectile dysfunction in men. A study of men with impotence as the result of pharmaceutical medications (such as antidepressants) found that 200 mg of ginkgo extract improved sexual function in 76 percent of the men.

A double-blind trial involving *Panax ginseng* taken for three months found that it significantly improved libido, the ability to maintain an erection, and patient satisfaction with sex.

A double-blind, randomized, placebo-controlled study involving forty men who were confirmed to have low DHEA levels were given either 50 mg of DHEA or a placebo for six months. Men taking DHEA had a significant improvement in libido and erectile function.

General Recommendations

A number of studies have shown that L-arginine improves erectile function and sexual satisfaction. It does this by increasing the activity of nitric oxide in the body. This leads to vasodilation and improved penile blood flow. Studies combining L-arginine with Pycnogenol or citrulline have shown improved male sexual function.

Niacin (vitamin B3) is a vasodilator and improves blood flow. Take 250 mg three times daily.

Zinc is a mineral that's required in the synthesis of testosterone. Take 30 mg twice daily, along with 3 to 5 mg of copper.

Tribulus terrestris (puncture vine) is a folk remedy for improving libido and erectile function. Take 500 mg three times daily.

Damiana (*Turnera diffusa*) is a traditional remedy for impotence that improves blood flow to the genitals. Take 400 to 800 mg or 2 to 3 cc of the tincture three times daily.

Ashwagandha (*Withania somniferum*) is an ancient Ayurvedic medicine used to treat stress and impotence. Take 1,000 mg three times daily.

Yohimbe (*Pausinystalia yohimbe*) increases blood flow to erectile tissue and increases libido. Take a product standardized to yohimbine hydrochloride at a dosage of 10 mg three times daily. It should be used under the supervision of a doctor and should be avoided by people with high blood pressure, any cardiovascular condition, or kidney disease; by pregnant women; or by individuals being treated for a psychological disorder.

Oatstraw (*Avena sativa*) relaxes the nervous system and is thought to increase libido. Take 300 mg three times daily.

Cordyceps has historically been used to treat low libido and impotence in men, and Chinese studies verify this effect. Take 800 mg twice daily of Cs-4 mycelium extract.

Potency wood (*Muira puama*) from South America improves sexual desire and impotency. Take 500 mg three times daily.

Homeopathy

A three-month study of middle-aged men suffering from mild erectile dysfunction found the combination of L-arginine and Pycnogenol achieved normal erectile function in 92.5 percent of users.

Agnus Castus is a remedy for men who were involved in frequent sexual activity for many years. There may be a cold sensation in the genitals. Men requiring this remedy are often anxious about their health and may have problems with memory and concentration.

Caladium is a remedy for men who have an interest in sexual relations, but the genitals are completely limp. There may be frequent wet dreams without an erection. Men who require this remedy often crave tobacco.

Lycopodium (*Lycopodium clavatum*) is for men who have erection problems as a result of worry and low self-confidence. Digestive problems, such as gas and bloating, are common, and symptoms are worse in the late afternoon.

Selenium Metallicum is a remedy for men who have decreased sexual ability, especially after a fever or an exhausting illness. They feel weak and exhausted, but interest is usually still present. There may be unusual hair loss.

Staphysagria is for mild-mannered, shy men with deep emotions, such as suppressed anger. Their problems with impotence often begin after an embarrassing event.

Acupressure

See pages 787–794 for information about pressure points and administering treatment.

- To relieve stress and encourage calm, deep breathing, work Lung 1 (Lu1).

- Bladder Points 23 and 47 (B23 and B47)—together known as the Sea of Vitality—will improve sexual potency and reduce fatigue.

Bodywork

Reflexology
See pages 804–805 for information about reflexology areas and how to work them.

Work the areas that correspond to the testes, the prostate, the pituitary and adrenal glands, and the solar plexus.

Hydrotherapy
Constitutional hydrotherapy can be used to improve circulation. See pages 795–796 for directions.

Some men find that hot baths and saunas lower their sex drive. Try taking warm—not hot—showers and baths. Stay away from saunas to see if your condition improves.

Aromatherapy

Several oils ease stress while stimulating sexual desire. Among the best are patchouli, ylang-ylang, sandalwood, and jasmine. Try a few drops in a bath or add them to a carrier oil, and use this in a sensual massage.

Stress Reduction

General Stress-Reduction Therapies
Regular meditation can fit nicely into the schedule of almost anyone, including people who are overworked. Try to set aside twenty minutes every night after work to detach yourself from the worries of the day.

Other Recommendations

- Regular exercise stimulates blood flow, reduces stress, and helps unclog arteries. Moderate daily exercise has been strongly linked to better sexual performance.
- Don't smoke or expose yourself to secondhand smoke. Nicotine is a well-known cause of impotence.

REFERENCES

Choi, H. K., D. H. Seong, and K. H. Rha. 1995. Clinical efficacy of Korean red ginseng for erectile dysfunction. *International Journal of Impotence Research* 7:181–86.

Cohen, A. J., and B. Bartlik. 1998. Ginkgo biloba for antidepressant-induced sexual dysfunction. *Journal of Sex and Marital Therapy* 24:139–43.

Cormio, L. 2011. Oral L-citrulline supplementation improves erection hardness in men with mild erectile dysfunction. *Urology* 77(1):119–22.

Reiter, W. J., A. Pycha, G. Schatzl, et al. 1999. Dehydroepiandrosterone in the treatment of erectile dysfunction: A prospective, double-blind randomized, placebo controlled study. *Urology* 53:590–95.

Stanislavov, R., V. Nokolova. 2003. Treatment of erectile dysfunction with Pycnogenol and L-arginine. *J Sex Marital Ther* 29(3):207–13.

Infertility

To many couples, pregnancy seems like a simple matter—so simple that not getting pregnant is their chief concern. But after years of protected sex, men and women who decide they want children may discover that conception is a far more complex process than they realized.

Here's an extremely simplified version of what must happen: First, a woman secretes several hormones—each at the correct time—that cause one of the eggs in her ovaries to mature and to be released into the fallopian tube. A man must then contribute enough sperm (tens of millions of them) that have the ability to travel up into the tube, where the egg is fertilized. The egg makes its way to the uterus and implants itself in the uterine wall. If anything goes wrong with any one of these events, the couple will not conceive. Because the process is so complicated, it often takes a number of months of trying before a woman can become pregnant. But if a couple has had regular, unprotected sex for at least a year and still cannot conceive, the partners are considered infertile.

For the last few decades, the rate of infertility in the United States has increased. No hard statistics are available, but experts estimate that between 16 and 25 percent of all couples have serious difficulty getting pregnant. As with most other conditions that have been on the rise, many of today's infertility cases can be attributed to lifestyle changes in the latter half of the twentieth century. Poor nutrition, stress, eating disorders, extremely intense exercise, and exposure to environmental toxins all take a grave toll on the body. When one or both members of a couple have weakened body systems, the chances increase that something will go awry in the conception process. People today also have more sex partners than they used to, and with increased sexual activity comes a greater risk of contracting diseases that damage the reproductive organs. Finally, many couples now choose to delay childbearing until their thirties or even forties, when a woman's fertility begins to decline.

If you're having trouble getting pregnant, it's wise for both of you to take a break and spend a few months restoring and nourishing your bodies. Good nutrition, herbal supplementation, hormone-balancing protocols, and effective stress management help a great many couples conceive; these strategies will also increase the chances that your baby will be healthy. (Not to mention that you'll need those stress-management techniques when you're a parent!)

Hormone balance is particularly important for both sexes. We find that women with infertility problems often have low ovulatory progesterone levels or low thyroid function. Both of these hormones can be a limiting factor in conception. With men, low thyroid, as well as low testosterone, can be problematic.

Many couples are confused about when, during the woman's menstrual cycle, conception can occur. It is important to understand that the best chance of conception happens one to two days before ovulation occurs, not on the day of ovulation. Over-the-counter LH (luteinizing hormone) test kits are readily available to help determine when ovulation is going to occur. LH levels in the body rise approximately forty-eight hours before an egg is released (ovulation). Basal body temperature can also be used to determine ovulatory patterns. This method must be used over many months to determine when a woman ovulates. Many practitioners and books explain how to properly use this technique.

Although a lot of focus with fertility is on the female partner, keep in mind that studies show that approximately 40 percent of infertility cases are due to men's sperm abnormalities. These include low sperm count, decreased sperm motility, or abnormal sperm shape.

One or both of you may have an anatomical abnormality; for example, many women suffer from blocked fallopian tubes, often as a result of a chlamydia infection, and men may have a varicose vein in the testicle, called a varicocele. In many cases, these conditions can be treated with surgeries and procedures. Couples that can't get pregnant any other way may eventually consider in vitro fertilization, and an increasing number of women with ovary problems are turning to egg donors. Unfortunately, however, all the medical techniques in the world—complementary, conventional, and cutting-edge—can't guarantee that every couple that wants a baby will conceive. Before you begin a series of invasive and expensive procedures, be sure to speak frankly with your doctor about the risks involved and the chances of success. And take heart: many people, exhausted from years of diagnostics and surgeries, give up trying—only to discover that they've finally become relaxed enough to conceive.

SYMPTOMS

- Failure to conceive after twelve months of regular, unprotected intercourse that is timed with ovulatory patterns.

ROOT CAUSES

Dozens of factors can cause infertility. Following are some of the most common:

- Poor nutrition and nutritional deficiencies
- Medical conditions such as endometriosis, polycystic ovary syndrome, varicocele
- Stress
- Sexually transmitted diseases
- Eating disorders, especially anorexia
- Environmental toxins such as xenoestrogens
- Overly intense exercise
- Congenital abnormalities
- Obesity
- Hormonal problems (especially low thyroid or low progesterone)
- Toxic metals

Testing Techniques

The following tests help assess possible reasons for infertility:

Hormone testing (thyroid, DHEA, cortisol, testosterone, IGF-1, estrogen, progesterone)—saliva, blood, or urine

Ovulation pattern—ovulation kit

Vitamin and mineral analysis—blood

Anemia—blood test (CBC, iron, ferritin, % saturation)

Food and environmental allergies/sensitivities—blood, electrodermal

Toxic metals—hair or urine analysis

Xenoestrogens—blood, urine

Gluten allergy/sensitivity—blood

TREATMENT

Diet

Recommended Food

In general, you should eat wholesome meals made with organic vegetables, grains, and soy products. Eat fish several times a week, but be sure it's from a clean water source.

Vitamin E nourishes the endocrine system, so use cold-pressed nut and seed oils for cooking or as a base for salad dressings. Wheat germ is another good source of vitamin E; add it to smoothies, cereals, or salads.

Essential fatty acids promote gland health and are often lacking in people who follow radical low-fat diets. Incorporate cold-water fish, flaxseeds, or flaxseed oil into your meals daily.

Men should snack regularly on pumpkin seeds. They're an excellent source of zinc, a nutrient that's an important part of male reproductive fluids.

Eat vegetables, fruits, beans, whole grains, and other sources of fiber at every meal, and drink a glass of clean, quality water every two waking hours. You'll promote your overall health and sweep away toxins that may be suppressing your reproductive system.

Food to Avoid

Don't eat anything that depresses body systems or causes nutrient depletion. Cut out refined sugar and white flour, along with fried or processed food.

Animal meats are loaded with chemicals that mimic the effects of estrogen, a hormone that in excess can decrease sperm count and fertility. If you must eat meat, make sure it's organic.

Avoid alcohol, which reduces the number of normal sperm in men and can damage egg quality.

Caffeine consumption has been linked to fertility problems, including miscarriage. Avoid coffee, soft drinks, chocolate, black and green teas, and pharmaceutical medications containing caffeine.

Gluten allergy has been shown to be a cause of infertility. Have your doctor test you for gluten allergy/sensitivity or avoid gluten-containing foods.

In one study, forty-eight women ages twenty-three to thirty-nine who were diagnosed with infertility took Vitex supplement once daily for three months. During the trial, seven women became pregnant and twenty-five experienced normalized progesterone levels, which, in theory, may increase the chances for conception.

℞ Super Seven Prescriptions—Infertility

Super Prescription #1 Vitex agnus-castus (chasteberry)
Women should take 160 to 240 mg of a 0.6 percent aucubin extract each morning. Vitex stimulates the ovaries to ovulate and normalizes progesterone levels.

Super Prescription #2 Natural progesterone cream
Women should apply ¼ teaspoon (20 mg) to the skin once daily. Make sure to start using this hormone after you ovulate. If you become pregnant, continue utilizing the progesterone until the third trimester or as directed by your doctor. *Note*: This treatment is best used under the guidance of a doctor who is knowledgeable about natural hormones.

Super Prescription #3 Vitamin C

Take 500 mg twice daily. Vitamin C prevents sperm agglutination in men and has been shown to be helpful with female infertility as well.

Super Prescription #4 Vitamin E

Take 400 IU daily. Animal and human studies have shown this vitamin to be important for fertility.

Super Prescription #5 L-arginine

Men should take 2,000 mg twice daily on an empty stomach. This amino acid has been shown to increase sperm quality and count.

Super Prescription #6 *Panax ginseng*

Men should take 300 mg of a product standardized to between 4 and 7 percent ginsenosides daily. This herb has been shown to increase sperm count and motility.

Super Prescription #7 Zinc

Men should take 30 mg twice daily, along with 3 to 5 mg of copper. Studies show that this mineral improves sperm quality, count, and motility.

General Recommendations

L-carnitine or acetylcarnitine improves sperm motility. Take 1,500 mg twice daily.

Coenzyme Q10 improves sperm motility. Take 100 mg daily.

Selenium improves sperm motility. Take a daily total of at least 100 mcg.

A high-potency multivitamin provides a base of the nutrients that are important for fertility. Take as directed on the container.

Iron is important for women if testing shows iron-deficiency anemia. Take 15 mg twice daily or as directed by your doctor.

PABA has been shown in studies to help women with chronic infertility. It is thought to improve the effects of estrogen. Take 100 mg four times daily for up to seven months.

Vitamin B12 has been shown to increase sperm count. Men should take 1,500 mcg of oral B12 or 400 mcg of the sublingual form daily.

Vicki, a thirty-six-year-old from Alabama, had tried one unsuccessful course of in vitro fertilization with her husband. Since they had spent four years trying to conceive, she sought a natural approach from our clinic. We diagnosed her with low thyroid and low progesterone. Vicki was placed on thyroid supplementation and the herb Vitex to support ovulation and progesterone levels. She was pregnant three months later. Her son is now almost two years old.

Homeopathy

Consult a homeopathic practitioner for a constitutional remedy.

Acupressure

You may need to use these points on a daily basis for several months before you see results. For information about pressure points and administering treatment, see pages 787–794.

In a study, 178 men with low sperm counts or abnormal sperm function were given 4,000 mg of L-arginine daily for at least two months. As a result, 62 percent of the men had a marked increase in sperm motility and count, and twenty-eight pregnancies occurred. Researchers also noted that men with very low initial sperm counts, of less than 20 million per ml, did not have as beneficial a response as men with higher counts did.

- Both men and women should work Bladder 23 and 47 (B23 and B47) to buildup vitality and encourage conception.
- To stimulate general wellness and the effective absorption of nutrients, work Stomach 36 (St36).
- If you need to relieve tension, use Lung 1 (Lu1). It will help you to breathe deeply and focus on the here and now.

Acupuncture

See a qualified practitioner for regular treatments, as studies have shown this therapy to be helpful for improving female fertility.

Bodywork

Massage

Massage won't magically make you fertile, but it is relaxing, and it has the additional benefit of stimulating blood flow to your entire body, including to your reproductive organs and endocrine system.

Reflexology

See pages 804–805 for information about reflexology areas and how to work them.

Work all the gland points to regulate hormone production.

Women should work the areas corresponding to the reproductive system. These points will help stimulate blood supply to the pelvis and will help relieve blockages.

To clear blockages, men should work the areas corresponding to the testes and the prostate.

For relief of tension and stress, both sexes should work the diaphragm/solar plexus point.

Hydrotherapy

Sitz baths, either hot or cold, will increase blood supply to the pelvic region.

Aromatherapy

Rose oil is said to improve sperm's ability to travel through the female reproductive organs to a waiting egg. Although no one has verified this via scientific method, it certainly can't hurt to use a little rose in a massage oil or a bath, especially since the essence has calming and sensuous qualities.

If months of trying to conceive have sapped you or your partner of sexual desire, try using ylang-ylang, sandalwood, or patchouli in a bath or a massage. Each of these oils is a renowned aphrodisiac and promotes a sense of quiet relaxation. *Note:* If you become pregnant, stop using essential oils.

Stress Reduction

Tension and stress, whether about fertility or any other issue, have long been linked to an inability to conceive. It doesn't matter which stress-reduction technique you use, as long you find one that works for you and employ it frequently.

Other Recommendations

- Smoke can dramatically reduce your fertility and will also harm a growing fetus. If you're trying to get pregnant, you must avoid smoke of all kinds.
- Exercise to improve your circulation and general health, but don't overdo it. People who overtrain find it difficult to conceive.
- Women who are obese need to focus on losing weight for optimal fertility. See the Obesity section.
- Men should know that sperm must stay relatively cool. That's why the testicles are located outside the body, not inside it. If the testicles are heated, sperm may die or be damaged. Stay away from saunas and hot tubs, and don't wear tight-fitting underwear.
- After sexual intercourse, a woman should lie in bed for fifteen to twenty minutes with her knees up. To keep conception from seeming like a science project, the man should stay with her and hold her gently.

REFERENCES

Propping, D., and T. Katzorke. 1987. Treatment of corpus luteum insufficiency. *Zeitschrift für Allgemeinmedizin* 63:932–33.

Schacter, A., et al. 1973. Treatment of oligospermia with the amino acid arginine. *Journal of Urology* 110:311–13.

Influenza. See Flu

Insomnia

Insomnia is our nation's silent health crisis. Up to 95 percent of Americans report having an episode of insomnia at some point in their life. About 50 percent of the senior population have chronic insomnia, compared to 25 percent of the general population. For 10 percent of the general population, insomnia is severe. And research shows that half of those diagnosed with insomnia have a cause not related to a psychiatric disorder.

Of course people who have chronic insomnia—a consistent inability to go to sleep or to stay asleep through the night—are at risk for far more than fatigue. Sleep deficiency suppresses the immune system and the libido, decreases productivity, and can lead to other disorders like depression, chronic fatigue, heart disease, and headaches.

Before the use of electric lighting, the average American got nine hours of sleep a night. Now the average is less than seven hours and still going down, as the distractions of twenty-four-hour shopping and entertainment become more widespread. Studies involving mental function show that most adults do best with eight hours; some may need as many as nine or even ten. Children and teens need more sleep than adults do, and older people often find that they simply sleep less than they used to. If you nod off to sleep very quickly—within five minutes of putting your head on the pillow—or if you feel an urge to nap during the day, you probably need more sleep than you're getting. Poor sleep has been shown to increase the risk of several diseases.

Stress, anxiety, depression, and medications are common causes of insomnia. Stimulants, heavy metals, chronic pain, breathing problems, and other disorders can also keep you from sleeping.

Sleep apnea affects 5 percent of adults, but many will never be diagnosed. During this condition, a person repeatedly stops breathing during the night and wakes up to catch his or her breath. The two consequences of this are a significant drop in the blood's oxygen and severe sleep deprivation. Be suspicious of this condition if you snore, have daytime sleepiness, have high blood pressure, or are overweight. This condition is best identified during a sleep study that your doctor can order. The recommendations in this section—especially the dietary ones—may help to treat sleep apnea. Weight loss can be an important component, as can avoiding sleeping on your back. One standard treatment is a CPAP machine, which involves a mask that is kept over your face while you sleep. It keeps constant pressure in the airway so that it does not collapse. Orthodontic devices that pull the lower jaw and the tongue forward are sometimes useful. In rare cases, extremely large tonsils or abnormalities in the throat structure may need to be surgically corrected.

Restless leg syndrome is a disorder characterized by unusual or painful sensations in the legs, accompanied by an irresistible urge to move the legs. It's often brought on by rest and occurs most often in the evening. It can produce difficulty falling asleep. Many studies have shown that restless leg sufferers have low or low-normal iron levels. Iron supplementation has helped many people, but three months of treatment is usually needed before improvement is noted.

Hormone imbalance can be a root cause of insomnia. This can involve several different hormones. It is common for many women experiencing menopause to develop insomnia. This is generally due to changes in estrogen and progesterone levels. The obvious solution is to follow a hormone-balancing program. See the Menopause section for more information. Likewise, younger women with premenstrual syndrome can experience the same. In addition, low or high thyroid can interfere with sleep. We also find that elevated levels of the stress hormone cortisol interfere with deep REM sleep, which studies confirm. It is not uncommon to find seniors with deficiencies in DHEA, testosterone, and growth hormone, which can be underlying causes as well. The sleep hormone melatonin can work wonders in selected cases, when supplemented correctly.

If you suffer from insomnia, you may find that the gentle treatments in this section help you get a good night's sleep. If they don't, talk to your doctor. He or she should review your general health and may also refer you to a sleep-disorder specialist. It is not recommended, under any circumstance, that you take over-the-counter sleeping aids. They do not promote deep, restful sleep, and they may create any of several side effects, including depression, confusion, and dry mouth. Worse, they can be addictive.

Medications that may cause insomnia include:

- Antidepressants
- Cardiovascular medications, such as those for the heart and blood pressure
- ADHD medication
- Sinus decongestants
- Corticosteroids
- Antihistamines

SYMPTOMS

- Inability to fall asleep or to sleep through the night

ROOT CAUSES

- Stress and anxiety
- Lack of exercise
- Aging
- Restless leg syndrome
- Stimulants, including caffeine, decongestants, and thyroid medications
- Hormonal changes (e.g., menopause)
- Vitamin/mineral deficiencies
- (e.g., B12, iron)
- Sugar
- Breathing disorders, including asthma and sleep apnea
- Indigestion
- Pain
- Other disorders, such as hypothyroidism and hypoglycemia
- Alcohol

Testing Techniques

The following tests help assess possible reasons for insomnia:

Sleep study—lab setting

Hormone testing (thyroid, DHEA, cortisol, testosterone, IGF-1, estrogen, progesterone)—saliva, blood, or urine

Vitamin and mineral analysis (especially magnesium, calcium, B12, iron)— blood

Anemia—blood test (CBC, iron, ferritin, % saturation)

Food and environmental allergies/sensitivities—blood, electrodermal

Blood sugar balance—blood

TREATMENT

Diet

Recommended Food

At dinner, eat foods that are high in tryptophan, a chemical that stimulates serotonin, which in turn helps you sleep. Turkey, chicken, tuna, soy products, live unsweetened yogurt, and whole-grain crackers are all good, low-sugar sources.

Complex carbohydrates are also relaxing, so incorporate whole grains, especially brown rice or pasta, into your dinners.

This book does not generally recommend dairy products, aside from yogurt, but a glass of milk before bedtime is a time-honored sleep aid. Try this only if you do not have a sensitivity or an allergy to dairy products.

Deficiencies of calcium and magnesium can lead to insomnia. Be sure your diet is high in leafy greens, sesame and sunflower seeds, oats, almonds, and walnuts.

The B vitamins are also essential for good sleep. Brewer's yeast is the best source. Sprinkle it on your dinner salad or add a teaspoon to a bedtime glass of water or a green drink.

Drink a glass of clean, quality water every two waking hours so you won't wake up at night with a dry mouth. Have your last glass two hours before bedtime, or you'll be up for other reasons.

The adrenal glands release cortisol as a response to stress. Cortisol is released in a natural rhythm with the sleep-wake cycle. Levels increase and peak in the early morning hours as part of the body's physiological response to awakening. An oversecretion of cortisol at nighttime can interfere with sleep. This is because rapid eye movement (REM) sleep, which takes place during deep sleep, occurs primarily when cortisol levels are decreasing. Conversely, the adrenal hormone DHEA has a balancing effect on high cortisol levels and has been shown to significantly increase REM time during sleep.

Food to Avoid

The first rule for insomniacs is to monitor caffeine intake strenuously. Do not have any products containing caffeine—such as coffee, black tea, or chocolate—for eight hours before you go to sleep.

Drink alcohol only in moderation, and don't have any within two hours of going to bed. While a drink might make you feel drowsy, the alcohol only disrupts the deep, late-night sleep that is so crucial to rest. If you have a chronic problem with insomnia, avoid alcohol completely.

Food allergies or sensitivities disrupt sleep for some people. See the Food Allergy section to identify possible offending foods.

Sugar is another common culprit in insomnia. After lunchtime, avoid sugary foods, even sweet fruits. Chocolate, with its double whammy of sugar and caffeine, should be considered an enemy of the sleep-deprived.

Rx Super Seven Prescriptions—Insomnia

Super Prescription #1 Melatonin
Take 0.3 to 3 mg half an hour before bedtime. This hormone promotes sleep. Sublingual melatonin works well for those who have trouble falling asleep. Time-released melatonin is a good choice for those who wake up during the night.

Super Prescription #2 Hydroxytryptophan (5-HTP)
Take 100 to 200 mg a half hour before bedtime. This supplement promotes serotonin production in the brain for relaxation. Do not use if you are currently taking pharmaceutical antidepressants.

Super Prescription #3 GABA
Take 250 to 500 mg a half hour before bedtime. GABA relaxes the brain to help one get into sleep mode.

Super Prescription #4 L-theanine
Take 200 to 500 mg a half hour before bedtime. L-theanine calms the brain and initiates a deeper sleep cycle.

Super Prescription #5 Calcium/magnesium
Take 500 mg of calcium and 250 mg of magnesium each evening. Both minerals help relax the nervous system. Some people have better results taking one of the minerals alone in the evening and the other earlier in the day. Experiment to see what works better for you.

Super Prescription #6 Valerian (*Valeriana officinalis*)
Take 600 mg or 2 ml a half hour before bedtime. Several studies show valerian to be effective for insomnia. *Note*: A small percentage of users may notice a stimulating effect from valerian.

Super Prescription #7 Passionflower (*Passiflora incarnata*)
Take 500 mg or 1 to 2 ml a half hour before bedtime. Passionflower is a great sleep aid that relaxes the nervous system and does not cause drowsiness in the morning.

A double-blind trial found that 600 mg of valerian extract taken thirty minutes before bedtime was comparable in efficacy to oxazepam (Serax), a commonly prescribed pharmaceutical for insomnia. Studies have also found that the combination of valerian and lemon balm (*Melissa officinalis*) works well to treat insomnia, with a comparable effect to the pharmaceutical sleep medication triazolam (Halcion). A hangover sensation was noted in people taking the triazolam but not in the lemon balm/valerian users.

General Recommendations

Lemon balm helps to relax the brain and promote sleep. It works well combined with valerian. Take as directed on the label.

Hops (*Humulus lupulus*) is a nervine that relaxes the nervous system. Take 500 mg or 1 to 2 ml a half hour before bedtime.

L-tryptophan promotes sleep, especially for those who wake up at night. Take 500 mg before bedtime.

Vitamin B6 is involved in the production of serotonin and other neurotransmitters that promote sleep. Take 50 mg daily.

Chamomile (*Matricaria chamomilla*) relaxes the nervous system. Drink a fresh cup of tea in the evening or take 300 mg of the capsule form.

Saint-John's-wort (*Hypericum perforatum*) acts as a nerve tonic and can ease mild cases of depression and related insomnia. Take 900 mg daily of a 0.3 percent hypericin extract. Do not take Saint-John's-wort if you are on medication for depression.

Vitamin B12 is more commonly deficient in seniors, and a deficiency may contribute to insomnia. Take 1,000 mcg sublingually or by capsule.

Homeopathy

Pick the remedy that best matches your symptoms in this section. Take a 6x, 12x, 6C, 12C, or 30C potency twice daily for two weeks to see if there are any positive results. After you notice improvement, stop taking the remedy, unless symptoms return. Consultation with a homeopathic practitioner is advised.

Aconitum Napellus is a remedy for people who have just experienced a terrifying situation and who develop insomnia. Restlessness, fear, and panic attacks may wake a person up.

Arsenicum Album is for people who have tremendous anxiety and restlessness. They often wake up between the hours of midnight and 2 A.M. They tend to be perfectionists and have many insecurities and fears.

Cocculus is a good remedy for people who can't sleep after staying up too long. As a result, they may feel weak and dizzy, have trouble thinking, and be irritable as well as sleepy.

Coffea Cruda is very specific for people with insomnia that's caused by over-stimulation. They are wide awake at 3 A.M. with a racing mind.

Ignatia (*Ignatia amara*) is a specific remedy for insomnia caused by emotional upset—usually grief or a loss. There can be uncontrollable crying, loss of appetite, and mood swings. The person often sighs a lot during the day, and muscles may twitch during sleep.

Kali Phosphoricum is for insomnia as a result of nervous exhaustion caused by overwork or mental strain. The person is extremely sensitive, and depression and anxiety are common.

Lycopodium (*Lycopodium clavatum*) is for people with insomnia as a result of fear and stress. They usually have poor confidence, which further worsens stress levels. Digestive problems, such as gas and bloating, are usually present. There is a craving for sweets.

Nux Vomica is for insomnia after indulging in rich, spicy food or alcohol. The sleep problem may be the result of overwork. The person is irritable and impatient, wakes at 3 A.M. thinking about business, and is highly sensitive to light, noise, sound, and other stimuli.

Sulfur is a good remedy for insomnia that comes on from itching at night or from feeling too heated at night. The person throws the covers off or sticks the feet out. There is a strong craving for ice-cold drinks and spicy foods.

Zincum Metallicum is for people who are very restless from being overworked. Their legs and arms are restless, and it's hard for them to lie still in bed.

Acupressure

See pages 787–794 for information about pressure points and administering treatment.
- Pericardium 6 (P6) and Lung 1 (Lu1) will reduce anxiety and heart palpitations.
- Another point to reduce tension is Conception Vessel 17 (CV17).
- If indigestion is a problem, you should make it a habit to avoid greasy and spicy foods. If you do indulge, Spleen 16 (Sp16) will help you digest the food properly.
- Large Intestine 4 (LI4) is a good general point for pain relief. Try it if arthritis or other aches keep you up at night.

Bodywork

Massage
Any kind of massage will help you relax and unwind. Most people with insomnia would benefit from a professional massage as well as home and self-care techniques. Use some relaxing essential oils for an even more potent effect.

Reflexology
See pages 804–805 for information about reflexology areas and how to work them.
To relax your nerves, work the diaphragm and the solar plexus.

Hydrotherapy
Before sleeping, take a ten-minute hot footbath to draw blood out toward your limbs and away from your head.

If you need to relax, take a hot bath—but make sure to do it at least two hours before bed. Otherwise, your body temperature will be too high to allow sleep.

Other Bodywork Recommendations
Many people who have trouble sleeping rub their heads in frustration. Try to avoid this temptation. You'll only increase the blood flow to your brain, which can make sleeping even more difficult.

Acupuncture and Chinese herbal therapy can be very effective for insomnia. See a qualified practitioner.

Aromatherapy

Essential oils can have a dramatic relaxing effect. Many can help you get to sleep, but lavender, neroli, chamomile, and ylang-ylang are some of the best. Add some to a bath or a massage, or sprinkle a few drops on your pillow. You might also like to add the oil to a diffuser in your bedroom.

Marjoram is another sleep-inducing oil that has the additional benefit of warming and relaxing the muscles. You can use it in any of the previous preparations, but it may be most effective in a bath or a massage.

Lavender sachets are a time-honored sleep aid. Tuck one under your pillow for all-night insomnia relief.

Stress Reduction

General Stress-Reduction Therapies

Make nightly prayer a habit. Try to devote twenty or thirty minutes (some of you may need even more) before bedtime to cultivating a relaxed focus and a sense of detachment from the day's worries. You'll find that you're much more likely to sleep.

Most of us have lain awake in bed at some point, trying to nod off by counting sheep. But, as you've probably experienced, unlimited counting can lead to panic, especially as you reach the higher numbers. By the time you've reached one hundred, you may be frantic with the awareness of how much sleepless time has passed since you've begun the exercise, and a sense of futility sets in. Instead, try this meditative technique when you can't sleep: Breathe calmly and deeply from your abdomen, and count each breath. Give one count to each inhalation and one count to each exhalation. When you reach ten, start again at one. Don't keep track of how many series of ten you've done; simply use the numbers as a means of focus, rather than as a means of marking time. This technique will help you avoid frustration and will often send even seasoned insomniacs off to sleep within minutes. And even if you can't get to sleep, you'll feel much more relaxed and rested than if you spent the night sweating over sheep counts.

Research shows listening to relaxing music such as classical music helps people with insomnia. Do this at least thirty minutes before bedtime.

Other Recommendations

- Get into a sleep routine. Create a bedtime ritual to help yourself quiet down and to signal your body that it's time to rest. Have a cup of herbal tea, or practice one of the relaxation techniques listed in this section. Go to bed at the same time every night, and wake up at the same hour each morning. Do not change this routine on the weekend.
- Keep your bedroom quiet, dark, and comfortable. Invest in a good mattress and pillow, and have several covers available to suit various nighttime temperatures.
- Use the bed for sleep and sex only. Everything else, including reading, writing letters, and making phone calls, should take place off the bed, preferably in another room.
- If you can't sleep, get out of bed and move to another room, if possible. Try not to dwell on your insomnia; instead, read a magazine or a light novel, or engage in some other quiet activity.
- Don't smoke or expose yourself to secondhand smoke. Nicotine, like alcohol, has an initial calming effect but ultimately disrupts sleep.
- Many nonaspirin pain relievers contain caffeine. If you have chronic pain and need relief to sleep, check for brands that don't list caffeine as an ingredient.

- Get exercise during the day, even if long nights awake have left you tired. People who exercise regularly report better and deeper rest than those who don't. Do not exercise within two hours before bed, however, as your body may be too stimulated to sleep.
- Listening to classical or other relaxing music for thirty minutes before bedtime can help those with insomnia. Do this nightly for at least two weeks.
- Avoid using cell phones, tablets, and other electrical devices at bedtime. Studies show this worsens sleep quality.

REFERENCES

Dorn, M. 2000. Valerian versus oxazepam: Efficacy and tolerability in non-organic and non-psychiatric insomniacs: A randomized, double-blind, clinical, comparative study. *Forsch KomplementärmedKlass Naturheilkd* 7:79–84 [in German].

Dressing, H., D. Riemann, H. Low, et al. 1992. Insomnia: Is valerian/balm combination of equal value to benzodiazepine? *Therapiewoche* 42:726–36 [in German].

Irritable Bowel Syndrome

Common Illnesses That Mimic IBS

- Cancer of the colon or the rectum
- Duodenal ulcer
- Diverticular disease
- Biliary tract disease
- Parasitic diseases, such as amebiasis, giardiasis, campylobacter
- Lactose intolerance
- Laxative abuse
- Ulcerative colitis
- Imbalanced intestinal flora
- Malabsorption conditions, such as celiac disease or pancreatic insufficiency

If you have irritable bowel syndrome (IBS), you are not alone. Once a relatively rare disorder, IBS now affects an estimated 10 to 20 percent of the US population. Although women are two times more likely than men to seek treatment for IBS, it is thought that men and women are affected in equal numbers. Research has shown that when looked at retrospectively, the onset of symptoms began in childhood for many sufferers. It is the most common reason for a referral to a gastroenterologist.

IBS is characterized by a malfunction in the digestive tract. Usually, waste material is delivered through the tract to the rectum by rhythmic contractions of the intestines. In IBS, those contractions become erratic and irregular. Bowel movements are unpredictable and painful, with attending constipation, diarrhea, or an alternation of both. The abdomen may be cramped or bloated, certain foods can no longer be tolerated, and other all-too-familiar signs of gastric distress develop. In some cases, waste matter is pushed through the tract with such force that stool incontinence results. Studies have found that people with IBS have increased sensitivity to pain in the digestive tract.

There are really five main fundamental causes of IBS. The modern-day, fast-food diet is definitely one of them. Refined foods that are hard to digest contribute to many symptoms of poor digestion. Second, poor stress-coping mechanisms trigger nervous-system reactions that contribute to IBS. Unresolved emotional traumas can have this negative effect as well. Third, chronic infections of the digestive tract with fungi, parasites, and bacteria can be causative factors. Fourth, poorly functioning digestive organs contribute to IBS symptoms. These include low stomach-acid production, low bile production, low pancreatic-enzyme production, and dysbiosis, in which there is a deficiency of the good bacteria that are involved with digestion and detoxification. The fifth cause, and the least common, is a structural abnormality of some type. Spinal misalignments, for example, impair nerve flow to the digestive tract, which contributes to digestive problems.

It is important that you consult with a doctor to find out whether you have IBS or some other condition that causes similar symptoms. However, in our opinion, natural therapies are the only sensible approach for the long-term control and the resolution of this condition, as they treat the underlying cause(s).

Although irritable bowel syndrome is now the standard term, there are many other names for this group of symptoms, including:

- Spastic colon
- Mucus colitis
- Gastric colitis
- Nervous indigestion
- Intestinal neurosis

SYMPTOMS

- Constipation
- Diarrhea
- Alternating constipation and diarrhea
- Spastic colon
- Mucus colitis
- Mucus in stools
- Gastric colitis
- Abdominal pain and cramping, usually either relieved by going to the bathroom or brought on by it
- Flatulence and abdominal rumblings
- Nausea
- Headache
- Intolerance to certain foods
- Fatigue
- Gurgling and rumbling of the abdomen
- Burping
- Heartburn
- Occasional vomiting
- Unpleasant taste in the mouth
- Feeling full easily
- Depression
- Anxiety
- Mental "fog"
- Frequent urination
- Painful sexual intercourse (dyspareunia)
- Painful periods
- Irritation of the rectum
- Insomnia

ROOT CAUSES

- A diet that's high in refined, man-made foods and sugars and low in fiber
- Food allergies or sensitivities
- Candida overgrowth, parasite infection, and dysbiosis
- Poor stress-coping mechanisms
- Small intestine bacterial overgrowth (SIBO)

Testing Techniques

The following tests help assess possible reasons for irritable bowel syndrome:

Hormone testing (thyroid, DHEA, cortisol, testosterone, estrogen, proges-terone)—saliva, blood, or urine

Intestinal permeability—urine

Detoxification profile—urine

Digestive function and microbe/parasite/fungal testing—stool analysis

Food and environmental allergies/sensitivities—blood, electrodermal

Breath test for small intestine bacterial overgrowth

TREATMENT

Diet

The most reliable way to calm an irritable bowel is to adhere to a good diet. You may find that the following suggestions advocate a drastic change from your present way of eating, but the difference in the way you feel will be worth it.

Even when eating the most healthful of foods, however, you must be careful not to eat just before going to bed.

Recommended Food

For IBS sufferers there needs to be a delicate balance of fiber. You should slowly increase the amount of fiber-rich foods in your diet so that your body can adjust. Consider psyllium, chia seeds, or ground flaxseeds along with sixty ounces or more of water a day to help bowel movements.

Drink a glass of clean, quality water every two waking hours to ease the transit of waste matter and to keep your whole body functioning smoothly.

Irritable bowel syndrome can deplete your intestines of friendly bacteria. Eat a cultured product such as live yogurt, kefir, or sauerkraut every day.

Food to Avoid

The first step in treating IBS is to determine whether your problem is actually a sensitivity to food. See Food Allergies, and follow the elimination diet there. If you can trace your symptoms to a particular food or foods, make it a priority to avoid those allergens. Keep a close eye on how dairy products affect you; lactose is often a trigger for IBS-like symptoms. Wheat, gluten, and sugar products are common offenders as well.

One of the more effective diets is a low-FODMAP (fermentable oligosaccharides, disaccharides, monosaccharides, and polyols) diet. These short-chain carbohydrates are poorly absorbed in the small intestine. The goal of the low-FODMAP diet is to cut back on, or eliminate, these readily fermentable foods, reducing both SIBO and IBS symptoms. SIBO sufferers should avoid the following foods that are high in FODMAPs:

- Fructose (fruits, honey, high fructose corn syrup [HFCS], etc.)
- Lactose (dairy)
- Fructans (wheat, garlic, onion, etc.)
- Galactans (legumes such as beans, lentils, soybeans, etc.)
- Polyols (sweeteners containing isomalt, mannitol, sorbitol, xylitol, etc.)
- Stone fruits (such as avocado, apricots, cherries, nectarines, peaches, plums)

Saturated, hydrogenated, and partially hydrogenated fats disturb the intestines and are hard to digest. Stay away from red meat, butter, margarine, and fried foods.

Avoid mucus-forming foods that encourage toxins to accumulate. Foods that promote mucus include all dairy products, fried and processed foods, refined flours, and chocolate.

Caffeine, alcohol, spicy foods, and tobacco all irritate the stomach lining, so eliminate them from your diet. Many of these items also contribute to stress.

Although a high intake of fiber is a necessity, steer clear of wheat bran. It often triggers allergies in IBS sufferers, and because the fiber is insoluble, it can propel waste matter through the intestines faster than is comfortable. Ground flaxseeds are a better choice.

Avoid ice-cold drinks, which inhibit digestion and may cause cramping.

Recent research shows that many people with IBS are sensitive to the sweetener fructose. It should be avoided or limited in the diet.

A vegetable-juice fast lasting three days is a good way to eliminate toxins that have built up as a result of improper bowel functioning; do this fast once a month for three consecutive months.

℞ Super Seven Prescriptions—Irritable Bowel Syndrome

Super Prescription #1 Peppermint oil (*Mentha piperita*)
Take 1 or 2 enteric-coated peppermint oil capsules twice daily between meals. This herb reduces gas and cramping, and studies show that it is effective for IBS.

Super Prescription #2 Gentian root (*Gentiana lutea*)
This improves overall digestive function. Take 300 mg or 10 to 20 drops five to fifteen minutes before meals. It works well as part of a "bitters" herbal formula.

Super Prescription #3 Digestive enzymes
Take 1 or 2 capsules of a full-spectrum enzyme product with each meal. Enzymes help you to digest food more efficiently.

Super Prescription #4 Probiotic
Take a product containing at least 20 billion active organisms and up to 150 billion daily. Friendly bacteria such as *Lactobacillus acidophilus* and *bifidus* are involved with digestion and prevent the overgrowth of candida and other harmful microbes.

Super Prescription #5 Ginger root (*Zingiber officinale*)
Drink 1 cup of fresh tea or take 500 mg of the capsule form with each meal. Ginger reduces gas, bloating, and diarrhea and improves the functioning of the stomach.

Super Prescription #6 Diamine oxidase (DAO) enzyme
Take 1 or 2 capsules within fifteen minutes of eating foods that cause a reaction. This reduces the histamine level in the body caused by food intolerance.

Super Prescription #7 Aloe vera juice
Drink ¼ cup twice daily or as directed on the container. Aloe is very soothing and healing to the digestive tract, and it fights intestinal infection.

A study of enteric-coated peppermint oil was shown to reduce IBS symptoms by over 50 percent in three-fourths of patients. Another study found eight weeks of supplementation significantly improved abdominal pain and discomfort and quality of life. Another study showed decreased bloating, flatulence, stomach growling, stool frequency, abdominal pain, and improved stool form.

General Recommendations

Peppermint tea (*Mentha piperita*) is a hallowed remedy for digestive troubles. Take peppermint tea after meals, instead of having dessert. Use it with caution if you have acid reflux.

A toxic liver can aggravate IBS, and IBS can put additional stress on the liver. Support yours with detoxifying milk thistle (*Silybum marianum*). For the best effect, you'll need to take this herb on a continuing basis. Take 250 mg daily of a product standardized for 80 to 85 percent silymarin content. Take it with each meal.

Slippery elm (*Ulmus fulva*) and pau d'arco (*Tabebuia avellanedae*) are both traditional soothers of an irritated bowel. Take 800 to 1,000 mg of slippery elm three or four times daily, or use 5 cc of a tincture three times daily. The dosage for pau d'arco is 100 mg of the powdered bark or 0.5 to 1.0 cc of a tincture three times a day.

Betaine hydrochloride supports stomach acid levels for better digestion. Take 1 or 2 capsules with each meal.

Skullcap (*Scutellaria lateriflora*) relaxes the nervous system and promotes digestion. Take 250 mg or 2 ml with each meal.

Melatonin has been shown in several trials to improve IBS symptoms better than placebo.

Homeopathy

Pick the remedy that best matches your symptoms in this section. Take a 6x, 12x, 6C, 12C, or 30C potency twice daily for two weeks to see if there are any positive results. After you notice improvement, stop taking the remedy, unless symptoms return. Consultation with a homeopathic practitioner is advised.

Argentum Nitricum is for bloating, gas, and diarrhea accompanied by anxiety and nervousness. Digestive upset comes on after eating sweets.

Arsenicum Album is for burning pains and diarrhea accompanied by great restlessness and anxiety. The person tends to be chilly and prefers sipping warm drinks. Symptoms are often worse from midnight to 2 A.M.

Colocynthis is a good remedy when one has constriction and cutting pains in the abdomen. Symptoms often come on after eating fruit or during diarrhea. Bending over, heat, and pressure make the symptoms better. Symptoms may come on after suppressed anger.

Lycopodium (*Lycopodium clavatum*) is the remedy when there are bloating, distension, and gurgling noises with abdominal pain. Symptoms are typically worse between 4 and 8 P.M. The person has a strong craving for sweets and feels better from warm drinks. The person has low self-confidence and is irritable.

Magnesia Phosphorica is for abdominal cramping and spasms that are better from warm drinks and warm applications to the abdomen.

Natrum Carbonicum is for people with multiple food allergies who experience indigestion and heartburn. They crave milk, potatoes, and sweets but experience irritable bowels when ingesting them. They desire to be left alone.

Nux Vomica is helpful for people with abdominal pains and bowel problems caused by stress and a poor diet. Constipation is common, and they feel as if they never complete a bowel movement. Spasms may occur in their digestive tracts. Symptoms are worse from anger or excitement. They have a strong craving for spicy foods, alcohol, tobacco, coffee, and other stimulants, which worsen the digestive symptoms.

Sulfur is a good choice for people who experience diarrhea that wakes them up early in the morning to rush to the bathroom. Diarrhea may occur frequently throughout the day, although constipation can be present as well. Often, the gas has a foul smell like rotten eggs. The rectum is often irritated, itchy, and burning. There is a craving for sweets, spicy foods, and alcohol.

Acupressure

See pages 787–794 for information about pressure points and administering treatment.

- The point of choice for relieving abdominal pain is Conception Vessel 12 (CV12); this point can also prevent indigestion when used before a meal.
- Conception Vessel 6 (CV6) soothes abdominal pain, constipation, and gas.
- Pericardium 6 (P6) has a calming effect and soothes an upset stomach.
- Large Intestine 11 (LI11) relaxes the colon if you are constipated.
- Stomach 36 (St36) is an overall toner and strengthens the digestive system in particular.

Bodywork

Massage

Some self-massage techniques are helpful for stimulating digestion and relaxing cramps.

Use your finger to massage your tongue and gums in the morning. This technique prepares the upper part of your digestive tract for the work of the day.

At night, or whenever you feel IBS pain or cramps, massage your abdomen. Lie down in bed, with your knees bent, and gently examine the area for regions of tension. When you find those regions, massage them with the flat of your hand, using firm but gentle pressure.

Reflexology

See pages 804–805 for information about reflexology areas and how to work them.

For diarrhea, work the areas that correspond to the liver, the ascending colon, the transverse colon, and the adrenal glands.

If you are constipated, massage the areas corresponding to the liver, the gallbladder, the colon, and the adrenal glands.

For flatulence, work the areas corresponding to the intestines, the liver, and the sigmoid colon.

Work the solar plexus to reduce tension.

Aromatherapy

Neroli, chamomile, and lavender will relax abdominal cramping and reduce pain. You can use them separately or together in a warm bath or a hot compress. You might also like to add one or more to a carrier oil to use in an abdominal self-massage.

Black pepper can relieve constipation and improve a sluggish digestion. Use it on a hot compress applied directly to the abdomen.

Stress Reduction

General Stress-Reduction Therapies

Any antistress technique can help, but positive mental imagery and deep breathing are particularly beneficial. It is helpful to work with a counselor who teaches stress-reduction techniques.

People with severe anxiety should consider EEG biofeedback, which will teach them how to control their brainwaves and relax their nervous system.

Other Recommendations

- When your intestines feel tight and cramped, lie down with a heating pad or a warm compress against your abdomen.
- Constitutional hydrotherapy is effective for reducing abdominal pain and bloating. You can do a treatment for acute symptoms, and regular treatments are effective for improving overall digestive function.

REFERENCES

Cappello, G., M. Spezzaferro, L. Grossi, et al. 2007. Peppermint oil (Mintoil) in the treatment of irritable bowel syndrome: A prospective double blind placebo-controlled randomized trial. *Dig Liver Dis* 39(6):530–36.

Merat, S., S. Khalili, P. Mostajabi, et al. 2010. The effect of enteric-coated, delayed-release peppermint oil on irritable bowel syndrome. *Dig Dis Sci* 55(5):1385–90.

Liu, J. H., G. H. Chen, H. Z. Yeh, et al. 1997. Enteric-coated peppermint-oil capsules in the treatment of irritable bowel syndrome: A prospective, randomized trial. *J Gastroenterol* 32(6):765–768.

Jet Lag

Jet lag occurs when the body's internal clock becomes disrupted from traveling across time zones. This leads to a temporary sleep problem in which one is awake when it is time to sleep. As a result, symptoms such as fatigue, poor focus, headache, and digestive issues can occur.

SYMPTOMS

- Insomnia
- Fatigue during the day
- Poor concentration
- Muscle soreness
- Digestive upset
- Headache
- Overall sensation of not feeling well

ROOT CAUSES

Traveling across multiple time zones disrupts one's sleep–wake cycle. The pineal gland in the brain releases melatonin when the eyes are exposed to darkness. So when people are exposed to darkness during the time of day that is normally day for them (and vice versa), it disrupts their internal clock. Changes in cabin pressure and dehydration at higher altitudes may also account for some symptoms.

TREATMENT

Diet

Recommended Food

Make sure to consume plenty of clean, quality water while flying to prevent dehydration. This can prevent jet lag symptoms.

Food to Avoid

Avoid foods that can be dehydrating, like caffeine and high-sugar beverages.

Testing Techniques

No tests are required, but for those who do not seem to recover, melatonin levels can be tested—saliva.

℞ Super Seven Prescriptions—Jet Lag

Super Prescription #1 Melatonin

Take 3 mg of sublingual or time-released melatonin half an hour before bedtime for the zone you have traveled to.

Super Prescription #2 Homeopathic Gelsemium

Take 2 pellets of a 30C potency every two hours while flying to prevent jet lag symptoms.

Super Prescription #3 Homeopathic rescue remedy

Take 5 drops every two hours while flying to prevent jet lag symptoms.

Super Prescription #4 B-complex

Take a 50 mg B-complex each morning and afternoon to improve your energy level.

Super Prescription #5 Ashwagandha

Take 125 to 250 mg of a 0.8 percent with anolide extract to prevent jet lag symptoms. This supplement supports your stress glands.

Super Prescription #6 Eleutherococcus

Take 300 mg of an extract twice daily to help your body combat the effects of flying.

Super Prescription #7 Psyllium

Take as directed on the container to prevent constipation caused by dehydration while flying.

General Recommendations

Work with a holistic doctor to try different natural approaches depending on your testing and health history.

Homeopathy

Pick the remedy that best matches your symptoms in this section. Take a 6x, 12x, 6C, 12C, or 30C potency three times daily to see if there is any improvement. If you notice improvement, stop taking the remedy unless the symptoms return. Consultation with a homeopathic practitioner is advised.

Cocculus Indicus is good if you are feeling very dizzy and have symptoms like vertigo.

Kali Phosphoricum is for poor concentration and the fatigue that accompanies jet lag.

Nux Vomica is for the symptoms of fatigue, stomach cramping, constipation, irritability, and insomnia associated with jet lag.

Bodywork

Reflexology

Work the area of your foot associated with brain function.

Hydrotherapy

If poor digestion and fatigue are present, follow the constitutional hydrotherapy treatment on pages 795–796.

Other Recommendations

Exercise during the day but not in the evening when you get to your new time zone.

Kidney Stones

Kidney stones have become an increasingly common medical problem in Western society, mainly due to poor dietary habits. Although many kidney stones are so small that they pass unnoticed, they may sometimes become very large, up to the size of a marble. It is not hard to imagine that as these large stones move through the urinary tract, they cause great—and often excruciating—pain. Kidney stones are most likely to affect white men over the age of the thirty. People of any race or sex who live in the southern United States also have a higher risk, probably because of dietary habits in that region.

Complementary therapies offer effective, natural pain relief for more minor cases, as well as strategies for keeping the stones from growing any larger, but on the whole, it is far easier to prevent kidney stones in the first place. History holds a clue to their prevention: Back in the early 1900s, when Americans ate natural, wholesome foods, kidney stones were largely unheard of. As the century wore on, and as diets became lower in fiber and higher in fat, sugar, dairy, and junk, the disorder became much more common. Now a man living in America has a 10 percent chance of passing a kidney stone at least once in his life. If you suffer from kidney stones, take heart in the knowledge that you can prevent a recurrence of this painful condition with changes in diet and lifestyle and by using specific nutritional supplements.

There are different types of kidney stones, with 80 percent being composed of calcium salts, especially the oxalate type. Some stones are also composed of calcium phosphate, uric acid, struvite, cystine, or other materials. If your stones are mainly composed of uric acid, please follow the recommendations in the Gout section. This section focuses on the prevention and the treatment of calcium-oxalate stones.

If you have been diagnosed with or suspect that you have kidney stones, then you should be under the care of a professional. Your doctor will rule out other conditions or underlying causes and will check for infection. In cases of very large stones or severe pain, you may need to be hospitalized. This condition can be a medical emergency when stones block the urinary tract for a long time, causing urine to back up and distend the kidney (hydronephrosis). You are also at more risk for a urinary tract infection during an acute kidney stone crisis. Conventional treatment may involve breaking the stones up with sound waves (lithotripsy) or surgical removal.

Smaller stones that are not causing symptoms or an infection will usually pass through without any problems if you follow our recommendations. People with a chronic susceptibility to this condition should remember that an effective prevention program generally requires the nutritional approach outlined in this chapter.

SYMPTOMS

- Pain on one side of the lower back, in the belly, or down into the groin
- Nausea and vomiting
- Chills and fever, if the stone causes a blockage and an infection
- A frequent urge to urinate
- Blood and sediment in the urine

ROOT CAUSES

- A poor diet
- Dehydration
- Urinary pH balance
- Allergies and food sensitivities
- Infections that disturb the flow of fluids
- Obesity
- Inactivity
- A magnesium and potassium deficiency
- An inherited inability to absorb calcium properly or an inherited tendency to excrete too much oxalic acid
- Metabolic disorders that increase the risk of kidney stone formation, such as hyperparathyroidism, Cushing's syndrome, sarcoidosis, cancer, and others
- Medications such as diuretics

Testing Techniques

The following tests help assess possible reasons for kidney stones:

Urine pH and type of crystals formed—urinalysis

X-rays, ultrasound, or CT scan

Detoxification profile—urine

Vitamin and mineral analysis (especially for magnesium, B6, vitamin D, calcium)—blood, urine

Food and environmental allergies/sensitivities—blood, electrodermal

Heavy-metal toxicity (especially cadmium)—hair or urine

TREATMENT

Diet

Recommended Food

Many people with kidney stones suffer from dehydration. A lack of fluids increases the mineral concentration in the kidneys and, with it, the chance that stones will crystallize. While you have a kidney stone, drink 2½ to 3 quarts of clean, quality water every day. Once the stone has passed, resume a normal daily dose of 1 glass every two waking hours. Hydration is the single most important tactic in the treatment and the prevention of kidney stones.

Vegetarians have a much lower risk of getting kidney stones than meat eaters do. Follow a diet based on fresh, raw vegetables and whole grains; eat beans, nuts and seeds, and fish for protein. If you must eat animal products, stick to lean, high-quality sources of white meat.

Consume oat and wheat bran daily, as they reduce the risk of kidney stones being formed.

Lemon juice mixed with a little hot water is another remedy that will help acidify the urine and ease the passage of calcium-oxalate stones. Drink some at breakfast and throughout the day. Orange juice has been shown to be helpful as well.

Vitamin A is healing to the urinary tract, so be sure to eat lots of orange-yellow and green vegetables.

Consume ¼ cup of pumpkin seeds daily. Studies show that consuming these seeds reduces risk factors for kidney stone formation.

A magnesium deficiency has been linked to recurring kidney stones. Boost your levels of this nutrient by eating green leafy vegetables, kelp, soybeans, almonds, and apples.

Food to Avoid

Eliminate foods that contain high amounts of oxalic acid from your diet. By far the worst offenders are spinach, rhubarb, tomatoes, collards, eggplant, beets, celery, summer squash, sweet potatoes, peanuts, almonds, blueberries, blackberries, strawberries, Concord grapes, parsley, and cocoa.

Avoid grapefruit juice, which studies show increases the risk of kidney stones.

Animal fat causes the body to excrete calcium, creating a buildup in the kidneys. Avoid all red meat, and limit your consumption of other animal products.

Avoid calcium overload by eliminating dairy products from your diet. The calcium from milk, cheese, ice cream, and the like is not easily absorbed by the digestive system and ends up as extra waste matter in your kidneys.

When you eat too much sugar, the resulting high levels of insulin leach calcium from the bones and divert it into the urinary tract. Stay away from all products that contain refined sugar. Of particular importance are soft drinks that contain phosphoric acid. They should be completely avoided, as some studies show that they cause an increase risk in kidney stones.

Salt, caffeine, and alcohol all conspire to dehydrate your body and increase the concentration of minerals in the urine. Cut out caffeine and alcohol, and dramatically restrict your salt intake.

R̶x̶ **Super Seven Prescriptions—Kidney Stones**

Super Prescription #1 Magnesium
Take 250 mg twice daily with meals. Magnesium prevents the formation of calcium-oxalate crystals.

Super Prescription #2 Vitamin B6
Take 50 mg daily. Vitamin B6 has been shown to reduce calcium-oxalate levels, and studies show that people with kidney stones tend to be deficient in B6.

Super Prescription #3 IP-6 (inositol hexaphosphate)
Take 120 mg daily. Studies show that this supplement reduces calcium-oxalate crystals in the urine.

Super Prescription #4 Vitamin E
Take 400 IU daily. Vitamin E may be helpful for people who have a history of elevated calcium-oxalate levels.

Super Prescription #5 Cranberry extract (*Vaccinium macrocarpona*)
Take 400 mg twice daily of a standardized extract or as directed on the container. Studies have shown that cranberry reduces urinary calcium levels in people with a history of kidney stones. It also is used to prevent urinary tract infections.

Super Prescription #6 Aloe vera
Drink ¼ cup daily or as directed on the container, as it reduces urinary crystals.

Super Prescription #7 Vitamin A
Take 5,000 IU daily. A deficiency of this vitamin is considered a risk factor for kidney stone formation.

General Recommendations

Uva ursi is a traditional herbal treatment for kidney stones. It relieves pain, cleanses the urinary tract, and fights infection. Take 250 to 500 mg three times daily. Do not take uva ursi for more than fourteen days at a stretch.

Dandelion root (*Taraxacum officinale*) is an effective kidney cleanser. Take 500 mg two times daily. Do not take dandelion root for more than a month at a time.

Horsetail (*Equisetum arvense*) has beneficial diuretic qualities. To make a tea, macerate horsetail leaves and steep them in cold water for twelve hours. Heat the mixture and drink 3 to 4 cups daily. If you prefer capsules or tablets, take 2 grams three times a day.

Juniper berry (*Juniperus communis*) tea is another strong diuretic kidney cleanser. Drink 3 or 4 cups every day until the stone passes.

Vitamin C supplementation has been shown to lower the incidence of kidney stone formation, when the level is below 4,000 mg daily. However, in certain individuals it may accelerate stone formation; therefore, people with a history of kidney stones should have their urinary oxalate levels monitored by a doctor.

Potassium citrate is used by doctors to prevent kidney stones. Speak to your doctor about its use.

Homeopathy

Pick the remedy that best matches your symptoms in this section. Take a 6x, 12x, 6C, 12C, or 30C potency twice daily for two weeks to see if there are any positive results. After you notice improvement, stop taking the remedy, unless symptoms return. Consultation with a homeopathic practitioner is advised.

Belladonna (*Atropa belladonna*) is for sudden, excruciating pain in the right kidney. Symptoms are worse with any jarring. A high fever and a flushed face may be present.

Berberis Vulgaris is helpful when there are sharp, stitching, or shooting pains that radiate throughout the ureters, the bladder, the testes, or the thighs.

Dioscorea helps when the kidney stone pain causes one to stretch or arch backward for pain relief.

Lachesis is for left-sided kidney pain. Hemorrhaging may occur from the kidney stone.

Lycopodium (*Lycopodium clavatum*) is for kidney stones that cause pain on the right side of the back or the belly. Symptoms are often worse between 4 and 8 P.M.

Nux Vomica is for stone pain (colic), accompanied by cramping, nausea, or vomiting. People who benefit from this remedy may have futile urges to empty their bowels or bladders and may feel very irritable.

Acupressure

See pages 787–794 for information about pressure points and administering treatment.

Work Large Intestine 4 (LI4) to relieve kidney stone pain.

Bodywork

Acupuncture is recommended to help combat the pain of a kidney stone and to promote a more effective passage.

Reflexology

See pages 804–805 for information about reflexology areas and how to work them.

To help pass kidney stones and ease the pain, work the following points daily: ureters, kidneys, bladder, diaphragm, parathyroid, and lower back. If you want to prevent the recurrence of stones, work these areas on a weekly basis.

Hydrotherapy

A hot sitz bath helps to relieve the pain. You can drink water or herbal tea while sitting in the water to encourage faster elimination of the stone. For some people, a constitutional hydrotherapy feels even better.

Aromatherapy

To relieve abdominal pain, use any of the following, either alone or in a combination that pleases you: chamomile, lavender, and marjoram. You can add them to a sitz bath (or a regular bath, if you like), or mix them with a carrier oil and rub it directly on your abdomen.

A study of 55 people with reoccurring kidney stones looked at the effect of supplementing 500 mg of magnesium daily for up to four years. The average number of recurrences of kidney stones dropped by 90 percent. Also, 85 percent of the people in the study remained stone free, as compared to 41 percent who did not supplement magnesium. Studies have also shown that the combination of magnesium and vitamin B6 supplementation is very effective in reducing kidney stone formation. One study of 149 people with recurrent kidney stones who supplemented B6 (10 mg) and magnesium (300 mg) had a 92.3 percent improvement in stone formation.

Other Recommendations

Antacids that contain aluminum may cause kidney stones, especially when taken along with dairy products. Choose an antacid made without this metal, or, better yet, simply avoid foods that give you indigestion.

REFERENCES

Johnson, G., et al. 1982. Effects of magnesium hydroxide in renal stone disease. *Journal of the American College of Nutrition* 1:179–85.

Prien, E. L., and S. N. Gershoff. 1974. Magnesium oxide-pyridoxine therapy for recurrent calcium oxalate calculi. *Journal of Urology* 112:509–12.

Lactose Intolerance

With lactose intolerance, one loses the ability to break down the sugar lactose into its components of glucose and galactose. Lactose is the primary sugar contained in dairy products. The disorder causes a variety of symptoms, including abdominal bloating and distention, loose stool, nausea, bowel sounds, and abdominal pain. Lactose intolerance is very common, affecting 25 percent of white and 75–90 percent of black, Native American, and Asian American populations. The statistic for the worldwide population is 75 percent.

The lactose-digesting enzyme lactase is produced in the portion of the small intestine known as the duodenum. Individuals who don't produce enough of this enzyme experience the digestive problems listed above after consuming dairy products. The undigested lactose causes water retention in the intestines, increasing intestinal contractions. The lactose is fermented by bacteria in the colon, producing hydrogen and methane gases, which explain the bloating. It also causes water to be retained in the colon, which can cause loose stool.

Beyond digestive symptoms, lactose intolerance also causes malabsorption of nutrients, which can contribute to osteopenia, or thinning of the bones.

Lactose intolerance is less common in infants but becomes more common when the infant is finished nursing. If colic is a problem then lactose intolerance should be suspected. There are other, secondary causes of lactose intolerance, including digestive disorders such as gastroenteritis, Crohn's disease, celiac disease, and chemotherapy.

We have also seen people become lactose intolerant after antibiotic use, especially when there is repeated use. According to research, the part of the small intestine that produces lactase is adversely affected by the antibiotics. The inability to produce lactase increases as one ages. This is why some people who never had a problem with milk products in childhood become lactose intolerant later in life. Research has shown that ethnic groups descended from northern Europe or northwestern India are less likely to have lactose intolerance.

TREATMENT

Diet

Recommended Food

Nondairy foods or lactose-free dairy products. All fruits, vegetables, grains, nuts, seeds, and fish are fine to eat. There is some research showing that unpasteurized yogurt improves lactose digestion since it naturally contains the enzyme lactase.

Food to Avoid

The biggest source of lactose is milk, including goat and sheep milk. Yogurt contains a fair amount of lactose but also contains friendly flora that can help digest it. Furthermore, unpasteurized yogurt has been shown to contain lactase. Cheese contains a low amount of lactose. The amount of lactose one can tolerate varies from person to person. There are lactose-free milks, cheeses, and yogurts available. Be aware that these alternative products contain the milk protein casein, which can trigger problems in people who are sensitive to it.

Lactose in Dairy Foods	
Food	**Grams of lactose**
Milk, regular/lowfat/nonfat (cow, goat, sheep), 1 cup	12–13 g
Yogurt, lowfat, 6 ounces	6–12 g
Cottage cheese, 2 percent, ½ cup	3 g
American cheese, 1 slice	1 g
Cheddar cheese, 1 ounce	<.01 g
Nondairy milk (almond, coconut, hemp, rice, soy)	0 g
Lactose-free milk, 1 cup	0 g

Testing Techniques

Breath-hydrogen test—After an overnight fast, one collects a breath sample and then is given a solution of lactose. Additional breath samples are collected over a period of three hours to assess hydrogen-gas concentrations. If the breath-hydrogen concentration increases beyond a certain quantity, then the diagnosis of lactase deficiency and thus lactose intolerance is made.

Elimination and reintroduction—Eliminate lactose-containing foods for several days and see if your digestive symptoms clear.

℞ Super Seven Prescriptions—Lactose Intolerance

Super Prescription #1 Lactase enzyme formula
Take 1 to 2 capsules when consuming lactose-containing dairy products. Reduces likelihood of diarrhea, gas, bloating, and other digestive symptoms when consuming dairy.

Super Prescription #2 Full-spectrum digestive enzyme
Take 1 to 2 capsules when consuming dairy products. Reduces the likelihood of diarrhea, gas, bloating, and other digestive symptoms. Helps to digest protein in dairy products.

Super Prescription #3 Probiotic
Take a probiotic with at least twenty billion organisms and one that contains *Lactobacillus acidophilus*. Stimulates the production of intestinal lactase.

Super Prescription #4 Calcium
Supplement 500 mg of a well-absorbed calcium supplement daily with a meal. It will help to offset the reduction of dietary calcium due to the avoidance of dairy products.

Super Prescription #5 Vitamin D
Take 2,000 IU to 5,000 IU daily with a meal to prevent deficiencies from avoiding dairy products.

Super Prescription #6 Vitamin K
Take 200 mcg to 500 mcg of vitamin K to aid in calcium utilization for bone production, important for those avoiding dairy products.

Super Prescription #7 Ginger root
Take 500 mg or 20 drops of tincture one to two times daily if one has digestive reactions to lactose.

REFERENCES

Marteau, P. 1990. Effect of the microbial lactase (EC 3.2.1.23) activity in yoghurt on the intestinal absorption of lactose: An in vivo study in lactase-deficient humans. *Br J Nutr* (1):71–79.

Roy, P. K. 2015. Lactose intolerance. Medscape. Accessed June 21, 2015. http://emedicine.medscape.com/article/187249-overview#a6.

Warren, Rachel. 2014. Lactose intolerant? Not all dairy is off limits. MedHelp. Accessed June 21, 2015. http://www.medhelp.org/nutrition/articles/Dairy-101-for-People-with-Lactose-Intolerance/1231.

Lupus

Lupus is an autoimmune disorder in which antibodies mistakenly identify the body's tissues as foreign substances and attack them, causing inflammation and pain. The disease most often strikes women in their childbearing years; only 10 percent of people with lupus are men. For reasons that are as yet unknown, African American women are three times more likely to receive a diagnosis than are their Caucasian counterparts, and American women of Asian or Hispanic descent are also more susceptible. Lupus is a rare condition, but, as with other autoimmune disorders, the number of incidents has been on the rise in recent years.

Lupus takes two related but quite distinct forms: discoid lupus erythematosus (DLE) and systemic lupus erythematosus (SLE). In DLE, the only symptom is a scaly red rash that spreads across the cheeks and the nose, and sometimes the forehead and the scalp. We tend to think of this rash as butterfly-shaped, but in a different era, the pattern reminded doctors of a wolf's face—hence the name lupus, which means "wolf" in Latin. The red patches usually come and go in cycles, but sometimes they leave disfiguring scars. Scars that occur on the scalp may prevent hair from growing in the area they cover. DLE can be distressing, but it does not pose a serious health threat. Since the rash is often triggered by exposure to sunlight, the most effective treatment is to remain inside during peak daylight hours and to shade the face and the head when outdoors.

Sufferers of SLE may also experience a rash, and their disease, like DLE, goes through periods of remission and activation, but the similarity between the two disorders stops there. Systemic lupus, as the name implies, affects not just the skin but the entire body. The process that produces the red rash spreads to the joints and the muscles, creating pain and inflammation very similar to that of rheumatoid arthritis. People with SLE suffer from frequent low-grade fevers that may spike when the disease cycle is at its peak. Not surprisingly, the fever and the pain leave their victims exhausted and sometimes depressed. For some people, the symptoms never progress beyond this point. In other cases, the inflammation spreads to the kidneys, the liver, the heart, or the spleen, creating dangerous and even life-threatening problems.

No one knows the exact cause of lupus. Conventional medicine focuses on factors that often trigger flare-ups; certain medications, viral and bacterial illnesses, birth-control pills, pregnancy, and periods of extreme stress are all suspects, but it is likely that there is no single culprit. Holistic doctors such as ourselves take a close look at other factors; addressing them can be quite helpful to people with this disease. The factors include food allergies, hormone balance, digestive function ("leaky gut syndrome") and detoxification, heavy-metal toxicity, and nutritional deficiencies.

Until the early twentieth century, lupus was fatal within a few years of its onset. Now almost all people with lupus live out a normal lifespan, provided that they and their doctors monitor the symptoms and control any threatening developments. Today, quality of life is the most pressing issue for the majority of lupus sufferers. Although some people experience very little inflammation and pain, others are nearly crippled by it. Doctors can help ease the worst flare-ups with medications for pain control and antibody suppression, but it's best to try to avoid the need for aggressive measures. An anti-inflammatory diet, adequate rest and stress control, and specific natural treatments can all help you to reduce the chance of flare-ups and minimize the symptoms when they do occur.

SYMPTOMS OF DLE

- A butterfly-shaped facial rash that may spread to the forehead or the scalp

SYMPTOMS OF SLE

- Facial rash
- Fever
- Fatigue and malaise
- Joint and muscle pain
- Weight loss
- Hair loss
- Sensitivity to the sun
- Mouth sores

- Vulnerability to illness
- Enlarged lymph nodes
- Nausea
- Constipation or diarrhea
- Recurring bladder infections
- Presence of lupus antibodies in the blood

ROOT CAUSES

- An allergic reaction to medications or vaccines
- Viruses
- Bacteria, especially streptococcus
- Extreme and prolonged emotional or physical stress
- Estrogen disruption related to pregnancy or birth-control pills

- Use of synthetic hormones
- Deficiency of certain hormones (especially DHEA, progesterone, testosterone, and growth hormone)
- Food allergies
- Poor digestion and detoxification
- Heavy-metal toxicity
- Vitamin D deficiency

Testing Techniques

The following tests help assess possible causes of lupus:

Hormone testing (thyroid, DHEA, cortisol, testosterone, IGF-1, estrogen, progesterone)—saliva, blood, or urine

Intestinal permeability—urine

Detoxification profile—urine

Vitamin and mineral analysis—blood

Essential fatty acid balance—blood or urine

Digestive function and microbe/parasite/candida testing—stool analysis

Food and environmental allergies/sensitivities—blood, electrodermal

Heavy-metal toxicity—hair or urine

Vitamin D—blood

TREATMENT

Diet

Recommended Food

Give your body optimal support by eating well-rounded, varied meals of whole foods. Buy organic products whenever possible, to reduce your exposure to toxins and pesticides. If you must buy conventional produce, wash it thoroughly in clean, quality water before eating.

Raw vegetables and citrus fruits will help return your body to an alkaline state. These foods are also high in fiber, which relieves digestive problems, and in antioxidants, which counteract inflammation.

For extra antioxidant protection, eat wheat germ and cold-pressed oils (like olive oil) for vitamin E.

Essential fatty acids are the "good" fats that actually help reduce inflammation. Eat cold-water fish from a clean water source several times a week, and add 1 to 2 tablespoons of ground flaxseeds or flaxseed oil to a daily salad.

During a flare-up of lupus, antibodies will attack your own joint cartilage. You can repair some of the damage by eating foods that are high in sulfur. Good sources include onions, garlic, and asparagus.

If you're prone to bladder infections, drink unsweetened natural cranberry juice every day.

Corticosteroid use is associated with bone loss and osteoporosis. If you must take these drugs, increase your intake of calcium by eating plenty of green leafy vegetables and soy products.

For good general health, drink a glass of clean, quality water every two waking hours. You'll also keep your joints lubricated: water makes their cartilage soft and flexible and maintains proper levels of joint fluid.

Food to Avoid

Saturated fats, hydrogenated fats, and partially hydrogenated fats make inflammation worse; in fact, some people find that their pain goes away completely when they eliminate animal meats and fried or greasy foods from their diet.

An internal acidic environment also promotes inflammation and pain. You already know to avoid saturated fats, but you'll also need to radically restrict your intake of eggs, sugar, refined carbohydrates, alcohol, and caffeine.

If you need another reason to avoid sugar and refined carbohydrates, here it is: these products damage the immune system and leave you even more susceptible to infection and illness.

Food allergies can mimic lupus symptoms or make them worse. Try the elimination diet on page 316 to determine whether there's a food or foods that you should avoid. Gluten, in particular, tends to cause problems in people with lupus.

You are highly vulnerable to microorganisms and toxins, so never drink tap water.

Be kind to your kidneys. Along with avoiding saturated fats and animal meats, restrict your salt intake.

Anyone with an autoimmune disorder should practice regular juice fasts to keep the body functioning at its peak. Try a three-day juice fast once a month. You can support the fast with plenty of green drinks and cleansing herbal teas.

℞ Super Seven Prescriptions—Lupus

Super Prescription #1 Fish oil
Take up to 20 grams of fish oil daily and a minimum of 8 grams. High doses of fish oil were shown to be of help in a human study. *Note*: High-potency fish oil formulas are available, meaning fewer capsules need to be taken.

Super Prescription #2 Plant sterols and sterolins

Take 20 mg three times daily on an empty stomach. These naturally occurring plant chemicals were shown to have a balancing effect on the immune system for people with autoimmune diseases.

Super Prescription #3 DHEA

Take up to 200 mg daily, under the supervision of a doctor. Studies have shown DHEA to improve symptoms of systemic lupus in women.

Super Prescription #4 Vitamin D

Take 2,000 to 5,000 IU daily with meals. Vitamin D modulates the immune system for those with autoimmune diseases.

Super Prescription #5 Methylsulfonylmethane (MSM)

Take 2,000 to 8,000 mg daily. MSM has natural anti-inflammatory benefits and contains the mineral sulfur, an integral component of cartilage. Reduce the dosage if diarrhea occurs.

Super Prescription #6 Enzymes

Take 1 or 2 capsules of a full-spectrum enzyme product with each meal. Enzymes help you to digest food more efficiently. Protease enzymes can be taken between meals for an anti-inflammatory effect.

Super Prescription #7 Boswellia *(Boswellia serrata)*

Take 1,200 to 1,500 mg of a standardized extract containing 60 to 65 percent boswellic acids two to three times daily. This herb has powerful anti-inflammatory effects.

In a double-blind trial, the combination of 20 grams of fish oil daily and a low-fat diet led to improvement in fourteen of seventeen people with systemic lupus in twelve weeks.

General Recommendations

Vitamin E may be helpful for people with discoid lupus. Take 800 to 2,000 IU daily.

Turmeric (*Curcuma longa*) has anti-inflammatory benefits. Take a product containing 450 mg of curcumin twice daily.

Take a super-green-food supplement, such as chlorella or spirulina, or a mixture of super green foods each day. Take as directed on the container.

A high-potency multivitamin contains a strong base of the antioxidants and other nutrients that protect against tissue damage. Take as directed on the container.

A probiotic contains friendly bacteria, such as *Lactobacillus acidophilus* and *bifidus*, that aid in digestion and detoxification. Take a product containing at least four billion active organisms daily.

Evening primrose oil, black currant oil, and borage oil contain the essential fatty acid GLA, which reduces joint inflammation. Take up to 2.8 grams of GLA daily.

Green tea (*Camellia sinensis*) contains a rich source of antioxidants and substances that assist detoxification. Drink the organic tea regularly (2 cups or more daily) or take 500 to 1,500 mg of the capsule form.

Milk thistle (*Silybum marianum*) improves liver function and protects against the potential damage of pharmaceutical medications. Take 250 mg of a standardized extract of 80 to 85 percent silymarin three times daily.

Ginkgo biloba improves circulation through the kidneys and has anti-inflammatory benefits. Take 60 to 120 mg twice daily of a product standardized to 24 percent flavone glycosides.

You can often avoid harsh conventional painkillers by using analgesic herbs. White willow bark (*Salix alba*) will soothe joint pain. Find a white willow extract that is standardized for salicin content, and take 30 to 60 mg twice daily. A lotion or a cream made with capsicum will also reduce the pain.

Devil's claw (*Harpagophytum procumbens*) root is a potent herb that will control inflammation. Take 2.5 to 5.0 grams twice a day, or use 1 to 2 cc of a tincture three times a day. Expect to take devil's claw root at least two months before you see results.

Teas made with burdock root (*Articum lappa*) or red clover (*Trifolium pratense*) have a detoxifying effect. Drink them during a fast or any time you want a little extra housecleaning.

Lupus can send stress levels soaring. If you've lost weight and are very slender, however, a very strong relaxant might be too much for you. Instead, try tea made with a moderately potent herb, like skullcap or hops. If neither of these herbs works, or if you have a larger frame, move on to valerian (*Valeriana officinalis*) or kava kava (*Piper methysticum*).

Gentian root (*Gentiana lutea*) and herbal bitters formulas improve overall digestive function. Take 300 mg or 10 to 20 drops five to fifteen minutes before meals.

Bioidentical hormone replacement can help those with lupus as it naturally balances the immune system.

Homeopathy

Pick the remedy that best matches your symptoms in this section. Take a 6x, 12x, 6C, 12C, or 30C potency twice daily for two weeks to see if there are any positive results. After you notice improvement, stop taking the remedy, unless symptoms return. Consultation with a homeopathic practitioner is advised.

Arsenicum Album will relieve burning joints that feel better with warm applications. The person tends to feel anxious and restless.

Belladonna (*Atropa belladonna*) works on joints that are hot, red, and burning and that feel worse with motion. Pain and swelling may come on suddenly.

Sepia is for women with lupus, who find that their symptoms flare up near their menstrual cycles. There are usually signs of hormone imbalance, such as PMS or extreme menopausal symptoms. There is a craving for sweet, salty, and sour foods. The person tends to be chilly, irritable, and depressed.

Pulsatilla (*Pulsatilla pratensis*) is helpful if your pains wander from joint to joint and if your symptoms improve in fresh, cool air or with cool applications.

Rhus Toxicodendron relieves lupus symptoms that are worse in the cold and the damp or with long periods of inactivity. Stiffness of the joints is the main symptom, which improves with some movement and warmth.

Sulfur is for burning pains that are better with cold applications. The person tends to get overheated easily and prefers a cool environment. There is a strong craving for spicy foods and ice-cold drinks.

Acupressure

Acupressure works wonders on rheumatic pains. As the following points are probably quite tender, don't massage them. Instead, use firm pressure. Plan to work the appropriate points two or three times a day for several months before you see results; it may take six months for the pain to subside completely. Once the pain has been significantly reduced, you can reduce your sessions to one a day. For more information about pressure points and administering treatment, see pages 787–794.

- Large Intestine 4 (LI4) is used for relief of pain anywhere on the body, but it is especially effective for pain in the hands, the wrists, the elbows, the shoulders, or the neck.
- For elbow and shoulder pain, use Large Intestine 11(LI11).
- If your ankles are affected, work Spleen 5 (Sp5) and Kidney 3 (K3).
- To relieve stress, work Lung 1 (Lu1) on a regular basis.
- For acute anxiety and nervousness, add Pericardium 6 (P6) to your daily practice or use as needed.

Bodywork

Acupuncture is worth trying for people with this condition, to reduce inflammation and pain.

Reflexology

See pages 804–805 for information about reflexology areas and how to work them.

Lupus is a systemic disorder, so if you have time, it's best to work the whole foot. If that's not possible, concentrate on the adrenals to reduce swelling and on any specific areas that are causing you pain.

To relieve tension, also work the area corresponding to the solar plexus.

Hydrotherapy

A hot bath with Epsom salts will temporarily reduce pain and draw toxins away from your joints and muscles.

Constitutional hydrotherapy is an excellent long-term therapy to minimize lupus symptoms. See pages 795–796 for directions.

Aromatherapy

Find a few relaxing oils that you like and use them regularly in a bath or a room diffuser. Some good choices to start with are lavender, rose, jasmine, and geranium.

Black pepper and ginger encourage blood flow and will help revive tired joints and muscles. If you're constipated, you can add a few drops of either essence to a carrier oil and rub it onto your abdomen.

If you want to detoxify your body, use lemon balm or juniper in a hot bath.

Stress Reduction

General Stress-Reduction Therapies

It doesn't matter how you reduce stress, just find a technique that you like and use it regularly—on a daily basis, if possible. If you're not sure where to start, a basic yoga class will help you relax and will give you the gentle exercise you need.

If your pain is intense, consider thermal biofeedback. This therapy will teach you to send warming, nourishing blood to your joints.

Many people with lupus find that support groups are as essential to their health as regular checkups are. Ask your doctor or local hospital for information about groups in your area.

Other Recommendations

- Avoid the bright sunlight, especially in the warm months or when snow (which reflects the sun) is on the ground. When you do go outside, always wear a hat and protective clothing. Your skin may be sensitive to some sunscreens; if so, talk to your doctor about a nonirritating prescription sunblock.
- Although you may not feel like exercising, gentle movement is highly recommended to reduce pain and promote good general health. A daily walk in the early morning sunlight is an excellent idea.
- Birth-control pills and synthetic hormones may trigger flare-ups, so it's wise to avoid them.
- Women with lupus were once counseled to avoid pregnancy, but pregnancy can sometimes actually lead to a remission of the disease. For many women, it's the stressful months after the baby is born that cause a flare-up. The decision regarding the safety of pregnancy must be made on a case-by-case basis, so talk to your doctor.
- Chinese herbal therapy can be helpful. See a qualified practitioner.

REFERENCES

Walton, A. J. E., M. L. Snaith, M. Locniskar, et al. 1991. Dietary fish oil and the severity of symptoms in patients with systemic lupus erythematosus. *Annals of Rheumatological Disease* 50:463–66.

Lyme Disease

Lyme disease is a bacterial infection transmitted by ticks. It affects many systems of the body. As it has become more widespread across the United States, it has developed into a national health care concern. Lyme-experienced doctors and the Centers for Disease Control and Prevention (CDC) disagree on the number of cases and on how to best diagnose and treat this feared disease. Doctors knowledgeable in the diagnosis, symptoms, and treatment of Lyme disease believe that this bacterial infection is vastly underdiagnosed and contributes immensely to chronic health problems. On the other hand the CDC and many mainstream physicians downplay the epidemic of Lyme disease. However, all agree it has become a much larger health problem than it was just a few years ago.

According to the CDC, "Lyme disease is the most commonly reported vector borne illness in the United States . . . and has a higher concentration in the northeast and upper Midwest including Connecticut, Delaware, Maine, Maryland, Massachusetts, Minnesota, New Hampshire, New Jersey, New York, Pennsylvania, Rhode Island, Vermont, Virginia, and Wisconsin." However, it is also quite common now in California and Texas. This means the most populated states in the country have a problem with Lyme disease.

That said, Lyme disease can be contracted anywhere in the country. The CDC reports that there are approximately three hundred thousand Americans diagnosed with Lyme disease each year. This is up to twelve times higher than what was reported in years past.

Classic symptoms of Lyme that start in the first thirty days after exposure may include include fever, headache, fatigue, muscle and joint pain, swollen lymph nodes, and a skin rash called erythema migrans. Often people will report flulike symptoms. Lyme disease should be considered when this occurs in the summer months.

The rash occurs in 50 to 80 percent of infected persons (this figures varies depending on which expert you consult) and begins at the site of the tick bite an average of seven days after being bitten. As the rash enlarges it may result in what is called a "bull's-eye" rash. It is usually warm to the touch but not painful or itchy.

If not treated early, Lyme can progress into a number of chronic symptoms. It is often referred to as the "great imitator." Since the inflammatory reactions that occur with Lyme affect so many body systems there are a number of symptoms it can cause and a number of conditions it resembles. For example, it can cause joint pain similar to that produced by many types of arthritis. It can also cause muscle and tendon discomfort similar to that of fibromyalgia. The relenting fatigue caused by Lyme disease is similar to that of chronic fatigue syndrome. Neurological symptoms such as numbness, pain, facial paralysis, mood changes, insomnia, and others mimic symptoms of autoimmune conditions like multiple sclerosis, rheumatoid arthritis, and lupus. Lyme disease can also lead to inflammation of the heart, known as carditis.

Lyme infection is caused by transmission of the bacterium *Borrelia burgdorferi* through the bite of the blacklegged tick, also known as the Ixodes tick. Yet research shows that only 50 percent of Lyme patients remember a tick bite, and only 17 to 25 percent of those who develop the rash remember a tick bite. This is why many experts believe that Lyme is transmitted by other carriers such as mosquitoes, mice mites, fleas, and flies. Animals that can carry the contagious ticks include birds, deer, mice, and other small mammals. Recent studies suggest it may also be transferred through sexual intercourse, pregnancy, and possibly breast-feeding. At this point it is not clear what other modes of transmission are occurring.

The tick presents quite a tricky problem for the immune system. Its saliva contains substances that suppress the immune response at the bite site, allowing the bacteria to penetrate more easily into the skin without dealing with an immune response. In the days and weeks that follow the tick bite, the bacteria spread through the lymphatics and blood to other skin sites and internal organs.

The diagnosis of Lyme disease is a clinical diagnosis that involves a patient's signs and symptoms. In some cases lab testing can be helpful. A physician should consider whether the patient was exposed to Lyme infection in an area known to have Lyme disease, whether the patient was involved in outdoor activities in a location where contact with a tick was possible (especially wooded, brushy, or grassy areas within thirty days prior to the onset of a rash), and whether the patient had a known tick bite. Also to be considered is whether the patient has symptoms typical of Lyme disease; whether a physical exam shows signs of Lyme disease, such as swollen lymph nodes, rash, swollen joints, bull's-eye rash (although many people do not have outward physical symptoms, and 50 percent of the time a patient does not have a classic bull's-eye rash); whether there are symptoms not caused by other conditions, such as fatigue, anxiety and other psychiatric symptoms, memory problems, joint pain, insomnia, neurological symptoms such as numbness and tingling; and whether lab testing can help to support the diagnosis (although lab tests should not be relied upon as diagnostic) or can attribute the symptoms to other illnesses.

A person should consider a diagnosis of Lyme disease if he or she has unexplained illnesses that affect many systems of the body, symptoms that migrate, symptoms that are unresponsive to good treatments, or symptoms that flare up every month (tracking the growth cycle of the Lyme bacteria).

An often unrecognized complication of Lyme disease is what is known as tick-borne coinfections. These are caused by microbes that can infect the body following a tick bite. They include babesia, bartonella, ehrlicia, and anaplasma. It is thought that most people with Lyme disease have one or more of these coinfections. They can be tested for with blood tests, although lab unreliability can be a problem. You should suspect one of these infections if your symptoms do not resolve with good treatment or if new symptoms pop up during treatment. Antibiotics and natural agents can be used to treat these coinfections.

The best treatment for Lyme disease involves an integrative approach combining antibiotic therapy and natural therapies. It is always best to treat Lyme disease as soon as possible if an infection is suspected or diagnosed.

SYMPTOMS

- Severe fatigue
- Arthritis in any joint
- Neurological problems
- Psychiatric problems
- Cognitive problems
- Muscle pain
- Joint pain
- Hearing problems
- Heart problems
- Skin rash

ROOT CAUSES

- Exposure to organisms transmitted primarily from tick bites
- Weak immune system

Testing Techniques

Conventional approaches to Lyme disease testing are fraught with accuracy problems. Most doctors follow the CDC recommendation to start with a blood test known as the enzyme immunoassay (EIA) or immunofluorescence assay (IFA). The CDC says that if this test is negative, health care providers should consider a different diagnosis. The test measures antibodies to proteins of the Lyme bacteria. It is a poor test, especially for those with chronic Lyme disease, and misses about 50 percent of positive cases.

According to the CDC if the first test yields positive or equivocal (uncertain) results, then one of two options should be considered. First, if the patient has had symptoms for fewer than or equal to thirty days, then an IgM Western blot should be performed. This measures for antibodies that suggest an acute infection. Second, if the patient has had symptoms for more than thirty days, the IgG Western blot should be performed. A positive test suggests a chronic Lyme infection. The right lab, especially one that specializes in Lyme testing, can pick up 80 percent of Lyme-positive cases. The best labs will test against a variety of different proteins. Unfortunately, most mainstream labs do not test for all the relevant proteins, which is why they miss many cases.

Another blood test that can help identify infection is CD-57. CD-57 is a type of white blood cell that, if low, may indicate that the patient is fighting off chronic Lyme disease, although it may be low from other infections as well. In addition, elevation of immune inflammation markers such as C4a and C3a may suggest Lyme but are not diagnostic.

No test is 100 percent accurate for Lyme disease, but there are labs that specialize in Lyme testing. This is why you need to work with an integrative doctor knowledgeable about the diagnosis and treatment of the disease. If a patient has symptoms and exposure that are suggestive of Lyme disease but no testing confirms it, that does not mean the patient does not need treatment. In cases like this a doctor can treat the patient, preferably with the integrative therapies discussed in this chapter.

If you live in an area known to have infectious ticks (which can cause more illnesses than just Lyme disease), it is important to have a family member perform regular inspections of your skin. If a tick is found on the skin, the following recommendations from the CDC are a valid way to remove it:

- Use fine-tipped tweezers to grasp the tick as close to the skin's surface as possible.
- Pull upward with steady, even pressure. Don't twist or jerk the tick; this can cause the mouth-parts to break off and remain in the skin. If this happens, remove the mouth-parts with tweezers. If you are unable to remove the mouth easily with clean tweezers, leave it alone and let the skin heal.
- After removing the tick, thoroughly clean the bite area and your hands with rubbing alcohol, an iodine scrub, or soap and water.
- Dispose of a live tick by submersing it in alcohol, placing it in a sealed bag/container, wrapping it tightly in tape, or flushing it down the toilet. Never crush a tick with your fingers.

Note: Your local health department as well as various labs can test the tick you have found for Borrelia burgdorferi and coinfections including bartonella, babesia, Rickersia ricketsii, Ehrlichia chaffeensis (HME), and Anaplasma phagocytophila (HGE). Place the tick in a container such as a sandwich bag with a moist cotton ball.

TREATMENT

Diet

Recommended Food

Eat clean, organic foods since the immune system is already stressed. Consume vegetables, fruit, beans, nuts, seeds, and grains such as brown rice, quinoa, and buckwheat. Drink 60 to 80 ounces of water daily to support detoxification. Consume fresh vegetable juices throughout the day to support immunity and detoxification.

Consume yogurt with live cultures and other fermented foods to increase levels of your good bacteria, which help immunity.

Food to Avoid

Avoid gluten-containing foods as they tend to cause inflammation. Restrict simple sugars as they suppress immunity and feed the microbes involved with Lyme disease.

℞ Super Seven Prescriptions—Lyme Disease

Super Prescription #1 Otoba bark extract (banderol)
Start with 5 drops twice daily and work up to 30 drops twice daily or as prescribed by your holistic doctor.

Super Prescription #2 Cat's claw
Start with 5 drops twice daily and work up to 30 drops twice daily or as prescribed by your holistic doctor.

Super Prescription #3 Curcumin
Take 500 mg three times daily. This extract from turmeric has anti-inflammatory benefits.

Super Prescription #4 Glutathione
Take 250 to 500 mg twice daily on an empty stomach to support detoxification during Lyme treatment.

Super Prescription #5 Probiotic
Take at least twenty billion organisms daily to support immunity, healthy flora, and good digestion during Lyme treatment.

Super Prescription #6 Multivitamin and -mineral formula
Take as directed to provide a base of nutrients often depleted by this disease.

Super Prescription #7 Oregano oil
Take 20 drops or 300 mg of the capsule form with each meal. It has antibacterial and antifungal properties that will help you recover from Lyme disease.

General Recommendations

Olive leaf extract supports immunity and destroys pathogenic organisms. Take 300 to 500 mg three times daily.

Milk thistle supports liver and kidney detoxification. Take 300 to 500 mg three times daily.

Super-green-food blend supports detoxification and immunity. Take as directed on the label.

Vitamin C improves immunity. Take 1,000 mg three times daily.

Colloidal silver attacks the microbes associated with Lyme disease. Take as directed on the label.

Vitamin D3 supports immunity and reduces inflammation. Take 5,000 IU daily with a meal.

Astragalus supports immunity. Take 500 mg three times daily.

Ashwagandha works to improve energy levels and reduce inflammation. Take 250 mg of an extract one to two times daily.

Other Recommendations

- For those who are on antibiotic therapy it is important to prevent fungal infection, which can set in when the good gut flora are destroyed by antibiotics. Probiotics, mentioned above, used in conjunction with antifungal agents such as grapefruit-seed extract, oregano, and medications like Nystatin and Diflucan are very effective. Following a low-sugar diet is also important.

- The digestive system is often impaired from Lyme infection and from antibiotic use. Besides probiotics, nutrients that help the gut to heal include aloe, the amino acid L-glutamine, N-acetylglucosamine, digestive enzymes, and deglycyrrhizinated licorice root (DGL).

- The use of intravenous therapy takes Lyme treatment to a higher level. For those undergoing antibiotic therapy or herbal therapy who experience Herxheimer reactions (periodic exacerbation of their symptoms), the use of intravenous glutathione can work wonders to help with symptoms and detoxification. Also, intravenous formulas that contain B vitamins and minerals such as magnesium, zinc, and selenium help with the fatigue that is so common with Lyme disease and also assist in detoxification. Other intravenous treatments such as ozone and ultraviolet radiation can provide significant benefit.

- Hormonal support is very important, particularly for the stress hormones DHEA and cortisol, which greatly affect the functioning of the immune system. Work with a holistic doctor to balance these hormones.

- A treatment for chronic Lyme disease that uses antibiotics only is often disappointing. It is imperative that natural therapies also be employed to support the immune system, kill the relevant bacteria, support detoxification, and balance the many systems of the body. For optimal health to return, the best treatments are not focused solely on killing the offending microbes but also work to balance bodily systems.

Eva Sapi, Ph.D., from the Department of Biology and Environmental Sciences at the University of New Haven, published a study in 2010 looking at the effects of the herbs samento and banderol against the three known forms of *Borrelia burgdorferi*. She also looked at doxycycline, an antibiotic commonly used to treat Lyme disease. The results were quite impressive: "Here we have provided evidence that two natural antimicrobial agents (Samento and Banderol [Otoba] extracts) had significant effect on all three known forms of *B. burgdorferi* bacteria in vitro. We have also demonstrated that doxycycline, one of the primary antibiotics used in the clinic to treat Lyme disease, only had significant effect on the spirochetal form of *B. burgdorferi*." In other words, they found this herbal combination to be more effective in killing all three forms of *Borrelia* than doxycycline. Those who undergo antibiotic therapy can use these and other anti-Lyme herbs as an adjunctive therapy.

REFERENCES

Akshita, D., et al. 2010. In vitro effectiveness of samento and banderol herbal extracts on the different morphological forms of *Borrelia burgdorferi*. Townsend Letter, July.

CDC website. Accessed June 14, 2015 at http://www.cdc.gov/lyme/stats/.

CDC website. Accessed June 20, 2015 at http://www.cdc.gov/media/releases /2013/p0819-lyme-disease.html.

CDC website. Accessed June 20, 2015 at http://www.cdc.gov/lyme/removal /index.html.

Macular Degeneration

The macula is the part of the eye that allows us to see detail in the center of our vision field. When the macula breaks down or is damaged, fine work like reading, sewing, or painting becomes difficult or impossible. Small objects—stitches on fabric, for example, or type on a page—may look wavy or bent, and there may be dark spots over the item you're trying to see. This visual impairment begins at the center of the vision and, if not halted, will slowly expand toward the periphery.

In the United States, macular degeneration is the leading cause of serious visual impairment in people over fifty-five, and in those sixty-five and older, it is the second-highest cause of blindness, next only to cataracts. There are two kinds of macular degeneration: atrophic (or "dry") and neovascular ("wet"). Atrophic is by far the more common of the two and accounts for 80 to 95 percent of all cases. Although its effects usually don't show until a relatively advanced age, atrophic macular degeneration happens over a lifetime, as cellular debris gradually accumulates under the retina. With aging one has a decline in the carotenoid concentration of the retina and increased damage from ultraviolet rays. Other factors leading to macular degeneration include inflammation, prediabetes and diabetes, poor circulation, and oxidative stress.

Neovascular macular degeneration isn't actually degeneration at all. Rather, it is caused by an abnormal growth of blood vessels under the retina. If these blood vessels leak, the fluid can scar the macula and impair central, detailed vision. Unlike atrophic degeneration, this form of the disease can frequently be reversed with laser treatment, as long as it's caught early enough. It can often be prevented altogether, with the same alternative therapies used to treat atrophic degeneration.

Major conventional risk factors for macular degeneration include smoking, atherosclerosis, aging, and high blood pressure. Research in recent years has proven that diet is a critical element in the prevention of this disease. A diet that's high in cholesterol and saturated fat appears to increase susceptibility, while a diet that's rich in fruits, vegetables, and fish is protective. Carotenoids, found in fruits and particularly in vegetables, are quite protective antioxidants against macular damage from sunlight. A holistic approach also considers the role of inefficient digestion and absorption, which can contribute to mineral deficiencies that play a role in this disease. Also, toxic metals can increase free-radical damage of the macula and the eye and should be dealt with, if a problem. Finally, several nutritional supplements, especially minerals and carotenoids, have proven to be effective in the prevention and the treatment of macular degeneration.

If you experience any kind of blurred vision, do not attempt to diagnose yourself. See a physician or an eye doctor to rule out an underlying disorder; if you do have macular degeneration, your doctor should run a test to discover whether you are affected by the atrophic or neovascular form. And since both kinds of macular degeneration—as well as many other eye problems—can be detected by a doctor long before the symptoms appear, you should always have regular eye exams, especially if you're age fifty-five or older.

SYMPTOMS

- Blurring, distortion, or dark spots at the center of the vision field, especially when looking at detail

ROOT CAUSES

Anything that causes free-radical damage or poor circulation can contribute to macular degeneration, including the following:

- Aging
- High blood pressure
- Smoking
- Exposure to ultraviolet light
- A diet that's low in antioxidants, which fight free-radical damage, especially the carotenoids lutein, zeaxanthin, and astaxanthin
- A diet that's high in total fat
- Environmental toxins (particularly toxic metals)
- Arteriosclerosis (hardening of arteries) and poor circulation
- Poor digestion and detoxification
- Nutritional deficiencies, including deficiencies of the B vitamins
- Inflammation
- Ethnicity (more common in Caucasian Americans than African Americans)
- Medications such as aspirin

Testing Techniques

The following tests help assess possible reasons for macular degeneration:

Blood pressure

Hormone testing (thyroid, DHEA, cortisol, testosterone, IGF-1, estrogen, progesterone)—saliva, blood, or urine

Intestinal permeability—urine

Detoxification profile—urine

Vitamin and mineral analysis (especially zinc, carotenoids, vitamins E and C, selenium)—blood

Digestive function and microbe/parasite/candida testing—stool analysis

Blood sugar balance—blood

Toxic metals (mercury, lead, arsenic, etc.)—hair or urine

TREATMENT

Diet

Recommended Food

Food sources of carotenoids, especially lutein and zeaxanthin, are very important. These include spinach, kale, collards, turnip greens, corn, green peas, broccoli, romaine lettuce, green beans, eggs, and oranges. Consume one or more of these daily. Also make fresh juices from these foods, and add carrots.

Omega-3 fatty acids as found in salmon, sardines, and flaxseeds decrease the risk of macular degeneration. Consume fish twice weekly.

Vitamin C and bioflavonoids work together against free radicals; they also strengthen the capillaries and the tissues of the eye. Eat red, blue, and purple fruits

One study involved over thirty-six hundred people, ages fifty-five to eighty years, who were at risk for age-related macular degeneration. Those who took antioxidants plus zinc were less likely than those who took only antioxidants or only zinc to lose their vision over the six-year study. Individuals who took a placebo were the most likely to develop advanced age-related macular degeneration and vision loss.

A survey of 876 elderly individuals found that people whose intake of lutein and zeaxanthin was in the top twentieth percentile were 56 percent less likely to have age-related macular degeneration, as compared with people who had a low intake of these two carotenoids.

A double-blind trial found that supplementation with 45 mg of zinc daily for one to two years significantly slowed the rate of vision loss in people with macular degeneration.

and vegetables—berries, cherries, tomatoes, and plums—for bioflavonoids, and enjoy citrus fruits as a source of vitamin C.

Powerful antioxidants are also found in camu camu, acai, amla, goji berry, mangosteen, and pomegranate. Incorporate these foods into the diet or take them in supplement form.

Food to Avoid

Stay far away from foods that contain free radicals. Fats that are hydrogenated or partially hydrogenated are problematic. Also avoid sugar, alcohol, and charred or grilled meats.

℞ Super Seven Prescriptions—Macular Degeneration

Super Prescription #1 Lutein
Take 15 mg daily with a meal. It prevents oxidative damage of the macula.

Super Prescription #2 Zeaxanthin
Take 3 mg daily with a meal. It prevents oxidative damage of the macula.

Super Prescription #3 Fish oil
EPA and DHA found in fish oil are associated with macular protection. Take 2,000 mg of these two components combined daily.

Super Prescription #4 Zinc
Take 45 mg daily, along with 2 mg of copper. Zinc is required for proper vision and is an antioxidant, and it was shown in studies to help macular degeneration.

Super Prescription #5 Astaxanthin
This powerful antioxidant protects against damage to the macula. Take 1,000 mcg or more daily.

Super Prescription #6 Bilberry (*Vaccinium myrtillus*)
Take 240 to 600 mg a day of a standardized formula containing 25 percent anthocyanosides. This herb contains flavonoids, phytochemicals that protect the eyes against oxidative damage. It also strengthens the capillaries and the connective tissues of the eye.

Super Prescription #7 *Ginkgo biloba*
Take 120 mg twice daily of a product standardized to 24 percent flavone glycosides. Ginkgo improves circulation and has potent antioxidant effects. One study found it helpful for early-stage macular degeneration.

General Recommendations

Betaine hydrochloride mimics stomach acid for the improved absorption of nutrients, especially minerals. Take 1 to 3 capsules with each meal or as directed by a health-care professional.

Fish oil contains DHA, which is concentrated in the retina of the eye. The consumption of fish has been shown to reduce the risk of macular degeneration. Take a fish-oil product containing 1,000 mg of DHA daily.

Vitamin E complex acts as an antioxidant and has been shown to improve vision in people with age-related macular degeneration. Take 400 IU daily with a meal.

A mixed carotenoid complex contains a blend of carotenoids that protects against ultraviolet light damage. Take 25,000 IU twice daily.

Digestive enzymes improve digestion and absorption. Take a full-spectrum complex with each meal.

Grapeseed extract or Pycnogenol extract scavenges free radicals from the eye and the brain and improves circulation. Take 150 to 300 mg daily.

Taurine is an amino acid that is believed to protect the retina from ultraviolet light damage. Take 500 mg twice daily on an empty stomach.

Intravenous nutrient therapy by a holistic doctor can be very helpful for this condition. See a local doctor for this treatment.

A high-potency multivitamin provides a base of antioxidants and nutrients for eye health.

Glutathione provides antioxidant protection for the eye. Take 250 mg twice daily.

B vitamins such as B12, folate, and B6 reduce the risk of macular degeneration. Take as part of a multivitamin.

Homeopathy

Homeopathy may be helpful for macular degeneration. See a homeopathic practitioner for a constitutional remedy.

Acupressure

See pages 787–794 for information about pressure points and administering treatment. Work Large Intestine 3 and 4 (LI3 and LI4) to improve circulation to your head.

Bodywork

An allover massage will improve circulation and help deliver oxygen to all parts of the body, including the eyes.

Reflexology

See pages 804–805 for information about reflexology areas and how to work them.

Work the eye/ear area of the foot, which is located at the base of the toes.

Hydrotherapy

Alternating hot and cold cloths to the eyes will improve circulation.

Stress Reduction

General Stress-Reduction Therapies

Vision problems can be alarming and discouraging. Cope with the stress by setting aside time to relax every day.

Other Recommendations

- Smoking is a potent way to deliver free radicals to your body. If you smoke, stop. If you don't, protect yourself from secondhand smoke.
- Regular, moderate exercise will help keep blood flowing properly to the eyes.
- Protect your eyes from the sun. In bright light, wear sunglasses that filter out 98 percent of the ultraviolet spectrum.

- For advanced cases of macular degeneration, consider a nutrition-oriented doctor who uses intravenous vitamin and mineral therapy.

REFERENCES

Newsome, D. A., M. Swartz, N. C. Leone, et al. 1988. Oral zinc in macular degeneration. *Archives of Ophthalmology* 106:192–98.

Seddon, J. M., et al. 1994. Dietary carotenoids, vitamins A, C, and E, and advanced age-related macular degeneration. *Journal of the American Medical Association* 272:1413–20.

Memory Problems

Misplaced documents. Forgotten names. Missed appointments. More than two-thirds of people over sixty-five say that they have trouble recalling old details and absorbing new ones. To some people, memory problems are just part of what used to be called "senility," an unfortunate but natural part of old age. For others, periodic forgetfulness sets off alarm bells: Is this Alzheimer's? Stroke? Dementia?

Poor memory is a problem but not an inevitable part of the aging process. While it's true that nerve cells in the brain do shrink a little with advanced age and that it's harder for them to form connections with one another, most researchers now believe that memory loss is caused mainly by lifestyle factors. Most cases can be prevented or reversed with some simple changes in diet, exercise, and habits.

Many people with memory problems are actually suffering from a malnourished brain. The brain, like the rest of the body, needs to receive its supply of oxygen and nutrients from the blood if it is to function at its best. Chemicals called neurotransmitters, which enable the brain cells to communicate and create memory links, are especially dependent on good nutrition. The brain also needs high doses of nutrients to fight damage from free radicals. Of particular importance are essential fatty acids, which are required for the cell walls of brain cells. These essential fatty acids, particularly DHA, impact memory and concentration in a positive fashion. When the circulation is sluggish and blood is low in "brain food," memory disturbances may well be the result.

Other factors can contribute as well. Several medications, alone or in combination, can cause memory loss, as can underlying illnesses like depression, thyroid problems and other hormone imbalances, and chronic fatigue. Sometimes even allergic reactions to food can impair memory. Poor digestion can be at the root of memory problems, as can a hormone imbalance. In particular, elevated levels of the stress hormone cortisol can impair memory. One must also consider hypoglycemia as a possible cause of poor memory. This makes sense, considering that glucose is the primary fuel source for the brain. Systemic candidiasis frequently causes a foggy or poor memory. Also, toxic metals such as lead, mercury, and others can impair mental function and should be chelated out, if they're a problem.

If you try the suggestions here and your problems don't improve within a couple of weeks, see your doctor.

SYMPTOMS

- Difficulty recalling details

Caution: If you have trouble recalling the names of close friends and family members, or if your memory problems began after a head injury, see your doctor immediately.

ROOT CAUSES

- A poor diet, especially one that's high in fat and low in nutrients
- Free radicals
- Inactivity, both physical and mental
- Medications
- Abuse of alcohol or street drugs
- Underlying disorders, such as candidiasis, heavy-metal
- poisoning, depression, dementia, thyroid disorders, and hypoglycemia
- Nutritional deficiencies (especially of DHA, vitamin B12, folate)
- Accumulation of calcium ions in the brain

Testing Techniques

The following tests help assess possible reasons for memory problems:

Toxic-metal testing for elements toxic to brain tissue, such as aluminum, mercury, lead, arsenic, and others. The best test is a toxic-element challenge urinalysis. The patient takes a chelating agent such as DMSA or DMPS, which pulls toxic metals out of tissue storage. Urine is then collected, usually for twenty-four hours. Hair analysis can also be used as a screening test.

Oxidative stress analysis—urine or blood testing

Antioxidant testing—urine, blood, or skin scanning

Digestive function and microbe/parasite/candida testing—stool analysis

Anemia—blood test (CBC, iron, ferritin, % saturation)

Hormone analysis by saliva, urine, or blood (estrogens, progesterone, testosterone, DHEA, cortisol, melatonin, IGF-1, thyroid panel)

TREATMENT

Diet

A good diet is crucial to brain health. Proper nutrition allows for optimal memory.

Recommended Food

Eat a wholesome diet of basic, unprocessed foods. Because conventionally grown foods often contain toxins, buy organic whenever possible. If organic food is unavailable or too expensive, wash your food thoroughly before eating.

The antioxidant vitamins A, C, and E will combat damage from free radicals. Fresh fruits and vegetables are among the best sources of antioxidants, so have a couple of servings at every meal. For vitamin E, add wheat germ to salads, cereals, or juices. Nuts and seeds are other good sources of this vital nutrient.

A deficiency of the B-complex vitamins can cause memory problems. Brewer's yeast is a potent source of B vitamins, as are wheat germ, eggs, and spirulina.

To improve circulation, increase energy levels, and detoxify your body, drink a glass of clean, quality water every two waking hours.

Eat plenty of fiber to keep toxins moving through your digestive tract and to prevent them from taking up residence in your body. Whole grains, oats, and raw or lightly cooked vegetables are good sources of fiber and are also nutritionally dense.

Consume fish, such as salmon, mackerel, and other clean fish, three times weekly for their essential fatty acids.

If you're older, your digestive system may not be able to absorb nutrients as well as it used to. Fresh fruit and vegetable juices are easily absorbable and packed with the vitamins you need, so have several glasses daily.

Food to Avoid

Determine whether your memory problems are caused or aggravated by food allergies. See the Food Allergies section and try the elimination diet on page 316; you may want to focus on cutting out wheat and dairy, as allergic responses to these items are most likely to lead to memory problems. If your memory improves when a food or foods are removed from your diet and worsens when they are reintroduced, banish those products from your diet.

Avoid refined carbohydrates and sugars. Even prediabetes has been shown to decrease cognitive function. Also, alcohol destroys brain cells, causes dehydration, and clouds the mind. Stay away from it.

R_X Super Seven Prescriptions—Memory Problems

Super Prescription # 1 Citicoline
Take 250 to 500 mg. A number of studies demonstrate that this natural nutrient improves age-related memory impairment.

Super Prescription # 2 Vitamin B12
Take 50 mcg to 200 mcg by capsule, or consider using a sublingual form. Vitamin B12 deficiency contributes to poor memory and is common in seniors.

Super Prescription #3 Acetyl-L-carnitine
Take 500 mg three times daily. It improves brain-cell communication and memory.

Super Prescription #4 Phosphatidylserine
Take 300 mg daily. This naturally occurring phospholipid improves brain-cell communication and memory.

Super Prescription #5 Club moss (*Huperzia serrata*)
Take a product standardized to contain 0.2 mg of huperizine A daily. This compound has been shown to increase acetylcholine levels in the brain and to improve memory in people with Alzheimer's disease.

Super Prescription #6 Essential fatty acids
Take 1 to 2 tablespoons of flaxseed oil or 2 to 5 grams of fish oil daily. It supplies essential fatty acids for proper brain function.

Super Prescription #7 *Ginkgo biloba* (**24 percent**)
Take 120 mg two or three times daily. It improves circulation to the brain, improves memory, and has antioxidant benefits.

General Recommendations

Jellyfish extract protects brain cells by binding the excess calcium ions that accumulate in the brain. It has been shown to improve memory. Take 10 to 20 mg daily.

Turmeric reduces inflammation of the brain. Take 250 to 500 mg daily.

Ashwagandha (*Withania somniferum*) is used as a brain tonic in Ayurvedic medicine. It reduces stress-hormone levels. Take 125 to 250 mg of 0.8 percent withanolide extract daily.

Phosphatidylcholine is a nutrient that increases acetylcholine levels to improve memory. Take 1,000 to 1,500 mg daily.

Panax ginseng improves memory and balances stress-hormone levels. Take a standardized product containing 4 to 7 percent ginsenosides at 100 to 250 mg twice daily. Do not use it if you have high blood pressure.

DHEA is an important hormone for cognitive function. If your level of DHEA is low, talk with your doctor about starting at a dosage of 15 mg.

Cordyceps sinensis is used in Chinese medicine for poor memory. Take 2 to 4 capsules daily.

DMAE helps the body produce acetylcholine for memory and has antioxidant properties. Take 100 mg daily.

Gotu kola is an Ayurvedic herb that historically has been used as a brain tonic. Take 120 mg daily.

B-complex contains the B vitamins that are involved with brain function. Take 100 mg daily.

Antioxidant formula: choose a formula that contains a wide range of antioxidants, such as selenium, carotenoids, vitamin C, and others.

There are a number of published studies demonstrating that citicoline improves memory. For example, when citicoline was given to groups of elderly people they saw improvements in memory, attention, behavior, reaction time, relational life, independence, and cooperation. In a study of older adults with memory deficits but without dementia, citicoline supplements significantly improved immediate and short-term memory. This suggests beneficial effects on the underlying cognitive processes of memory retrieval and storage. Also, a review of double-blind, randomized human trials on citicoline and cognitive function found that citicoline modestly improves memory and behavioral outcomes. And lastly, three months of citicoline supplementation was found to improve verbal memory in a group of healthy older adults who were free of any medical, neurological, or psychiatric illness but who had relatively inefficient memories.

Reishi (*Ganoderma lucidum*) extract improves mental alertness. Take 800 mg twice daily.

Chlorella improves the detoxification of toxic metals that may be causing free-radical damage. Take as directed on the container.

A high-potency multivitamin/-mineral supplies most of the vitamins and the minerals involved with memory. Take as directed on the container.

Bacopa (*Bacopa manniera*) is a nutrient that has been shown to improve memory and recall. Take 300 mg daily.

Homeopathy

Pick the remedy that best matches your symptoms in this section. Take a 6x, 12x, 6C, 12C, or 30C potency twice daily for two weeks to see if there are any positive results. After you notice improvement, stop taking the remedy, unless symptoms return. Consultation with a homeopathic practitioner is advised.

Alumina can clear confusion and reduce memory impairment. Constipation is often present in people who can benefit from alumina.

Calcarea Carbonica is for a shortened attention span, confusion, childish behavior, and difficulty recalling words (not just names). The person tends to be flabby and chilly and perspires easily on the back of the head and the feet.

Kali Phosphoricum is for poor memory and mental fatigue.

Lycopodium (*Lycopodium clavatum*) is helpful if you're fearful and have trouble recalling words. You often have digestive problems, such as gas and bloating.

Sulfur will help people who have problems remembering names and who generally have better recall after resting during the day. They tend to be very warm and crave spicy foods and ice-cold drinks.

Acupressure

See pages 787–794 for information about pressure points and administering treatment.

- If you're getting older and need an all-around tune-up, set aside a few minutes each day to work Stomach 36 (St36). It benefits all the systems of the body and also helps you absorb nutrients from your food.
- If you're under stress, work Lung 1 (Lu1) to encourage deep, calming breaths.
- Work Large Intestine 4 (LI4) to encourage circulation to the brain.

Bodywork

Massage
An allover massage will stimulate blood flow to each part of the body, including the brain. Add one of the essential oils listed under Aromatherapy in this section for an even more potent effect.

Reflexology
See pages 804–805 for information about reflexology areas and how to work them. To clear out mental cobwebs and stimulate brain function, work the areas corresponding to the head and the neck. The liver point will aid in detoxification of the blood.

Hydrotherapy
Constitutional hydrotherapy is effective in promoting circulation to the brain. See pages 795–796 for directions.

Aromatherapy

A rosemary and lavender combination has been shown to improve memory.

Stress Reduction

General Stress-Reduction Therapies
Set aside time every morning to meditate. Meditation helps you weed out mental distractions so that you begin your day with focus and clarity.

Other Recommendations

- When it comes to brain function, more and more evidence shows that the old adage "Use it or lose it" is good advice. If you don't work your brain, it will grow lazy and bored. By contrast, people who continue to engage in intellectual and social activities throughout old age retain their brainpower and general health much longer than people who retire to the easy chair. Crosswords, chess, checkers, and reading are all examples of daily mind-exercising events.
- Regular, moderate exercise will keep the blood circulating to your brain. Consider taking up a sport, such as tennis or golf, that has a social component; that way, you'll stimulate your mind as well as your body.

REFERENCES

Alvarez, X. A., et al. 1997. Citicoline improves memory performance in elderly subjects. *Methods and Findings in Experimental & Clinical Pharmacology* 19(3):201–10.

Fiorvanti, M., and Yanagi, M. 2006. The Cochrane Library, Oxford, England. Issue 4.

Secades, J. J., and J. L. Lorenzo. 2006. Citicoline: pharmacological and clinical review, 2006 update. *Methods Find Exp Clin Pharmacol* 27(Suppl B):1–56.

Spiers, P. A., et al. 1996. Citicoline improves verbal memory in aging. *Arch Neurol* 53:441–48.

Menopause

A woman has officially entered menopause when she has gone twelve months without a menstrual cycle. Typically occurring around age fifty, menopause is a transitional time in a woman's life. With the baby-boom generation reaching middle age, approximately six thousand women enter menopause every day, or over two million a year.

The period of time leading up to menopause is known as perimenopause or premenopause. During this time the menstrual cycle begins to change; periods may occur closer together, they may be irregular, or they may be longer or heavier than normal. During perimenopause the ovaries do not ovulate as regularly. Ovarian production of hormones decreases, particularly of progesterone. Other hormones such as estrogen and testosterone begin to decrease as well.

Perimenopausal and menopausal women may experience a variety of symptoms. The most common is hot flashes. An estimated 75 percent of menopausal women endure hot flashes for about two years, and another 25 percent have them for five years or more. Other menopausal symptoms include depression, fatigue, vaginal dryness, heart palpitations, and mood swings. Some of these can last for years.

Women's reactions to menopause vary widely. Some enjoy the change and others suffer from severe symptoms. If a woman is healthy, active, and well nourished, her adrenal glands will usually respond to menopause by creating precursor hormones such as pregnenolone and DHEA, which are then converted into estrogen, progesterone, and testosterone. And if she takes natural steps to encourage this process, it is likely that she can avoid harsh and possibly dangerous medications altogether.

Synthetic hormones are less commonly prescribed by conventional doctors than they used to be. However, many doctors now commonly prescribe antidepressants to relieve hot flashes. These medications come with a host of potential side effects such as agitation, suicidal thoughts, nausea, diarrhea, insomnia, decreased sexual desire, and delayed orgasm or inability to have an orgasm. They have even been linked to bone loss and increased risk of breast cancer.

Occasionally, menopause results from a disorder or a serious problem. If menopause arrives due to unnatural causes, such as anorexia, bulimia, or extremely intense exercise, the root cause must be treated so that the cycle returns. When menopause is brought about by a hysterectomy or removal of the ovaries, natural hormonal-replacement therapy may be necessary to counter the sudden depletion of estrogen and progesterone and the resulting bone loss and increased heart disease risk.

We believe that every woman must be treated individually. Optimally, it is best to undergo a hormone test to find out which hormone imbalances you may have. For women with mild to moderate symptoms of menopause, we generally recommend the use of diet, exercise, and nutritional supplements, especially herbal and homeopathic remedies. The beauty of this approach is that these natural supplements balance the hormones that are already present in the body. In addition, the use of natural progesterone appears to be very safe and effective when a stronger approach is needed. Likewise, precursor hormones, such as pregnenolone and DHEA, may be helpful.

For women with extreme symptoms that are unresponsive to nutritional supplements, the use of natural hormone replacement is very effective. This is particularly true of women who had their ovaries removed at an early age or others with moderate to severe osteoporosis. Hormone therapy is, of course, best done under the care of a doctor who is knowledgeable in natural hormones.

SYMPTOMS

- Cessation of periods
- Hot flashes
- Vaginal dryness and thinning
- Night sweats
- Insomnia
- Dizziness
- Heart palpitations
- Headaches
- Memory problems and difficulty concentrating
- Cold hands and feet
- Reduced libido
- Bladder problems, including incontinence
- Mood swings
- Depression and anxiety
- Fatigue
- Joint pain
- Skin changes (acne, facial hair, scalp hair loss)

ROOT CAUSES OF EARLY MENOPAUSE

- Eating disorders
- Surgical removal of the ovaries, usually as part of a hysterectomy
- Extraordinarily intense exercise
- or physical training
- Hypofunctioning adrenal glands
- Ovarian disease

Testing Techniques

The following tests help assess hormone balance and other issues related to menopause:

Hormone testing (thyroid, DHEA, cortisol, testosterone, IGF-1, estrogen, progesterone, FSH)—saliva, blood, or urine

Complete blood count and chemistry profile—blood

Thyroid panel—blood or saliva or urine

Cardiovascular profile—blood (see Cardiovascular Disease section for more detail)

Bone resorption assessment—urine

Bone density—DEXA scan (X-ray)

TREATMENT

Diet

If you begin to incorporate these suggestions into your diet at the onset of perimenopause, you will likely experience far fewer problems when menopause begins in earnest.

Recommended Food

Increase your intake of plant foods such as legumes, vegetables, fruits, whole grains, nuts, and other seeds as they contain hormone-balancing plant chemicals known as phytoestrogens. Ground flaxseeds also contain phytoestrogens and have been shown in studies to reduce hot flashes. In one positive study women consumed 40 grams of ground flaxseed daily. Fermented soy foods such as tofu, miso, and tempeh can help reduce hot flashes.

Essential fatty acids protect the heart and promote smooth, radiant skin. Good sources are cold-water fish like salmon, cod, and tuna, as well as flaxseeds.

Vitamin E regulates estrogen production. Make sure to include cold-pressed nut and seed oils in your diet, perhaps as a dressing for a green salad.

Food to Avoid

Eat hormone-free animal products to avoid causing a hormone imbalance. Reduce your intake of spicy foods and alcohol, which may worsen hot-flash frequency and intensity.

℞ Super Seven Prescriptions—Menopause

Super Prescription #1 Black cohosh (*Cimicifuga racemosa*)
Take 80 mg one or two times daily. This herb has been shown in numerous studies to alleviate a multitude of menopausal symptoms, including hot flashes.

A study involving 131 doctors and 629 female patients revealed that black cohosh (*Cimicifuga racemosa*) alleviated several menopausal symptoms in 80 percent of women within six to eight weeks. Symptoms that were improved included hot flashes, headaches, vertigo, heart palpitations, nervousness, ringing in the ears, anxiety, insomnia, and depression. Another study of 80 women going through menopause found that black cohosh (*Cimicifuga racemosa*) had the best results in alleviating symptoms, as compared to Premarin or a placebo.

Pueraria mirifica is a member of the legume family and common in warm climates such as Thailand. It contains hormone-balancing phytoestrogens. One study found that 50 or 100 mg a day of PM for six days effectively reduced hot flashes and night sweats.

Super Prescription #2 Natural progesterone cream
Perimenopausal women should apply ¼ teaspoon (20 mg) to the skin on the inside of their wrists and forearms one or two times daily, from days fourteen to twenty-five of the menstrual cycle or as directed by their health care practitioner.

Menopausal women should apply ¼ teaspoon (20 mg) to the skin on the inside of their wrists and forearms two times daily, three to four weeks of the month or as directed by their health-care practitioner.

Postmenopausal should women apply ⅛ teaspoon (10 mg) to the skin on the inside of their wrists and forearms once daily, three weeks of the month. Natural progesterone alleviates a multitude of menopausal symptoms and may help bone density.

Super Prescription #3 Vitex (chasteberry)
Take 160 to 240 mg of a 0.6 percent aucubin extract daily. Vitex relieves hot flashes and prevents a heavy menses for perimenopausal women. Do not use it if you are taking the birth control pill.

Super Prescription #4 Maca (*Lepidium peruvianum*)
Take 500 mg twice daily of an extract. Research shows this herbal extract relieves common menopausaul symptoms such as hot flashes.

Super Prescription #5 *Pueraria mirifica*
Take 50 to 100 mg daily of an extract. It reduces hot flashes and nightsweats.

Super Prescription #6 American ginseng (*Panax quinquefolius*)
Take 600 to 1,200 mg daily. This herb supports adrenal function, improves energy, relaxes the nervous system, and has a cooling effect.

Super Prescription #7 Rehmania (*Rehmania glutinosa*)
Take 25 to 100 mg daily. This Chinese herb has a cooling effect and reduces hot flashes, night sweats, heart palpitations, and other common menopause symptoms.

General Recommendations

DHEA supports memory, libido, and mood. If your level of DHEA is low, take 5 to 15 mg as a starting dosage.

Hops (*Humulus lupulus*) reduces anxiety and tension and has mild hormone-balancing properties. Take 250 mg two or three times daily.

Pregnenolone is a precursor hormone to make estrogen and progesterone. Take 30 mg twice daily. Use DHEA and pregnenolone only under the guidance of your doctor.

Adrenal-glandular extract supports the hormone-producing adrenal glands. Take 1 or 2 capsules twice daily on an empty stomach.

For memory and concentration problems, take *Ginkgo biloba*. It increases blood flow to the brain. Take 120 to 240 mg daily of an extract standardized to 24 percent flavone glycosides.

Hormone-replacement therapy puts a great stress on the liver. If you choose to take this medication, detoxify with milk thistle (*Silybum marianum*). Find a formula that's standardized to 70 to 80 percent silymarin content, and take 250 mg twice a day.

Saint-John's-wort (*Hypericum perforatum*) has been shown to fight depression that comes on with menopause. Take 900 mg daily of a 0.3 percent hypericin extract.

If you have heart palpitations, take motherwort (*Leonurus cardiaca*) at a dosage of 200 mg or 2 ml three times daily.

Sage (*Salvia officinalis*) helps control the sweating associated with hot flashes. Take a daily dose of 4 to 6 grams.

Red clover (*Trifolium pratense*) has been shown in some studies to reduce the symptoms of menopause. Take 40 mg one or two times daily.

If you need to unwind and destress, find a quiet moment to drink a cup of tea made from chamomile, peppermint, or passionflower. Each of these herbs is relaxing and calming.

Vitamin E complex (containing tocopherols and tocotrienols) may help reduce the symptoms of menopause. Take 800 to 1,200 IU daily. Do not use this high a dosage if you're on blood-thinning medications.

For mild vaginal dryness, use a lubricant from your health food store or pharmacy. For severe vaginal dryness, have your doctor prescribe vaginal estriol cream. Insert 1 gram nightly, containing 0.5 mg, for two weeks and then as needed.

A high-potency multivitamin/-mineral provides a base of vitamins and minerals for overall health.

Take a daily total of 1,000 mg of calcium and 500 mg of magnesium, or a bone formula for bone health.

For a more powerful relaxing effect, especially if you need to sleep, drink valerian tea.

Soy protein powder (preferably fermented) up to 60 grams a day reduces hot flashes. Do not use it if you have a soy allergy.

Homeopathy

Pick the remedy that best matches your symptoms in this section. Take a 6x, 12x, 6C, 12C, or 30C potency twice daily for two weeks to see if there are any positive results. After you notice improvement, stop taking the remedy, unless symptoms return. Consultation with a homeopathic practitioner is advised.

Belladonna (*Atropa belladonna*) is a remedy for sudden hot flashes that cause a flushing of the face. Throbbing symptoms may occur in the head or other areas of the body, accompanied by heat. Heart palpitations, restlessness, and right-sided headaches are common symptoms.

Calcarea Carbonica will help menopausal symptoms such as night sweats, heavy flow, and hot flashes even though the woman is chilly. There is often a sense of anxiety, fatigue, and a feeling of being overwhelmed. Women may also experience leg cramps and crave both eggs and sweets. There is weight gain with the menopausal transition.

Lachesis will ease a variety of menopausal complaints, including hot flashes, anxiety, headaches, insomnia, memory problems, and lack of concentration. It is a specific remedy for heart palpitations that are worse from lying on the left side. The woman is often very talkative and may have strong emotions such as jealousy,

For every synthetic hormone prescription, there exists a natural version that is identical to what is found in your body. If you need hormone-replacement therapy, consult a doctor who is knowledgeable in natural hormone replacement. These hormones are available from a compounding pharmacy in your area. *Note*: Most hormones require a prescription.

A double-blind trial found that transdermal natural progesterone cream reduced hot flashes in 83 percent of women, compared with improvement in only 19 percent of those given a placebo. Transdermal natural progesterone has also been shown to prevent the buildup of the endometrium (lining of uterus) among post-menopausal women who take synthetic estrogen (Premarin).

suspiciousness, or anger. Tight clothing around the neck is avoided. The libido often increases with menopause.

Natrum Muriaticum is for women who experience backaches and migraines, along with a craving for salt and cold drinks. It is also used for hot flashes and vaginal dryness. Symptoms are worse in the sun. Depression and aversion to people may be present. The woman cries easily.

Oophorinum is a specific remedy for hot flashes in women who have had their ovaries removed.

Pulsatilla (*Pulsatilla pratensis*) is for women who feel much worse in a warm room and who strongly desire fresh air. Mood swings and weepiness are characteristic symptoms. They may have a strong craving for sweets, pastries, and chocolate.

Sepia is for menopausal women who experience pain or anxiety during intercourse, usually because of vaginal dryness. If periods still occur, there may be heavy bleeding. This remedy may help uterine prolapse and incontinence. Women who benefit from this remedy usually feel irritable and exhausted. They have a strong craving for chocolate, sweets, or sour foods and have an aversion to sex.

Sulfur is a good remedy for hot flashes and night sweats. The woman perspires easily and throws the covers off at night. She has a strong thirst for ice-cold drinks.

Acupressure

See pages 787–794 for information about pressure points and administering treatment.
- Governing Vessel 24.5 (GV24.5) regulates glands and will minimize headaches and hot flashes.
- Work Governing Vessel 20 (GV20) for improved concentration and memory, as well as for relief from headache pain.
- Conception Vessel 17 (CV17) will soothe tension and help you sleep. It also helps reduce hot flashes.
- If you suffer from anxiety that leads to heart palpitations, work Pericardium 6 (P6). You can use this point as part of a daily practice, or you can press it whenever you feel tension coming on.
- To strengthen the urinary tract, work Bladder 60 (B60).

Bodywork

Massage
Massage therapy is a terrific stress reliever. If you don't already receive regular massage treatments, this is a good time in your life to start.

If you're feeling less sexual desire than you used to, you may be suffering from touch deprivation. Keep up physical contact with your partner by learning a few simple massage techniques for the head, the shoulder, or the back.

Reflexology
See pages 804–805 for information about reflexology areas and how to work them.

If you have only a short amount of time, concentrate on the area corresponding to the uterus. You can also work the ovaries, the fallopian tubes, and all glands.

For stress relief, work the solar plexus.

The chest and lung area will strengthen your heart.

Hydrotherapy

A warm sitz bath will increase circulation to the pelvic area and will improve vaginal dryness and decreased libido.

Aromatherapy

Geranium and rose oils have a gentle balancing effect on hormone levels. They have the additional benefit of reducing stress. Add these oils to a bath or use them in a massage.

If you want to lift your spirits, you can try several oils. Bergamot, rose, and jasmine are some of the best; use them in any preparation you like.

Patchouli and ylang-ylang instill a sense of calm, while arousing sexual desire. Try a few drops in the bath or a room diffuser, or use in a massage.

Add chamomile to a lotion, and apply to dry skin for a softening, smoothing effect.

Stress Reduction

General Stress-Reduction Therapies

For some women, menopause is difficult. Any of the techniques in the Exercise and Stress Reduction chapter can help you relieve stress. The key is to pick one or two and do them regularly. Walking has been shown in studies to alleviate hot flashes.

Other Recommendations

- Remember that one year without a single period must pass before menopause can officially be declared. If a full year has not passed since your last cycle, it's possible that you could still get pregnant. Take appropriate precautions.
- Don't smoke. Smoking is linked to premature menopause, as well as to heart disease.
- Regular exercise improves general health, as well as many symptoms of menopause. Nonimpact workouts like swimming and cycling are good for your cardiovascular system, but to prevent bone loss you'll need to include weight-bearing exercise as well. Walking is one of the best allover conditioners, and weight lifting has been shown to increase bone density and vitality even for people in their nineties.
- Acupuncture can be helpful for alleviating a variety of menopausal symptoms, as can Chinese herbal therapy. See a qualified practitioner.

REFERENCES

Anasti, J. N., H. B. Leonetti, and K. J. Wilson. 2001. Topical progesterone cream has antiproliferative effect on estrogen-stimulated endometrium. *Obstetrics and Gynecology* (4 Suppl 1):S10

Chandeying, V., and S. Lamlertkittiku. 2007. Challenges in the conduct of Thai herbal scientific study: Efficacy and safety of phytoestrogen, pueraria mirifica (*Kwao Keur Kao*), phase I, in the alleviation of climacteric symptoms in perimenopausal women. *Journal of the Medical Association of Thailand* 90(7):1274–80.

Leonetti, H. B., S. Long, and J. N. Anasti. 1999. Transdermal progesterone cream for vasomotor symptoms and postmenopausal bone loss. *Obstetrics and Gynecology* 94:225–28.

Stoll, W. 1987. Phytopharmacon influences atrophic vaginal epithelium: Doubleblind study—Cimicifuga vs. estrogenic substances. *Therapeutikon* 1:2–30.

Stolze, H. 1982. An alternative to treat menopausal complaints. *Gyne* 2:4–16.

Menstrual Cramps

Any woman will tell you that it is not fun dealing with painful cramps every month. Fifty percent of menstruating women in America suffer with varying degrees of menstrual cramps.

The medical term for menstrual cramps is dysmenorrhea, derived from the Greek phrase for "difficult monthly flow." There are two classes of dysmenorrhea: primary and secondary. The primary type refers to painful menstrual cramps that are not related to a physical abnormality or pelvic disease. Secondary refers to painful menstrual cramps caused by a pelvic abnormality such as structural abnormalities or adhesions, or by other diseases such as endometriosis, ovarian disease, celiac disease, thyroid conditions, uterine polyps, or fibroids.

Primary dysmenorrhea usually starts within six months from when a woman starts her menses (known as menarche). Pelvic exams will show no structural abnormalities or infections.

Secondary dysmenorrhea usually begins later, in a woman's twenties or thirties. The woman may experience heavy menstrual flow or irregular bleeding. She finds very little pain relief from pain medications or birth-control pills. There may also be problems with infertility, painful intercourse, and vaginal discharge.

Conventional treatment of menstrual cramps focuses on two classes of drugs. The first is birth-control pills, also known as oral contraceptives. Birth-control pills work by inhibiting ovulation, which reduces the levels of pain-causing prostaglandins in the uterus, and by reducing the amount of menstrual fluid. Birth-control pills can take several months to be effective but overall have a high effectiveness rate. They contain synthetic hormones that are foreign to the human body. Side effects may include spotting between periods, nausea, breast tenderness, headaches, weight gain, mood changes, missed periods, decreased libido, vaginal discharge, visual changes, heart attack, stroke, blood clots, breast cancer, and Crohn's disease.

Similarly, Mirena, the popular long-acting birth control, is an intrauterine device (IUD) implanted in the uterus that contains the synthetic hormone levonorgestrel. It has been shown to prevent menstrual cramps. We are not fans of this device because it contains a synthetic hormone. Risks can be life threatening, including perforation of the uterus, pelvic inflammatory disease, and ectopic pregnancy. Other side effects are the same as those listed earlier for birth control pills.

The second class of drugs commonly recommended for menstrual cramps includes nonsteroidal anti-inflammatory drugs, also known as NSAIDs. Common examples include ibuprofen (Motrin, Advil) and naproxen (Aleve). These medications are available over the counter and can be very effective for acute menstrual pain. Aspirin has not been shown to be effective and should be avoided. NSAID side effects may include nausea, vomiting, diarrhea, constipation, decreased appetite, rash, dizziness, headache, drowsiness, fluid retention, shortness of breath, bleeding of the digestive tract, blood clots, liver damage, and kidney damage.

At a physiological level there can be a few different causes of primary dysmenorrhea. For example, there can be an imbalance between the hormones and the pain-inducing chemicals produced by the body known as prostaglandins. More specifically, the levels of the prostaglandin known as PgF can be up to thirteen times higher in women with dysmenorrhea than in women without dysmenorrhea. Additionally, there are often low levels of progesterone one to two weeks before menses. Progesterone acts as a relaxant for the uterus and muscles.

There are a variety of effective natural approaches that can reduce the severity of dysmenorrhea and in some cases clear it dramatically.

SYMPTOMS

- Labor-like or cramping pain of the lower abdomen
- Lower abdominal pain that radiates to the back or thigh
- Fatigue, backache, headache, nausea, vomiting, and diarrhea (these symptoms are experienced by about half of women with menstrual cramps)

ROOT CAUSES

- Smoking
- Obesity
- Heavy or prolonged menstrual flow
- Genetics
- No pregnancies
- Hormone imbalance, particularly low progesterone

Testing Techniques

The condition is diagnosed based on symptoms.

Ultrasound, MRI, or other diagnostic imaging can be used to identify structural abnormalities and diseases associated with secondary dysmenorrhea.

TREATMENT

Diet

Besides the conventional treatments outlined above, a holistic approach considers various approaches for body balancing. A healthy diet is a foundation for improving prostaglandin and hormone balance in treating menstrual cramps.

Recommended Food

A diet rich in omega-3 fatty acids works to increase anti-inflammatory and antispasmodic prostaglandins such as PgE1 and PgE3. Examples include ground flaxseeds, walnuts, wild salmon, sardines, hempseeds, and pumpkin seeds. Oils from these foods added to salads are excellent choices. A high intake of vegetables is important to promote good hormone balance.

Food to Avoid

It is generally recommended to reduce foods high in arachidonic acid such as red meat, poultry, and eggs. Arachidonic acid acts as a precursor to the prostaglandins that cause uterine spasming. Also, decrease sugar and refined-carbohydrate intake, particularly before the menses. Sugars worsen inflammation.

℞ **Super Seven Prescriptions—Menstrual cramps**

The B vitamins thiamine (B1) at 100 mg daily and niacin at 100 mg twice daily have been shown in studies to have approximately an 87 percent effectiveness rate for alleviating menstrual cramps.

Super Prescription #1 Crampbark (*Viburnum opulus*)

Take 250 to 500 mg of the capsule form or a half teaspoon of the tincture every two waking hours when one is having menstrual cramps. This herb is great for relieving acute uterine cramping.

Super Prescription # 2 Natural progesterone

Apply 20 to 40 mg of transdermal natural progesterone or take 100 mg of the oral form one to two times daily from approximately ten days before menstrual flow. Stop when menstrual flow starts. Best used under the guidance of a holistic doctor.

Super Prescription #3 Combination Homeopathic Cramp Formula

Take as directed for the acute relief of menstrual cramps.

Super Prescription #4 Pycnogenol

Take 100 mg twice daily every day of the month. Several studies have demonstrated that Pycnogenol alleviates menstrual pain. It is best used for several months in a row for a cumulative effect.

Super Prescription #5 Vitex

Take 300 to 500 mg of an extract every day of the month for at least five months. Vitex enhances ovarian production of progesterone and has other hormone-balancing qualities.

Super Prescription #6 B vitamins

Take 100 mg daily of thiamine and 100 mg twice daily of niacin, as research shows this duo is effective in reducing menstrual cramps.

Super Prescription #7 Vitamin D3

Take 5,000 IU daily with a meal, or a higher dose as directed by a holistic doctor.

A study by Italian researchers published in the *Archives of Internal Medicine* looked at a single dose of vitamin D3 of 300,000 international units given five days before the beginning of the menstrual cycle in women with a history of primary dysmenorrhea. Over the next two months they found significant reduction in pain scores compared to those who took a placebo. The authors noted that vitamin D regulates genes involved in the prostaglandin pathways and decreases inflammatory chemicals known as cytokines.

General Recommendations

Vitamin E has been used by holistic practitioners for decades to help this condition. A typical dosage is 400 IU to 1,200 IU daily.

A calcium deficiency can lead to more spasming of the uterus and increased pain. Studies have shown that calcium supplementation helps premenstrual syndrome and can help symptoms of cramping. Supplement 500 mg daily of a chelated form.

Fish oil and the omega-3 fatty acids it contains help to balance the prostaglandins that cause cramping and pain. Krill oil has also been effective. In addition, supplement GLA (gamma linoleic acid), which is often extracted from evening primrose or black currant seed oil. GLA supports progesterone production. For fish oil take 2,000 mg of EPA and DHA combined daily and 1,000 to 1,500 mg of GLA daily.

Homeopathy

Homeopathic remedies can often give a woman the quickest relief from cramping pain. Following are remedies to consider for quick, acute relief. Take two pellets of a 30C potency every thirty to sixty minutes until relief is noticed. If there is no improvement within three doses try a different remedy.

Belladonna is for throbbing pains that are worse on the right side and that come on suddenly. Flushes of heat may accompany the cramping.

Chamomilla is helpful when there is extreme cramping or pain causing anger and irritability.

Cimicifuga is a good choice when there are shooting pains that radiate down the thighs or across the pelvis.

Magnesia phosphorica is for cramping and spasmodic pain that is better from warm applications. If you do not know what homeopathic remedy to use, start with Magnesia phosphorica.

Sabina is for painful cramps accompanied by large blood clots.

Other Recommendations

- One of the most underrated ways to prevent and treat menstrual cramps is exercise. Various studies have shown that exercise reduces the intensity of menstrual cramps, and in some studies quite effectively.
- Chiropractic treatments can be helpful as they normalize nerve and blood flow to the pelvis. In addition, acupuncture can be used for pain control and for hormone balancing.
- You should be aware that smoking is a risk for dysmenorrhea and should be discontinued.
- Some women find that hot water bottles or warm towels applied over the lower abdomen provide quick relief. Another option is to alternate a warm towel (three minutes) and cold towel (three minutes) several times over the lower abdomen to provide relief of cramping pain.

REFERENCES

Gokhale, L. B. 1996. Curative treatment of primary spasmodic dysmenorrhea. *Indian J Med Res* 103:227–31.

Hudgins, A. 1952. Niacin for dysmenorrhea. *Am Pract Digest Treat* 3:892–93.

Lasco A., et al. 2012. Improvement of primary dysmenorrhea caused by a single oral dose of vitamin D: Results of a randomized, double-blind, placebo-controlled study. *Arch Intern Med* 172(4):366–367. doi: 10.1001/archinternmed.2011.715

Mercury Toxicity

Mercury toxicity is one of the least recognized health concerns in America and around the world. Elevated levels of this toxin are linked to heart disease, diabetes, autoimmunity, impaired cognitive function, chronic fatigue syndrome, immune-system dysfunction, hormone imbalance, and even attention-deficit/hyperactivity disorder. In short, mercury disrupts the function of all the cells in the body. Unfortunately, the average physician and dentist don't have a clue about the devastating damage this poison can cause in the human body.

Mercury has no known role in human metabolism and can be difficult for the body to get rid of. The metal has an affinity for sulfur-containing groups in cells known as sulfhydryl groups, as well as for a number of amino acids and enzymes. This means it adversely affects nutrients such as N-acetylcysteine, alpha lipoic acid, and glutathione. These nutrients are important antioxidants that can aid with mercury detoxification, further complicating the situation.

Mercury also targets the energy-producing warehouses of the cells known as the mitochondria. This damage can lead to a variety of health problems, ranging from neurological issues to fatigue. Since mercury affects every cell, it affects the entire body. Several studies have linked mercury toxicity to high blood pressure, coronary heart disease, heart attacks, kidney dysfunction, and an overall increase in total mortality.

The fact is, there's a mountain of evidence showing that mercury is a dangerous toxin that can harm both the human body and the environment. Even the World Health Organization acknowledges this. For years they've published guidelines for acceptable mercury levels. Their publication "Exposure to Mercury: A Major Public Health Concern" says it all in its title and clarifies the risk in the first sentence: "Mercury is highly toxic to human health."

Mercury occurs naturally in the environment in several different forms. Human beings can neither create it nor destroy it. It's found in the earth's crust and in rocks, including coal. According to the Environmental Protection Agency, "Coal-burning power plants are the largest human-caused source of mercury emissions to the air in the United States." It's also released into the atmosphere as a by-product of gold and mercury mining, and in the manufacturing of cement, pesticides, chlorine, mirrors, medical equipment, and through dentistry (amalgam fillings), industrial leaks, and corpse and waste incineration.

The most common forms of mercury are elemental mercury, methyl mercury, and inorganic mercury compounds. The elemental form is commonly used in medical equipment, such as thermometers, blood pressure cuffs, barometers, and some types of light bulbs. However, if the elemental mercury isn't enclosed in a container, it will give off vapor. High levels of this vapor breathed in over a short period of time can be fatal. The two other forms are what we're most commonly affected by.

Elemental mercury is not safe when it's released into the environment as a by-product of coal-burning power plants. In fact, it's a major source of human exposure to the toxic metal. According to the WHO, "It can stay for up to a year in the atmosphere, where it can be transported and deposited globally. It ultimately settles in the sediment of lakes, rivers or bays where it is transformed into methyl mercury, absorbed by phytoplankton, ingested by zooplankton and fish, and accumulates especially in long-lived predatory species, such as shark and swordfish." And, of course, fish that eat the toxic methyl mercury pass that mercury on to humans when we eat the fish, which explains why fish are ultimately the biggest source of mercury toxicity in the human body. The more methyl mercury a fish feeds on and the longer it lives determine how much mercury it passes on to us.

A recent study found that between 43 percent and 100 percent of the fish from nine countries (including the United States) contained mercury at levels so high that eating them more than once per month would be unsafe. The biggest risk is to children, especially those who are still developing in the womb and being exposed to mercury when the mother consumes unsafe fish (mercury passes through the placenta into the bloodstream of the fetus).

Dental amalgams (silver fillings), which contain approximately 50 percent mercury, are a source of exposure to the troublesome inorganic mercury. A study in the *Journal of Dental Research* analyzed mercury-vapor concentration in forty-six people, thirty-five of whom had amalgam fillings. Researchers found that participants with amalgam fillings produced mercury vapors that were nine times greater than baseline levels in participants with no amalgams. Chewing increased their mercury concentration sixfold compared to nonchewing mercury levels and by fifty-four-fold over people without amalgam fillings. To make matters worse, some of the mercury from fillings that enters the digestive tract is transformed into methyl mercury, the type of mercury commonly found in fish.

Mercury salts are another form of inorganic mercury compound. They have long been used in folk medicine and in herbal formulas developed by practitioners of traditional Chinese medicine and Ayurvedic medicine. It would be rare for Chinese or Ayurvedic medicine herbalists in the United States to use formulas that contain this very toxic form of mercury. However, herbal supplements and teas imported from China and India have been found to contain mercury and other contaminants. Therefore, we recommend using only herbal products that are harvested and manufactured in the United States, or at least independently tested for toxic metals and other contaminants.

SYMPTOMS

- Mood swings, nervousness, irritability, and other emotional changes
- Insomnia
- Headache
- Abnormal sensations (such as numbness or tingling)
- Muscle twitching
- Tremors
- Weakness
- Muscle atrophy
- Decreased cognitive function
- Peripheral vision impairment
- Stinging or needle-like sensations in the extremities and mouth
- Loss of coordination
- Muscle weakness
- Impairments of speech and hearing
- Diabetes
- Autoimmune conditions
- Decreased white blood cell activity
- Shortness of breath
- Low testosterone level
- Dizziness
- Neuropathy

Researchers from the Indiana University School of Public Health found that adults who were exposed to higher mercury levels when they were younger had a whopping 65 percent increased risk of developing type 2 diabetes later in life. The study tracked 3,875 American men and women between the ages of twenty and thirty-two for eighteen years. Even after controlling for dietary and lifestyle factors such as omega-3 fatty acids and magnesium—both of which can help with blood sugar metabolism and can help reduce the toxic effects of mercury—researchers found that the jump in risk remained.

- Increased salivation
- Abdominal pain
- Joint pain

- Hearing loss
- Skin rashes, itching
- Kidney function

ROOT CAUSES

The two main sources include:

- Amalgam fillings

- Fish consumption

Other less common sources may include:

Of elemental mercury:

- Thermometers
- Barometers
- Batteries
- Bronzing
- Calibration instruments
- Chloralkali production
- Dental amalgams
- Electroplating
- Ethnomedical practices
- Fingerprinting products
- Fluorescent and mercury lamps/

bulbs
- Infrared detectors
- Jewelry industry
- Manometers
- Neon lamps
- Paints
- Paper pulp production
- Photography
- Silver and gold production
- Semiconductor cells

Of organic mercury:

- Antiseptics
- Bactericidals
- Embalming agents
- Farming chemicals
- Fungicides
- Germicidal agents
- Insecticidal products
- Laundry products

- Diaper products
- Paper manufacturing
- Pathology products
- Histology products
- Seed preservation
- Wood preservatives
- Exposure to chemicals used in the paper and pulp industries

Of inorganic mercury:

- Antisyphilitic agents
- Acetaldehyde production
- Chemical laboratory work
- Cosmetics
- Disinfectants
- Explosives
- Embalming
- Fur hat processing
- Ink manufacturing
- Mercury vapor lamps
- Mirror silvering

- Perfume industry
- Photography
- Spermicidal jellies
- Tattooing inks
- Taxidermy production
- Vinyl chloride production
- Wood preservation
- Exposure to the manufacturing of mirrors, thermometers, fluorescent lights, radiography machines, and gold mining

---

Testing Techniques

Mercury—urine, hair, blood

TREATMENT

Diet

Recommended Food

Fresh vegetable juicing with a variety of greens, carrots, cilantro, and beets is recommended on a daily basis to aid in detoxification of mercury. A high-fiber diet rich in fruits and vegetables is important to bind gut mercury. Additional fiber from chia, psyllium, or ground flaxseeds is also recommended to aid detoxification. Adequate water intake of 60 to 80 ounces daily is important to support mercury detoxification.

Food to Avoid

Make sure to avoid all fish known to be laden with mercury. This list includes:

- Mackerel (king)
- Marlin
- Orange roughy
- Shark
- Swordfish
- Tilefish
- Tuna
- Bluefish
- Grouper
- Mackerel
- Sea bass
- Carp
- Cod (Alaskan)
- Croaker (white Pacific)
- Halibut
- Jacksmelt
- Lobster
- Mahimahi
- Monkfish
- Perch
- Sablefish
- Skate
- Snapper
- Weakfish

℞ Super Seven Prescriptions—Mercury Toxicity

Super Prescription #1 Glutathione
Take 250 to 500 mg twice daily. This super antioxidant pulls mercury out of the cells and supports liver and kidney detoxification.

Super Prescription #2 Selenium
Take 200 mcg daily. This mineral increases mercury excretion and prevents its absorption.

Super Prescription #3 Chlorella
Take 3,000 g daily to bind mercury in the digestive tract and promote its elimination.

Super Prescription #4 Modified citrus pectin
This special type of fiber has been shown to bind and help excrete several metals, including mercury.

Glutathione is a valuable antioxidant that supports the body's ability to metabolize mercury. It works on a cellular level. There are several ways to increase glutathione levels, including oral, transdermal, and intravenous supplementation.

Super Prescription #5 Alpha lipoic acid
Take 300 mg twice daily to support mercury detoxification.

Super Prescription #6 N-acetylcysteine
Take 500 mg twice daily on an empty stomach to support mercury detoxification.

Super Prescription #7 Vitamin C
Take 1,000 mg two to three times daily to support liver and kidney detoxification.

General Recommendations

Probiotics are the good bacteria in the digestive tract that also help to metabolize mercury. They are an important part of the detoxification activity in the gut. Take twenty billion organisms or more of a quality probiotic daily.

Multivitamin and mineral formulas provide a base of nutrients that aid your organs and cells in eliminating mercury. Take as directed.

Other Recommendations

- Intravenous chelation therapy is available from holistic doctors. Consult with a local practitioner.
- Sauna therapy of various types works to mobilize toxic metals like mercury from fat tissue so it can be more readily eliminated. The body uses sweating as a means of elimination through the skin.

REFERENCES

BioDiversity Research Institute website. Global Mercury Hotspots. Accessed online April 14, 2013, at http://www.briloon.org/uploads/documents/hgcenter/gmh/gmhSummary.pdf.

CBS Evening News Website. Accessed online April 14, 2013, at http://www.cbsnews.com/8301-18563_162-57563739/study-finds-unsafe-mercury-levels-in-84-percent-of-all-fish/.

Emedicine health website. Mercury poisoning. Accessed online April 14, 2013, at http://www.emedicinehealth.com/mercury_poisoning/page3_em.htm.

EPA website. Mercury. Accessed April 14, 2013, online at http://www.epa.gov/hg/about.htm.

He, K., et al. 2013. Mercury exposure in young adulthood and incidence of diabetes later in life: The CARDIA trace element study. *Diabetes Care* 36(6):1584–9.

Natural Resources Defense Council website. Mercury Contamination in Fish. Accessed June 28, 2015, at http://www.nrdc.org/health/effects/mercury/guide.asp.

Olson, David. Mercury Toxicity. Medscape website. Accessed June 28, 2015, at http://emedicine.medscape.com/article/1175560-overview#a4.

Preventing Disease through Heal Thy Environment Exposures to Mercury: A Major Public Health Concern. World Health Organization. Accessed April 24, 2013, online at http://www.who.int/ipcs/features/mercury.pdf.

The Proceedings from the 13th International Symposium of The Institute of Functional Medicine. Managing Biotransformation: The Metabolic, Genomic, and Detoxification Balance Points. Alternative Therapies website. Accessed online April 20, 2013, at http://www.alternative-therapies.com/at/web_pdfs/ifm_proceedings_low.pdf.

Vimy, M. J., F. L. Lorsheider. 1985. Intra-oral air mercury released from dental amalgams. *J Dent Res* 64(8):1069–71.

Motion Sickness

Repeated acceleration and deceleration in stop-and-go traffic inside a car; heavy waves slapping against a boat during a sail; the spinning, climbing, and diving of a roller coaster ride: whether a person is traveling by car, boat, or airplane or participating in an amusement-park ride, motion sickness can occur.

Motion sickness happens when the brain receives conflicting messages from the inner ears and the eyes. The inner ears are responsible for controlling the body's balance and equilibrium. The eyes are responsible for conveying back to the brain what is being seen. Abrupt, irregular body movements and postures inside moving objects can set off this conflict between the inner ears and the eyes. This inner battle can cause a person to become pale, dizzy, nauseous, and clammy. He or she may complain of a headache or a feeling of uneasiness and may even vomit.

SYMPTOMS

- Queasiness
- Rapid breathing
- Nausea
- Fatigue

- Cold sweats
- Vomiting
- Dizziness
- Loss of coordination

ROOT CAUSES

- Disturbance of inner ear
- Overeating
- Conflicting messages sent to the brain from the eyes and the inner ears

- Eating heavy foods before or during travel
- Dehydration
- Anxiety and stress
- Poor ventilation

Testing Techniques

The following tests help assess possible reasons for motion sickness:

Inner-ear or vision testing by your doctor

Food and environmental allergies/sensitivities—blood, electrodermal

---

TREATMENT

Diet

Recommended Food

Consume live foods that are easy to digest. Fresh vegetable juices may be helpful for some people. Consume dry crackers to help an upset stomach.

Food to Avoid

Avoid greasy and fried foods before traveling because they are more likely to upset the stomach. Some people feel less motion sickness on an empty stomach, whereas others do better on a full stomach.

℞ **Super Seven Prescriptions—Motion Sickness**

Super Prescription #1 Homeopathic Cocculus

Take 2 pellets of a 30C potency every fifteen minutes for up to three times to see if the motion sickness dissipates. If there is no improvement, try another therapy.

Super Prescription #2 Ginger root (*Zingiber officinale*)

Take 500 mg in capsule or tablet form before traveling and again every two hours while traveling. Another alternative is the tea form.

Super Prescription #3 Chamomile (*Matricaria recutita*)

Take 300 mg in capsule form or drink 1 cup of tea to calm an upset stomach from motion sickness.

Super Prescription #4 Peppermint (*Mentha piperita*)

Take 300 mg in capsule form or drink 1 cup of tea to calm an upset stomach from motion sickness.

Super Prescription #5 Black horehound

Take 1 ml before traveling and every three hours. This herbal extract is recommended by herbalists for this condition.

Super Prescription #6 Fennel (*Foeniculum vulgare*)

Take 300 mg in capsule form or drink 1 cup of tea to calm an upset stomach from motion sickness.

Super Prescription #7 Chinese herbal formula

Take as directed on the label for motion sickness.

One study found that those who took 940 mg of ginger in capsule form experienced less motion sickness than those who took the common motion-sickness medication dimenhydrinate (Dramamine).

Homeopathy

Pick the remedy that best matches your symptoms in this section. Take a 6x, 12x, 6C, 12C, or 30C potency every fifteen minutes up to three times to see if there is any improvement. If you notice improvement, stop taking the remedy unless your symptoms return. Consultation with a homeopathic practitioner is advised.

Borax is for those who experience vertigo from tilting the head downward.

Nux Vomica is for vertigo accompanied by great nausea and vomiting. The patient is irritable and feels better lying down.

Petroleum is for motion sickness accompanied by heartburn that is relieved by eating.

Sepia is for motion sickness from reading while traveling.

Tabacum is for vertigo characterized by nausea and a cold clammy feeling. This remedy is commonly used for seasickness.

Acupressure

Pericardium 6 (P6) relieves nausea. A special wristband (Seabands) can be used to prevent nausea. The band, available from a pharmacy or an acupuncturist's office, gently pushes on the acupressure point Pericardium 6 (P6).

Other Recommendations

- Acupuncture has been shown to be effective in the treatment of motion sickness. See a qualified practitioner.
- If you are in a car, open the windows. Fresh air is helpful for some.
- If you are in a car, look out the window at a fixed point, such as a distant sign or hill. Looking out the window instead of at books or toys may prevent motion sickness.

REFERENCE

Mowrey, D. B., et al. 1982. Motion sickness, ginger, and psychophysics. *Lancet* 1:655–57.

MRSA

One infection that has been in the news headlines in recent years is methicillin-resistant *Staphylococcus aureus* (MRSA), pronounced "mersa." This infection is caused by a strain of staphylococcus bacteria that has developed resistance to antibiotics frequently used to treat staph infections.

There are two main types of MRSA infections. The first occurs in hospitals, nursing homes, and other heath-care facilities. The second type occurs in the community among healthy people, such as wrestlers or child-care workers or in gyms and sports facilities. It is transmitted by skin-to-skin contact or contact via shared athletic equipment.

MRSA can be very serious and even fatal if it spreads through the bloodstream and into the body. It requires immediate medical attention. The holistic therapies described in this chapter work well early in the disease or combined with conventional therapy. Certain antibiotics are still effective against MRSA.

Rinse nostrils with tea tree oil wash and wash the body with a tea tree oil soap. Other important hygienic steps to prevent MRSA include washing hands throughout the day; covering wounds with sterile bandages; not sharing personal items such as clothing, towels, razors, and equipment; showering after exercise; and cleaning linens regularly.

SYMPTOMS

- Small red bumps that often look like pimples, spider bites, insect bites, or boils that can turn into pus-filled abscesses

ROOT CAUSES

- Weak immunity
- Poor hygiene

Testing Techniques

The following tests help assess the causes of MRSA:

Culture of infected tissue or nasal swab for the presence of the staphylococcus bacteria

Testing for weak immunity—blood

TREATMENT

Diet

Recommended Food

Increase your intake of fluids such as water, herbal teas (especially ginger, cinnamon, and peppermint), soups, and broths. Drink 80 ounces of clean, quality water daily. Chicken soup and miso are often soothing. Warm water mixed with honey and lemon can relieve pain as well as the coughing that may be present with a sore throat.

A two- to three-day juice fast can improve immunity.

Food to Avoid

Dehydrating substances such as alcohol and caffeine should be avoided. Restrict sugar products, which suppress the immune system. Fruit juices should be highly diluted because of their sugar content. Avoid dairy products, which tend to increase mucus production.

℞ **Super Seven Prescriptions—MRSA**

Super Prescription #1 Colloidal silver
Apply topically as a spray or a gel and take internally as directed on the label.

Super Prescription # Tea tree oil
Apply to the affected area three times daily. This powerful antibacterial essential oil, derived from a tree native to Australia, is effective against all types of *Staphylococcus aureus* bacteria, including MRSA.

Super Prescription #3 Garlic oil
Apply to the affected area three times daily. Long known for its antibacterial effects, garlic has dozens of infection-fighting compounds and has been found to be effective against MRSA. It is also available in spray form.

Super Prescription #4 Oregano oil
Apply topically and take internally as directed on the label. Small amounts have been shown to kill MRSA.

Super Prescription #5 Vitamin C
Take 1,000 mg five to six times daily for immune support.

In a randomized study published in the *Journal of Hospital Infection*, treatment with an ointment containing 10 percent tea tree oil successfully cleared 41 percent of MRSA infections.

In a Taiwanese study published in the journal *Colloids and Surfaces B: Bio-Interfaces*, colloidal silver was found to kill the potentially deadly superbug methicillin-resistant *Staphylococcus aureus* (MRSA) and *Pseudomonas aeruginosa*, another dangerous super-bug, on surfaces such as doorknobs and light switches, where they are known to colonize and spread among people.

> **Super Prescription #6 Essential oil combo**
> Take a combo essential oil product with components such as myrhh and frankincense. Use as directed.
>
> ---
>
> **Super Prescription #7 Probiotic**
> Take twenty billion colony-forming units daily for immune-system support.

General Recommendations

Intravenous vitamin C can help bolster immunity This is available from a holistic doctor.

Various essential oils besides tea tree oil can be helpful. Work with a holistic doctor to see what works for you.

Homeopathy

Pick the remedy that best matches your symptoms in this section. Take 2 pellets of a 30C potency four times daily for three days. If you notice any improvement, stop taking the remedy unless the symptoms return. If your symptoms do not improve within twenty-four hours, try another remedy.

Apis is recommended when there is stinging or burning pain.

Graphite is indicated for a honey-colored discharge from the infection.

Hepar Sulphuris is often used when there is sharp sticking pain and the lesion feels better with cold applications.

Silica is helpful when there is pus formation that should discharge or that continuously discharges.

Acupressure

Points Kidney 27 (K27), Bladder 23 (B23), and Bladder 47 (B47) enhance the immune response to MRSA.

Bodywork

Acupuncture can be used to enhance the immune response to MRSA.

Reflexology
Massage the lymph areas.

Aromatherapy

Other essential oils that are effective against MRSA include lemongrass, lemon, cinnamon, and white thyme. Use under the direction of a holistic health care provider.

Other Recommendations

- Intravenous vitamin C by a holistic doctor can fight MRSA infection.
- Echinacea (*Echinacea purpurea*) and goldenseal (*Hydrastis canadensis*) enhance immune function and have antibacterial properties. Take a 500 mg capsule or 2 to 4 ml of a tincture four times daily.

- Vitamin A improves immune function. Take 25,000 to 50,000 IU daily for five days. Do not use if pregnant or nursing.
- Thyme extract optimizes immunity. Take 1 or 2 capsules twice daily or as directed on the container.

REFERENCES

Dryden, M. S., et al. 2004. A randomized, controlled trial of tea tree topical preparations versus a standard topical regimen for the clearance of MRSA colonization. *Journal of Hospital Infection* 56:283–86.

Ehre-Dror, A., et al. 2009. Silver nanoparticle-E. coli colloidal interaction in water and effect on E. coli survival. *Journal of Colloid and Interface Science* 339:521–26.

MTHFR Mutation

One of the exciting fields of medicine is known as nutritional genomics, also referred to as nutrigenomics. This is the study of how foods and nutrient affects our genes. It is amazing to contemplate the fact that each of the seventy trillion cells that make up your body contains twenty thousand genes. They're like the "software" of the body—they control how the body works the way software controls a computer. However, our genes are not perfect, and we all inherit some gene mutations or variations from the norm. Often mutations are not problematic, but some can be very serious.

One gene in particular (and two of its variations) plays an essential role in cellular health. Mutations in the methylenetetrahydrofolate reductase gene (abbreviated MTHFR) can increase your risk for several health problems that can range from heart disease, stroke, cancer, birth defects, hormone imbalances, chronic fatigue, fibromyalgia, and even mood disorders.

MTHFR gene controls the MTHFR enzyme, which initiates essential chemical reactions in your body. One of these essential chemical reactions is called methylation. Methylation uses a single carbon and three hydrogens (methyl group) in cellular processes such as energy production, forming immune cells, regulating genes, processing chemicals from your body and the environment, forming and metabolizing brain chemicals (neurotransmitters), metabolizing hormones, nerve formation, cell replication and repair, and many others.

One can have different variations or mutations of the MTHFR gene. If you have the normal version of the gene, typically referred to as MTHFR 677CC, things function pretty smoothly, as long as you have all the nutrients on board that methylation depends on. But if you happen to have one of two common variations of the gene—MTHFR C677T (CT) or MTHFR A1298C—the activity of the enzyme is reduced and you have a much higher risk of developing certain diseases. It's a little like putting poor-quality gasoline in a high-performance car. It will run, just not very well.

MTHFR gene mutations are inherited from your parents. If you have just one mutated copy of the gene from one of your parents, you are heterozygous for that gene. If you have two mutated copies of the gene, one from *each* parent, you are homozygous for the gene. Functioning of the gene is more affected if you have inherited two mutated MTHFR genes. Research has also shown that the MTHFR *enzyme* can be greatly affected as well, depending on which mutations you inherit.

Overall it's been estimated that 45 percent of the population has one copy of the CT gene mutation. And your ethnicity may play a role. Researchers tested more than seven thousand newborn babies from sixteen regions around the world and found:

Half of Italians from Sicily and Campania (a region that includes Naples and Salerno) had the CT variation.

Half of Mexican babies had the CT version.

Around half of the babies from southern China, Hungary, and the Strasbourg area of France had the CT variation.

Half of the Caucasian babies in the Atlanta area had the normal CC variation.

MTHFR mutations make a person predisposed to B-vitamin deficiencies, and that's a problem because efficient methylation depends on the B-complex vitamins. They help make a host of important substances, including some essential proteins, fats, and brain chemicals. The B vitamin most affected by MTHFR mutations is folate. In fact, folate is so critical to the methylation process and to the proper functioning of the MTHFR gene that drives methylation that the word *folate* can be found within the full name of the gene: methylenetetrahydrofolate reductase.

If you're born with either of the variations of the MTHFR gene you're much more likely to be deficient in folate, even if you eat a healthy diet. And although it's possible that your blood may be lower in folate, the bigger problem is that your *intracellular* level will be low. You see, folate has to go through several steps to be converted into the active form that your cells can use. This means that having a high blood folate level could actually be a sign you have a MTHFR problem. Because the gene variations lead to lower activity of the MTHFR enzyme, people with the mutation usually do need extra folate. And it is certainly possible that such individuals are not getting enough in their diet or are not taking a quality folate supplement.

It is important to understand the terms *folate* and *folic acid*, as they are different substances. Folic acid is a *synthetic* form of folate that isn't found in nature. This fake folate is commonly added to foods and used in bargain dietary supplements. It isn't the best type to use. The problem is that folic acid must go through several additional steps in your body before it's ready to be converted into a usable form; it can actually keep your cells from using folate effectively. People with the MTHFR mutation will have problems metabolizing folic acid into a usable form.

Folate, on the other hand, is immediately ready to be converted into the active form that your cells can use. Many leading supplement makers have replaced folic acid with the methylfolate form of folate, so finding a supplement should be easy. And leafy green vegetables are a good food source of natural folate.

SYMPTOMS

- Hypertension
- Delayed speech
- Muscle pain

- Insomnia
- Irritable bowel syndrome
- Fibromyalgia

- Chronic fatigue syndrome
- Hand tremor
- Memory loss
- Headaches
- Brain fog

CONDITIONS RELATED TO MTHFR MUTATION

Cardiovascular diseases: Homocysteine is an amino acid found in blood plasma. Normally, homocysteine is created in one of the many biochemical steps that occur during methylation, but when you have a CT mutation and the MTHFR enzyme isn't working up to par your homocysteine levels start climbing. We get concerned whenever a patient has a homocysteine level above 10 μmol/L. Elevated homocysteine levels are a risk factor for cardiovascular diseases such as heart disease and stroke. That's because homocysteine can damage blood vessel walls.

The link between homocysteine and heart-related conditions is strongest for peripheral artery disease (PAD) and stroke. PAD leads to poor blood flow to the legs, producing pain and resulting in thousands of leg amputations each year. The evidence supporting a link between the TT mutation and PAD is very strong.

Research has also found a solid connection between MTHFR mutations, elevated homocysteine, and stroke risk. In one study researchers examined ninety-one newborns whose mothers had the TT gene variation. They found that 20 percent of the babies had abnormalities in their brain structure, putting them at a higher risk for perinatal strokes.

Alzheimer's and Parkinson's disease: Although the research hasn't always been consistent, there's compelling evidence linking one MTHFR gene variation to both Alzheimer's and Parkinson disease. Research on pesticides, for example, has found that they lower your folate levels and can trigger Alzheimer's or Parkinson's. But if you inherited this variation and aren't taking supplements, you may already be dealing with a similar folate deficiency.

Cancer: Folate assists with several biochemical processes, including the replication of new DNA (our genetic code) and the repair of damaged DNA. Variations of MTHFR have been linked to many different types of cancer, including breast and colorectal cancers and some types of leukemia.

In addition, people with mutations react poorly when they're given the drug methotrexate for cancer or rheumatoid arthritis. We recommend that anyone who might receive this drug first be tested for the type of MTHFR gene they have.

Birth defects: The original link between folate deficiency and neural-tube defects (which include spina bifida, anencephaly, encephalocele) dates back to 1991. These birth defects are typically severe and affect the central nervous system of the growing fetus. Folate deficiency was eventually also recognized as a risk factor for cleft lip and cleft palate. Later research revealed that elevated homocysteine levels were associated with several birth defects.

Many countries, including the United States, now fortify bread with folic acid. As a result, the incidence of neural-tube defects has dropped. But results would likely be even better if the methylfolate form of the vitamin were used.

Chronic fatigue syndrome (CFS) and fibromyalgia: Dr. Paul Anderson, a naturopathic doctor and researcher with an expertise in MTFHR therapy, conducted an interesting study in patients diagnosed with CFS and fibromyalgia. When the patients' MTFHR status was tested all of them were found to have some degree of abnormality. In addition, participants who received a naturopathic therapy of intravenous B-complex vitamins (including the active form of folate—methylfolate) had a 55 to 75 percent increase in positive outcomes.

Hormone balance: Folate is involved in the metabolism of several hormones, including thyroid and estrogen. Your MTHFR status can affect the balance of these—and other—hormones. For example, methylation problems are a known risk factor for the buildup of toxic estrogens that increase the risk of breast cancer and possibly prostate cancer. If you improve methylation you can lower the levels of these toxic estrogens.

Mood disorders: Since 1943 doctors have known that not getting enough B vitamins can lead to mood disorders such as depression and anxiety. Folate, vitamin B6, vitamin B12, L-tryptophan, L-methionine, and S-adenosylmethionine (SAMe) all play essential roles in methylation reactions. Research has found a relationship between MTHFR defects and the risk of depression, bipolar disorder, and schizophrenia. One study found that men with one variation had double the risk of bipolar disorder or schizophrenia, compared to men who had a normal version of the MTHFR gene.

Testing Techniques

MTHFR gene mutations—blood or saliva

Medications That Disrupt MTHFR

- Acid-reflux medications
- Antimalarials
- Bactrim
- Carbamazepine
- Cholestyramine
- Colestipol
- Cyclosporin A
- Ethanol
- Metformin
- Methotrexate
- Niacin (high dose)
- Nitrous Oxide
- Oral contraceptives
- Phenytoin
- Sulfasalazine
- Theophylline
- Triamterene
- Trimethoprim

TREATMENT

Diet

Recommended Food
Consume a diet plentiful in folate-rich foods, including lentils, garbanzo beans, pinto beans, spinach, asparagus, black beans, kidney beans, turnip greens, brussels sprouts, romaine lettuce, and broccoli.

Food to Avoid
Avoid or limit foods enriched with folic acid, including commercial wheat flour and cereals.

℞ Super Seven Prescriptions—MTHFR Mutation

Super Prescription #1 Methylfolate
  Take 400 mcg daily or more as your holistic doctor prescribes.

Super Prescription #2 Vitamin B12 (methylcobalamin)
  Take 500 mcg daily or more as your holistic doctor prescribes. B12 (methylcobalamin form) works synergistically with methylfolate.

Super Prescription #3 B-complex

Take a B-complex with methylfolate and methylcobalamin and the other B vitamins for B-vitamin balance and detoxification-pathway support.

Super Prescription #4 Glutathione

People with MTHFR mutations are more likely to be low in the super antioxidant glutathione. Take 250 mg twice daily on an empty stomach.

Super Prescription #5 Multivitamin

Take as directed on the label for a full spectrum of nutrients involved in cellular pathways.

Super Prescription #6 Digestive enzymes

Take as directed on the label with meals to support digestion and absorption for optimal cellular nutrition.

Super Prescription #7 Super-green-food blend

Take as directed on the label to provide a blend of super green foods such as chlorella, wheat grass, barley grass, spirulina, and others that support cellular function.

REFERENCES

Anderson, P. S. 2012. Active comparator trial of addition of MTHFR specific support versus standard integrative naturopathic therapy for treating patients with diagnosed Fibromyalgia (FMS) and Chronic Fatigue Syndrome (CFS). Poster Presentation, presented at the California Association of Naturopathic Doctors Webinar, February 2014.

Coppedè, F., P. Tannorella, I. Pezzini, et al. 2012. Folate, homocysteine, vitamin B12, and polymorphisms of genes participating in one-carbon metabolism in late-onset Alzheimer's disease patients and healthy controls. *Antioxid Redox Signal* 17(2):195–204.

Czeizel, A. E., and I. Dudas. 1992. Prevention of the first occurrence of neural-tube defects by periconceptional vitamin supplementation. *New England Journal of Medicine* 327:1832–35.

Czeizel, A. E. 1995. Folic acid in the prevention of neural tube defects. *Journal of Pediatric Gastroenterology and Nutrition* 20:4–16.

Elhawary, N. A., D. Hewedi, A. Arab, et al. 2013. The MTHFR 677T allele may influence the severity and biochemical risk factors of Alzheimer's disease in an Egyptian population. *Dis Markers* 35(5):439–46.

Gilbody, S., S. Lewis, T. Lightfoot. 2007. Methylenetetrahydrofolate reductase (MTHFR) genetic polymorphisms and psychiatric disorders: a HuGE review. *Am J Epidemiol* 165(1):1–13.

Kempisty, B., A. Mostowska, I. Górska, et al. 2006. Association of 677C>T polymorphism of methylenetetrahydrofolate reductase (MTHFR) gene with bipolar disorder and schizophrenia. *Neurosci Lett* 400(3):267–71.

Khandanpour, N., G. Willis, F. J. Meyer, et al. 2009. Peripheral arterial disease and methylenetetrahydrofolate reductase (MTHFR) C677T mutations: A case-control study and meta-analysis. *J Vasc Surg* 49:711–18.

Lee, S. A. 2009. Gene-diet interaction on cancer risk in epidemiological studies. *J Prev Med Public Health* 42(6):360–70.

Lynch, B. 2011. MTHFR A1298C mutation: Some information on A1298C mutations. MTHFR.net. Accessed June 29, 2015 at http://mthfr.net/mthfr-a1298c-mutation-some-information-on-a1298c-mthfr-mutations/2011/11/30/.

Mansouri, L., N. Fekih-Mrissa, S. Klai, et al. 2013. Association of methylenetetrahydrofolate reductase polymorphisms with susceptibility to Alzheimer's disease. *Clin Neurol Neurosurg* 115(9):1693–96.

MRC Vitamin Study Research Group. 1991. Prevention of neural tube defects: results of the Medical Research Council Vitamin Study. *Lancet* 338:131–37.

Folate. 2012. National Institutes of Health website. Accessed October 26, 2014. http://ods.od.nih.gov/factsheets/Folate-HealthProfessional/#h3.

Pogliani, L., C. Cerini, F. Penagini, et al. 2014. Cerebral ultrasound abnormalities in offspring of women with C677T homozygous mutation in the MTHFR gene: a prospective study. *World J Pediatr* Epub ahead of print.

Shaw, G. M. 1995. Risks of orofacial clefts in children born to women using multivitamins containing folic acid periconceptionally. *Lancet* 346:393–96.

Van Allen, M. I., et al. 1993. Recommendations on the use of folic acid supplementation to prevent the recurrence of neural tube defects. *Canadian Medical Association Journal* 149(9):1239–43.

Wilcken, B., F. Bamforth, Z. Li, et al. 2003. Geographical and ethnic variation of the 677C>T allele of 5,10 methylenetetrahydrofolate reductase (MTHFR): findings from over 7000 newborns from 16 areas world wide. *J Med Genet* 40(8):619–25.

Yan, J., M. Yin, Z. E. Dreyer, et al. 2012. A meta-analysis of MTHFR C677T and A1298C polymorphisms and risk of acute lymphoblastic leukemia in children. *Pediatr Blood Cancer* 58(4):513–18.

Zintzaras, E. 2006. C677T and A1298C methylenetetrahydrofolate reductase gene polymorphisms in schizophrenia, bipolar disorder and depression: a meta-analysis of genetic association studies. *Psychiatr Genet* 16(3):105–15.

Multiple Sclerosis

Multiple sclerosis (MS) is a chronic, progressive, degenerative disease of the central nervous system. Because nerves are delicate, highly sensitive structures, they are sheathed in a protective material known as myelin. In a person with MS, the myelin degenerates, leaving sections of the nerves bare and vulnerable. If nerves are damaged and scarred over, the areas of the body that are controlled by the affected nerves will malfunction. Although MS is not a common disorder, it does strike more frequently than most other neurological diseases, and in recent years the percentage of cases has increased. It's estimated that between 250,000 and 350,000 Americans currently suffer from MS. Multiple sclerosis can develop at any age, but onset usually occurs between the ages of twenty and forty. About two-thirds of MS victims are women.

The course of MS is highly individual and depends mainly on which nerves are affected and on the extent of the damage. Nevertheless, the disease does exhibit some general symptom patterns. Multiple sclerosis always occurs in cycles of flare-ups, called exacerbations, and remissions. The first attack and the exacerbations that follow may consist of nothing more than some blurred vision or unexplained fatigue. Because the symptoms are vague and disappear after a short time—sometimes after just days—and because a person may spend years in remission, MS often goes undiagnosed in these extremely early stages. Exacerbations get progressively worse, however, and when a person experiences more obviously alarming symptoms like facial paralysis, weak or numb limbs, or slurred speech, it's likely that a doctor will investigate the possibility of MS.

How the disease moves on from this stage varies from person to person. Some people will go into complete, lifelong remission. Just as rare is the case in which the disease hits with more force, causing significant, lasting damage after the very first attack. The vast majority of sufferers fall somewhere between these two extremes. Many will recover from the first major exacerbation and will experience only mild recurrences every ten years or so. Some will suffer from more frequent relapses that slowly become more severe and leave permanent disability in their wake. As the decades go on, a person may have trouble with movement, balance, and coordination and eventually develop the classic staggering gait. In the advanced stages, there may be blindness, incontinence, paralysis, or difficulty breathing. Because MS affects the brain's functions, many sufferers also experience mood alterations, swinging up to euphoria and then plunging down into a deep depression.

Why the sheaths of myelin degenerate in some people remains a mystery, but there's no shortage of theories. The prevailing hypothesis is that MS is an autoimmune disorder in which a person's white blood cells mistake myelin for an invader and attack it. Another popular theory is that MS is caused by a virus or another latent infection, and indeed, the symptoms of MS are similar to those of some viral infections—so similar that doctors are often not able to distinguish a viral attack from MS in its early stages. Possibly, MS is caused by a combination of these factors, and the virus somehow causes the formation of antibodies that attack myelin.

Although multiple sclerosis is appearing with increasing frequency in the United States, the disease is rare in Eastern and developing countries and in the tropics. Any time this kind of geographical discrepancy occurs, it makes sense to investigate lifestyle and environmental factors as potential causes. Also, MS occurs more frequently in higher latitudes. High-risk areas include the northern United States, Canada, Great Britain, Scandinavia, Tasmania, and northern Europe, as examples. The reason for this is unclear, although studies show that people who had a higher sun exposure between the ages of six and fifteen have a significantly reduced risk of the disease. This may have something to do with vitamin D from sun exposure.

It's well known that extreme stress and poor nutrition can bring on an exacerbation, so it's quite possible that they also contribute to the onset of the disease. Environmental toxins, especially heavy metals, can produce symptoms similar to those of MS and may damage both DNA and myelin. Food allergies or sensitivities appear to be a factor for some people with this condition. Many researchers are currently looking into the relationship between an allergy to wheat or dairy and the incidence of MS. One must also look at the possibility of toxic-metal accumulation, such as mercury, as a causative or aggravating factor. Good digestion is important, as there is a link between autoimmune diseases and malabsorption. Several nutritional deficiencies, especially of essential fatty acids and vitamin B12, are critical, as they are involved with a healthy myelin sheath.

Compounding the frightening symptoms of MS is the inability of many patients to receive a definitive diagnosis, especially in early stages of the disease. Doctors can perform spinal taps, testing the cerebrospinal fluid, or do MRI scans to look for abnormal antibodies and myelin damage, but because MS may cause damage much like that from a virus or other autoimmune disorders, the tests are often inclusive. In most cases, a diagnosis is made only when all other possibilities are ruled out.

If you have MS or MS-like symptoms, it's critical that you find a good specialist and work closely with him or her. Despite the common perception, many people with MS live long, productive lives. Disabilities caused by severe attacks, when they happen at all, often occur several decades after a diagnosis and can often be managed quite well. It is crucial that you also work with a holistic doctor to address the underlying reasons for your illness. We have had several patients with MS remain relatively symptom-free by following a comprehensive natural approach, as described in this section.

SYMPTOMS

Multiple sclerosis occurs in cycles of remission and exacerbation. Symptoms may occur singly at first, but later on, they usually appear in groups of two or more.

- Deep fatigue
- Blurred vision
- Dizziness
- Impaired speech
- Facial paralysis
- Numbness or weakness in the limbs
- Loss of balance
- Poor coordination
- Nausea and vomiting
- Constipation
- Staggering gait
- Tremors
- Bowel and bladder incontinence
- Blindness
- Paralysis

ROOT CAUSES

- Chronic infection (viral, bacterial, candida)
- Long periods of extreme stress
- Stress-hormone imbalance
- Poor nutrition (especially vitamin D deficiency)
- Environmental toxins
- Toxic metals
- Food allergies
- Free-radical damage
- Immunizations

Testing Techniques

The following tests help assess possible reasons for multiple sclerosis:

Immune-system imbalance or disease—blood

Hormone testing (thyroid, DHEA, cortisol, testosterone, IGF-1, estrogen, progesterone)—saliva, blood, or urine

Intestinal permeability—urine

Detoxification profile—urine

Vitamin and mineral analysis (especially magnesium, B12)—blood

Essential fatty-acid balance—blood or urine

Amino acid balance—blood or urine

Digestive function and microbe/parasite/candida testing—stool analysis

Food and environmental allergies/sensitivities—blood, electrodermal

---

TREATMENT

Diet

Recommended Food

Eat meals and snacks made with whole, unprocessed foods. Try to prepare meals yourself so you know what goes into them. Buy organic products as often as possible.

Roy Swank, M.D., a professor of neurology at the University of Oregon Medical School, prescribed a special diet for 150 patients with MS. This included the elimination of margarine, hydrogenated oils, and shortenings. Saturated fat was limited to 20 grams per day or less. The diet included vegetable oils that are rich in polyunsaturated fatty acids and 5 grams per day of cod liver oil. Patients were to eat fish three or more times a week and consume a normal amount of protein. Results showed that 95 percent of the people who started this regimen and had minimal disability to begin with showed very little or no progression of the disease over a thirty-year period. Also, people who followed the diet had a death rate significantly lower than a study group with MS who didn't follow the diet (31 percent versus 80 percent).

Have several helpings of deeply colored fresh fruits and vegetables every day. These foods are high in antioxidants, which fight free-radical damage to your cells. They're also high in fiber, which will keep your colon free of wastes and will help you avoid constipation.

Essential fatty acids reduce inflammation of the nerve fibers and strengthen myelin. Eat fish from a clean water source three or more times a week, and have a tablespoon of flaxseeds or flaxseed oil every day.

Lecithin may also help to strengthen the myelin sheath. Good sources include tofu and other soy products, bean sprouts, and cabbage.

To reduce stress, add whole grains, wheat germ, and brewer's yeast to your meals. The B vitamins in these foods are calming to the nervous system.

Food to Avoid

Reduce your exposure to chemicals and pesticides by eating organic foods. Do not eat junk food or packaged food that contains artificial flavoring, colorings, or preservatives.

If you're allergic to any food, you need to find out now. Read the Food Allergies section in this book and follow the elimination diet presented there. You should make it a priority to look for allergies to gluten (wheat and other grains) or dairy, but corn, yeast, sugar, peanuts, soy, and eggs are also common sensitivities.

Eliminate inflammatory foods from your diet that may make your nerve damage and muscle problems worse. If you've stopped eating red meat and dairy, you've already made great strides toward this goal. You should also avoid other foods that are fatty, fried, or greasy.

Keep up your resistance to infection by restricting your sugar consumption. If you're feeling well, the occasional treat is fine, but for the most part, you should avoid colas, sweet baked goods, candies, cakes, and other items made with refined sugar.

If you want to fight MS, you need all the nutritional support you can get. Avoid alcohol and caffeine, which deplete vitamins and minerals from your body and worsen inflammation.

℞ Super Seven Prescriptions—Multiple Sclerosis

Super Prescription #1 Fish oil
Take a minimum of 5 grams daily and up to 20 grams daily. Omega-3 fatty acids reduce inflammation and are required for healthy nerve functioning. Dr. Swank used 5 grams of cod liver oil in his thirty-year study, while other studies have used up to 20 grams.

Super Prescription #2 Vitamin B12
Take 1,000 to 1,500 mcg of the sublingual form daily or receive the injectable form from your doctor. Vitamin B12 is involved in the formation of the myelin sheath, and nutrition-oriented doctors such as ourselves find B12 helpful for people with this condition.

Super Prescription #3 Vitamin D
Take 2,500 to 5,000 IU daily. Vitamin D works to modulate the immune system and reduce inflammation.

Super Prescription #4 High-potency multivitamin
Take as directed on the container. It contains a base of the nutrients needed for healthy immune and nervous systems.

Super Prescription #5 Plant sterols and sterolins
Take 20 mg three times daily on an empty stomach. These naturally occurring plant chemicals have been shown to have a balancing effect on the immune systems of people with autoimmune diseases.

Super Prescription #6 Digestive enzymes
Take 1 or 2 capsules of a full-spectrum enzyme product with each meal. Enzymes help you to digest food more efficiently and lessen autoimmune reactions. Protease enzymes can be taken between meals to reduce autoimmune complexes and inflammation.

Super Prescription #7 Gamma linoleic acid (GLA)
Take 300 to 500 mg daily. It is found in evening primrose and borage oil. GLA is a fatty acid that has an anti-inflammatory effect.

A population study reported in the *Journal of the American Medical Association* found that among whites, the risk of multiple sclerosis significantly decreased with increasing levels of vitamin D.

General Recommendations

Ginkgo biloba has potent antioxidant activity for the nerves and improves circulation. Take 60 to 120 mg twice daily of a standardized product containing 24 percent flavone glycosides and 6 percent terpene lactones.

Vitamin E is a potent antioxidant. Take 400 IU of a mixed complex (tocopherols and tocotrienols) daily.

Ashwagandha (*Withania somniferum*) balances the stress hormones. Take 125 to 250 mg of 0.8 percent withanolide extract daily.

Take a super-green-food supplement, such as chlorella or spirulina, or a mixture of super green foods, each day for detoxification and pH balance. Take as directed on the container.

DHEA is a stress hormone that is helpful for many autoimmune diseases. Have your levels tested, and if they are low, start with 15 mg daily under the supervision of a doctor. Higher doses of up to 100 mg are sometimes necessary.

It's important to avoid stress, so keep a stash of calming herbal teas on hand. Skullcap, hops (*Humulus lupulus*), and passionflower are all good choices.

Homeopathy

Pick the remedy that best matches your symptoms in this section. Take a 6x, 12x, 6C, 12C, or 30C potency twice daily for two weeks to see if there are any positive results. After you notice improvement, stop taking the remedy, unless symptoms return. Consultation with a homeopathic practitioner is advised.

Agaricus is helpful when there are symptoms of twitching, muscle spasms, poor coordination, and uncontrolled eye movement.

Alumina is for symptoms of progressive paralysis and confusion and the legs feel very heavy. Weakness and paralysis of the lower extremities may occur. There is delayed nerve conduction. Constipation is common.

Argentum Nitricum is for loss of balance and poor coordination that is progressing to paralysis.

Arsenicum Album is for progressive paralysis and burning sensations. The person tends to be anxious and restless.

Causticum is indicated when there is slow, progressive paralysis of the limbs, as well as of muscles that control speech, swallowing, and respiration. There may be numbness of the hands and the feet. Incontinence is common.

Cocculus is helpful when there is progressive paralysis, as well as dizziness when looking at moving objects. The vision is slow to accommodate.

Conium is for ascending paralysis that begins with weakness in the thighs. There is heaviness in the lower limbs. The person drops things easily.

Gelsemium (*Gelsemium sempervirens*) is helpful when there is great weakness and trembling of the muscles. There may also be numbness of the face and the tongue and double vision. The eyelids feel heavy. The symptoms are better after urination.

Ignatia (*Ignatia amara*) will help when multiple sclerosis, especially paralysis, comes on after grief. There is twitching and muscle spasms.

Lachesis is for left-sided symptoms, such as numbness or paralysis. Jealousy or anger worsens symptoms.

Natrum Muriaticum helps when there are symptoms of awkwardness, such as dropping things. Optic neuritis is usually present, as well as numbness throughout the body. The person wants to be alone and feels depressed. The symptoms may come on after grief. The symptoms are worse in the sun.

Nux Vomica is helpful when there is paralysis, along with muscle spasms, cramps, and twitching. The person is highly driven and irritable and craves alcohol and stimulants.

Phosphorus is for numbness in the hands and the feet. The person has problems with incontinence and vision. There is a craving for ice-cold drinks.

Plumbum is for progressive paralysis and wasting of the muscles. There is a tremendous heaviness of the legs.

Bodywork

Massage
Regular massage is highly recommended for MS sufferers. It will help keep the muscles functioning and may hasten recovery time after an exacerbation, and it will also improve circulation and reduce stress.

Reflexology
See pages 804–805 for information about reflexology areas and how to work them.

To stimulate blood supply to the nerves, work the entire spinal area.

Work the diaphragm and the solar plexus to reduce tension and support the central nervous system.

It's also a good idea to work the area corresponding to any part of the body affected by MS.

Acupuncture from a qualified practitioner can be helpful for many of the symptoms of MS.

Hydrotherapy
Avoid saunas and hot baths. They may sound relaxing, but high heat often aggravates the symptoms of MS. A cool or cold bath or shower, however, will stimulate your blood flow and even lift your spirits.

Aromatherapy

Experiment with relaxing oils until you find a few you like, and then rotate them so that you don't become immune to the effects of any single oil. Lavender, jasmine, geranium, ylang-ylang, and rose are all good choices to start with. Use them in any preparation you like.

Stress Reduction

Make stress reduction a priority. Biofeedback, deep breathing, prayer, and yoga are all good choices.

A diagnosis of MS, or an attack of MS-like symptoms, can be a shock. Professional counseling can assist you as you try to understand your disorder and make sense of its place in your life.

Other Recommendations

- Gentle exercise will keep your muscles in good shape, improve circulation, keep your digestive system regular, and help you release stress. Swimming and walking are especially helpful for MS patients, as are stretching exercises.
- Rest whenever you feel the need. If you think you might be getting ill or experiencing the beginning of an exacerbation, get to bed right away and stay there for a few days. You might be able to head off the worst of the symptoms.
- Don't forget that tobacco smoke is an environmental toxin best avoided.
- Consult with a holistic dentist to make sure there are no chronic root canal infections, mercury-filling problems, or other dental issues that may be triggering the immune system.
- Get fifteen minutes of sunlight exposure daily.
- Intravenous nutrients can make a big difference for those with MS. Vitamin B12, magnesium, and vitamin C are important.
- The use of low-dose naltrexone has published studies showing benefit for those with MS, particularly the problem of spasticity. Consult with your holistic doctor about its use.

REFERENCES

Munger, K. L., et al. 2006. Serum 25-hydroxyvitamin D levels and risk of multiple sclerosis. *Journal of the American Medical Association* 296:2832–38.

Swank, R. L. 1991. Multiple sclerosis: Fat-oil relationship. *Nutrition* 7:368–76.

Swank, R. L., et al. 1990. Effect of low saturated fat diet in early and late cases of multiple sclerosis. *Lancet* 336:37–39.

Muscle Aches and Cramps

You might experience back soreness after a long day playing with the kids, have aching shoulders after overdoing it in the swimming pool, or feel calf pains during the night. Occasional muscle aches and cramps often accompany the rigors of life. They are rarely a cause to worry.

Muscle aches can affect an active child, as well as a sedentary child who sits in front of the television playing video games and watching programs. The pain often occurs when muscles are overused and pulled or strained, particularly after a vigorous workout that didn't follow a warm-up or stretching session. The pain can range from mild to severe and usually dissipates after a few restful days. Lingering or recurrent pain, especially when accompanied by a fever, decreased muscular strength, or joint swelling, could suggest a severe strain, possibly injury.

The feeling of a muscle turning into a knot indicates a muscle cramp. Muscle cramps could afflict any child, regardless of fitness or diet. Heat cramps, which are common to the calves, the thighs, and the abdomen, can strike a person who exercises in hot weather or a hot gymnasium and who needs water. Night cramps often knot up the muscles of the calves, the feet, and the thighs, causing sharp pains and tightened muscles, which commonly awaken people from a sound sleep.

Nutritional deficiencies of calcium, magnesium, potassium, and the B vitamins are often the root cause of muscle aches and cramps. Lack of sleep can also contribute to this problem.

SYMPTOMS

- Muscle contractions or spasms, usually in the legs

ROOT CAUSES

- Mineral imbalance (calcium, potassium, magnesium, zinc)
- Poor sleep
- Poor circulation
- Impinged nerve

Testing Techniques

The following tests help assess possible reasons for chronic muscle cramps and aches:

Hormone testing (thyroid, DHEA, cortisol, testosterone, IGF-1, estrogen, progesterone)—saliva, blood, or urine

Intestinal permeability—urine

Vitamin and mineral analysis (especially magnesium, calcium, potassium, zinc)—blood, hair

Digestive function and microbe/parasite/candida testing—stool analysis

Food and environmental allergies/sensitivities—blood, electrodermal

Toxic metals—hair or urine

TREATMENT

Diet

Recommended Food

Eat foods that are high in calcium: kelp, cheese, collards, kale, turnip greens, almonds, yogurt, milk, broccoli, and calcium-enriched rice and soymilk.

Also eat foods that are high in magnesium: whole grains, nuts, legumes, soy, and green leafy vegetables.

Foods that are high in potassium are beneficial as well: fruits and vegetables, especially apples, bananas, carrots, oranges, potatoes, tomatoes, cantaloupes, peaches, plums, strawberries, meat, and fish.

Electrolyte drinks can help you quickly restore lost minerals. We recommend these drinks only on a short-term basis, though. Many contain artificial colorings and large amounts of sugar, although more healthful alternatives are available.

Drinking clean, quality water on hot days or after physical activity is important.

Food to Avoid

Avoid products that lead to the loss of minerals, such as soda pop, candy, and refined breads and pastas.

R Super Seven Prescriptions—Muscle Aches and Cramps

Super Prescription #1 Magnesium

Take 250 mg twice daily. Magnesium is a muscle relaxer, and a deficiency contributes to cramping, aching, and tightness.

Super Prescription #2 Calcium

Take 500 mg twice daily. Calcium is required for muscle and nerve relaxation. It works in tandem with magnesium to relax muscles.

Super Prescription #3 Potassium

Take up to 300 mg daily. A potassium deficiency can lead to muscle cramping. *Note*: If you are on blood pressure medication, use under the guidance of your doctor.

Super Prescription #4 Homeopathic Magnesia Phosphorica

Take 3 pellets of a 6x potency three to five times daily. This remedy is specific for muscle cramping.

Super Prescription #5 High-potency multivitamin /-mineral

Take a high-potency multivitamin and -mineral formula daily, as it will contain a strong base of the nutrients that protect against muscle cramping.

Super Prescription #6 Super-green-food supplement

Take an organic super green food, such as chlorella or spirulina, or a mixture of super green foods each day. Take as directed on the container. It contains a variety of minerals for muscle relaxation.

Super Prescription #7 Methylsulfonylmethane (MSM)

Take 500 mg three times daily. This nutrient has natural antispasmodic properties. It is especially good for muscle cramps and aches related to an injury. Reduce the dosage if diarrhea occurs.

General Recommendations

B vitamins can become depleted due to the effect of stress, causing muscle cramps and aches. Take a 50 mg complex twice daily.

Protease enzymes reduce muscle aching and inflammation. Take 1 capsule three times daily between meals.

Black cohosh (*Cimicifuga racemosa*) reduces spasms of the muscles. Take 40 mg of a 2.5 percent triterpene glycoside extract twice daily.

Arnica (*Arnica montana*) oil relieves muscle pain and tenderness. Apply the oil to painful areas twice daily.

Horse chestnut (*Aesculus hippocastanum*) is helpful for spasms in the legs due to poor circulation. Take 300 mg twice daily.

Homeopathy

Pick the remedy that best matches your symptoms in this section. Take a 6x, 12x, 6C, or 30C potency twice daily for two weeks to see if there are any positive results.

After you notice improvement, stop taking the remedy, unless symptoms return. Consultation with a homeopathic practitioner is advised.

Arnica (*Arnica montana*) is the top choice for pain that feels deep and bruised and for allover tenderness. The symptoms are worse after exertion.

Calcarea Carbonica is for people who get muscle cramps and soreness from exertion and from cold, damp climates. They are usually chilly, with clammy hands and feet. They crave sweets and eggs. They often feel anxious, overwhelmed, and easily fatigued.

Causticum is helpful when the muscles and the joints become stiff and sore from overuse and from the cold or in dry weather. The symptoms are improved with warm applications. The muscles and the joints feel contracted.

Cimicifuga is for muscles that feel sore, bruised, and worse in the cold. The back of the neck is sore and stiff. The person is prone to depression and hormone imbalance.

Ignatia Amara is for tight, spasmodic, or cramping muscles or for muscle spasms and cramps that begin after an emotional upset or stress.

Magnesia Phosphorica is for cramping or spasming muscles that feel better from warm applications.

Nux vomica (*Strychnos nux vomica*) is for tight muscles that spasm. The person is chilly, and the symptoms are worse in cold weather and better with warm applications. Digestive problems, such as stomachache or heartburn, are often present. The person is irritable and fatigued.

Rhus Toxicodendron is for pain and stiffness that are worse in the early morning or after resting and in cold, rainy weather. The symptoms ease with continued movement and warm applications. The person feels restless.

Acupressure

See pages 787–794 for information about pressure points and administering treatment.

To relax cramped muscles and soothe your nerves, use Liver 3 (Lv3).

Bodywork

Massage
Massage is excellent to work the cramps out by improving the circulation.

Other Bodywork Recommendations
Stretching is important to relax the muscles and prevent overtightening. Spinal alignment by a chiropractor, an osteopath, or a naturopathic doctor can be helpful for cases of chronic muscle spasm and aches.

Aromatherapy

Add 1 drop of lavender and 1 drop of peppermint to a carrier oil and massage onto the muscle. If the muscle aches or cramps occur at night, use black pepper instead of peppermint.

Obesity

Obesity is the single most common problem that doctors see in their practices. According to data from the National Health and Nutrition Examination Survey, more than two-thirds of adults in the United States are overweight or obese. Unfortunately, it's also a risk factor for a host of disorders. The risk factors for those who are overweight or obese are type 2 diabetes, coronary heart disease, high LDL ("bad") cholesterol, stroke, hypertension, nonalcoholic fatty liver disease, gallbladder disease, osteoarthritis (the degeneration of the cartilage and the bone of the joints), sleep apnea and other breathing problems, some forms of cancer (breast, colorectal, endometrial, and kidney), complications of pregnancy, and menstrual irregularities. And since heavy people are likely to consume high quantities of toxic food, their immune systems are depressed, leaving them susceptible to any virus or bug that happens to be going around at home or in the office.

In fact, the rising occurrence of obesity can be traced in part to our attempts to fight it. Take the low-protein, high-carbohydrate diet that in the early 1990s was universally espoused as healthful: people filled up their plates with so much pasta, bread, and fat-free sweets that they actually ended up eating more calories—and, of course, gaining more weight. Other strategies, such as appetite suppressants and extreme diets, do indeed help people lose weight short-term. But they're also too dangerous to use for long, so at some point those people have to return to a lifestyle that is healthful. Because many "diet gurus" haven't taught people how to put healthful eating in the context of their daily routines, they soon put the weight right back on.

There are several reasons why a person is susceptible to obesity. Genetics is an obvious factor that makes it more difficult for some people to lose weight. This inherited condition makes some people more likely to put on weight from simple-carbohydrate consumption. Insulin levels spike upward and result in fat deposition. This problem is compounded by the fact that the average American consumes 150 pounds of sugar each year! In addition, some researchers feel that the body has a genetically programmed "set point." This refers to the theory that the body tries to maintain a set metabolic rate at which calories are burned, especially the fat cells. For people with a genetic susceptibility, it is even more important to be diligent with the diet and lifestyle recommendations we make. Also, nutritional supplements can help to lessen genetic tendencies.

The amount of calories someone consumes is an obvious reason for weight gain. Consuming too many calories without burning them results in a simple mathematical reality—weight gain. To stay within a certain parameter for your metabolism, it is helpful to grasp the concept of general calorie amounts of commonly consumed foods.

The second important concept, after calorie consumption, is the calories expended through movement and exercise. The more calories that are utilized for energy, the fewer that will go toward fat accumulation. In this technologically advanced and television-addicted society, people are expending far fewer calories than they used to.

Hormone balance is also important for the prevention and the treatment of obesity. Many hormones in the body have an effect on metabolism. The most notable are thyroid hormones, which greatly influence the metabolic rate in our cells. However, several others hormones, such as DHEA, testosterone, and growth hormones, have powerful effects as well. We have also found that an estrogen and progesterone imbalance contributes to fat deposition and water retention, and thus to weight gain. This seems to be particularly true for women who use synthetic hormones. A hormone balance must also take into account the level of the brain hormone serotonin. Low levels of this neurotransmitter contribute to feelings of hunger and to sugar/

carbohydrate cravings. There are natural ways to optimize this neurotransmitter, as discussed in this section and in the section on Depression. Further research in this field will shed more light on the role of neurotransmitters and obesity.

Toxins in the body also pose a problem for people who are overweight. Many of the chemicals that people are exposed to interfere with normal cell function, including metabolism. Pesticides, heavy metals such as mercury, and other toxins are a part of our polluted world. Interestingly, many of these toxins are stored in fat tissue in order to prevent damage to vital body organs, such as the brain and the heart.

In addition, a diet that is devoid of nutrients leads to nutritional deficiencies. The body does not burn fat by magic but requires several vitamins, minerals, and enzymes to do so efficiently. It appears that certain nutrients can help in the prevention and the treatment of obesity. While none should be considered "magic bullets," they can in some cases be quite helpful as part of a comprehensive weight or fat-reduction protocol.

The mental and the emotional, as well as the spiritual, well-being of a person cannot be ignored in regard to obesity. Imbalances in these areas often supersede genetic and physical reasons for weight gain. For example, many people with depression and anxiety consume comfort foods as a way to feel a false sense of love or worth. Some patients with obesity first began to have problems with weight after experiencing an unresolved emotional trauma. Treating the whole person is of paramount importance with obesity.

Determining a Healthy Body Size: Two Tests

Test #1: Body Mass Index
The body mass index, or BMI, helps you determine the appropriate weight for your frame. For most people, the BMI test is more reliable than scales or height/weight charts are, but you should know that people with very muscular physiques may come up with a misleading reading. Because muscle weighs more than fat, many professional athletes have high BMIs—although, clearly, they don't need to lose weight.

Here's how to calculate your BMI. After each step are sample calculations, made for a person who is 5'8" and 150 pounds:

1. Write down your height in inches:

   _____
   (5'8" = 68 inches)

2. Multiply the number in Line 1 by .025:

   _____
   (68 X .025 = 1.70)

3. Square the number in Line 2: _____
   (1.70 X 1.70 = 2.89)

4. Write down your weight in pounds:

   _____
   (150)

5. Multiply the number in Line 4 by .45:

   _____
   (150 X .45 = 67.50)

6. Divide the number in Line 5 by the number in Line 3: _____
   (67.50/2.89 = 23.36)

Interpreting the Results
If your BMI is between 18.9 and 24.9, you are considered to be of a healthy weight. Like everyone else, you need to eat well and exercise, but if you take the second test here and it doesn't indicate a health risk, you don't need to lose pounds. If your BMI is 25 or higher, there's a good chance that you need to lose weight. If you have any weight-related health problems like heart disease, high blood pressure, high cholesterol, joint or back pain, or diabetes, you should make

a concerted effort to burn more calories than you take in. People who smoke, who drink heavily, or who have a family history of the diseases listed previously would also be wise to lose weight. If you don't have any of these concerns, it's possible that you are simply a large but healthy person. Take the second test to further assess your health risk.

If your BMI is below 18.9, you may be underweight. If you're an otherwise healthy adolescent who does not have an eating disorder, you're probably just going through a phase. When you get a little older, your metabolism will likely right itself. Adults, however, should talk to a doctor about what a low BMI means for them as individuals. And anyone who suffers from an eating disorder should get professional help right away.

Test #2: Waist Circumference
Measure your waist circumference, using your navel as the defining point of your waist. For men, a waist circumference of more than forty inches is considered a health risk. Women should not have a waist circumference of more than thirty-five inches.

Since fat cells produce hormones that affect metabolism and inflammation, large waists are an indicator of possible future health problems, especially of cardiovascular conditions like heart disease and high blood pressure. If you have a large waist circumference, you should read these pages for advice about losing weight.

If you have a high BMI but have a normal waist circumference, are healthy, have no family history of weight-related disease, and don't drink excessively or smoke, your weight is probably just fine. If it bothers you, or if you sense that your weight is slowing you down or affecting your health, see your doctor for an individual assessment. And remember: Even if you don't need to lose weight, you should still eat well and exercise on a regular basis.

SYMPTOMS

- Weight gain and fat deposition
- Difficulty breathing
- Increased sweating

ROOT CAUSES

Obesity is almost always caused by a combination of the first two items listed here: taking in more calories than are expended. But, as we described, there can be many factors at work.

- Poor diet (high in calories and simple carbohydrates)
- Inactivity
- Hormone imbalance (particularly thyroid)
- Toxins
- Neurotransmitter imbalance (serotonin)
- Mental, emotional, or spiritual issues
- Preexisting medical conditions (e.g., hypothyroidism)
- Genetics
- Side effects of pharmaceutical medications (e.g., antidepressants)

Testing Techniques

The following tests help assess possible reasons for weight gain:

Hormone testing (thyroid, DHEA, cortisol, testosterone, IGF-1, estrogen, insulin, progesterone, adiponectin, leptin)—saliva, blood, or urine

Intestinal permeability—urine

Detoxification profile—urine

Vitamin and mineral analysis (especially magnesium, L-carnitine, chromium, and CoQ10)—blood

Digestive function and microbe/parasite/candida testing—stool analysis

Food and environmental allergies/sensitivities—blood, electrodermal

Blood sugar balance—blood

Toxic metals—hair or urine

TREATMENT

Diet

Your best bet for health and weight loss is to focus on eating foods that are fresh, whole, and nutritionally dense.

Recommended Food

Don't rely on someone else: start cooking for yourself. Shop for a variety of basic, whole foods. You can eat vegetables, fruits, nuts, and seeds raw for their fiber and digestive enzymes; the rest of the time, use light cooking methods like broiling, steaming, roasting, or grilling.

Make sure you get enough protein every day. Otherwise, you'll feel deprived and downright hungry. Fish is an excellent source of protein, but few of us can eat it every single day. Plan on having beans, lean poultry, soy products, nuts, or yogurt with every meal. High-quality protein drinks from whey, eggs, or rice are good choices.

Whole, complex carbohydrates like brown rice, whole-grain bread, and oats are necessary for a healthful eating plan. They're also high in fiber, which helps you feel full and keeps you free of toxins. Use common sense, though; carbohydrates are meant to be one part of your diet, not all of it. Many overweight people benefit from reducing their carbohydrate intake.

Essential fatty acids are just what their name implies: fats that are good for you. Cold-water fish, flaxseeds, and cold-pressed oils like olive oil are necessary for proper functioning of almost every body system, and they help you feel satisfied after a meal. As with everything else, however, use EFAs in moderation. Extra helpings of anything, even of salmon fillets, contribute to your waistline but not to your health. Sauté your vegetables in a tablespoon, not a cup, of olive oil.

Low levels of serotonin, a neurotransmitter, may increase your desire for refined and complex carbohydrates, including for sugar. Eat foods that are high in tryptophan—turkey, chicken, tuna, soymilk, and live unsweetened yogurt. This chemical encourages the production of serotonin and may stave off cravings.

A double-blind study by the University of Rome included twenty obese people for two phases of time. The first phase involved a nonrestrictive diet, and the second phase focused on a calorie-restricted diet. During both phases, people receiving 900 mg of 5-HTP had a reduction in carbohydrate intake and the consistent presence of an early sensation of fullness.

Vegetable juice is healthful and filling. Drink a glass a half hour before meals to keep your appetite in check.

Water also takes the edge off your hunger. Plan on drinking a glass of clean, quality water every two waking hours.

Eat a balanced ratio of the major food groups. Many people do well on a diet that is a Paleo style, with greatly reduced quantities of grains and dairy products.

Eat more small, regular meals throughout the day to quench your appetite and balance blood sugar levels.

Do not skip meals, particularly breakfast. This puts the body into a starvation mode that can increase fat accumulation.

Food to Avoid

Americans are addicted to sugar. Sugar is high in calories and causes mood swings and blood sugar crashes that may only increase your cravings. If you're trying to lose weight, your first priority should be to reduce or, in some cases, eliminate refined sugar from your diet. No cookies, cakes, candy, ice cream, sodas, white breads, pastas, and crackers, and especially no low-fat sweets, which contain extra sugar to make up for the missing richness. It's also wise to limit your intake of natural sugars. Fruit sugars, honey, and molasses are less damaging to your body than refined products are, but in large quantities they can still lead to weight gain. Eat them only in moderation.

Avoid processed and junk food. Food made with artificial flavors, colors, and preservatives offers you little in the way of real sustenance. Their toxins are also highly addictive. As most of us know, even one fast-food cheeseburger or a handful of greasy, salty potato chips is enough to derail your body from its natural sense of what's healthful.

Refined flours are another example of the proverbial "empty calories." Pasta, white bread, and white rice are stripped of most of their nutrients, leaving you with nothing but a plate full of calories, insulin surgers, and weight gain.

You've heard it a thousand times, and it's still true: you must radically cut back on your consumption of "bad" fats. If you stop eating processed food (including margarine and shortening), you'll go a long way toward this goal. Naturally sweetened baked goods are also high in saturated fats. If you enjoy any of these items, reserve them for the occasional treat.

℞ Super Seven Prescriptions—Obesity

Super Prescription #1 Indian sphaeranthus (*Sphaeranthis indicus*) and mangosteen extract (*Garcinia mangostana*) combination
Take 400 mg each morning and evening on an empty stomach to help with metabolism.

Super Prescription #2 *Caralluma fimbriata*
Take 500 mg thirty to forty-five minutes before meals twice a day, usually at breakfast and dinner. This herbal extract suppresses appetite.

Super Prescription #3 *Irvingia gabonensis*
Take 150 mg twice daily of a standardized extract.

In a clinical study, a standardized seed extract of the Irvingia gabonensis plant at a dosage of 150 mg twice daily for ten weeks reduced weight in subjects by twenty-eight pounds, compared to 1.5 pounds in similar subjects taking a placebo.

A randomized, double-blind study involving sixty overweight and obese people demonstrated that people supplementing conjugated linoleic acid (CLA) had a significantly higher reduction in body fat mass, as compared to people taking a placebo.

Super Prescription #4 Green tea (*Camellia sinensis*) extract

Take 1,500 mg of green tea extract standardized to 80 to 90 percent polyphenols and 35 to 55 percent epigallocatechin gallate. Studies have shown that green tea extract increases thermogenesis, the body's ability to burn energy. *Note*: Green tea contains caffeine, which may account for some of this benefit.

Super Prescription #5 Conjugated linoleic acid (CLA)

Take 3.4 grams daily. Studies show that this fatty acid reduces body-fat composition.

Super Prescription #6 Soluble fiber

Take 2 to 4 capsules before or with each meal and with 8 ounces of water. Studies show that it makes one feel full and reduces insulin levels that contribute to weight gain.

Super Prescription #7 Resveratrol

Take 125 to 250 mg daily. This helps with glucose metabolism in cells.

In an eight-week randomized, placebo-controlled study sixty obese volunteers were divided into two groups. One group of thirty received 800 mg of the two extracts Indian sphaeranthus and mangosteen extract. The other group got a placebo. Both groups followed a 2,000-calorie-per-day diet and were instructed to walk for a half hour five days a week. Those taking the combined extracts averaged a 4.6-pound weight loss after just two weeks, dropped an average of 11.74 pounds total (3.7 times more than those on the placebo), and shaved an average 4.7 inches off their abdomen (2 times more than those on the placebo). The extract users also averaged an impressive 3.9 times greater drop in body mass index and a 2.2 times greater reduction in waist-to-hip ratio compared to the unlucky placebo group.

In a study at Western Geriatric Research Institute in Los Angeles, overweight patients took a regular dose of Caralluma or a placebo for four weeks. The participants were instructed not to change their daily activity pattern (exercise) or their food intake for four weeks before starting the trial and during the trial. Out of eighteen patients who took the Caralluma and completed the trial, fifteen lost weight. Eleven patients lost an average of six pounds, with the highest loss at nine pounds. The other four participants lost one to two pounds. Of the patients taking a placebo who completed the trial, three gained one pound each, one lost one pound, and the other two dropped out due to minor digestive upset.

General Recommendations

A high-potency multivitamin/-mineral provides a base of vitamins and minerals required for people on a restricted diet.

Take 100 to 300 mg of 5-hydroxytryptophan (5-HTP) three times daily; 5-HTP reduces carbohydrate cravings and improves satiety. *Note*: Do not take 5-HTP if you are currently using pharmaceutical antidepressants or antianxiety medications.

Studies show that pyruvate (pyruvate acid) may aid weight loss when combined with a low-fat diet and/or exercise.

L-carnitine is involved with burning fat as a fuel source for the cells. Take 500 to 1,000 mg three times daily.

Essential fatty acids are required to burn fat as fuel. Take 1 tablespoon of flaxseed oil or 3 grams of fish oil daily, along with 100 mg of GLA (gamma linoleic acid).

Supplementing 7-KETO (3-acetyl-7-oxo-dehydroepiandrosterone) has been shown in a study of overweight people to help with weight and fat loss. Take 100 mg twice daily.

Dandelion root (*Taraxacum officinale*) improves liver metabolism and detoxification, which may support weight loss. Take 300 mg or 2 ml with each meal.

Bladderwrack (*Fucus vesiculosus*) supports thyroid function. Use it if you have suboptimal thyroid activity. Take 100 mg or 1 ml twice daily.

Homeopathy

Pick the remedy that best matches your symptoms in this section. Take a 6x, 12x, 6C, 12C, or 30C potency twice daily for two weeks to see if there are any positive results. After you notice improvement, stop taking the remedy, unless symptoms return. Consultation with a homeopathic practitioner is advised.

Calcarea Carbonica is for people who tend to be flabby and chilly. The palms, the feet, and the back of the head sweat easily. They have a strong craving for eggs, sweets, and dairy products. They tend to feel easily overwhelmed.

Ignatia (*Ignatia amara*) is for highly sensitive people who use food to make themselves feel better. There is often a recent history of acute grief or an emotional trauma.

Pulsatilla (*Pulsatilla pratensis*) is helpful when there is a strong craving for sweets. The person gets warm easily and strongly desires the windows to be open or wants to be outside. There is a sense of sadness, with a desire to be consoled.

Staphysagria is for people with a history of abuse, leading to overeating as a way to deal with suppressed anger. The anger tends to build over time. They have a craving for sweets.

Acupressure

See pages 787–794 for information about pressure points and administering treatment.
- Conception Vessel 6 (CV6) stimulates digestion and increases your metabolism.
- Use Spleen 16 (Sp16) to return an out-of-control appetite to a more normal state.

Bodywork

Reflexology

See pages 804–805 for information about reflexology areas and how to work them.

Work the liver to increase metabolism and stimulate detoxification. For additional cleansing, work the colon.

Instead of eating when you're nervous, work the diaphragm and the solar plexus areas to calm down.

Aromatherapy

Bergamot blunts hunger pangs. For an immediate effect, hold the vial of oil directly under your nose and inhale.

Try using essential oils instead of sugar to lift your mood. Lavender, rose, geranium, and orange will make you feel more cheerful.

Stress Reduction

General Stress-Reduction Therapies

Every day, take some time out for deep breathing and visualization. Imagine yourself making healthful food choices and turning down less-nutritious offers. See yourself doing the things you'd like to do but can't because of your excess weight: running a mile, playing with your grandkids, even climbing a mountain.

Yoga, a technique that encourages control of the senses, will help you learn to handle stress without turning to the refrigerator. It's also a good gentle exercise for people who haven't been active for a while.

Stress can make you eat, but sticking to a weight-loss plan can be stressful itself. Find a couple of friends who will lend a sympathetic ear; it helps if they're also trying to lose weight. Or you could join a support group.

Other Recommendations

Exercise. It's more effective than dieting alone. But you don't have to run a marathon to reap the benefits of activity; in fact, it's far better for you to take a brisk walk every day than to engage in more strenuous activity once or twice a week. Overall, it is best to pick an exercise that you really enjoy. If you're very out of shape or have heart problems, contact your doctor before starting an exercise program. And whatever you're doing, ease into it gradually.

REFERENCES

Blankson, H., J. A. Stakkestad, H. Fagertun, et al. 2000. Conjugated linoleic acid reduces body fat mass in overweight and obese humans. *Journal of Nutrition* 130(12):2943–48.

Cangiano, C., F. Ceci, A. Cascino, et al. 1992. Eating behavior and adherence to dietary supplements in obese adult subjects treated with 5-hydroxytryptophan. *American Journal of Clinical Nutrition* 56(5):863–67.

Lau, F. C., et al. 2011. Efficacy and tolerability of Merastin: A randomized, double-blind, placebo-controlled study. *FASEB J* 25:(Meeting Abstract Supplement) 601.9. Presented at Experimental Biology 2011, Washington, DC. April 10, 2011. Program No. 601.9, Poster No. A278.

Lawrence, R., and S. Choudhary. 2004. Caralluma fimbriata in the treatment of obesity. Presented at the 12th Annual Congress on Anti-Aging Medicine, Las Vegas, NV, December 5.

Ngondi, J. L., et al. 2009. IGOB131, a novel seed extract of the West African plant *Irvingia gabonensis,* significantly reduces body weight and improves metabolic parameters in overweight humans in a randomized double-blind placebo controlled investigation. *Lipids in Health and Disease* 8:4–12.

Osteoporosis

In the United States, nearly 50 percent of all women between the ages of forty-five and seventy suffer from some degree of osteoporosis. This disorder, which translates literally as "porous bones," is so common that we tend to think of its effects—frailty, broken bones, back pain, a stooped posture, and the so-called dowager's hump—as the normal results of aging. In reality, osteoporosis is a condition brought on by faulty dietary and lifestyle habits. Studies of cultures that have more healthful lifestyles than Americans do find that its occurrence is much more rare.

Childhood, adolescence, and early adulthood are the prime opportunities for building healthy bones. Bones reach their greatest mass and density at around age thirty; after that, they begin to weaken. Some bone loss is entirely normal and not terribly worrisome, but when the process is accelerated, the bones turn frail and brittle. Unfortunately, the disorder rarely rings any warning bells until serious damage is already done. The first sign may be a minor fall or an accident that results in a broken bone, or back pain caused by a collapsed vertebra.

Researchers have found that there is a connection between a dysfunctional immune system and osteoporosis. A group of immune cells known as cytokines can initiate a type of inflammatory response that leads to bone breakdown. Fortunately, a healthful diet and lifestyle, hormone balance, and specific nutritional supplements, as described in this chapter, contribute to normal cytokine activity.

Hormone balance is critical for good bone density. A good example is a premenopausal woman who has her ovaries removed. Studies show that this can lead to a sudden drop in bone density, due to low estrogen and progesterone levels. Many hormones are important for bone-cell (osteoblast) activity, including estrogen, progesterone, testosterone, DHEA, growth hormone, and calcitonin. On the other hand, excessive levels of cortisol, thyroid, and parathyroid hormones can lead to bone loss.

Diet is important for strong bones. A healthy eating plan should include foods that are rich in bone-building minerals, such as green leafy vegetables, nuts and seeds, flax, soy, and fish. On the other hand, soda pop, caffeine, salt, and alcohol all contribute to bone breakdown when consumed in excess. Research has shown that a diet that tends toward alkalinity improves bone density.

One of the best ways to prevent bone loss or halt its progress is to engage in weight-bearing exercise. This stimulates bone-cell formation.

Many vitamins and minerals are required for healthy bones. Calcium is the obvious one, but several others, such as magnesium, vitamin D, boron, silicon, vitamin C, strontium, vitamin K, and others, play important roles in bone metabolism.

A combination of a good diet, exercise, and nutritional supplements is important for healthy bones. Exposure to sunlight is important as well. More severe cases of osteoporosis may require natural-hormone therapy and, in some cases, drug therapy.

SYMPTOMS

Osteoporosis is largely asymptomatic, but watch out for the following danger signs:

- A stooped posture
- Dowager's hump
- Sleeves and hems that used to fit but that now are too long
- Backache
- Easily broken bones

ROOT CAUSES

- Inactivity
- Poor diet
- Hormone imbalance
- Long-term use of certain medications (anticonvulsants, prednisone, heparin, methotrexate, lithium, isoniazid, furosemide [Lasix], antacids, chemotherapy, thyroid, and others)
- Smoking
- Hormone deficiencies
- Nutritional deficiencies
- Lack of sun exposure
- Eating disorders
- Prolonged stress
- Toxic metals
- Medical conditions (diabetes, Cushing's disease, homocystinemia, hyperthyroidism, malabsorption, and others)
- Heredity
- Acidic pH balance
- Chronic inflammation

Testing Techniques

The following tests help assess possible reasons for osteoporosis:

Immune system imbalance or disease—blood

Hormone testing (thyroid, DHEA, cortisol, testosterone, IGF-1, estrogen, progesterone)—saliva, blood, or urine

Intestinal permeability—urine

Vitamin and mineral analysis (especially magnesium, calcium, vitamin K, vitamin D3)—blood, hair

Toxic metals—urine or hair

Digestive function and microbe/parasite/candida testing—stool analysis

Food and environmental allergies/sensitivities—blood, electrodermal

Bone resorption (pyridinium and deoxypyridinium)—urine

TREATMENT

Diet

Recommended Food

Osteoporosis is less common in cultures that eat unprocessed foods. Since osteoporosis is caused in part by inflammation, consume anti-inflammatory foods such as vegetables, fruits, nuts, seeds, fish rich in omega-3 (such as wild salmon), sardines, and lean poultry. Avoid inflammatory foods such as caffeine, alcohol, soda, and other simple sugars.

Fermented soy foods and protein powders have been shown to increase bone formation. Sea vegetables high in calcium are also helpful and have become more readily available. Consider wakame (½ cup contains 1,700 mg), agar (¼ cup contains 1,000 mg), nori (½ cup contains 600 mg), and kombu (¼ cup contains 500 mg). It should be noted that sardines with bones are a good source not only of omega-3 fatty acids but also of calcium, with 500 mg per ½ cup.

Vitamin K is important for proper bone formation. This nutrient is abundant in

The gold standard for testing your bone density is an X-ray known as the DEXA (dual energy X-ray absorptiometry) scan. Yet by the time this test shows a decrease in bone density, you may have had a significant loss of bone. A good test to monitor current bone metabolism is a urine test that measures bone breakdown. When bone (and cartilage) breaks down, it releases two substances known as deoxypyridinium and pyridinium, which are excreted in the urine. The rate of excretion parallels the degree of bone turnover. A high level signifies that there is likely too much bone breakdown, which is imbalanced with bone building. This test is helpful as a way to assess the protocol currently being used to prevent or treat your osteoporosis.

Swiss researchers looked at the effects of potassium citrate supplements on blood pH and bone density. Published in the *Journal of the American Society of Nephrology*, the study involved 161 postmenopausal women, average age fifty-nine, who were known to have low bone mass. One group of women received tablets of potassium citrate—which is slightly alkaline—at a daily dose of 30 millimoles (1,173 mg). The other group got an equal dose of potassium chloride, which is nonalkaline. Bone-mineral-density (BMD) measurements were performed at the start of the study, after six months, and after one year on the supplements. At the end of the study, the women taking potassium chloride showed an average bone-density loss at the lower spine of 1 percent—a significant loss. However, the group taking potassium citrate had a 1 percent increase in BMD at the lower spine, plus an increase in density of almost 2 percent at the hip. This group also excreted less calcium in the urine. We recommend people eat a diet rich in potassium as found in fruits and vegetables.

dark-green leafy vegetables such as lettuce, spinach, and broccoli. The form in these foods is vitamin K1.

Vitamin K2 is also effective for bone formation. The best food source of vitamin K2 is natto (fermented soybeans) and, to a lesser degree, fermented cheeses (the type with holes, such as Swiss and Jarlsberg), butter, beef liver, chicken, and egg yolks.

Eat a pH-balanced diet rich in vegetables and fruits.

Food to Avoid

One reason Westerners have such a high rate of osteoporosis is their consumption of foods that are high in sugar. Eliminate sugar, refined grains, and soda pop from your diet. Higher blood glucose and insulin levels with diabetes or insulin resistance often benefit from high protein and reduced simple-carbohydrate intake. The lower one's insulin level, the lower the inflammatory response.

Reduce your intake of red meat. A high intake may contribute to bone loss in some individuals.

A high salt intake is linked to bone loss. Do not eat processed foods, which are usually loaded with salt, and never add conventional table salt to your meals.

Moderate your use of caffeine and alcohol as they contribute to bone loss.

It may surprise you to learn that countries where people drink the most milk are also those with the highest rates of osteoporosis. This may be due to the fact that lactose intolerance and casein (protein found in cow's milk) allergy are very common and lead to malabsorption. Also, calcium from cow's milk is not well absorbed, at a rate of 25 percent. Milk products lead to other health problems as well, so don't rely on them as a source of calcium. Unsweetened, cultured yogurt is an exception.

Calcium Content

Wakame (sea vegetable), ½ cup—1,700 mg	Almonds, 1 cup—300 mg
Agar (sea vegetable), ¼ cup—1,000 mg	Spinach, 1 cup—280 mg
Nori (sea vegetable), ½ cup—600 mg	Yogurt, 1 cup—270 mg
Kombu (sea vegetable), ¼ cup—500 mg	Sesame seeds, ½ cup—250 mg
Sardines with bones, ½ cup—500 mg	Kale, 1 cup—200 mg
Collard greens, 1 cup—355 mg	Broccoli, 1 cup—180 mg
Tempeh, 1 cup—340 mg	Tofu, 1 cup—150 mg
Milk, 1 cup—300 mg	Walnuts, ¼ cup—70 mg
Calcium-enriched rice milk or soymilk, 1 cup—300 mg	Black beans, 1 cup—60 mg
	Lentils, 1 cup—50 mg

R̲X̲ **Super Seven Prescriptions—Osteoporosis**

Super Prescription #1 Calcium

Take 500 to 600 mg twice daily in divided doses of well-absorbed calcium complexes, such as citrate, citrate-malate, chelate, or hydroxyapatite. Calcium is the main mineral that composes bone.

Super Prescription #2 Magnesium

Take 250 to 350 mg twice daily in divided doses. Magnesium is required for proper calcium metabolism, through parathyroid-hormone production and vitamin D activation. Some researchers believe that it is as important as calcium. *Note*: Reduce the dosage if loose stools occur.

Super Prescription #3 Vitamin D3

Take 5,000 IU daily with a meal if you have osteoporosis (or more if your doctor is monitoring your level with a blood test). This vitamin improves intestinal calcium absorption and reduces the urinary excretion of calcium.

Super Prescription #4 Vitamin K

Take 2 to 10 mg daily and up to 500 mcg daily for preventative purposes. Vitamin K is needed to form the protein osteocalcin, a substance that attracts calcium into the bone matrix. Low levels of vitamin K are associated with osteoporosis and fractures. *Note:* Do not use if you are taking blood-thinning medications.

Super Prescription #5 Strontium

Take 680 mg daily. Studies show strontium improves bone density.

Super Prescription #6 Essential fatty acids

Take 4 grams of fish oil daily, along with 3,000 mg of evening primrose oil (*Oenothera biennis*). Studies show that these essential fatty acids improve calcium absorption and deposition into the bone.

Super Prescription #7 Silicon

Take 50 to 20 mg daily. Silicon is a mineral that is involved in collagen and calcification.

General Recommendations

High-potency multivitamin provides a base of nutrients required for healthy bones. Take as directed on the container.

Boron is a mineral that activates vitamin D3 and supports estrogen levels for effective calcium metabolism. Take 3 to 5 mg daily.

Vitamin C is used to manufacture collagen, an important component of bones. Take 500 to 1,000 mg twice daily.

Some, but not all, studies of ipriflavone have shown this supplement to increase bone density when combined with calcium, vitamin D3, or hormone replacement. Take 600 mg daily with food. *Note*: Have your lymphocyte (a type of white blood cell) levels monitored by your doctor when using this supplement, as one study found that it lowered the levels in 29 out of 132 women.

A twelve-year study of more than seventy-seven thousand women found that those who drank more than fourteen glasses of milk a week had 45 percent more hip fractures, as compared to women who consumed one glass a week or less.

According to a number of studies, including a review in the *American Journal of Cardiology*, 30 to 50 percent of the general US population has a vitamin D deficiency.

A study in the *American Journal of Clinical Nutrition* reported that a low intake of vitamin K was associated with an increased risk of hip fracture. The data from the study came from reviewing the diets of more than seventy-two thousand women. Studies have also shown that vitamin K supplementation improves bone density.

A study in the *Journal of Aging* found that the combination of the essential fatty acids EPA (fish oil) and GLA (evening primrose oil [*Oenothera biennis*]), along with 600 mg of calcium, improved bone density in senior women. During the first eighteen months, the lumbar-spine density remained the same with the treatment group but decreased 3.2 percent overall in the placebo group. Thigh-bone density increased 1.3 percent in the treatment group, but decreased 2.1 percent in the placebo group. During the second period of eighteen months, with all patients receiving the essential fatty acid combination, lumbar-spine density increased 3.1 percent in patients who remained on active treatment, and 2.3 percent in patients who switched from placebo to active treatment. Thigh-bone density in the latter group showed an increase of 4.7 percent.

Zinc is required for enzymatic reactions that build bone. Take a daily total of 30 mg, along with 2 to 3 mg of copper.

Manganese is involved with bone calcification. Take 15 to 30 mg daily.

Vitamins B12, B6, and folic acid prevent the buildup of homocysteine, a by-product of protein metabolism that can cause osteoporosis. See the Cardiovascular Disease section.

Betaine hydrochloric acid improves stomach acid levels for digestion and absorption. Take 1 to 3 capsules with each meal. *Note*: Do not use if you have an active ulcer.

A greens formula that contains super green foods, such as chlorella, spirulina, and others, has an alkalinizing effect and is rich in minerals. Take as directed on the container.

Soy protein powder has been shown to protect against bone loss. Take 40 grams daily, containing 90 mg of isoflavones.

Strontium is a nutrient shown to be helpful in increasing bone density when combined with calcium. Take 340 to 680 mg daily.

Homeopathy

Pick the remedy that best matches your symptoms in this section. Take a 6x, 12x, 6C, 12C, or 30C potency twice daily for four weeks to see if there are any positive results. After you notice improvement, stop taking the remedy, unless symptoms return.

Homeopathy is best used in conjunction with the modifications in diet, lifestyle, and other areas covered in this chapter. Although you cannot "feel" bone-density improvement, symptoms such as bone aching or pain or slow healing of fractures can be observed. Consultation with a homeopathic practitioner is advised.

Calcarea Carbonica is a remedy for people with signs of calcium imbalance, such as osteoporosis, aching bones, muscle cramps, and swollen joints. People who require this remedy are generally chilly and flabby and feel worse in the cold and the dampness. They are easily fatigued and get overwhelmed. They crave sweets, milk, and eggs.

Calcarea Phosphorica is a good remedy for osteoporosis or fractures. This remedy stimulates bone building. Symptoms of neck and back pain and stiffness, which feel worse from cold drafts, are often present. Calcium deposits may occur, even with bone loss. People who require this remedy often have a feeling of discontent and a strong desire for travel or a change. Calcarea Phosphorica is a remedy that can be used for bone support even if you don't have any particular symptoms.

Phosphorus is a remedy for weak bones or fractures that heal slowly. People who require this remedy tend to be tall, thin, and very social and suggestible. They have a strong craving for ice-cold drinks.

Silica (*Silicea*) is for people who have poor bone density and tend to be very thin. People who need this remedy are often nervous, easily fatigued, and chilly and have a low resistance to infection.

Symphytum is a specific remedy for healing fractures and reducing their pain more quickly.

Acupressure

See pages 787–794 for information about pressure points and administering treatment.

- To increase your ability to absorb nutrients (including calcium), work Stomach 36 (St36). With regular practice, your digestion will improve, and you'll find that you have more energy than before.
- To reduce stress, work Lung 1 (Lu1) on a daily basis.
- If you have pain, work Large Intestine 4 (LI4). Do not use this point if you are pregnant.
- For pain in the ankles, use Spleen 5 (Sp5) and Kidney 3 (K3).
- Governing Vessel 24.5 (GV24.5) will help bring about hormonal balance.

Bodywork

Massage
Massage is a good wellness measure, especially for the elderly. Don't let fear of pain or injury prevent you from receiving massage treatment; instead, find a reputable therapist with experience in degenerative diseases.

Reflexology
See pages 804–805 for information about reflexology areas and how to work them.

If you have osteoporosis, reflexology can help ease pain. Be careful, however. Do not treat the foot or the hand roughly or with too much pressure.

Work the areas corresponding to the vertebrae; the hip, the back, and the sciatic areas; and the lower back.

Aromatherapy

Black pepper and rosemary both have warming qualities that soothe aching bones and joints. Use them in a massage, a lotion, or a bath.

If bone loss leads to stress, try any of several oils that have a relaxing, uplifting effect. You may want to start with lavender, geranium, or rose; use them in any preparation that suits you.

Stress Reduction

General Stress-Reduction Therapies
It can be difficult to handle the restricted motion and the fear that often accompany osteoporosis. If you're in the early or middle stages of the disorder, try taking a yoga or Pilates class from an experienced instructor. In addition to relieving your stress, you'll strengthen your bone and muscle mass. You'll also improve your balance, which reduces your chances of falling and breaking a bone.

Other Recommendations

- Undertake a regular weight-bearing exercise. Although swimming and cycling are excellent for cardiovascular toning, they are not as aggressive for building bone mass. Instead, try an aerobic workout with gentle impact (walking is a good idea). Then supplement that exercise with weight lifting. You don't have to join a gym and pump heavy iron—even very small hand weights can make a real difference in bone strength. If you've never lifted weights before, you should make an appointment with a trainer to get yourself started.

- Don't smoke or expose yourself to secondhand smoke. Smoking makes bones brittle and weak and is also a cause of many other "age-related" diseases.
- Natural hormone replacement should be considered if you have moderate to severe osteoporosis, especially if testing shows your levels to be deficient. Work with a doctor who is knowledgeable in natural hormones. Important ones include estrogen, progesterone, testosterone, DHEA, and growth hormone.

REFERENCES

Feskanich, D. et al. 1997. Milk, dietary calcium, and bone fractures in women: A 12 year prospective study. *American Journal of Public Health* 87:992–97.

Feskanich, D., P. Weber, W. C. Willett, et al. 1999. Vitamin K intake and hip fractures in women: A prospective study. *American Journal of Clinical Nutrition* 69(1):74–79.

Iwamoto, I., S. Kosha, S. Noguchi, et al. 1999. A longitudinal study of the effect of vitamin K2 on bone mineral density in postmenopausal women: A comparative study with vitamin D3 and estrogen-progestin therapy. *Maturitas* 31:161–64.

Jehle, S., et al. American Society of Nephrology 43rd Annual Meeting. Abstract FC223. Presented November 19, 2010.

Kruger, M. C., H. Coetzer, R. de Winter, et al. 1998. Calcium, gamma-linolenic acid and eicosapentaenoic acid supplementation in senile osteoporosis. *Aging* (Milano) 10(5):385–94.

Lee, J. H., et al. 2008. Vitamin D deficiency: an important, common, and easily treatable cardiovascular risk factor? *Journal of the American College of Cardiology* 52:1949–56.

Shiraki, M., Y. Shiraki, C. Aoki, and M. Miura. 2000. Vitamin K2 (menadione) effectively prevents fractures and sustains lumbar bone mineral density in osteoporosis. *Journal of Bone and Mineral Research* 15:515–21.

Parasites (Intestinal)

Microorganisms naturally inhabit and move through the body. Some are harmless, while others cause sickness. Infections can occur when parasites make their homes in your skin, gastrointestinal tract, lungs, liver, and other organs. Parasites require a host (e.g., human cells) to live and thrive.

Parasitic infections were once thought of as a problem that existed mainly in underdeveloped countries. After all, diarrheal disease (from parasites and bacteria) is the greatest worldwide cause of death. Global travel has been a major contributor to the spread of parasitic infections in North America. Contaminated water and food are also major contributors. In addition, better diagnostic techniques have provided a more accurate identification of parasites and have led researchers to conclude that parasitic infections are much more common than previously thought. One laboratory that specializes in stool analysis states that "almost 30 percent of specimens examined are positive for a parasite."

Diarrhea and abdominal pain are the most common symptoms of a parasitic infection. However, in many cases of a parasite infection, these symptoms may not be present. A whole list of symptoms and conditions could be related to a parasitic infection. Examples include loss of appetite, fatigue, constipation, depressed immunity, food allergy, fever, chills, heartburn, stomach pain, inflammatory bowel disease, lower back pain, itchy anus, rash and skin itching, hives, weight loss, arthritis, bloody stools, mucus in the stool, colitis, Crohn's disease, flatulence, foul-smelling stools, malabsorption, rectal bleeding, mood changes (depression, irritability), and vomiting.

Parasites interfere with the normal activities of the cells they infect, which may lead to symptoms and disease. The secretions released by a parasite can trigger a bodily response in which the immune system attacks its own tissues. This is known as an autoimmune reaction. Examples include rheumatoid arthritis and Crohn's disease. Not all parasites are necessarily harmful. Some parasites live symbiotically in the digestive tract. It is thought that certain parasites become a problem only when the environment of the body changes. For example, dysbiosis—the imbalance between friendly and potentially harmful bacteria in the digestive tract—can lead to certain parasites becoming pathogenic (disease causing). The nutritional status of a person, as well as a compromised immune system, dictates whether a parasite can become a problem.

Parasites are commonly transmitted through food that is contaminated with fecal matter (e.g., from food preparers who do not wash their hands after going to the restroom), through waste, and through the water supply.

There are many different types of parasites. Following are some of the more common ones in North America.

Blastocystis hominis. This parasite is detected in a high number of stool tests. Researchers are unclear whether it is a pathogen, because many people carry it but do not have symptoms. However, it can cause various digestive symptoms, such as cramps, nausea, weight loss, bloating, and others. It is also associated with conditions like irritable bowel syndrome, chronic fatigue, and arthritis.

Dientamoeba fragilis. Symptoms of this parasite, which resides in the large intestine, include diarrhea and abdominal pain.

E. histolytica. This amoeba is linked to diarrhea and a variety of digestive symptoms.

Giardia. This is one of the most common parasites found in humans. It is transmitted through water, in food, between children in day-care centers, via a fecal-oral route, or through sexual intercourse. Epidemics from contaminated streams and community water systems occur every year in the United States.

Cryptosporidium. This is transmitted through contaminated food and water and from person-to-person contact. Explosive diarrhea is a common symptom. This parasite is of particular concern for children who are HIV-positive, as their immune systems may not be able to fight off the parasite, making it a life-threatening condition.

Ascaris lumbricoides. This parasite causes the most common human worm infection in the world. Infection is common in the southeastern United States. In children, it can cause abdominal cramps and malnutrition. Fecal-oral transmission often occurs via uncooked or unwashed vegetables.

Hookworm. Hookworm is not as common in the United States as in other parts of the world, yet cases do occur. It usually causes no symptoms, although a skin itch may be present. Acute symptoms can include abdominal pain, diarrhea, weight loss, anemia, and many others. These worms can live up to ten years. They are transmitted via direct contact with soil containing the eggs of hookworms.

Strongyloides. The eggs of these worms can penetrate the skin and migrate to the lungs and the intestines. Most infections occur via the fecal-oral route. Infected people may be asymptomatic or may have various digestive problems. Liver and nervous system infection can also be a serious problem.

Trichinosis. Infection occurs from eating undercooked or processed meat. There may be no symptoms, or else nausea, abdominal cramps, fever, and muscle pain (larvae can invade muscle tissue) can occur.

The conventional treatment focuses on antiparasitic medications to eradicate the infection. Toxicity and side effects vary for each medication.

The first step in treating a parasitic infection is to get a proper diagnosis. This is mainly dependent on a stool analysis. We highly recommend using a laboratory that specializes in comprehensive parasitology testing. Many of the stool tests done by clinics are not sensitive enough to pick up all of the different forms of parasites. Certain blood tests by your doctor can also help to pinpoint a diagnosis. In some cases, we treat patients for a parasite infection when they have the symptoms and the history that match a parasite infection, even though lab testing does not show a positive result. Some parasitic infections are hard to detect, but when diagnosis is uncertain, they should be treated. Natural therapies work well and should be used for a minimum of two months. One standard that many natural health practitioners follow is to treat for one additional month after the symptoms of a parasite infection have cleared. In some cases, conventional antiparasitic medication may also be required. Please note that natural treatment of parasitic infections should be done under the guidance of a knowledgeable health-care practitioner or doctor. Pregnant women should not follow the parasitic protocol in this section.

SYMPTOMS

- Loss of appetite
- Fatigue
- Constipation
- Depressed immunity
- Food allergy
- Fever
- Chills
- Heartburn
- Stomach pain
- Inflammatory bowel disease
- Colitis
- Lower back pain
- Crohn's disease
- Itchy anus

- Flatulence
- Rash and skin itching
- Foul-smelling stools
- Hives
- Malabsorption
- Weight loss
- Rectal bleeding
- Arthritis
- Mood changes (depression, irritability)
- Bloody stools
- Mucus in stool
- Vomiting

Surprising Fact: Approximately 25 percent of the world's population is infected with hookworms.

Surprising Fact: It is estimated that more than one billion people are infected with ascariasis worldwide, of whom twenty thousand die each year.

ROOT CAUSES

- Contaminated food or water
- Dysbiosis (imbalanced gut flora)
- A weakened immune system

Testing Techniques

The following tests help assess a parasite infection:

Immune-system imbalance or disease—blood

Parasite testing—stool analysis and blood work

TREATMENT

Diet

Recommended Food

Fresh garlic, ginger, and onions are excellent as prepared foods, because they have been shown to have antiparasitic effects.

Raw pumpkin seeds kill worms and parasites. They can be ground up if desired. Consume ¼ cup to ½ cup daily with 8 ounces of water.

Papaya juice has anti-worm effects.

Food to Avoid

Sugar products should be reduced or avoided to optimize the health of your immune system.

Make sure that all fruits and vegetables are washed properly. Meat and seafood products need to be thoroughly cooked. Avoid giving raw seafood to children.

℞ Super Seven Prescriptions—Parasites

Super Prescription #1 Black walnut (*Juglans nigra*)

Adults should take 30 drops or 250 mg three times daily. This herb has a long history of use by herbalists and naturopathic doctors for the treatment of parasites.

Super Prescription #2 Wormwood (*Artemisia absinthium*)

Take 20 drops or 200 mg three times daily with meals. Wormwood is a common herbal therapy for parasites and is generally used in a combination formula.

Super Prescription #3 Coptis (gold thread)

Take 20 drops or 200 mg three times daily with meals. This Chinese herb has antiparasitic effects.

Super Prescription #4 Oregano oil (*Origanum vulgare*)

Take 500 mg of the capsule form four times daily or as directed on the container. Oregano oil has powerful antibacterial and antiparasitic effects.

Super Prescription #5 Grapefruit seed extract

Take as directed on the container for a powerful antiparasitic effect.

> **Super Prescription #6 Goldenseal (*Hydrastis canadensis*)**
> Take 30 drops or 300 mg four times daily. Goldenseal helps fight infections in the digestive tract.
>
> ---
>
> **Super Prescription #7 Ginger (*Zingiber officinale*) root**
> Take 500 mg, 20 drops of the tincture, or 1 cup of fresh tea four times daily. Ginger has antiparasitic effects and reduces intestinal bloating and cramping.

General Recommendations

Peppermint (*Mentha piperita*) has been shown to be effective against some parasites. Take 2 ml or drink a fresh cup of tea four times daily.

Take a probiotic containing at least four billion active organisms twice daily, thirty minutes after meals. It supplies friendly bacteria such as *Lactobacillus acidophilus* and *bifidus*.

A combination parasitic homeopathic remedy helps stimulate the immune system to fight off an infection. Take as directed on the container.

Propolis has been shown to fight certain parasitic infections, such as giardia. Take 500 mg or 30 drops four times daily.

Rhubarb (*Rheum officinale*) is often used in parasite formulas as a stimulating laxative to help clear the intestines of a parasite. Take as directed on the container.

Homeopathy

Pick the remedy that best matches your symptoms in this section. For acute parasitic infections, take a 30C potency four times daily. For chronic infection, take a 6x, 12x, 6C, 12C, or 30C twice daily for two weeks to see if there are any positive results. After you notice improvement, stop taking the remedy, unless symptoms return. Consultation with a homeopathic practitioner is advised.

Cina is a specific remedy for pinworm or threadworm infections. The child is very irritable, does not want to be touched, and picks at the nose and the rectum. The child's appetite is very great. There may be pale, dark circles under the eyes. The child grinds his or her teeth at night.

Filix Mas is a specific remedy for tapeworms. The person has swollen glands, an itchy nose, and dark circles around the eyes and feels irritable and anxious.

Natrum Phosphoricum is a remedy that can be used for all types of worms. The person has signs of overacidity, such as belching and heartburn. There is often a yellow, creamy coating on the tongue.

Sabadilla is for a person with pinworms or tapeworms, characterized by itching of the rectum that alternates with itching of the nose or the ears.

Spigelia is a homeopathic remedy for worms. The person has an itchy rectum and pain around the navel. Bad breath is common.

Teucrium is a good remedy for pinworms, threadworms, and round worms. The child has itching and a crawling sensation in the nose and the rectum and feels very irritable and nervous.

Bodywork

Chinese herbal therapy and moxibustion treatments from a qualified practitioner can be helpful in the treatment of parasites.

REFERENCES

Great Smokies Diagnostic Laboratory Functional Assessment Resource Manual. 1998. Asheville, N.C.

Parkinson's Disease

Parkinson's disease is a chronic, degenerative disorder of the nervous system, in which voluntary movement is impaired or lost. Although the disease may come to affect your entire body, it most noticeably weakens your ability to control motions categorized as semivoluntary: keeping your jaw in place so that the mouth stays closed; swinging your arms as you walk; moving your tongue so that your speech is clear and precise. Parkinson's disease rarely affects people under sixty years of age, and men are about 30 percent more likely to develop it than women are.

Although muscle movement is an extraordinarily complex process that involves millions of nerve cells, this disease pinpoints relatively small sections of the brain, called the basal cell ganglia. When the nerve cells there begin to deteriorate, they create a chemical upset that can ultimately render the whole body disabled. In a healthy brain, two neurotransmitters, acetylcholine and dopamine, work in tandem to regulate muscle actions. Acetylcholine helps muscles contract—without it, we'd be limp, unable to stand or even sit down—while dopamine tempers acetylcholine's effect. But the brain deterioration of Parkinson's throws this chemical duo off balance, reducing the quantities of dopamine and resulting in muscles that are too tightly contracted.

The symptoms of Parkinson's develop gradually, usually over a period of ten or fifteen years. The first sign is usually a tremor in one hand, which disappears when you move the hand or go to sleep. As the disorder progresses, the trembling is more pronounced and spreads to other parts of the body, usually the arms, the legs, and the head. The arms and the legs, in addition to shaking, may feel heavy and rigid, and you gradually lose the ability to write smoothly and speak clearly. As your muscles tighten, you may have trouble moving your bowels regularly. You may shuffle as you walk, with your head, neck, and shoulders hunched over and your arms held to your sides. One or both hands develop the characteristic "pill-rolling" movement, in which the thumb and the forefinger rub against each other, one making a clockwise circular motion, the other moving counterclockwise. Parkinson's often keeps the facial muscles in a nearly constant state of contraction; the face may take on a mask-like appearance, with staring, unblinking eyes and a drooling mouth. Eventually, everyday tasks become difficult to manage. Simply getting out of a chair or speaking a clear sentence may be impossible. Although the muscular debility in these advanced stages is overwhelming, the person's mind is unaffected, and the affected body parts usually don't hurt or even feel numb.

Scientists still haven't determined exactly what causes the nerve cells of the basal cell ganglia to deteriorate, resulting in low dopamine levels, but we can base some tentative theories on several clues. For one, the incidence of Parkinson's is rising at an extraordinary rate: the percentage of cases in the United States has increased tenfold since the 1970s. This soaring rate suggests that the disease is strongly influenced

A study published in the *International Journal of Epidemiology* that analyzed data concerning pesticide use in California counties reported that there was an increased mortality rate from Parkinson's disease in counties that used agricultural pesticides. The same study also reported that California growers use approximately 250 million pounds of pesticides annually, accounting for a quarter of all pesticides used in the United States.

by environmental factors. Finally, medications—both prescription and illicit—and environmental toxins are known to induce tremors in individuals. Given these facts, it seems likely that a poisoned body system greatly increases the risk of incurring Parkinson's. Bodies can be made toxic from exposure to heavy metals, carbon monoxide, pesticides, insecticides, and drugs; they can also be poisoned by a poor diet or allergic responses to food. Finally, free radicals, which destroy or damage cells, are a suspect in any degenerative disease.

The most common therapy for this disease is levodopa (L-dopa), which is sold in the United States under the brand name Sinemet. Levodopa is taken up by the brain and changed into dopamine. For some patients, it significantly improves mobility and allows them to function more normally. As Parkinson's disease worsens over time, larger doses must be taken. The drug can have debilitating side effects for some patients, such as involuntary movements, tics, and hallucinations. Carbidopa, the other active ingredient (besides levodopa) in the drug Sinemet, works to prolong the effects of levodopa and help reduce its side effects. Carbidopa works by slowing the conversion of levodopa to dopamine in the bloodstream so that more of it reaches the brain. Another common drug is Comtan (entacapone), which has the same effect as carbidopa when taken along with levodopa. It blocks a key enzyme that is responsible for breaking down levodopa before it reaches the brain. Similarly, the drug deprenyl (Eldepryl) can enhance and prolong the levodopa response by delaying the breakdown of levodopa-formed dopamine. Other medications such as Parlodel (bromocriptine), Requip (ropinirole), Permax (pergolide), and Mirapex (pramipexole dihydrocholoride) work directly on cells of the substantia nigra in the brain in a way that imitates dopamine. Still other drugs like Artane (trihexyphenidyl), Symmetrel (amantadine), and Cogentin (benztropine) are used to help improve tremors. The most common side effects of drugs for Parkinson's disease are hallucinations, mental confusion, and dyskinesia. Surgery is generally used as a last resort. This involves destroying certain parts of the brain that are overactive in this disease. A less invasive option than destroying certain brain tissues is deep brain stimulation, where a thin electrode is implanted into the brain to block signals that cause symptoms of Parkinson's disease, especially tremors.

If you've been diagnosed with Parkinson's, you should be under the care of an experienced neurologist. He or she will usually want to place you on medications that reduce the symptoms of the disease. Sometimes these drugs are highly effective, but they almost always have strong side effects, so it's important to choose a doctor who listens to your concerns and helps you make informed decisions about the medications or the procedures you try. You should also support your body with good nutrition and take up a cleansing regime to rid yourself of possible toxins. Specific supplements, such as coenzyme Q10, should also be highly considered. In addition, holistic doctors report impressive results with intravenous glutathione therapy.

SYMPTOMS

- Tremors
- Rigid or heavy-feeling arms and legs
- A "pill-rolling" motion of the hand and the thumb
- Constipation
- Difficulty speaking
- A shuffling gait, with the arms close to the body
- A stooped posture

- A masklike facial expression
- Drooling
- Eventually, an inability to perform most voluntary and semivoluntary movements

ROOT CAUSES

There are no definitive causes known for Parkinson's disease. Suspect causes or aggravating factors may include:

- Insecticides, pesticides, and herbicides
- Inflammatory brain disorder
- Free radicals
- Heavy metals
- Poor nutrition
- Carbon-monoxide poisoning
- Food allergies

Testing Techniques

The following tests help assess possible reasons for Parkinson's disease:

Hormone testing (thyroid, DHEA, cortisol, testosterone, IGF-1, estrogen, progesterone)—saliva, blood, or urine

Intestinal permeability—urine

Detoxification profile—urine

Vitamin and mineral analysis (especially CoQ10)—blood

Digestive function and microbe/parasite/candida testing—stool analysis

Food and environmental allergies/sensitivities—blood, electrodermal

Toxic metals—hair or urine analysis

Pesticides and other environmental toxins—urine or blood

TREATMENT

Diet

Recommended Food

Studies have found that eating most of the day's protein intake at dinner and keeping protein levels low earlier in the day is helpful. This type of diet should be supervised by a health-care professional.

Raw foods (fruits, vegetables, nuts, and seeds) are high in fiber, which will keep you regular, and contain antioxidants that fight free-radical damage. Follow a diet that is composed of 50 to 75 percent raw, organic foods. If you can't find or afford organic products, make sure to wash everything in clean, quality water before eating.

When you do eat protein, focus on beans, legumes, soy products, or fish (from a clean water source). *Note*: The consumption of beans has been found to lower the risk of Parkinson's disease.

Use cold-pressed oils in salad dressings. They're high in vitamin E, a powerful antioxidant that's important in the prevention and the treatment of Parkinson's disease.

Fresh vegetable juices are excellent for their mineral content.

Eat live unsweetened yogurt or another cultured product every day. The "friendly" bacteria in cultured foods will help your digestive system to work smoothly.

Drink a glass of clean, quality water every two waking hours. Clean, quality—not tap—water will flush toxins and other impurities from your body and will also lend general support to every body system.

Food to Avoid

It has been observed that a high percentage of people with Parkinson's have an overabundance of protein in their diets. Many patients who stop eating animal meats have noted an improvement in muscle control and coordination.

Do not eat processed or junk food, which contains high levels of chemicals and other toxins. Avoid artificial sweeteners and preservatives that are known as "excitotoxins." These include aspartame and monosodium glutamate.

Avoid alcohol, caffeine, and sugar, as they can disrupt neurological function. Overeating leads to a dangerous number of free radicals in your body. It's never a good idea to stuff yourself at mealtimes, but people with Parkinson's should try to keep caloric intake low, while maintaining an excellent nutritional status. Following the recommendations to avoid animal meats and processed food will go a long way toward keeping your calorie count down.

Food allergies are a possible aggravator of Parkinson's disease. Read the Food Allergies section, and follow the elimination diet there. If you feel better after abstaining from certain foods, keep them out of your diet.

> In a trial of people with early Parkinson's disease, the combination of vitamins C (750 mg four times daily) and E (800 IU four times daily) was able to delay the need for drug therapy (i.e., L-dopa) by an average of about two and a half years, when compared with people not taking the vitamins.

℞ Super Seven Prescriptions—Parkinson's Disease

Note: These supplements should be used under the supervision of a doctor.

Super Prescription #1 Coenzyme Q10
Take 1,200 mg daily. Coenzyme Q10 is an antioxidant that has been shown in one preliminary study to reduce the progression of early-stage Parkinson's disease.

Super Prescription #2 Vitamin C
Take 750 mg four times daily. Vitamin C is an important antioxidant that prevents free-radical damage.

Super Prescription #3 Vitamin E-complex
Take 800 IU four times daily. Vitamin E (tocopherols and tocotrienols) is an important antioxidant that prevents free-radical damage.

Super Prescription #4 Glutathione
Take 250 mg three times daily. This antioxidant prevents cellular damage.

Super Prescription #5 Essential fatty acids
Take a fish oil product that will provide at least 1 gram of DHA and EPA daily. Flaxseed oil and evening primrose oil (*Oenothera biennis*) are additional options.

Super Prescription #6 Nicotinamide adenine dinucleotide (NADH)
Take 5 mg twice daily. Preliminary research has found that this supplement improves brain function and reduces symptoms in people with Parkinson's disease.

Super Prescription #7 N-acetylcysteine (NAC)

Take 500 mg three times daily. NAC increases levels of glutathione, an important antioxidant.

General Recommendations

Ginkgo biloba improves blood flow and has potent antioxidant properties. Take a standardized extract containing 24 percent flavone glycosides, and take 60 to 80 mg twice daily.

Milk thistle (*Silybum marianum*) is another detoxifying herb that allows your liver to throw off accumulated toxins and prevents damage from pharmaceutical treatment. Take 250 mg three times daily of an 80 to 85 percent silymarin extract.

Green tea (*Camellia sinensis*) contains a rich source of antioxidants and substances that assist detoxification. Drink the organic tea regularly (2 cups or more daily), or take 500 to 1,500 mg of the capsule form.

Calcium and magnesium are important for nervous system function. Take 1,000 mg of calcium and 500 mg of magnesium.

Calming teas can help you deal with the stress produced by a degenerative disorder. Try passionflower (*Passiflora incarnata*), skullcap, or valerian.

Consult with a holistic doctor for intravenous glutathione treatment. Glutathione is one of the body's most potent antioxidants, and some doctors report benefit for people with Parkinson's disease from this nontoxic therapy.

Homeopathy

Pick the remedy that best matches your symptoms in this section. Take a 6x, 12x, 6C, or 12C potency twice daily for two weeks to see if there are any positive results. After you notice improvement, stop taking the remedy, unless symptoms return. Consultation with a homeopathic practitioner is advised.

Argentum Nitricum is for people who lose their balance and have uncoordinated movement as early symptoms. Tremors of the hands may prevent them from writing. It is also helpful for tremors that appear periodically.

Causticum is for slow paralysis, with the right side being more affected, and hand tremors that are worse when writing.

Gelsemium (*Gelsemium sempervirens*) is for tremors, difficulty controlling the tongue and the eyes, and a staggering walk.

Helleborus is for very slow speech. The patient appears to be in a deep fog.

Mercurius Solubilis or Vivus is helpful if your hands are trembling so much that it is difficult to eat or drink. You have slow or stammering speech.

Natrum Muriaticum is for hand tremors that occur when you write. You constantly nod your head and drop things easily. You suppress your emotions.

Plumbum is for progressive paralysis and muscle wasting. Cramping accompanies the paralysis.

A placebo-controlled, multicenter clinical trial led by Clifford Shults, M.D., of the University of California, San Diego School of Medicine, looked at a total of eighty people with Parkinson's disease at ten centers across the country to determine whether coenzyme Q10 is safe and whether it can slow the rate of functional decline. During the study period, the group that received the largest dose of coenzyme Q10 (1,200 mg/day) had 44 percent less decline in mental function, motor (movement) function, and ability to carry out activities of daily living, such as feeding or dressing themselves. The greatest effect was on activities of daily living. The side effects of supplementing CoQ10 were mild, and no one had to reduce his or her dosage. Researchers believe that coenzyme Q10 (CoQ10) works by improving the mitochondria, the energy-production unit of cells. Mitochondria function is impaired in people with this disease. Coenzyme Q10 also has potent antioxidant effects.

Rhus Toxicodendron will ease muscle stiffness (usually accompanied by little or no trembling) that feels better when the affected body part is in motion. You find it hard to walk on first attempt but are successful once motion is started.

Acupressure

Current research is underway for the use of the mucuna bean. Mucuna beans (*Mucuna pruriens*) have been used in Brazil and India by traditional healers for people with Parkinson's disease. These beans are a natural source of L-dopa, as well as a rich source of vitamin E. They appear to have similar benefits to L-dopa pharmaceutical treatment, but further research will clarify their effectiveness.

Acupressure or acupuncture from a qualified practitioner is highly advised for improved nerve function.

- Gallbladder 20 (GB20) will stimulate better coordination of the nerves and the muscles.
- Stomach 36 (St36) helps you digest and absorb food properly.

Bodywork

Massage

Enjoy a lymphatic massage on a daily basis. It will drain toxic buildup from fatty deposits; better still, a massage can keep you in touch with your body during a time when you may feel estranged from it.

Reflexology

See pages 804–805 for information about reflexology areas and how to work them.

As with most body-wide disorders, it's best to work the entire foot for Parkinson's treatment. If you have limited time or want to concentrate on a few specific areas, work the brain and the spine regions to stimulate blood flow and strengthen the central nervous system.

Aromatherapy

Lavender, jasmine, rose, and geranium all help reduce stress. Use them in baths, diffusers, massages, or in any way you like.

Stress Reduction

General Stress-Reduction Therapies

In the early stages of Parkinson's, yoga is a good choice for stress reduction, because it offers the additional benefit of stretching your muscles and improving coordination.

Meditation is a perfect technique for people who are more sedentary.

After a diagnosis of Parkinson's, you may feel like withdrawing. Although some quiet, private time may be helpful for a while, try to stay engaged with your usual activities. If that becomes impossible, at least try to keep meeting with friends and family members. Their support is crucial to your health.

Other Recommendations

- Some form of regular movement is quite beneficial during all the stages of Parkinson's. Walking is appropriate for the early and the middle stages; for a more advanced case, passive stretching and movements, usually carried out by a physical therapist, keep the body in the best shape possible.
- Plan ahead. Install guardrails and banisters in your house, and invest in a few chairs with high arms to help keep yourself mobile as long as possible.

- Intravenous nutrients, particularly intravenous glutathione, help the symptoms of some patients.

REFERENCES

Fahn, S. 1992. A pilot trial of high-dose alpha-tocopherol and ascorbate in early Parkinson's disease. *Annals of Neurology* 32:S128–32.

Ritz, B., and F. Yu. 2000. Parkinson's disease mortality and pesticide exposure in California 1984–1994. *International Journal of Epidemiology* 29:323–29.

Shults, C. W., D. Oakes, K. Kieburtz, et al., and the Parkinson Study Group. 2002. Effects of coenzyme Q10 in early Parkinson disease: Evidence of slowing of the functional decline. *Archives of Neurology* 59(10):1541–50.

Poisoning

Poisoning can occur in a number of ways. It can result from a dangerous mixture of medications, from an overdose, from swallowing dangerous household chemicals or insecticides, and from ingesting poisonous plants, food, or nicotine.

A person's reaction can vary, dependent on the type and the amount of toxins ingested, with possible emergency and fatal outcomes. Reactions can include inflammation or burning around the lips, if the substance was taken orally; difficulty swallowing; nausea; sudden behavior changes; extreme thirst; breathing difficulties; unconsciousness; headaches; convulsions; vomiting; and death.

Improper use of medications, such as an overdose or the mixture of one medication with another without the doctor's recommendation, can trigger an adverse reaction. Many prescription medications can have negative effects when combined with others. Also, some people unknowingly harbor allergies to medications, which could lead to poisonous predicaments.

Children with access to household chemicals, detergents, and cleaners that are poorly capped and stored are vulnerable to sampling these poisons. The immediate response could include vomiting or gagging. Also, children may accidentally lick, chew, or swallow poisonous plants or nicotine patches, which could induce dizziness or possibly only transitory distress.

Another, more common form of poisoning comes from the ingestion of tainted food that was improperly cleaned, cooked, or refrigerated. These foods can contain dangerous bacteria and contaminants that create a feeling of pain, bloating, and nausea for three to six hours after consumption, as well as diarrhea, stomach cramps, and vomiting (see the Food Poisoning section).

The most serious type of food poisoning, particularly with improperly canned foods and seafood, is a potentially fatal form known as botulism. Generally, the longer it takes for the symptoms of food poisoning to appear, the more serious the poisoning.

Lead

The ingestion of dust from deteriorating lead-based paint is the most common cause of lead poisoning among children. Currently, more than 80 percent of public and privately owned housing units built before 1980 contain some lead-based paint.

Among children ages five and under, 60 percent of poisoning exposures are by nonpharmaceutical products, such as cosmetics, cleaning substances, plants, foreign bodies and toys, pesticides, art supplies, and alcohol. The remaining 40 percent are from pharmaceuticals.

SYMPTOMS

- Difficulty swallowing
- Nausea
- Sudden behavior changes
- Extreme thirst
- Breathing difficulties
- Unconsciousness
- Headaches
- Convulsions
- Vomiting

ROOT CAUSES

- Ingestion of a toxic substance

Testing Techniques

The following tests help assess poisons that have accumulated in the body:

Variety of different poisons, as ordered by your doctor—blood

Digestive function and microbe/parasite/candida testing—stool analysis

Toxic metals—hair or urine

Millions of poisoning exposures occur each year in the United States, resulting in nearly nine hundred thousand visits to emergency rooms. About 90 percent of poisonings happen in the home, and more than half of these involve children under age six.

Prevention is the key. Following are recommendations from the American Association of Poison Control Centers that can help you protect children from poisons:

- Post the telephone number for your poison control center near your phone, in a place where all family members will be able to find it quickly in an emergency.

- Remove all nonessential drugs and household products from your home. Discard them according to the manufacturer's instructions.

- If you have small children, avoid keeping highly toxic products, such as drain cleaners, in the home, the garage, the shed, or any other place that children can access.

- Buy medicines and household products in child-resistant packaging, and be sure that caps are always on tight. Do not remove child-safety caps. Avoid keeping medicines, vitamins, or household products in anything but their original packaging.

- Store all of your medicines and household products in a locked closet or cabinet—including products and medicines with child-resistant containers.

- Crawl around your house, including inside your closets, to inspect it from a child's point of view. You'll likely find a poisoning hazard that you hadn't noticed before.

- Never refer to medicine or vitamins as "candy."

- Make sure that visiting grandparents, family members, friends, or other caregivers keep their medications away from children. For example, if Grandma keeps pills in her purse, make sure the purse is out of the children's reach.

- Keep a bottle of syrup of ipecac in your home—this can be used to induce vomiting. Use it only when the poison control center tells you to.

- Avoid products such as cough syrup or mouthwash that contain alcohol—these are hazardous for young children. Look for alcohol-free alternatives.

- Keep cosmetics and beauty products out of

children's reach. Remember that hair permanents and relaxers are toxins as well.

Carbon monoxide (CO) is an invisible, odorless, poisonous gas that can cause sickness and death. The incomplete burning of fuels such as natural gas, oil, kerosene, propane, coal, and wood produce carbon monoxide. Fuel-burning appliances that are not working properly or are installed incorrectly can produce fatal concentrations of carbon monoxide in your home. Other hazards include burning charcoal indoors and running a car in the garage, both of which can lead to dangerous levels of CO in your home.

The following simple tips from the Centers for Disease Control and Prevention will prevent carbon monoxide poisoning.

- Install carbon monoxide alarms near the bedrooms and on each floor of your home. If your alarm sounds, the U.S. Consumer Product Safety Commission suggests that you press the reset button, call emergency services (911 or your local fire department), and immediately move to fresh air (either outdoors or near an open door or window). If you learn that fuel-burning appliances were the most likely cause of the poisoning, have a serviceperson check them for malfunction before turning them back on. Refer to the instructions on your CO alarm for more specific information about what to do if your alarm goes off.

- Symptoms of CO poisoning are similar to those of the flu, only without a fever (headache, fatigue, nausea, dizziness, shortness of breath). If you experience any of these symptoms, get fresh air immediately and contact a physician for a proper diagnosis. Open windows and doors, turn off combustion appliances, contact emergency services, and take the steps listed previously to ensure your home's safety.

- To keep carbon monoxide from collecting in your home, make sure that any fuel-burning equipment, such as a furnace, a stove, or a heater, works properly, and never use charcoal or other grills indoors or in the garage. Do not leave your car's engine running while it's in the garage, and consider putting weather stripping around the door between the garage and the house.

TREATMENT

Basic Plan

Acute Poisoning (Internal)

If you suspect that your child has ingested a poison, first get the poisonous substance away from your child. If there is still some in his or her mouth, have the child spit it out into a bowl, so that you have the substance if a doctor needs to examine it. Next, check your child for these signs:

- Severe throat pain or discomfort
- Excessive drooling
- Trouble breathing
- Convulsions
- Drowsiness

If your child has any of these signs, call an ambulance or get the child to an emergency room immediately. If there is no sign of these serious symptoms, call your local poison control center. The number is usually listed on the inside cover of your phone book (it's best to have it near your phone for emergency use). If you cannot find the number, call 911 and ask for poison control. You can also call your

> ### Iron Poisoning from Supplements or Medicines
>
> From 1986 through 1997, more than 218,000 children, ages five and under, ingested iron preparations, and 46 died. Again, make sure that medicines and supplements are out of the reach of children.

pediatrician. Do not make your child vomit unless instructed to do so by the poison control center or your doctor.

Poison on the Skin

If a chemical is spilled on your skin, remove your clothes and rinse the skin with lukewarm water for fifteen minutes. Then call the poison control center for further advice. Do not apply any topical treatment unless instructed to do so.

Poison in the Eye

Immediately flush your eye with lukewarm water. Aim for the inner corner of the eye. Flush for fifteen minutes, and call the poison control center for further directions.

℞ Super Seven Prescriptions—Poisoning

Note: These recommendations are not to be used instead of conventional/emergency therapy for poisoning.

Super Prescription #1 Activated charcoal capsules
Take 3 capsules three times daily for two days. Charcoal binds toxins in the digestive tract so that they can be excreted in the stool.

Super Prescription #2 Homeopathic Nux Vomica (*Strychnos nux vomica*)
Take a 30C potency four times daily. It is specific for poisoning from foods, medications, recreational drugs, or alcohol. The person is irritable and constipated.

Super Prescription #3 Homeopathic Arsenicum Album
Take a 30C potency four times daily. It is specific for the symptoms of food poisoning, such as vomiting and diarrhea.

Super Prescription #4 Milk thistle (*Silybum marianum*)
Take 250 mg of an 85 percent silymarin extract three times daily. It protects the liver and the kidneys from being damaged and improves detoxification.

Super Prescription #5 Alpha lipoic acid
Take 100 mg three times daily to prevent liver damage, especially from a medication overdosage.

Super Prescription #6 Vitamin C
Take 1,000 mg three times daily, or request the intravenous form from your doctor. Vitamin C aids in detoxification and prevents organ damage.

Super Prescription #7 N-acetylcysteine (NAC)
Take 500 mg three times daily. NAC improves detoxification and increases the level of the antioxidant glutathione.

General Recommendations

Reishi (*Ganoderma lucidum*) extract supports liver and kidney detoxification. Take 800 mg twice daily.

Bodywork

Acupuncture
Acupuncture is recommended to reduce the side effects of poisoning. See a qualified practitioner.

Other Bodywork Recommendations
Talk with your doctor about using these complementary therapies along with conventional therapy to recover from poisoning.

Pregnancy-Related Problems

Pregnancy is a joyful time, but it's rarely a comfortable one. There are probably as many different combinations of pregnancy-related problems as there are pregnant women. Nevertheless, most uncomfortable conditions are caused by one of three factors: hormonal changes; nutritional deficiencies, whether preexisting or brought on by the additional needs of the baby; or the pressure placed on bones and internal organs by the weight of the growing child.

If you're pregnant, it's essential to have regular checkups. Your doctor should monitor your health, as well as your baby's, and should remain vigilant for any signs of trouble. Good conventional care has saved the lives of many women and their developing babies, and serious problems can often be successfully treated when caught early enough. But as valuable as conventional medicine can be for pregnant women, it rarely offers ways to handle the daily discomfort. During this time, a woman may come to fully appreciate the gentle power of natural therapies. Although some highly potent herbs and other treatments are too strong for the baby, there are still many complementary strategies that will minimize the less-serious problems that accompany pregnancy. Each of the following recommendations is safe to use during pregnancy, but always alert your doctor or midwife to what you are using as nutritional supplements.

When to Call the Doctor

During pregnancy, your body goes through an astounding number of changes. Some will seem normal to you, but you may worry about others. It's wise to develop a good relationship with your doctor long before you get pregnant, so that you are well-informed and comfortable with asking questions. No matter how often you see or talk to a doctor, however, you should always call a medical professional right away if you experience any of the following:

- Vaginal bleeding
- Persistent abdominal pain or cramping

- Continuous or intense morning sickness during the first trimester
- Nausea and vomiting that occur after the first trimester is over

In rare cases, water retention and swelling are signs of a potentially dangerous condition. While most women do experience these symptoms during the course of a normal, healthy pregnancy, it's always a good idea to have them checked out by your doctor, just to be on the safe side.

ANEMIA

During pregnancy, your body needs more iron than usual. A deficiency can result in anemia, a disorder in which the body's cells don't receive enough oxygen. As a result, you feel tired and drained, and you may be more vulnerable to illness.

TREATMENT

Diet

Recommended Food

To overcome pregnancy-induced anemia, consume foods that are high in iron. Organic calf's liver is by far the best source, but if you're a vegetarian or just can't hold organ meats down right now, you do have some other options. Molasses, green leafy vegetables (with the exception of spinach), leeks, cashews, cherries, strawberries, dried fruits, figs, and eggs are all rich in iron.

Food to Avoid

- Spinach, rhubarb, tomatoes, and chocolate are high in oxalic acid, a substance that blocks the absorption of iron.
- If you're pregnant, you've already been advised to stay away from caffeine, which can harm the baby. Caffeine also inhibits iron absorption, as do carbonated sodas and dairy products.
- Do not take iron pills with meals that are high in fiber. The fiber will sweep the iron out of your system before you've had a chance to digest it.

℞ Super Seven Prescriptions—Anemia

Super Prescription #1 Iron
If you have been diagnosed with iron-deficiency anemia by your doctor, take 50 to 200 mg (or the amount recommended by your doctor, depending on the severity) of an easily absorbed form of iron, such as iron citrate, gluconate, glycinate, or fumarate, one to two times daily. Also, iron chelate is generally well absorbed. Avoid the use of iron sulfate (ferrous sulfate), which is poorly absorbed and can cause digestive upset.

Super Prescription #2 Prenatal multivitamin
Take as directed on the container. It supplies a wide range of nutrients for healthy red blood cells.

Super Prescription #3 Ferrum Phosphoricum
Take 5 pellets of the 3x or 6x potency three times daily. This homeopathic remedy improves iron utilization in the cells.

Super Prescription #4 Yellow dock (*Rumex crispis*)
Take 1 (300 mg) capsule or 20 drops of the tincture with each meal. It contains iron and improves iron absorption.

Super Prescription #5 Nettles (*Urtica diocia*)
Take 2 ml of the tincture twice daily or 300 mg of the capsule form, or drink 1 cup of the tea twice daily (organic source). This herb is a source of iron and other blood-building minerals.

Super Prescription #6 Chlorella
Take as directed on the container for a host of iron-building nutrients, including chlorophyll.

Super Prescription #7 Vitamin C
Take 100 mg with each dose of iron. It provides an acidic environment for enhanced iron absorption.

General Recommendations

See the chapter on Anemia for further details.

BACK PAIN

Most pregnant women experience some degree of back pain, thanks to the extra weight and the shifting center of gravity.

TREATMENT

Diet

Constipation, to which pregnant women are especially vulnerable, makes back pain worse. See the chapter on Constipation.

When back pain strikes, try drinking a glass or two of water immediately. If the pain is caused by dehydration, water will help.

R͓x **Super Seven Prescriptions—Back Pain**

Super Prescription #1 Calcium and magnesium
Take a complex of these two minerals that contains 500 mg of calcium and 250 mg of magnesium. Take it twice daily. These minerals reduce muscle spasms.

Super Prescriptions #2–#7 (Homeopathic remedies)
Pick the remedy that best matches your symptoms in this section. For acute back pain, take a 30C potency four times daily. For chronic back pain, take it twice daily for two weeks to see if there are any positive results. After you notice improvement, stop taking the remedy, unless symptoms return. Consultation with a homeopathic practitioner is advised.

Aesculus Hippocastanum is for lower back or sacral pain that is worse when you are sitting. The pain often radiates into the right hip.

Arnica (*Arnica montana*) is for an injury that leaves your back feeling bruised and sore and when you have difficulty moving around.

Bryonia (*Bryonia alba*) is for lower back pain and stiffness that feel worse with any movement and in cold, dry weather and that feel better when the area is rubbed.

Calcarea Carbonica is for chronic lower back pain and weakness in overweight individuals who also are chilly. Symptoms are worse in the cold and the dampness.

Cimicifuga Racemosa is for a stiff, aching neck and back. Muscles feel bruised but feel better with warmth. Also, it's used for menstrual cramps, with lower back pain radiating to the thighs.

Ignatia (Ignatia amara) is for back spasms and cramping, as the result of emotional stress.

Magnesia Phosphorica is for muscle spasms in the back that feel better from warmth.

Nux Vomica is for back spasms and cramping, especially of the lower back. The person may also have constipation and may feel chilly and irritable. Symptoms are worse from cold and better with warmth.

Rhus Toxicodendron is for a stiff lower back that is worse in the cold and the damp and better with movement. It is specific for sprained back muscles or ligaments.

Ruta Graveolens is for pain near the neck or in the lower back. The area of the injury feels lame, and the pain is worse at night. It's useful for back sprains and strains.

Bodywork

Massage

A pregnancy massage can provide temporary but welcome relief from back pain. Make an appointment with a therapist who is experienced in working with pregnant women.

Other Bodywork Recommendations

Acupressure and acupuncture can be helpful when performed by an experienced practitioner.

Reflexology

See pages 804–805 for information about reflexology areas and how to work them.

Work the base of the heel, which corresponds to the spine, the hips, and the tailbone.

Hydrotherapy

Floating in water makes you feel weightless and takes the pressure off your back (at least for the duration of your swim). You don't need much in the way of special equipment, just a pool or, in good weather, a lake or other body of clean water.

Alternating hot and cold towels over the back or the use of a hot pack for five minutes or less can be helpful.

Other Recommendations

- Prenatal yoga or stretching classes can be effective.

- At night, support your back and belly with pillows.
- When you're pregnant, the last thing you may think about is your posture. Make an extra effort to check that your back is straight, even when you're sitting down.
- Use common sense: don't wear high heels, and don't lift heavy objects.

BLEEDING GUMS

Increased estrogen production can make your gums soft, swollen, and prone to bleeding. Proper diet and supplements will reduce the severity of bleeding gums.

TREATMENT

Diet

Recommended Food
Good sources of calcium include sea vegetables, green leafy vegetables (with the exception of spinach), soybeans, and unsweetened cultured yogurt.

Enjoy citrus fruits and green vegetables for vitamin C.

Food to Avoid
Spinach, rhubarb, tomatoes, and chocolate inhibit your body's ability to absorb calcium.

℞ Super Seven Prescriptions—Bleeding Gums

Super Prescription #1 Vitamin C
Take 200 mg twice daily. Try a nonacidic vitamin C to prevent digestive upset.

Super Prescription #2 Homeopathic Ferrum Phosphoricum
Take 3 pellets of a 6x potency twice daily. This homeopathic remedy safely reduces bleeding and inflammation. Take until the bleeding stops, then discontinue.

Super Prescription #3 Bioflavonoid complex
Take 250 mg twice daily. Bioflavonoids reduce inflammation of the gums.

Super Prescription #4 Prenatal multivitamin
Take as directed on the container. It supplies a variety of nutrients that are required for gum health.

Super Prescription #5 Calendula (*Calendula officinalis*)
Put 15 drops of calendula tincture in 2 ounces of water. Swish it in your mouth, and spit it out. Calendula is healing to the mucosa of the gums.

Super Prescription #6 Homeopathic Mercurius Solubilis
Take a low potency (6x, 12x, 6C, 12C, or 30C) twice daily for swollen, bleeding gums that are accompanied by heavy salivation and bad breath. Stop using it when the bleeding stops.

> **Super Prescription #7 *Myrrh cerifera***
> Put 15 drops of myrrh tincture in 2 ounces of water. Swish it in your mouth, and spit it out. Myrrh is healing to the mucosa of the gums.

Bodywork

Massage

In the morning and before you go to bed, use your finger to massage your gums lightly.

CONSTIPATION

The hormonal changes of pregnancy, along with the positioning of the baby and fiber and fluid intake, make pregnant women more susceptible to constipation. Iron pills (ferrous sulfate) can also lead to constipation.

TREATMENT

Diet

Recommended Food

Eat plenty of fiber—fresh fruits and vegetables, whole grains, and beans—to encourage regularity. Dried fruits—especially that old standby, prunes—are another good choice.

Drink a glass of clean, quality water every two waking hours. That will keep food moving through your digestive system.

A hot beverage at breakfast will often wake up a sluggish digestive system. Try herbal tea or hot water with a little lemon juice.

Food to Avoid

Do not eat fatty, greasy, or fried foods, which travel slowly through the intestines.

℞ Super Seven Prescription—Constipation

> **Super Prescription #1 Psyllium**
> Take 1 teaspoon or 5 grams of psyllium husks twice daily or as directed on the container. Take it with 10 ounces of water. Psyllium acts as a bulk-forming laxative.
>
> **Super Prescription #2 Probiotic**
> Take a product containing at least four billion active organisms daily. Friendly bacteria such as *Lactobacillus acidophilus* and *bifidus* help with digestion and elimination.
>
> **Super Prescription #3 Chlorella**
> Take 1,500 mg of organic chlorella daily. This algae supplement provides a healthy source of fiber.
>
> **Super Prescription #4 Homeopathic Sepia**
> Take a 6x, 12x, 6C, 12C, or 30C potency twice daily for three days to see if there are any positive results. After you notice improvement, stop taking the remedy, unless symptoms return. Consultation with a homeopathic practitioner is advised.

Sepia is indicated for pregnant women who feel irritable and chilly and have stools that are hard to pass. A heavy sensation in the rectum and the lower abdomen is present. There is a strong craving for chocolate.

Super Prescription #5 Homeopathic Nux Vomica

Take a 6x, 12x, 6C, 12C, or 30C potency twice daily for three days to see if there are any positive results. After you notice improvement, stop taking the remedy, unless symptoms return. Consultation with a homeopathic practitioner is advised. Nux Vomica is indicated when one has an urgent feeling but can't pass stools or stools are never completed. The person feels irritable and overstressed. Nux Vomica works well for people who work too hard, exercise too little, and eat and drink too much.

Super Prescription #6 Homeopathic Natrum Muriaticum

Take a 6x, 12x, 6C, 12C, or 30C potency twice daily for three days to see if there are any positive results. After you notice improvement, stop taking the remedy, unless symptoms return. Consultation with a homeopathic practitioner is advised. This is a remedy for women with constipation who have strong cravings for salt and water. They may suffer from depression and are often sensitive to the sun or to light.

Super Prescription #7 Homeopathic Lycopodium (*Lycopodium clavatum*)

Take a 6x, 12x, 6C, 12C, or 30C potency twice daily for three days to see if there are any positive results. After you notice improvement, stop taking the remedy, unless symptoms return. Consultation with a homeopathic practitioner is advised. This remedy is for a woman who has constipation and problems with gas and bloating. She craves sweets, and her symptoms are worse in the late afternoon. Her digestive system feels better with warm drinks.

Bodywork

Reflexology

See pages 804–805 for information about reflexology areas and how to work them. Work with a knowledgeable therapist.

Exercise can stimulate bowel contractions. If you're feeling sluggish, take a brisk walk.

FLUID RETENTION (EDEMA)

Hormonal changes and increased fluids can cause your hands, legs, and feet to swell, especially in the later months of pregnancy. Although many women experience fluid retention, you should always have it checked out by a doctor, as it may be a symptom of a serious disorder.

TREATMENT

Diet

Recommended Food

As you lower your intake of salt, you must also increase your consumption of potassium. A combination of excess sodium and a deficiency in potassium has been found in many people with hypertension. Good sources of potassium include apples, asparagus, cabbage, oranges, tomatoes, bananas, kelp, and alfalfa.

Food to Avoid

Restrict your intake of salt. Obviously, you should avoid table salt, but you should also stay away from processed or junk food, both of which contain alarming amounts of sodium.

℞ Super Seven Prescriptions—Fluid Retention

Super Prescription #1 Dandelion leaf (*Taraxacum officinale*)
With your doctor's supervision, take 3 ml or 300 mg twice daily. Dandelion leaf is a gentle diuretic.

Super Prescription #2 B-complex vitamins
Vitamin B6 and other B-complex vitamins may help reduce edema. Take 50 mg twice daily.

Super Prescription #3 Homeopathic Natrum Muriaticum
Take 3 pellets of a 6x potency three times daily. It is particularly indicated if you have a strong desire for salt and the fluid retention is worse from being in the sun or from heat.

Super Prescription #4 Vitamin C
Take 500 mg twice daily. Vitamin C improves the lymph flow.

Super Prescription #5 Vitamin B6
Take 50 mg daily under the guidance of a doctor. Vitamin B6 has been found to reduce water retention, most likely due to its function in helping liver metabolism.

Super Prescription #6 Quercitin
Take 500 mg twice daily. Quercitin is a flavonoid that improves circulation.

Super Prescription #7 Garlic
Take 200 mg twice daily. Garlic has mild anti-edema properties.

Bodywork

Reflexology

See pages 804–805 for information about reflexology areas and how to work them.
  Work the lymph areas to reduce swelling.

Other Recommendations

- Regular exercise will minimize swelling. A daily walk or swim is a good idea.
- Swollen feet are uncomfortable, but tight shoes make them feel even worse. For the duration of your pregnancy, you may want to wear shoes that are larger than your usual size.

GAS

Even women with normally hardy digestive systems may find themselves suffering from gas and flatulence when pregnant. This bothersome condition is usually due to the slower movement of food through your intestines. Sometimes women also find that they are upset by certain foods for the duration of the pregnancy.

TREATMENT

Diet

Recommended Food
Papaya soothes the intestinal tract and is high in enzymes that help you digest food properly.

Instead of taxing your digestive system with large meals, eat several small ones throughout the day.

If your digestion is not as efficient as usual, try incorporating more easily digestible foods into your diet, such as soups, broths, and steamed vegetables.

Food to Avoid
If you suspect that a particular food is giving you gas, your body is trying to tell you something. Avoid that food until after you've delivered your child and finished nursing. Common offenders include beans, cow's milk, sugar, and spicy foods.

Keep a record of the food you eat during the day, and take note of when gas occurs. (Do not, however, try an elimination diet. It's too severe during pregnancy.) If you can isolate the food that irritates you, avoid it until the baby arrives and is weaned.

℞ Super Seven Prescriptions—Gas

Super Prescription #1 Ginger (*Zingiber officinale*)
Drink a cup of ginger tea when you feel bloated or after meals. You can also use 300 mg of the capsule form or 2 ml of the tincture.

Super Prescription #2 Chamomile (*Matricaria chamomilla*)
Drink a cup of chamomile tea when you feel bloated or after meals. If you prefer to use an extract, take 500 mg twice a day, or use 2 ml of a tincture twice daily.

Super Prescription #3 Homeopathic Magnesia Phosphorica
Take 3 pellets of a 6x potency up to three times daily for gas and cramping.

> ### Super Prescription #4 Homeopathic Carbo Vegetabilis
> Take a low potency (6x, 12x, 30x, 6C, or 30C) as needed, for gas and bloating that are accompanied by belching.
>
> ### Super Prescription #5 Homeopathic Pulsatilla (*Pulsatilla pratensis*)
> Take a low potency (6x, 12x, 30x, 6C, or 30C) as needed, for gas and bloating that occur from eating rich or fatty foods.
>
> ### Super Prescription #6 Homeopathic Lycopodium (*Lycopodium clavatum*)
> Take a low potency (6x, 12x, 30x, 6C, or 30C) as needed, for gas and bloating that occur in the evening. Warm drinks improve the symptoms as well.
>
> ### Super Prescription #7 Homeopathic Nux Vomica
> Take a low potency (6x, 12x, 30x, 6C, or 30C) as needed, for gas and bloating that occur from stress and spicy foods. Heartburn is also a common symptom treated by this remedy.

General Recommendations

Take a probiotic supplement that contains at least four billion organisms, thirty minutes after breakfast and dinner. These good bacteria reside in the digestive tract and aid digestion.

HEARTBURN

The position of the baby may cause stomach acid to back up into the esophagus, leaving you with a burning pain in your chest. You may also experience some regurgitation of acid into your throat and mouth.

TREATMENT

Diet

Recommended Food
Whenever you feel heartburn pain, drink a glass of clean, quality water to flush the gastric acids back down into your stomach.

Eat papaya for its healing qualities, or drink its juice.

Eat small meals throughout the day, instead of three large ones. If your stomach isn't completely full, there's less of a chance that its contents will back up.

Food to Avoid
Some foods are more challenging to digest than others are. If you stay away from fried and greasy foods, spicy foods, and heavy sauces, you may find that your problem resolves itself.

Avoid minty foods, such as peppermint, which can aggravate heartburn.

Allow a few hours between your last meal or snack and bedtime. You'll give your stomach a chance to process its contents before you lie down.

Food allergies are linked to heartburn. If a food causes you trouble, eliminate it from your diet. You may find that your symptoms improve significantly or even disappear.

℞ **Super Seven Prescriptions—Heartburn**

Super Prescription #1 Licorice root (DGL)

Chew one 400 mg tablet (or take it in powder form) for the relief of heartburn. DGL is a special type of licorice extract that soothes and heals the stomach and the esophagus. It does not cause high blood pressure.

Super Prescription #2 Homeopathic Nux Vomica

Take a low potency (6x, 12x, 30x, 6C, or 30C) as needed, for heartburn that occurs from stress and spicy foods.

Super Prescription #3 Slippery elm (*Ulmus fulva*)

Take 1 teaspoon, 300 mg of the capsule form, or 3 ml of tincture three times daily. This herb is used to soothe and reduce inflammation of the lining of the esophagus and the stomach.

Super Prescription #4 Marshmallow root (*Althea officinalis*)

Take 300 mg of the capsule or 3 ml of tincture three times daily. Marshmallow root soothes and reduces inflammation of the lining of the esophagus and the stomach.

Super Prescription #5 Digestive enzymes

Take 1 or 2 capsules of a full-spectrum blend with each meal. Enzymes help you to digest foods more effectively so that they are less likely to cause irritation *Note*: Some people may need to use a formula that contains no protease, as this protein-digestive enzyme may irritate the stomachs of some individuals.

Super Prescription #6 Probiotic

Take a product containing at least four billion active organisms daily. It contains friendly bacteria, such as *Lactobacillus acidophilus* and *bifidus*, that improve digestive function.

Super Prescription #7 Calcium

Liquid calcium is soothing to the stomach. Take a formula containing 500 mg of calcium and 250 mg of magnesium twice daily. Magnesium helps to relax tightened muscles of the esophagus and the stomach.

General Recommendations

A super-green-food supplement, such as chlorella or spirulina, or a mixture of super green foods in a drink, helps to neutralize acidity. Take as directed on the container.

Chamomile tea is soothing to the digestive tract. Drink 1 to 2 cups daily.

Homeopathy

Pick the remedy that best matches your symptoms in this section. For chronic acid reflux, take a 6x, 12x, 6C, 12C, or 30C twice daily for two weeks to see if there are any positive results. After you notice improvement, stop taking the remedy, unless symptoms return. Consultation with a homeopathic practitioner is advised.

Arsenicum Album is for a burning sensation in the esophagus or the stomach that is alleviated by drinking milk or by frequently sipping warm water and sitting up. The person feels anxious and restless

Carbo Vegetabilis will help people whose sluggish digestion leads to flatulence, belching, and bloating in the upper abdomen. People who benefit from this remedy are often pale and cold. Despite their chilliness, they feel better with cool air and drinks.

Lycopodium (*Lycopodium clavatum*) is also for gas and bloating, but in this case the symptoms are usually brought on by anxiety and lack of confidence. The person feels worse when wearing tight clothes and better when sipping warm drinks. There may be a sour taste in the mouth. Symptoms are often worse in the late afternoon and the evening.

Natrum Carbonicum is for people who have trouble digesting most foods, especially milk.

Nux Vomica is for people with heartburn and reflux that occur from stress, spicy foods, and alcohol. They generally feel chilly, irritable, and oversensitive to stimuli (noise, light). Constipation is often a problem as well.

Pulsatilla (*Pulsatilla pratensis*) is helpful if you feel worse after eating rich and fatty foods. Symptoms are worse in a warm room and better with fresh air. You also tend to feel tearful when ill, and you greatly desire to be comforted.

Phosphorus helps when you have a burning pain in the stomach that feels better from cold drinks. However, soon after drinking, you are nauseous and may vomit.

Sulfur is for burning pain and belching, accompanied by diarrhea. You tend to be very warm and get relief from ice-cold drinks.

Other Recommendations

Structure your day so that you don't have to bend over, lie down, or perform any strenuous activity within a couple of hours after eating.

HEMORRHOIDS

During pregnancy, both constipation and pressure on the lower part of the body can produce hemorrhoids.

TREATMENT

Diet

Recommended Food

Fiber will soften your stool and make it easier to pass. Eat whole grains, fresh or dried fruits and vegetables, or beans with every meal.

Another way to soften stools is to drink a glass of clean, quality water every two waking hours.

Food to Avoid

Don't eat foods that are difficult for your body to process. Greasy, fried, and junk foods are all off-limits; so are any other items that are high in saturated fat.

Cow's milk is constipating for some pregnant women.

℞ **Super Seven Prescriptions—Hemorrhoids**

Super Prescription #1 Psyllium

Psyllium is a good fiber supplement and has been shown to reduce the pain and the bleeding associated with hemorrhoids. Take 5 to 7 grams daily, along with 10 ounces of clean, quality water.

Super Prescription #2 Flaxseed oil

Take 1 to 2 tablespoons daily. Flaxseed oil improves regularity and reduces straining. It also contains essential fatty acids that promote tissue healing. *Note*: Reduce the dosage if diarrhea occurs.

Super Prescription #3 Bilberry (*Vaccinium myrtillus*)

Take a standardized extract containing 25 percent anthocyanosides at 160 mg twice daily. Bilberry improves circulation and strengthens capillary walls.

Super Prescription #4 Witch hazel (*Hamamelis virginiana*)

Apply it as a gel or a cream to external hemorrhoids, or add 1 ounce to a sitz bath daily.

Super Prescription #5 Probiotic

This contains friendly bacteria, such as *Lactobacillus* and *Bifidobacterium*, which improve digestion and constipation. Take a product that contains at least four billion active organisms daily.

Super Prescription #6 Bioflavonoid complex

Take 1,000 mg two or three times daily. Various flavonoids, such as rutin and hesperidin, have been shown to be effective in treating hemorrhoids. They reduce swelling and prevent bleeding.

Super Prescription #7 Greens drink

Consume a greens drink that contains a blend of super green foods, such as chlorella, spirulina, and so on. It provides fiber. Take as directed on the container.

A study of fifty-one pregnant women found that supplementation of bilberry significantly improved the pain, the burning, and the itching associated with their hemorrhoids.

Homeopathy

Pick the remedy that best matches your symptoms in this section. Take a 6x, 12x, 6C, 12C, or 30C potency twice daily for two weeks to see if there are any positive results. After you notice improvement, stop taking the remedy, unless symptoms return. Consultation with a homeopathic practitioner is advised.

Aesculus Hippocastanum is for a pain that feels as if the rectum is being poked with sticks. The pain extends to the back.

Aloe Vera is for large, painful hemorrhoids. Your doctor states that the hemorrhoids look like a "bunch of grapes." They feel better with cold compresses. You may be prone to diarrhea.

Calcarea Fluorica is helpful when bleeding and itching occur with the hemorrhoids. Often, lower back pain is present. You may have problems with flatulence and constipation.

Ignatia (*Ignatia amara*) is for hemorrhoids that cause a stabbing or sticking pain, along with rectal spasms. Symptoms feel worse from emotional upset.

Nux Vomica is for painful hemorrhoids that come on as a result of chronic constipation and straining with bowel movements. The woman feels irritable.

Ratanhia helps when one experiences a lot of pain after a bowel movement. There is a cutting pain that feels as if one is sitting on broken glass.

Sulfur is for large, itching, burning hemorrhoids that tend to be worse at night. The anal area is red and inflamed, and there is often flatulence with a foul odor.

Bodywork

Hydrotherapy

A sitz bath, if it's comfortable for you, offers temporary relief of pain and swelling.

Other Recommendations

Keep moving. A daily walk will improve your circulation and keep you regular.

INSOMNIA

In the last trimester, it may be difficult to find a comfortable position to sleep in. Changing moods can also make it hard to get a good night's sleep.

TREATMENT

Diet

Recommended Food

Pregnant women are often deficient in B vitamins, which are healing to the nerves and necessary for good sleep. Incorporate whole grains, green leafy vegetables, and wheat germ into each meal.

Try to have at least one of the following at dinner: turkey, chicken, tuna, tofu, soymilk, or live unsweetened yogurt. Each of these foods stimulates serotonin, a neurotransmitter that helps you get to sleep. They're also low in sugar.

For a bedtime snack, have some turkey or chicken on a whole-grain cracker.

Pregnant women are often low in calcium and magnesium, two nutrients that encourage restful sleep. Eat lots of leafy greens, sesame and sunflower seeds, oats, almonds, and walnuts.

Food to Avoid

You should already be avoiding caffeinated beverages, a common cause of insomnia, but now you need to add refined-sugar products to your list of foods to eliminate. Chocolate, which contains both sugar and caffeine, should be at the top of that list.

℞ Super Seven Prescriptions—Insomnia

Super Prescription #1 Calcium and magnesium
Take 500 mg of calcium and 250 mg of magnesium each evening. Both minerals help relax the nervous system. Some people have better results taking

one of the minerals alone in the evening and the other earlier in the day. Experiment to see what works better for you.

Super Prescription #2 Chamomile (*Matricaria chamomilla*)

This relaxes the nervous system. Drink a fresh cup of tea in the evening, or take 300 mg of the capsule form.

Super Prescription #3 Homeopathic Coffea Cruda

Take a low potency (6x, 12x, 30x, 6C, or 30C), as needed, for insomnia. This homeopathic remedy is very specific for people with insomnia caused from overstimulation. You find yourself wide awake at 3 A.M., with a racing mind.

Super Prescription #4 Homeopathic Ignatia (*Ignatia amara*)

Take a low potency (6x, 12x, 30x, 6C, or 30C), as needed, for insomnia. This is a remedy for insomnia caused by emotional upset—usually grief or a loss. There can be uncontrollable crying, loss of appetite, and mood swings. The person often sighs a lot during the day, and the muscles may twitch during sleep.

Super Prescription #5 Homeopathic Kali Phosphoricum

Take a low potency (6x, 12x, 30x, 6C, or 30C), as needed, for insomnia. It is helpful for insomnia that results from nervous exhaustion caused by overwork or mental strain.

Super Prescription #6 Homeopathic Arsenicum Album

Take a low potency (6x, 12x, 30x, 6C, or 30C), as needed, for insomnia. This remedy is for pregnant women who have tremendous anxiety and restlessness. They often wake up between the hours of midnight and 2 A.M. They tend to be perfectionists and have many insecurities and fears.

Super Prescription #7 Sulfur

Take a low potency (6x, 12x, 30x, 6C, or 30C), as needed, for insomnia. This remedy is for insomnia that comes on from itching at night or from feeling too hot at night. One throws the covers off or sticks one's feet out. There is a strong craving for ice-cold drinks and spicy foods.

Bodywork

Reflexology

See pages 804–805 for information about reflexology areas and how to work them.

If nervous tension is keeping you up, work the diaphragm and the solar plexus.

Hydrotherapy

About twenty minutes before bedtime, soak your feet in a hot bath. Not only will your burdened soles appreciate the attention, but you'll also draw blood away from your head and promote sleepiness.

Stress Reduction

Change, even when it comes in the welcome form of a new child, is always stressful. Spend twenty minutes before bedtime with positive mental imagery and prayer. You'll unwind, destress, and prepare yourself for deep sleep.

Other Recommendations

Use pillows under your back and belly or between your knees to get more comfortable at night.

If you simply can't sleep, lying in bed will only make you frustrated and angry. Instead, have some light reading or another easy activity on hand that you can enjoy during the night. (When the baby comes, you may look back on these idle hours as a gift.)

LEG AND FOOT CRAMPS

Poor circulation, due to hormonal changes and mineral deficiency (usually, calcium and/or magnesium), can cause painful cramps in the leg and the foot. As the baby grows and the pressure on the lower half of your body increases, the cramps may get worse.

TREATMENT

Diet

Recommended Food

Eat sea vegetables, green leafy vegetables (except spinach), soy products, and live unsweetened yogurt for calcium.

Food to Avoid

Avoid caffeine, alcohol, and high-sugar products that deplete the body of minerals.

℞ Super Seven Prescriptions—Leg and Foot Cramps

Super Prescription #1 Calcium and magnesium
Take a complex of these two minerals that contains 500 mg of calcium and 250 mg of magnesium, twice daily. These minerals reduce muscle spasms and cramps.

Super Prescription #2 Homeopathic Magnesia Phosphorica
Take 3 pellets of a 6x potency three times daily. This homeopathic remedy is very helpful and safe in the treatment of cramps and spasms.

Super Prescription #3 Prenatal multivitamin
Take as directed on the container. It provides a base of nutrients involved in relaxing the muscles.

Super Prescription #4 Super green foods
Take a single super green food, such as chlorella or spirulina, or try a blended mixture. These foods provide minerals that prevent cramping and spasms.

Super Prescription #5 B-complex vitamins
Take a 50 mg B-complex to ensure proper nerve and muscle function.

Super Prescription #6 Fish oil
Take 4,000 mg of fish oil daily, for essential fatty acids that support proper blood flow.

Super Prescription #7 Essential fatty acids
Take 1,000 mg of borage, evening primrose oil (*Oenothera biennis*), or black currant oil for essential fatty acids that support proper blood flow.

Bodywork

Massage
Rubbing the legs and the feet will stimulate blood flow and reduce cramping. A regular full-body massage will improve circulation throughout the entire body.

Other Recommendations

- Exercise daily to keep your blood moving. Walking and water aerobics are good, gentle choices.
- A hot compress on the cramped area will relax the muscles.
- Elevate your legs as often as possible, so that blood can flow back up to the heart.

MORNING SICKNESS

Many pregnant women experience nausea and vomiting in their first trimester, as a result of hormone changes. Morning sickness, the traditional term, is a misnomer, as the symptoms may occur at any time of the day or the night. If the nausea and the vomiting are continuous or severe, talk to your doctor; you need to be sure that you stay hydrated and that you and the baby are receiving adequate nutrition. While morning sickness during your first trimester is generally considered normal, nausea and vomiting after the twelfth or thirteenth week may be indicative of a serious problem.

TREATMENT

Diet
Your body is telling you what to eat and what not to eat, so it's probably best to follow its advice. Following are some additional dietary suggestions.

Recommended Food
B vitamins ward off queasiness, so start your day with whole-grain toast or crackers. Brown rice, oats, and wheat germ are other good options.

Although it's important to take in lots of nutrients during pregnancy, don't try to force yourself to eat large meals. Instead, plan on several small meals throughout the day.

Leafy greens are rich in vitamin K, which helps prevent nausea.

If you feel nauseated, try chewing a piece of fresh ginger or sucking on a slice of lemon or lime.

℞ Super Seven Prescriptions—Morning Sickness

Super Prescription #1 Ginger root (*Zingiber officinale*)
Drink a fresh cup of tea two or three times daily, or take 300 mg of the capsule form three times daily.

A study in the *Journal of Obstetrics and Gynecology* reported that twenty-eight of thirty-two pregnant women supplementing ginger had improvement in nausea symptoms, compared with ten of thirty-five in the placebo group. Researchers found no adverse effects of ginger on pregnancy outcome.

Super Prescription #2 Vitamin B6

Take 25 mg three times daily. Double-blind studies have found this to be effective. Vitamin B6 injections or intravenous administration by your doctor may be even more effective.

Super Prescription #3 Homeopathic Ipecacuanha

Take a low potency (6x, 12x, 30x, 6C, or 30C), as needed, for relief of nausea and vomiting. A characteristic symptom for this remedy is constant nausea that is not relieved by vomiting.

Super Prescription #4 Homeopathic Nux Vomica

Take a low potency (6x, 12x, 30x, 6C, or 30C), as needed, for relief of nausea and vomiting. Women who require this remedy feel irritable. Along with the nauseousness and the vomiting may be constipation and heartburn.

Super Prescription #5 Homeopathic Colchicum

Take a low potency (6x, 12x, 30x, 6C, or 30C), as needed, for relief of nausea and vomiting. Women who benefit from this remedy feel nauseous from the smell or the sight of food, especially eggs and fish.

Super Prescription #6 Homeopathic Tabacum

Take a low potency (6x, 12x , 30x, 6C, or 30C), as needed, for relief of nausea and vomiting. Women who benefit from this remedy have tremendous nausea and a sinking feeling in their stomachs. Any movement makes them nauseous.

Super Prescription #7 Vitamin K

Take 5 mg daily or receive injections or intravenous administration from your doctor. Vitamin K has been shown to relieve morning sickness.

General Recommendations

Chamomile (*Matricaria chamomilla*) and red raspberry (*Rubus idaeus*) tea help some women with morning sickness. Drink the tea throughout the day.

Homeopathy

Homeopathic Lacticum Acidum is for women who feel morning sickness as soon as they wake up. There is increased salivation and a burning sensation in the stomach. They feel better after eating.

Homeopathic Pulsatilla (*Pulsatilla pratensis*) is for women who crave sweets and creamy foods but get digestive upset from them. They tend to be weepy and easily upset. They should take a low potency (6x, 12x, 30x, 6C, or 30C), as needed, for relief of nausea and vomiting.

Homeopathic Sepia is helpful when odors trigger morning sickness. The woman craves sweets, vinegar, and sour foods. Emotionally, she is irritable and feels worn out.

Other Recommendations

Acupuncture and acupressure have been found to be effective for morning sickness. Commercial acupressure wristbands that relieve nausea are available.

PREECLAMPSIA

Preeclampsia, also referred to as toxemia, is a problem that occurs in some women during pregnancy. It can happen during the second half of pregnancy and involves the combination of high blood pressure, swelling, and large amounts of protein in the urine. Preeclampsia is more common in a woman's first pregnancy and in women whose mothers or sisters had preeclampsia. The risk of preeclampsia is higher in women carrying multiple babies, in teenage mothers, and in women older than age forty. Other women at risk include those who had high blood pressure or kidney disease before they became pregnant. The cause of preeclampsia isn't known, although nutritional deficiencies appear to be a major factor.

TREATMENT

Diet

Recommended Food
Plenty of clean, quality water is important, as is adequate protein.

Essential fatty acids, as found in fish, nuts and seeds, and ground flaxseeds, are recommended.

Food to Avoid
Avoid foods that are high in trans-fatty acids, as found in fried food (cooked vegetable oils), margarine, and some packaged foods.

℞ Super Seven Prescriptions—Preeclampsia

Super Prescription #1 Calcium
Take 500 mg three times daily. Several studies have found that calcium supplementation reduces the risk of developing preeclampsia, especially in women who are at high risk.

Super Prescription #2 Magnesium
Take 500 mg twice daily. Some studies have shown magnesium to reduce the risk of developing preeclampsia, plus it helps to lower blood pressure.

Super Prescription #3 Homeopathic Apis (*Apis mellifica*)
Take a 30C potency twice daily if you have swelling of the lower limbs or protein in your urine.

Super Prescription #4 Homeopathic Natrum Muriaticum
Take a 30C potency twice daily if you have swelling and water retention, as well as a strong craving for salt and an intolerance of warm rooms.

Super Prescription #5 Homeopathic Sepia
Take a 30C potency twice daily if you have preeclampsia, feelings of chilliness, and irritability. You have a strong craving for chocolate.

Super Prescription #6 Homeopathic Lachesis
Take a 30C potency twice daily if you have very high blood pressure, accompanied by great heat and flushing of the skin.

> **Super Prescription #7 Prenatal multivitamin**
> A high-quality prenatal multivitamin is recommended to provide a base of nutrients that promote good health. Particularly important are vitamins B2 and B6.

General Recommendations

Vitamins E-complex and C may be helpful as antioxidants. Take 400 IU daily of vitamin E and 500 mg of vitamin C.

STRETCH MARKS

When your body expands to accommodate the baby, the fibers of the skin can tear, leaving thin, red lines that eventually turn white or silver. There are a few ways to prevent stretch marks, but once you have them, they won't go away (although with time, they do fade significantly).

TREATMENT

Diet

Recommended Food

Eat wheat germ and use cold-pressed oils in your salad dressings and cooking. The vitamin E in these products promotes skin elasticity.

Essential fatty acids (EFAs) also keep the skin healthy and pliant. Fish, flaxseeds, and flaxseed oil are all high in EFAs, as are the cold-pressed oils mentioned earlier.

℞ Super Prescription—Stretch Marks

> **Super Prescription Vitamin E oil**
> Apply the oil to the stretch marks each morning and evening.

VARICOSE VEINS

These enlarged veins on the surface of the leg are caused by the weight of the baby and by hormonal changes. Straining to have bowel movements also places pressure on the veins. If you're having trouble passing stools, consult the recommendations for constipation during pregnancy. See the Varicose Veins section (pages 650–655).

TREATMENT

Diet

Recommended Food

Vitamin E-complex will prevent blood clots, a possible side effect of varicose veins. Wheat germ and cold-pressed oils are good sources of this nutrient. Red- or blue-colored berries are an ideal dessert or snack for you. They fortify vein walls and improve their elasticity. Buckwheat strengthens capillaries.

℞ Super Seven Prescriptions—Varicose Veins

Super Prescription #1 Bilberry (*Vaccinium myrtillus*)
Take a standardized extract containing 25 percent anthocyanosides at 160 mg twice daily. Bilberry improves circulation and strengthens capillary walls.

Super Prescription #2 Flaxseed oil
Take 1 to 2 tablespoons daily. Flaxseed oil improves regularity and reduces straining. It also contains essential fatty acids that promote tissue healing. *Note*: Reduce the dosage if diarrhea occurs.

Super Prescription #3 Witch hazel (*Hamamelis virginiana*)
Apply it as a gel or a cream to external varicose veins.

Super Prescription #4 Bioflavonoid complex
Take 1,000 mg two or three times daily. Bioflavonoids reduce swelling and inflammation.

Super Prescription #5 Homeopathic Hamamelis
Take a low potency (6x, 12x, 30x, 6C, or 30C) twice daily for varicose veins that are large, sore, and easily irritated and that sting.

Super Prescription #6 Homeopathic Arnica (*Arnica montana*)
Take a low potency (6x, 12x, 30x, 6C, or 30C) twice daily for varicose veins that are large, sore, and easily irritated and that sting. It's also helpful for varicose veins that are swollen and look bruised.

Super Prescription #7 Homeopathic Pulsatilla Nigrans
Take a low potency (6x, 12x, 30x, 6C, or 30C) twice daily for varicose veins in the legs that are hot and painful at nighttime. The legs feel better out of the covers and with the windows open.

Bodywork

Massage
Although a regular massage is usually an excellent tonic for pregnant women, do not rub varicose veins directly. Instead, ask your therapist to work around the affected area.

Reflexology
See pages 804–805 for information about reflexology areas and how to work them.

Work the colon, the liver, and the kidneys to keep your points of elimination open and to reduce the pressure on your legs.

Hydrotherapy
To minimize inflammation, make a wet compress using witch hazel, and apply it to the affected area.

Other Bodywork Recommendations
Make time every day to lie down with your feet higher than your head. Even if you

don't suffer from varicose veins, this will improve other pregnancy-related discomforts and will reduce the chances that varicose veins will develop later.

Other Recommendations

- Bicycling is usually recommended to improve circulation, but if you're pregnant, you may find it uncomfortable to ride a bike. Instead, try swimming or aqua-aerobics, which are good nonimpact exercises.
- Maternity support hose are available in many department and specialty stores. It's best to put them on first thing in the morning or after a period of rest, when your legs aren't already swollen. Make sure to get a good fit—anything that's too tight will make varicose veins worse.

REFERENCES

Sahakian, V., D. Rouse, S. Sipes, et al. 1991. Vitamin B6 is effective therapy for nausea and vomiting of pregnancy: A randomized, double-blind placebo-controlled study. *Obstetrics and Gynecology* 78:33–36.

Teglio, L., et al. 1987. Vaccinium myrtillus anthocyanosides (Tegens) in the treatment of venous insufficiency of lower limbs and acute piles in pregnancy. *Quaderni di Clinica Obstetrica e Ginecologica* 42(3):221–31.

Vutyavanich, T., S. Wongtra-ngan, and R. Ruangsri. 1995. Pyridoxine for nausea and vomiting of pregnancy: A randomized, double blind, placebo-controlled trial. *American Journal of Obstetrics and Gynecology* 173:881–84.

Premenstrual Syndrome (PMS)

Premenstrual syndrome, more commonly known as PMS, is a disorder that affects high numbers—almost 75 percent—of menstruating women. It usually occurs a week or two before bleeding begins and is characterized by a wide range of symptoms, including (but not limited to) bloating, breast tenderness, emotional changes, cramps, and fatigue. Some women with PMS experience just one or two of these symptoms and find them quite mild and tolerable; others are hit with several symptoms, each so intense as to be incapacitating. Most women's symptoms exist somewhere between the two extremes, producing a moderate level of discomfort and at least some disruption of daily activities.

Because so many women experience PMS, Western medicine long considered most PMS symptoms a normal part of womanhood. If a woman had debilitating PMS, she was likely to be dismissed—to a Western doctor, her symptoms were clearly "all in her head." We now know that PMS is a physical disorder—and a highly treatable one, at that.

Each month, a woman's hormones follow a predictable cycle of change. Some fluctuation is absolutely normal and necessary, but when the ups and downs become severe, or when the different kinds of hormones needed to regulate body functions are knocked out of balance, the result is water retention, cramps, fatigue, or any of the other symptoms of PMS. Hormone imbalance is a common problem with PMS. While excessive estrogen and progesterone deficiency (or an imbalanced ratio between the two) are believed by many practitioners and researchers to be the key imbalance, there can also be issues with elevated prolactin (pituitary hormone), increased aldosterone (adrenal gland dysfunction), serotonin deficiency, and thyroid abnormality (usually, low thyroid). One must also consider the role of the liver with PMS, as it is responsible for metabolizing hormones. Improving liver function with natural therapies often helps to lessen the symptoms of PMS.

Poor diet and nutritional deficiencies can be root problems of PMS as well. One must also consider the role of "hormone disrupters" in the environment, such as pesticides and herbicides.

In addition, PMS can be caused or aggravated by food allergies, seasonal affective disorder, stress, and depression; a wise course of treatment will address each of these potential triggers. If you have severe PMS that is not resolved by using the home treatments suggested here, consult with a holistic doctor. You may have an underlying disorder, such as hypoglycemia or an underactive thyroid.

SYMPTOMS

Psychological
- Irritability
- Tension
- Anxiety
- Mood swings
- Aggression
- Loss of concentration
- Depression
- Forgetfulness
- Mental confusion and fatigue
- Insomnia
- Change in libido
- Crying spells

Physiological
- Bloating
- Weight gain (fluid)
- Breast tenderness
- Headache
- Pelvic discomfort and pain
- Change in bowel habits
- Increased appetite
- Sugar cravings
- Generalized aches and pains
- Physical tiredness
- Weakness
- Clumsiness

ROOT CAUSES

- Hormonal imbalances
- Poor diet
- Food allergies
- Seasonal affective disorder
- Stress
- Depression
- Hypoglycemia
- Thyroid problems
- Environmental toxins (e.g., pesticides)
- Poor liver function
- Nutritional deficiencies

Testing Techniques

The following tests help assess possible reasons for PMS:

Hormone testing (thyroid, DHEA, cortisol, testosterone, IGF-1, estrogen, progesterone, prolactin)—saliva, blood, or urine

Detoxification profile—urine

Vitamin and mineral analysis (especially magnesium, calcium, B6, B12)—blood

Food and environmental allergies/sensitivities—blood, electrodermal

Blood sugar balance—blood

TREATMENT

Diet

A diet that's high in meat, fat, sugar, and salt will make hormones fluctuate out of control and will intensify the symptoms of PMS. It has been shown that vegetarian women have much less circulating free estrogen in their blood than nonvegetarian women do. This does not mean you have to become totally vegetarian. However, it does suggest that a diet that focuses on plant foods leads to less circulating estrogen, thus decreasing one's susceptibility to PMS. A good, wholesome diet can significantly reduce or even eliminate problems altogether.

Recommended Food

Meals based on whole, high-fiber foods will balance your blood sugar, ease digestive problems, and reduce stress on your liver. Vegetables, fruits, whole grains, legumes, herbs, nuts, and seeds should be plentiful in the diet.

Fermented soy products, such as tofu, tempeh, and miso, can also help prevent PMS, due to their hormone-balancing phytonutrients.

Make sure your animal products (meat, poultry, etc.) are hormone free.

Eat at least two servings of green leafy vegetables every day. They're a good source of calcium, which supports and calms the nervous system, and they also have a diuretic effect.

Essential fatty acids, found in cold-water fish, flaxseeds, and flaxseed oil, will reduce inflammation.

Consume 1 tablespoon of ground flaxseeds daily, along with 10 ounces of water, to promote healthy estrogen metabolism.

Vitamin B6 has been shown to significantly reduce the symptoms of PMS. Add wheat germ or brewer's yeast to one of your meals every day.

Every month, plan a vegetable-juice fast for one to two days before your symptoms usually begin. If they don't begin at a predictable time, do the fast two weeks before your period starts. The fast will help eliminate the toxins, especially the environmental estrogens, that make PMS worse, and it also gives your liver a break from processing hormonal imbalances.

Food to Avoid

A diet that's low in saturated fat (the type found in red meat and dairy products) helps reduce excess estrogen levels. It is also important to avoid harmful fats, such as trans-fatty acids, which occur in margarine and partially hydrogenated oils. Studies have shown that women who follow a low-fat diet experience a reduction in PMS symptoms.

Food allergies often mimic the symptoms of PMS or make existing symptoms worse. Consult the Food Allergies section, and use the elimination diet on page 316.

If you can identify foods that give you trouble, eliminate them from your diet completely.

Sugar throws blood sugar levels off balance, promoting mood swings and tension. Excessive consumption of highly refined sugar can deplete valuable reserves of chromium, magnesium, zinc, manganese, and B vitamins. These nutrients are necessary for the metabolism of sugar. Sugar also worsens symptoms of hypoglycemia (low blood sugar), especially premenstrually, resulting in symptoms of irritability, poor concentration, sugar cravings, and headaches. Restrict your intake of sugary food throughout the month, and eliminate it during the two weeks before your period.

If you retain water, drastically restrict your consumption of sodium. Processed and junk foods are the highest sources of salt in the American diet.

Restrict caffeine-containing products, such as coffee, soft drinks, chocolate, and some pain relievers. Caffeine worsens PMS symptoms, such as anxiety, depression, and breast tenderness. Instead of coffee, we recommend that you focus on herbal teas, such as peppermint and chamomile.

Alcohol has a dehydrating effect, which only makes many PMS symptoms worse. It also wreaks havoc on your blood sugar levels. Avoid it during the two weeks before your period.

℞ Super Seven Prescriptions—PMS

Super Prescription #1 Vitex (chasteberry)
Take 40 drops of tincture or 180 to 240 mg in capsule form of a standardized extract of 0.6 percent aucubine or 0.5 percent agnuside. Take it daily for four to six months. Vitex is the most well-studied herbal treatment for PMS. Improvements are usually noted within two cycles. Do not take it if you are using the birth control pill.

Super Prescription #2 Homeopathic Combination PMS Formula
Take as directed on the container. It contains a blend of the most common homeopathic remedies for PMS. It's very effective for acute relief or can be used preventatively.

Super Prescription #3 Vitamin B6
Take 50 mg daily. Numerous studies have found vitamin B6 to help PMS. It works synergistically with magnesium as a cofactor for estrogen metabolism by the liver.

Super Prescription #4 Magnesium
Take 250 mg twice daily. Magnesium is a cofactor required for the metabolism of estrogen, and it relieves cramping.

Super Prescription #5 Natural progesterone cream
Apply ¼ teaspoon (10 mg) twice daily to areas of thin skin, such as the insides of your forearms and your wrists, beginning after ovulation (approximately day fifteen if you have a regular twenty-eight-day cycle) until one day before your period begins. Natural progesterone is a stronger therapy for women with severe PMS.

Super Prescription #6 Calcium
Take 500 mg twice daily. Studies have shown that this mineral prevents PMS.

Super Prescription #7 Dong quai (*Angelica sinensis*)
Take 300 to 500 mg twice daily, on the last seven days of your cycle. Dong quai reduces the painful cramps and the breast tenderness that are associated with menses. It is thought to relax the smooth muscles of the uterus, thereby relieving cramps.

Studies show that women who consume more sugar also suffer from more severe PMS symptoms. A study in the *Journal of Reproductive Medicine* that included 853 female university students investigated the impact of a high-sugar diet. Researchers found a strong correlation between high sugar consumption and PMS.

Vitex has a balancing effect on progesterone levels, as well as on the hormone prolactin. A two-month study compared the effects of vitex to those of the pharmaceutical antidepressant Prozac. Both were found to be beneficial overall. Researchers noted that vitex was more helpful for physical complaints and Prozac more beneficial for psychological symptoms.

Numerous double-blind, clinical trials on vitamin B6 have been conducted over the last twenty years. In one six-month, double-blind, crossover trial, 84 percent of the women undergoing vitamin B6 treatment reported greater improvement than they did during treatment with a placebo. Another study found that vitamin B6 supplementation improved premenstrual acne flare-ups in approximately 75 percent of women.

One double-blind study looked at 497 women who were given either 1,200 mg of calcium or a placebo for three menstrual cycles. By the third month, a significant improvement in four PMS symptoms (negative mood, water retention, food cravings, and pain) was experienced by the group taking calcium.

General Recommendations

Passionflower (*Passiflora incarnata*) gently relaxes the nervous system and improves symptoms of restlessness, irritability, and insomnia. Take 2 ml or 300 mg three times daily for anxiety and irritability.

Dandelion leaf (*Taraxacum officinale*) lessens the water retention that is associated with PMS. Take 3 ml or 300 mg three times daily for the one to two weeks before your cycle when you experience water retention.

Zinc has been shown to be low in women with PMS. Take 15 to 30 mg daily as part of a multivitamin.

Vitamin E-complex helps to effectively reduce the breast tenderness that is associated with PMS. It has also been shown to significantly reduce other PMS symptoms. We recommend 400 to 800 IU daily. Natural vitamin E (d-alpha-tocopherol), with a blend of tocopherols and tocotrienols, is best.

Evening primrose oil (*Oenothera biennis*) is an excellent dietary source of GLA. This essential fatty acid is a precursor to prostaglandins, which have a regulating effect on hormones and other systems of the body. Some studies have shown the benefits of evening primrose oil supplementation for PMS-related depression, irritability, breast pain and tenderness, and fluid retention. Take 2,000 mg (200 mg of GLA) to 3,000 mg (300 mg of GLA), along with an oil blend that includes omega-3 fatty acids (flaxseed oil and fish oil).

D-glucarate is a phytonutrient that assists the liver in metabolizing estrogen. Take 500 mg twice daily.

Indole-3-carbinol assists the liver in metabolizing estrogen. Take 300 mg daily.

Milk thistle (*Silybum marianum*) improves liver detoxification. Take 250 mg of an 80 to 85 percent silymarin extract three times daily.

Dandelion root (*Taraxacum officinale*) also promotes good liver detoxification. Take 300 mg three times daily.

Crampbark (*Viburnum opulus*) is an herb that alleviates menstrual cramps. Take 3 ml or 500 mg every thirty to sixty minutes for acute menstrual cramps.

A high-potency multivitamin provides a base of nutrients that promotes hormonal health. Take as directed on the container.

The supplement 5-HTP reduces depression and anxiety associated with PMS. Take 50 to 100 mg three times daily for relief of symptoms. Do not use it if you are taking a pharmaceutical antidepressant or an antianxiety medication.

Homeopathy

Pick the remedy that best matches your symptoms in this section. Take a 6x, 12x, 6C, 12C, or 30C potency three times daily for acute symptoms or two weeks before the menses to prevent reoccurring symptoms. Consultation with a homeopathic practitioner is advised.

Bovista is a good choice when there is PMS accompanied by puffiness in the extremities and swelling. Another peculiar symptom is diarrhea that occurs before or during menses. The woman may feel very awkward and clumsy and have a tendency to drop things.

Calcarea Carbonica is indicated when a woman experiences fatigue, anxiety, and a feeling of being overwhelmed, along with PMS. Other common symptoms include water retention and breast tenderness. The period often comes early and lasts a long time. These women are usually chilly and have clammy feet and hands. They have a strong desire for eggs, dairy products, and sweets.

Chamomilla (*Matricaria chamomilla*) is a great remedy to relieve unbearable, painful menses. The woman feels irritable, angry, and very sensitive to pain. The symptoms are better with motion and worse with warm applications.

Cimicifuga (*Actaea racemosa*) is a remedy for a painful menses that gets worse as the flow increases. The woman experiences cramping and shooting pains that go across the legs or the thighs. Headache stiffness in the neck and the back are common.

Lachesis is specific for the emotional symptoms of PMS, which include jealousy, irritability, suspiciousness, and rage. The symptoms improve once the menstrual flow starts. The woman feels hot and is intolerant of anything touching her throat.

Lilium Tigrinum is a remedy for a premenstrual syndrome that's characterized by great irritability, along with a sensation that the woman's internal organs will prolapse through her pelvis. She crosses her legs to get relief from this sensation. Fresh air brings relief.

Lycopodium (*Lycopodium clavatum*) is for women who experience digestive upset, such as gas and bloating, especially in the late afternoon. They feel irritable and want to boss others around, although they lack self-confidence. They crave sweets and have a large appetite.

Natrum Muriaticum is for a woman who feels depressed and lonely. She feels worse when given consolation or sympathy. Migraine headaches or lower back pain that accompany the menses are common symptoms. There is a strong craving for salt and an aversion to being in the sun.

Nux Vomica is for emotional symptoms of PMS that include impatience, anger, and irritability. Constipation becomes worse with the period. There is a craving for alcohol, coffee, spicy, or fatty foods. The woman often feels chilly and improves from warmth and rest.

Pulsatilla (*Pulsatilla pratensis*) is a great hormone balancer for women with PMS who experience mood swings, weepiness, and irritability. Their symptoms improve when they receive consolation and attention. They desire to be in the fresh air and feel worse in warm rooms. They have a strong craving for chocolate and sweets.

Sepia is for symptoms of irritability and fatigue that accompany PMS. There is a bearing-down sensation in the uterus, as if it is going to fall out, and painful breast tenderness that occurs before or with the menses. Exercise improves the symptoms. There is a strong craving for chocolate and sweets.

Acupressure

See pages 787–794 for information about pressure points and administering treatment.

- Conception Vessel 4 and 6 (CV4 and CV6) will reduce the pain of menstrual cramps.
- Conception Vessel 6 (CV6) also relieves diarrhea and constipation.
- For lower back pain, work Bladder 25, 31, and 40 (B25, B31, and B40).
- Liver 3 (Lv3) eases tension and stress.

Bodywork

Massage

For back pain and cramps, have a massage that incorporates deep kneading. It will relax your muscles and improve blood flow. If you have cramps or digestive problems, try this self-massage: Lie down with your knees bent, and press the surface of your abdomen until you find the spots that are most tender. Massage these points with the flat of your hand, using firm but gentle pressure.

Reflexology

See pages 804–805 for information about reflexology areas and how to work them.

Work the areas corresponding to the uterus, the fallopian tubes, the endocrine glands, and the lower spine.

Hydrotherapy

To improve circulation to the pelvic region and to ease cramps, you can use the constitutional hydrotherapy method. See pages 795–796 for directions.

Aromatherapy

Black pepper and rosemary have a warming, soothing effect on cramped abdominal muscles. Use either of these oils in a bath or a massage for best results.

Geranium and rose oils are known to balance female hormones. They also have an uplifting emotional effect. Add them to a massage oil or use them in a bath.

If you want to reduce stress, use geranium or rose oils, as mentioned earlier, or try lavender, bergamot, or jasmine. Use these oils in any preparation you like.

Patchouli and ylang-ylang are traditionally used to ignite sexual desire. If PMS has depressed your sex drive, add a few drops of these oils to a bath or a room diffuser. You could also add them to a massage.

Stress Reduction

Although PMS is largely a physical problem, the techniques here will help you address any emotional components of your disorder.

General Stress-Reduction Therapies

Yoga serves a triple purpose for women with PMS: It relieves cramps, improves digestion, and releases stress.

Other Recommendations

- Women who exercise regularly experience fewer PMS symptoms than their sedentary counterparts do. A daily half-hour walk, even on days when you feel at your worst, can do wonders to both reduce symptoms and prevent them in the first place.
- Place a hot compress on your abdomen to relieve menstrual cramps and gastrointestinal troubles.
- Seasonal affective disorder has been linked to PMS. If your symptoms are worse in the winter, take walks in the morning sunshine, as suggested earlier,

and try to spend your daylight hours near a sunny window. See Seasonal Affective Disorder on pages 575–581 for more information and suggestions.

REFERENCES

Atmaca, M., S. Kumru, and E. Tezcan. 2003. Fluoxetine versus Vitex agnus castus extract in the treatment of premenstrual dysphoric disorder. *Human Psychopharmacology* 18(3):191–95.

Rossignol, A. M., et al. 1991. Prevalence and severity of the premenstrual syndrome: Effects of foods and beverages that are sweet or high in sugar content. *Journal of Reproductive Medicine* 36(2):131–36.

Snider, B. L., and D. F. Dieteman. 1974. Letter: Pyridoxine therapy for premenstrual acne flare. *Archives of Dermatology* 110(1):130–31.

Thys-Jacobs, S., P. Starkey, D. Bernstein, and J. Tian. 1998. Calcium carbonate and the premenstrual syndrome: Effects on premenstrual and menstrual symptoms. Premenstrual Syndrome Study Group. *American Journal of Obstetrics and Gynecology* 179(2):444–52.

Prostate Enlargement (Benign Prostatic Hyperplasia)

The prostate is a male reproductive gland that sits at the outlet of the urinary bladder, surrounding the urethra (the channel that carries urine away from the bladder). Normally, the prostate is about the size of a walnut. In many men, however, especially those who are middle-aged or older, the gland becomes inflamed or enlarged. When this happens, the prostate compresses the urethra, obstructing the flow of urine and causing other problems (e.g., infection, bladder stones, urinary retentions).

Benign prostatic hyperplasia (BPH) is the medical term, but the disorder is more commonly known as enlarged prostate. When a man reaches middle age, the prostate often starts growing. There can be several reasons why this growth occurs, but it appears to be mainly caused by hormonal changes associated with aging.

Almost half of all men over forty-five suffer from at least some degree of prostate enlargement. At first, an enlarged prostate produces no symptoms, but as it grows and puts increased pressure on the urethra, urinary problems develop. It may be difficult to start urinating, and once the flow has begun, it may be hard to stop. There may be dribbling in between urination, along with a sense that the bladder isn't completely empty. Many men find that they awaken several times a night to urinate. Although the symptoms are uncomfortable and disruptive, benign enlargement is usually not a sign of a more serious disease. In some cases, however, the prostate can become so enlarged that the bladder can rarely empty itself completely. This urine retention can lead to an infection of the bladder or the kidneys; in severe cases, a constantly full bladder can place a dangerous level of pressure on the kidneys and even cause them to fail. A poor diet, especially one that's low in fiber and high in saturated fat, likely contributes to prostate enlargement as well.

As men age, their hormone balance changes. Testosterone levels decline, while levels of the estrogen class of hormones increase. One prevailing theory as to why the prostate enlarges centers around the increased conversion of testosterone to one of its metabolites, known as dihydrotestosterone (DHT). The enzyme responsible for this conversion of testosterone to DHT is 5-alpha reductase. It is believed that the activity of this enzyme increases as men age, so that DHT levels increase. DHT is implicated in prostate growth. Recent studies show that there is more to the story than just DHT. In recent years, there has been growing evidence that estrogen plays a role in prostate enlargement. A man's body contains the hormone estrogen, albeit in lesser amounts than in women. Some research shows that the balance between estrogen, testosterone, and DHT is the main issue with prostate cell growth. It is interesting to note that the enzyme aromatase converts testosterone to a potent form of estrogen known as estradiol. Estradiol causes prostate cells to grow and multiply. Keep in mind that pesticides, herbicides, and other environmental pollutants mimic estrogen in the body. It is also postulated that a rise in the estrogen-to-testosterone ratio amplifies the effects of DHT on the cell receptors of the prostate, which leads to cell growth. This relative increase in estrogen also reduces the ability of the prostate cells to clear out DHT. It makes some sense that DHT may not be the major villain in prostate enlargement. Rather, it is the balance between estrogen, testosterone, and DHT—and, likely, even progesterone—that really matters. The point is that proper hormone balance through diet, exercise, nutritional supplements, and detoxification is the key to helping this condition.

Prostatic enlargement responds well to natural treatment. Dietary and herbal therapies are especially effective at reducing the swelling and balancing the hormones. It's wise, however, to have any urinary or prostate problems checked out by a doctor, preferably a urologist, just to rule out any underlying cause. And if you experience weight loss, bone pain, or bloody urine, call your doctor right away.

SYMPTOMS

- Frequent urination
- Increased nighttime urination
- Urination that is hard to start or stop
- Burning pain with urination
- Reoccurring bladder infections
- Dribbling
- The sensation of an incompletely emptied bladder

ROOT CAUSES

- Hormonal changes
- Nutritional deficiencies
- A diet that's high in fat and low in fiber

Testing Techniques

The following tests help assess possible reasons for prostate enlargement:

Hormone testing (thyroid, DHEA, cortisol, testosterone, DHT, estrogen, progesterone)—saliva, blood, or urine

Intestinal permeability—urine

Detoxification profile—urine

Vitamin and mineral analysis—blood

Digestive function and microbe/parasite/candida testing—stool analysis

Food and environmental allergies/sensitivities—blood, electrodermal

Toxic metals—hair or urine

Essential fatty acid balance—blood or urine

TREATMENT

Diet

Recommended Food

A diet of basic, whole foods will provide plenty of fiber and will regulate hormone levels. Eat lots of whole grains and fresh vegetables, and get your protein from beans, fish, and soy products. To keep chemicals and pesticides out of your system, buy organic whenever possible.

Tomatoes are an excellent source of lycopene, a phytochemical that has an important protective effect on the prostate. This book usually recommends fresh food, but when it comes to lycopene, there's an important exception: cooked tomato products are actually a more potent source of this phytochemical than fresh ones are. Incorporate both into your meals daily.

Pumpkin seeds are a traditional remedy for prostate problems, and for good reason. They're full of zinc, a nutrient that's necessary for good prostate health. You can snack on raw pumpkin seeds throughout the day, but resist the urge to toast and salt them. You'll just add unwanted fat and sodium.

To reduce swelling, eat cold-water fish, flaxseeds (1 or 2 tablespoons daily, along with 10 ounces of water), and flaxseed oil. These foods are high in essential fatty acids, which are known for their anti-inflammatory properties. Flaxseeds also contain phytonutrients known as lignans, which balance estrogen levels.

Drink green tea (decaffeinated) instead of coffee, as it promotes healthy detoxification.

Drink a glass of clean water every two waking hours to keep fluid moving through the urinary tract.

Food to Avoid

Eliminate all fats that are saturated, hydrogenated, or partially hydrogenated. These fats lead to inflammation and have been closely linked with several prostate disorders.

Sugar wreaks havoc on hormone levels and worsens inflammation. Radically restrict your consumption of refined sugar, or, better yet, banish it from your diet altogether.

Processed food is full of chemicals that may cause or contribute to prostate problems. Stay away from it.

Avoid alcohol and caffeine. They are irritants to the prostate gland.

℞ Super Seven Prescriptions—Prostate Enlargement

Super Prescription #1 Saw palmetto (*Serenoa repens*)
Take 320 mg daily of a product standardized to 80 to 95 percent fatty acids. Saw palmetto has been shown in numerous studies to improve the symptoms of this condition. It appears to reduce hormone stimulation of the prostate tissue.

Super Prescription #2 Beta-sitosterol
Take 60 to 130 mg daily. Studies show that this phytonutrient improves the symptoms of benign prostatic hyperplasia.

Whirl a cup of pumpkin seeds in the food processor for a few minutes, and you'll have pumpkin-seed butter. It makes a delicious spread for sandwiches or crackers.

A study involving three urology centers looked at the effects of *Pygeum africanum* extract (50 mg twice daily) on the symptoms of BPH. Researchers concluded through urine-flow measurements that pygeum induced significant improvements, including with nighttime urination.

Super Prescription #3 Rye pollen extract

Take as directed on the container (generally, 3 tablets twice daily). Several studies have shown that this extract lessens the symptoms of BPH.

Super Prescription #4 Nettle (*Urtica dioica*) root

Take 120 mg twice daily. Nettles are commonly used in prostate formulas, along with other nutrients. Studies have shown that they lessen BPH symptoms.

Super Prescription #5 *Pygeum africanum*

Take 160 to 200 mg daily of a product standardized to 13 percent total sterols. Pygeum is an extract from the bark of an African tree that has a long history of use, as well as scientific validation, for reducing prostate enlargement.

Super Prescription #6 Zinc

Take 100 mg daily for two months and then 50 mg as a maintenance dosage, and take 3 mg of copper along with the zinc.

Super Prescription #7 Essential fatty acids

Take 1 tablespoon of flaxseed oil or 3,000 mg of fish oil daily. Essential fatty acids reduce inflammation.

Saw palmetto (*Serenoa repens*) has been found to have many favorable effects on the prostate, including:

- Inhibiting the activity of the enzyme 5-alpha reductase, which reduces the conversion of testosterone to DHT
- Blocking DHT from binding to prostate cells
- Reducing the effects of estrogen and progesterone on the prostate cells
- Causing smooth-muscle relaxation (theoretically allowing the urethra to open more effectively and preventing the back up of urine)
- Reducing inflammation and edema by inhibiting the effects of inflammation-producing chemicals called prostaglandins
- Altering cholesterol metabolism in the prostate
- Modifying the levels of sex hormone–binding globulin (SHBG)

General Recommendations

Amino acids relieve urinary symptoms of BPH. Take glycine, alanine, and glutamic acid, as this was the combination used in one successful study. Take 750 mg three times daily for two weeks and then 375 mg three times daily as a maintenance dose.

Pumpkin seed oil is often used in combination with saw palmetto (*Serenoa repens*) for the relief of BPH symptoms. Take 160 mg three times daily with meals.

A high-potency multivitamin provides a base of nutrients for prostate health. Take as directed on the container.

D-glucarate is a phytonutrient that assists the liver in metabolizing estrogen. Take 500 mg twice daily.

Indole-3-carbinol assists the liver in metabolizing estrogen. Take 300 mg daily.

Milk thistle (*Silybum marianum*) improves liver detoxification and, indirectly, hormone balance. Take 250 mg of an 80 to 85 percent silymarin extract three times daily.

Natural progesterone can be helpful. Apply a transdermal cream that contains 20 mg per dose to the skin of the inner arm each evening.

Homeopathy

Apis Mellifica is for prostate enlargement when stinging pain accompanies urination. There may also be urinary retention present.

Causticum is indicated when one loses urine from coughing or sneezing. There can be a pressure sensation extending from the prostate to the bladder. Causticum is also indicated when sexual pleasure during orgasm has diminished.

Chimaphilla Umbellate is a remedy that helps with urine retention. There is often a sensation that one is sitting on a ball. The person may feel as if a ball is lodged in the pelvic floor or may experience pressure, swelling, and soreness that feel worse when sitting down.

Clematis is a specific remedy for swelling of the prostate that leads to slow urine passage or a dribbling of urine.

Lycopodium (*Lycopodium clavatum*) may be helpful for prostate enlargement accompanied by sexual dysfunction, such as impotence. Men who need this remedy often have digestive problems, such as gas and bloating. They tend to feel chilly and crave sweets.

Pulsatilla (*Pulsatilla pratensis*) is for prostate problems with bladder pain at the end of urination. Men who require this remedy tend to get warm easily and feel better in the fresh air.

Sabal Serrulata is a good remedy for urine retention, especially in elderly men. There may be a cold sensation in the prostate or the bladder. It is useful for men with prostate enlargement who are prone to bladder infections.

Selenium is for an enlarged prostate and the involuntary dribbling of urine or prostatic fluid. Symptoms are worse after walking or urination. Impotence is another indication for this remedy.

Staphysagria is for urinary retention and the chronic dribbling of urine. There can be a burning sensation in the urinary tract and the prostate. Men who require this remedy may have suppressed emotions, as well as impotence.

Thuja (*Thuja occidentalis*) is for an enlarged prostate and a frequent urge to urinate. Sometimes a forked stream of urine is seen.

Acupressure

See pages 787–794 for information about pressure points and administering treatment.

- All the bladder points along the groin (B27–B34) regulate the reproductive organs and increase circulation to the prostate. With regular work, they will help reduce inflammation, as well as lower back pain.

The *Journal of the American Medical Association* reported a review on the therapeutic efficacy and the safety of saw palmetto extract in men with symptomatic BPH. The authors reviewed eighteen randomized controlled trials involving 2,939 men with BPH. They concluded that saw palmetto was as effective as Proscar (finasteride), a commonly prescribed pharmaceutical medication for BPH. The benefit of saw palmetto, compared to that of a pharmaceutical treatment, was the absence of side effects, such as impotence or loss of libido.

Another study, using before- and after-treatment ultrasound images, demonstrated that the combination of saw palmetto and nettle root reduced the size of prostate swelling in men with BPH.

Bodywork

Reflexology
See pages 804–805 for information about reflexology areas and how to work them. Work the areas corresponding to the prostate, the lower back/bladder, and the lymph/groin area.

Hydrotherapy
Hot and cold hydrotherapy in the pelvic region stimulates circulation to the genitals and the urinary tract. Splash first hot water, then cold, onto your lower abdomen. Repeat three times.

Constitutional hydrotherapy is a good long-term treatment for this condition. See the directions on pages 795–796.

Aromatherapy

Bergamot and chamomile reduce inflammation. Add them to a bath, or use them in a full-body massage.

If you have prostatitis, use a few drops of tea tree oil in a bath to fight the infection. This oil can sometimes be irritating, so start by adding just 2 or 3 drops under the tap. If you do not have a reaction, you can add a few more drops the next time around.

For a constant urge to empty the bladder, use sandalwood for its diuretic effect. A bath or a full-body massage is the best means of delivering this treatment.

Stress Reduction

General Stress-Reduction Therapies
Excess unresolved stress can alter your hormones, so keep tension in check by practicing any of the therapies discussed in the Exercise and Stress Reduction chapter on a regular basis.

Other Recommendations

Exercise to keep your cholesterol down and to work off stress. Low-impact workouts are best, as a jarring exercise like jogging may be painful if you have an enlarged prostate. Avoid bicycling, which puts too much pressure on the prostate.

REFERENCES

Breza, J., O. Dzurny, A. Borowka, et al. 1998. Efficacy and acceptability of tadenan (Pygeum africanum extract) in the treatment of benign prostatic hyperplasia (BPH): A multicentre trial in central Europe. *Current Medical Research and Opinion* 14(3):127–39.

Overmyer, M. 1999. Saw palmetto shown to shrink prostatic epithelium. *Urology Times* 27(6):1, 42.

Wilt, J., et al. 1998. Saw palmetto extracts for treatment of benign prostatic hyper plasia: A systematic review. *Journal of the American Medical Association* 280(18):1604–9.

Prostatitis

Prostatitis is an infection or a chronic inflammation of the prostate gland. Unlike an enlarged prostate, it strikes men of all ages. The most common form is chronic non-bacterial prostatitis (NBP), also called chronic abacterial prostatitis. This condition is caused by a fungus, a virus, or a mycoplasma infection and often cannot be resolved by antibiotics (especially for the fungal and viral infections). An acute bacterial infection, usually by E. coli, is another cause. An enlarged prostate gland predisposes one to this condition since urine flow is not as efficient and microbes are more likely to accumulate. In addition, pain in the pelvic-floor muscles can cause pain in the prostate region.

When infected, the prostate becomes inflamed and tender, and the man has difficulty producing a constant flow of urine. The infection produces other symptoms as well, which may include a fever, chills, a pain in the lower back, and bloody urine. The greatest danger of prostatitis is that it will become a chronic problem, in which the bladder cannot empty itself. As with benign enlargement, this constant urine retention can cause an infection or kidney disorders. We have successfully treated several men who had chronic prostatitis who were unresponsive to previous doctors' treatments with antibiotics. Many of the natural therapies mentioned in this chapter work at the root causes of prostatitis, which include nonbacterial infections and prostate enlargement. Homeopathy can be particularly effective for this condition, as can certain nutritional therapies, such as rye pollen extract.

SYMPTOMS

- Urination problems, as with an enlarged prostate
- Urine with blood or pus
- Pain in the region between the genitals and the anus
- Fever
- Chills
- Impotence
- Lower back pain

ROOT CAUSES

- Infection
- Prostate enlargement (contributing to infection)
- Food allergies
- Dehydration

Testing Techniques

The following tests help assess possible reasons for prostatitis:

Urine culture—determine whether there is a fungal or bacterial growth

Intestinal permeability—urine

Detoxification profile—urine

Vitamin and mineral analysis—blood

Digestive function and microbe/parasite/candida testing—stool analysis

Food and environmental allergies/sensitivities—blood, electrodermal

Toxic metals—hair or urine

Essential fatty acid balance—blood or urine

TREATMENT

Diet

Recommended Food

Eat lots of whole grains and fresh vegetables, and get your protein from beans, fish, and soy products. To keep chemicals and pesticides out of your system, buy organic produce whenever possible.

Pumpkin seeds are a traditional remedy for prostate problems, and for good reason. They're full of zinc, a nutrient that's necessary for good prostate health. You can snack on raw pumpkin seeds throughout the day, but resist the urge to toast and salt them. You'll just add unwanted fat and sodium.

To reduce swelling, eat cold-water fish, flaxseeds (1 to 2 tablespoons daily, along with 10 ounces of water), and flaxseed oil. These foods are high in essential fatty acids, which are known for their anti-inflammatory properties.

Drink green tea (decaffeinated) instead of coffee, as it promotes healthy detoxification.

Take the aforementioned flaxseeds daily, along with 10 ounces of water. Flaxseeds contain a phytonutrient known as lignans, which balance estrogen levels.

Drink a glass of clean, quality water every two waking hours to keep fluid moving through the urinary tract.

Food to Avoid

Eliminate all fats that are saturated, hydrogenated, or partially hydrogenated. These fats lead to inflammation and have been closely linked with several prostate disorders.

Sugar wreaks havoc on hormone levels and worsens inflammation. Radically restrict your consumption of refined sugar, or, better yet, banish it from your diet altogether.

Processed food is full of chemicals that may cause or contribute to prostate problems. Stay away from it.

Avoid alcohol and caffeine. They are irritants to the prostate gland.

℞ Super Seven Prescriptions—Prostatitis

Super Prescription #1 Rye pollen extract
Take as directed on the container (generally, 2 tablets twice daily). Several studies have shown that this extract improves the symptoms of prostatitis.

Super Prescription #2 Quercitin
Take 500 mg twice daily. Quercitin is a type of flavonoid that reduces inflammation.

Super Prescription #3 Echinacea (*Echinacea purpurea*) and goldenseal (*Hydrastis canadensis*)
Take 500 mg of the capsule form or 4 ml of the tincture four times daily. These herbs enhance immune function to combat infection.

Super Prescription #4 Oregano oil (*Origanum vulgare*)
Take 500 mg of the capsule form four times daily for acute prostatitis and twice daily for chronic problems. Oregano oil has powerful antifungal, antibacterial, and antiviral effects.

Several studies have demonstrated that rye pollen extract improves the symptoms of chronic prostatitis, including prostate pain. One study published in the *British Journal of Urology* looked at the effects of a commercial rye pollen extract and ninety men with chronic prostatitis. These men were given 1 tablet three times daily for six months. Patients' symptoms, as well as laboratory tests and doctor evaluations after three and six months, found favorable results in 78 percent of the men; 36 percent were reported cured and 42 percent improved.

Super Prescription #5 *Pygeum africanum*

Take 160 to 200 mg daily of a product standardized to 13 percent total sterols. It has been shown to be helpful for this condition.

Super Prescription #6 Zinc

Take 100 mg daily for two months and then 50 mg as a maintenance dosage. Take 3 mg of copper along with the zinc. Zinc improves immune function and reduces prostate congestion.

Super Prescription #7 Saw palmetto (*Serenoa repens*)

Take 320 mg daily of a product standardized to 80 to 95 percent fatty acids. Saw palmetto reduces the prostate enlargement that often underlies chronic prostatitis.

General Recommendations

Thuja (*Thuja occidentalis*) is a great herb for nonbacterial prostatitis since it has antiviral and antifungal properties. Take 10 drops three times daily of the herbal tincture form.

Vitamin A enhances immune function. Take 25,000 to 50,000 IU daily for one week.

D-mannose is a special type of sugar that prevents bacteria from being able to attach to the urinary tract and the bladder wall. Take 500 mg four times daily.

Uva ursi can be helpful for bacterial prostatitis. Take a standardized capsule containing 250 mg of arbutin or 5 ml of the tincture four times daily.

A probiotic should be taken in the form of a product containing at least four billion organisms daily. It contains friendly bacteria that prevent the overgrowth of harmful bacteria and yeast, which contributes to prostatitis. It is especially important to take if you are using antibiotics. Take it at a separate time during the day, and continue use for two months.

Vitamin C enhances immune function, inhibits the growth of *E. coli*, and makes the urine more acidic so that bacteria cannot grow as easily. It also has anti-inflammatory properties that may benefit men with prostatitis. Take 1,000 mg four or five times daily.

Bromelain has a natural anti-inflammatory effect and has been shown to be helpful for prostatitis when combined with vitamin C. Protease enzyme products also have this benefit. Take 500 mg three times daily between meals. Look for products standardized to 2,000 MCU (milk-clotting units) per 1,000 mg or 1,200 GDU (gelatin-dissolving units) per 1,000 mg.

Cranberries (*Vaccinium macrocarpona*) prevent bacteria from adhering to the bladder wall. This plant is best used for the prevention of urinary tract infections but can be used as part of a comprehensive protocol for acute infection. Take 400 to 500 mg twice daily of cranberry extract capsules.

Homeopathy

Apis Mellifica is for prostatitis accompanied by stinging or burning pain during urination. Urinary retention may also be present.

Quercitin has been shown to be helpful for non-bacterial prostatitis, as well as for prostate pain (prostadynia). One study found that 500 mg taken twice daily for two weeks significantly improved symptoms in 59 percent of men with chronic prostatitis. A separate double-blind study showed that quercitin supplementation for one month improved symptoms in 67 percent of men with nonbacterial prostatitis. The effects of quercitin may be improved with the supplementation of bromelain and papain, two protease enzymes.

Causticum is indicated when one loses urine from coughing or sneezing. There can be a pressure sensation extending from the prostate to the bladder. Causticum is also indicated when sexual pleasure during orgasm has diminished.

Chimaphilla Umbellate is a remedy that helps acute prostatitis and urinary retention. There is often a sensation that one is sitting on a ball. The person may feel as if a ball is lodged in the pelvic floor or may experience pressure, swelling, and soreness that feel worse when sitting down.

Clematis is a specific remedy for swelling of the prostate that leads to slow urine passage or a dribbling of urine.

Lycopodium (*Lycopodium clavatum*) may be helpful for men who have a painful stream of urine. Symptoms are worse after urination. There can also be sexual dysfunction, such as impotence. Men who need this remedy often have digestive problems, such as gas and bloating. They tend to feel chilly and crave sweets.

Medorrhinum is for men with prostatitis that occurs after having gonorrhea or a new sexual partner.

Pulsatilla (*Pulsatilla pratensis*) is for prostate problems accompanied by bladder pain at the end of urination. Men who require this remedy tend to get warm easily and feel better in the fresh air.

Sabal Serrulata is a good remedy for urine retention, especially in elderly men. There may be a cold sensation in the prostate or the bladder. It's useful for men with prostatitis who are prone to bladder infections.

Selenium is for an enlarged prostate and the involuntary dribbling of urine or prostatic fluid. Symptoms feel worse after walking or urination. Impotence is another indication for this remedy.

Staphysagria is for urinary retention and the chronic dribbling of urine. There can be a burning sensation in the urinary tract and the prostate. Men who require this remedy may have suppressed emotions as well as impotence.

Sulfur is for prostatitis characterized by burning in the urethra or the prostate. Lower back pain is common. Symptoms are worse while standing and after sexual activity.

Thuja (*Thuja occidentalis*) is for prostatitis that develops after being treated for gonorrhea or other sexually transmitted diseases. Sometimes a forked stream of urine is seen.

Acupressure

See pages 787–794 for information about pressure points and administering treatment.

All the bladder points along the groin (B27–B34) regulate the reproductive organs and increase circulation to the prostate. With regular work, they will help reduce inflammation, as well as lower back pain.

Bodywork

Acupuncture and Chinese herbal therapy offered by a qualified practitioner can be helpful for chronic prostatitis.

Reflexology

See pages 804–805 for information about reflexology areas and how to work them.

Work the areas corresponding to the prostate, the lower back/bladder, and the lymph/groin area.

Hydrotherapy

Hot and cold hydrotherapy in the pelvic region stimulates circulation and reduces inflammation. First sit in a warm tub for two minutes, then sit in cool water for thirty seconds. Repeat three times.

Constitutional hydrotherapy is a good long-term treatment for this condition. See the directions on pages 795–796.

Aromatherapy

Bergamot and chamomile reduce inflammation. Add them to a bath or use them in a full-body massage.

If you have prostatitis, use a few drops of tea tree oil in a bath to fight the infection. This oil can sometimes be irritating, so start by adding just 2 or 3 drops under the tap. If you do not have a reaction, you can add a few more drops the next time around.

For a constant urge to empty the bladder, use sandalwood for its diuretic effect. A bath or a full-body massage is the best means of delivering this treatment.

Stress Reduction

General Stress-Reduction Therapies

Excess unresolved stress can alter your hormones, so keep tension in check by practicing any of therapies in the Exercise and Stress Reduction chapter on a regular basis.

Other Recommendations

Avoid bicycling, which puts too much pressure on the prostate.

REFERENCES

Rugendorff, E. W., W. Weidner, L. Ebeling, et al. 1993. Results of treatment with pollen extract (Cernilton N) in chronic prostatitis and prostatodynia. *British Journal of Urology* 71:433–38.

Shoskes, D. A., S. I. Zeitlin, A. Shahed, et al. 1999. Quercetin in men with category III chronic prostatitis: A preliminary prospective, double-blind, placebo-controlled trial. *Urology* 54:960–63.

Psoriasis

Psoriasis, a common skin disorder, occurs when skin cells replicate too quickly. The skin produces new cells at about ten times its normal rate, but it also continues to slough off old ones at its usual, slower pace. With nowhere else to go, the new cells pile up under the surface, creating patches of red, swollen skin covered with silvery or whitish scales. Psoriasis can appear anywhere on the body, but it most often surfaces on the scalp, the knees, the elbows, the buttocks, and the backs of the wrists. The rash usually doesn't itch, but if you scratch, it may bleed. Psoriasis comes and goes in cycles and leaves no scars, although the area may be thick and dry even in times of remission. The nails may also be affected and may develop stipples and pitted areas.

Occasionally, in a condition known as pustular psoriasis, blisters will rise on the palms of the hands or the soles of the feet. Psoriasis has also been linked to inflammatory arthritis of the fingers and the toes.

Psoriasis can cause a type of arthritis that resembles rheumatoid arthritis in some individuals. The nails are affected in 30 to 50 percent of people with psoriasis, resulting in a pitting, a discoloration, and a thickening of the nails' plates.

The exact cause of psoriasis remains unknown, but the prevailing theory connects the high rate of cell replication to a genetic flaw. This theory is backed up by the large number of cases that run in families. As with most genetic disorders, however, it's also likely that people simply inherit a predisposition to psoriasis. Lifestyle choices play an important part in determining the severity and the frequency of the condition or whether you'll even experience it at all. A poor diet, for example, often worsens this condition. The identification and the treatment of food allergies is the key for some individuals. The digestive tract is a focal point for many people with psoriasis. Poor digestion, especially incomplete protein digestion, leads to the creation of toxins known as polyamines, which contribute to excessive skin proliferation. In addition, the overgrowth of *Candida albicans* and various bacteria by-products is thought to worsen this condition. Along with the overgrowth of these microbes is often an imbalance or a deficiency of friendly flora, the good bacteria that help detoxify the body. Liver function is of critical importance, as it is the body's main filtering system. Optimizing liver function with sound nutrition and nutritional supplements can be helpful.

We have also found a connection between psoriasis and a low intake of essential fatty acids (EFAs). Finally, stress, fluctuating hormones, sunburn, and other environmental factors can contribute to flare-ups.

SYMPTOMS

- Red, inflamed patches of skin, covered with silvery or white scales
- Dull, distorted nails
- Blisters on the palms of the hands or the soles of the feet (in cases of pustular psoriasis)
- Thick, dry skin in times of remission

ROOT CAUSES

- Genetics
- A poor diet, especially one that's low in fiber and EFAs
- Difficulty digesting protein
- Overgrowth of fungi and other microbes
- Poor liver function
- Stress
- Hormonal changes
- Sunburn
- Illness or infection
- Certain medications
- Vitamin D deficiency

Testing Techniques

The following tests help assess possible reasons for psoriasis:

Hormone testing (thyroid, DHEA, cortisol, testosterone, IGF-1, estrogen, progesterone)—saliva, blood, or urine

Intestinal permeability—urine

Detoxification profile—urine

Vitamin and mineral analysis—blood

Digestive function and microbe/parasite/candida testing—stool analysis

Food and environmental allergies/sensitivities—blood, electrodermal

Toxic metals—urine or hair

TREATMENT

Diet

As with all skin disorders, psoriasis is best treated by encouraging the body to eliminate toxins through the bowels and the urinary tract, rather than through the skin.

Recommended Food

Get your protein from fish and vegetarian sources like tofu and beans. These foods are much easier to digest than animal proteins are.

Increase your intake of fiber. Eat fresh, whole foods and include whole grains, raw fruits and vegetables, or beans at every meal.

Essential fatty acids reduce inflammation and have been shown to greatly improve psoriasis. Cold-water fish like mackerel and salmon are excellent sources of EFAs, and so are both flaxseeds and flaxseed oil. (Flaxseeds are also a concentrated source of the fiber you need. Take 1 to 2 tablespoons daily, along with 10 ounces of water.)

Many psoriasis sufferers are deficient in zinc and vitamin A. Eat pumpkin seeds for zinc; for vitamin A, eat orange, yellow, or green vegetables.

Drink a glass of clean, quality water every two waking hours to improve digestion, flush away toxins, and reduce inflammation.

Food to Avoid

Avoid red meat, poultry, and milk. People with psoriasis often have difficulty digesting protein, and these foods are the hardest on your intestines. In addition, both red meat and milk contain arachidonic acid, which aggravates inflammation.

Do not eat other foods that are difficult to digest. Fatty, fried, and junk foods all fall into this category, as do products that are high in refined sugar.

Alcohol causes inflammation and triggers psoriasis in many people. Drink only in moderation and monitor your intake; if alcohol leads to a flare-up, you should stop drinking altogether.

In some people, psoriasis is brought on by allergic reactions to food. Read the Food Allergies section, and follow the elimination diet there. If a certain food triggers an episode of psoriasis or makes an existing one worse, remove it from your diet. Gluten, cow's milk, sugar, and citrus fruits are common offenders.

Make sure to avoid caffeine.

℞ **Super Seven Prescriptions—Psoriasis**

Super Prescription #1 Turmeric
Take 1,000 mg two to three times daily of a highly absorbable turmeric extract.

Super Prescription #2 Fish oil
Take 10 grams daily of a high-quality fish oil. Fish oil contains a substance known as EPA that has anti-inflammatory effects.

Super Prescription #3 Vitamin D
Take 2,500 to 5,000 IU daily with meals. Low levels of this nutrient are associated with psoriasis in some people.

Super Prescription #4 Milk thistle (*Silybum marianum*)
Take 250 mg three times daily of an 80 to 85 percent silymarin extract. Milk thistle improves liver detoxification and reduces cellular proliferation.

Super Prescription #5 Vitamin B12
Get a 1 cc injection from your doctor daily for ten days and then twice weekly. Some patients notice an improvement in their psoriasis after six weeks of treatments. Sublingual B12 may also be helpful, at 400 to 800 mcg daily.

Super Prescription #6 Sarsaparilla
Take 500 mg or 4 ml three times daily. This herb reduces the effects of bacterial toxins that aggravate psoriasis.

Super Prescription #7 Digestive enzymes
Take 1 or 2 capsules of a full-spectrum enzyme product with each meal. Enzymes help you to digest food more efficiently.

In a double-blind study, researchers examined the effect of people with psoriasis supplementing 10 grams of fish oil daily for eight weeks versus the results in another group taking a placebo. The fish-oil group had a significant lessening of itching, redness, and scaling.

General Recommendations

Take an organic super green food, such as chlorella or spirulina, or a mixture of super green foods, each day. Take as directed on the container.

Flaxseed oil contains the omega-3 fatty acids that reduce inflammation of the skin. Take 1 to 2 tablespoons daily.

Reishi (*Ganoderma lucidum*) extract improves liver detoxification. Take 800 mg twice daily.

A probiotic supplement provides friendly bacteria, such as *Lactobacillus acidophilus* and *bifidus*, which are important for detoxification and skin health. Take a product containing at least four billion active organisms daily.

Gentian root (*Gentiana lutea*) improves overall digestive function. Take 300 mg or 10 to 20 drops five to fifteen minutes before meals.

A high-potency multivitamin provides a base of nutrients for skin health. Take as directed on the container.

Drink a quarter cup of aloe vera juice for its cooling, anti-inflammatory effect, or apply aloe vera gel directly to the affected area.

Homeopathy

Arsenicum Album is for psoriasis characterized by dry, scaly, itching, and burning skin. Symptoms are better with warm applications. People who require this remedy are usually restless and anxious.

Calcarea Carbonica is recommended when there are dry, scaly plaques that often crack open. People who are helped by this remedy are usually overweight and chilly and have clammy hands and feet. They crave sweets, dairy products, and eggs. They have a sensation of being overwhelmed, anxious, and easily fatigued.

Graphites is for psoriasis that has lesions that ooze, often in a yellow-brown color. Lesions mainly occur on the backs of the hands and the ears, on the head and the scalp, and on the genitalia. Symptoms are usually worse at night.

Mercurius Solubilis may benefit people who seem introverted and formal but are very intense internally, with strong emotions and impulses. They tend to have swollen lymph nodes and moist or greasy-looking skin and are very sensitive to changes in temperature. The areas affected by psoriasis may become infected easily.

Mezereum is for a person who has fine, white, scaly plaques that cover large areas. The skin may itch intensely and crust easily and feels better with cold applications.

Petroleum is a remedy for psoriasis characterized by extreme dryness of the skin all over the body. People who benefit from this remedy usually have very dry skin in general. Itching will be worse at night and from getting warm in bed. Symptoms are much worse in the winter and in cold, dry weather.

Rhus Toxicodendron is for psoriasis characterized by dry, red, chapped, raw skin that itches intensely. Symptoms are better from hot applications or baths. The person is restless and often has a craving for cold milk.

Sepia is one of the most common homeopathic remedies for psoriasis. There is a thickening of the skin, with circular eruptions and dryness. This remedy is recommended for women with a hormonal imbalance. They feel chilly and irritable.

Staphysagria is for persistent psoriasis that erupts after suppressed grief or emotions. The scalp is most commonly affected.

Sulfur is a good choice for intense itching and burning and inflamed eruptions that are worse from warmth and bathing. The lesions are often moist and oozing. It is also commonly used for psoriatic arthritis.

Acupressure

See pages 787–794 for information about pressure points and administering treatment.
- Work Stomach 36 (St36) to strengthen your digestive tract.
- For psoriasis related to stress, use Bladder 10 (B10).

Bodywork

Reflexology

See pages 804–805 for information about reflexology areas and how to work them. The thyroid, which controls the rate of skin-cell replacement, is the most important area of the foot to work. Work the kidneys and the liver to purify the blood. For hormone regulation, stimulate the endocrine glands.

Hydrotherapy

Constitutional hydrotherapy is a good long-term therapy for psoriasis, as it promotes detoxification. See pages 795–796 for details.

Aromatherapy

Lavender oil reduces inflammation and relieves stress. Add a few drops to a lotion or a cream, and rub it gently into the affected areas of skin, while breathing deeply to inhale the scent.

Stress Reduction

General Stress-Reduction Therapies

If stress brings on your psoriasis, you may actually be lucky: People with stress-induced psoriasis have a much greater chance of controlling their condition than do people with other triggers. Any stress-reduction technique will help; choose one you are comfortable with.

Other Recommendations

- Many people find that mild sunlight greatly improves psoriasis. Try taking a walk in the morning sun; the exercise will reduce stress and improve your digestion.
- If you have patches of psoriasis on your scalp, do not use a blow dryer. Let your hair dry naturally instead.
- Your doctor may prescribe a topical agent for psoriasis. Although these drugs improve the condition temporarily, the problem will return when you stop using them. It's better to rely on measures that address the root of the problem.
- Sometimes other medications can trigger psoriasis. If you're taking nonsteroidal anti-inflammatories, lithium, chloroquine, or beta-blockers, talk to your doctor about possible substitutions.
- See the Candidiasis section. Treatment of underlying Candida problems can be helpful.
- We have seen low thyroid function be an aggravator of this condition. See the Hypothyroidism section for more information. In addition, the use of synthetic hormone replacement in menopausal women may be an irritant to the skin. See the Menopause section for natural ways to balance your hormones.
- Topical curcumin extract has been shown to be effective for psoriasis.

REFERENCES

Bittiner, S. B., W. F. G. Tucker, I. Cartwright, et al. 1988. A double-blind, randomised, placebo-controlled trial of fish oil in psoriasis. *Lancet* 1:378–80.

Restless Leg Syndrome

If you have an unpleasant sensation in your legs that makes you want to move them at night when you are trying to go to sleep, then you may be one of the millions of Americans that suffer from restless leg syndrome (RLS). Research shows that up to 10 percent of the US population may have this condition. It occurs in both men and women, although it is about twice as common in women. It usually occurs in middle-aged or older adults. Since people with RLS are forced to move their legs to get relief, it is classified as a movement disorder.

There are two types of RLS, primary and secondary. The exact cause of primary RLS is unknown, but there seems to be a genetic susceptibility, and the central and peripheral nervous systems seem to play a role. Those with primary RLS exhibit symptoms before the age of forty-five.

To treat RLS, conventional doctors rely on medications such as anticonvulsants that affect the brain and nervous system, which in turn controls the muscles. Another class of conventional drugs for RLS treatment works by augmenting dopamine activity in the brain. Certain natural substances also help dopamine production, including the amino acid N-acetyl tyrosine. Some patients respond well to taking 5-hydroxy-trytophan, which boosts serotonin, at bedtime.

SYMPTOMS

- Discomfort in the legs such as pulling, crawling, throbbing, or other abnormal sensations that lead to an uncontrollable urge to move them
- Symptoms occurring on both sides, and, less often, affecting other body parts, such as arms, trunk, or head
- In 80 percent of sufferers, an involuntary jerking or twitching of the legs during sleep, causing disrupted sleep and daytime fatigue

ROOT CAUSES

Genetics is thought to be the cause of primary RLS. Secondary causes include:

- Iron deficiency (approximately 25 percent of sufferers)
- Folate deficiency (or a MTHFR gene mutation)
- Magnesium deficiency
- Amyloidosis
- Diabetes
- Kidney disease
- Lumbosacral radiculopathy
- Lyme disease
- Monoclonal gammopathy
- Pregnancy
- Rheumatoid arthritis
- Sjogren's syndrome
- Venous disorder
- Certain pharmaceuticals, e.g., antihistamines such as diphenhydramine (Benadryl), antidepressants, lithium, beta-blockers, and antipsychotics

---

Testing Techniques

Nutrient deficiencies (iron and low iron stores, folate, B12, magnesium)—blood work

    Toxic metals—urine, blood, hair analysis

    Genetic metabolic imbalances such as MTHFR mutation—blood or saliva

    Hormone balance (thyroid)—blood

A secondary cause of RLS can be chronic venous disorders, which lead to poor circulation, particularly in the lower legs. Studies have shown that a majority of patients with chronic venous disease who receive treatment notice an improvement in RLS symptoms.

TREATMENT

Diet

Recommended Food

Eat a whole-food, plant-based diet that is rich in antioxidants.

Cold-water fish and their omega-3 fatty acids reduce brain inflammation.

Food sources of magnesium are important. Consume more magnesium-rich foods such as pumpkin seeds, spinach, quinoa, black beans, and navy beans.

If your potassium is low then good food sources include tomatoes, tomato juice, bananas, avocados, yogurt, and broccoli.

Food to Avoid

It is important to avoid caffeine and alcohol, which can worsen symptoms.

Iron supplementation can significantly ameliorate RLS in patients with low-normal levels of iron in their blood. Have your iron levels checked by your doctor. If you're deficient or on the low end of normal, then iron supplementation may be quite beneficial.

℞ Super Seven Prescriptions

Super Prescription #1 Iron
Take iron supplements if your doctor has determined your iron or ferritin (iron stores) is low. A typical dose is 50 to 100 mg of chelated iron daily.

Super Prescription #2 Folate
Take 400 mcg of methylfolate if your level is low or you have a MTHFR gene mutation. Work with a holistic doctor to optimize your dosage.

Super Prescription # 3 5-hydroxytryptophan (5-HTP)
Take 100 to 200 mg at bedtime. This amino acid increases serotonin, which relaxes the nervous system.

Super Prescription #4 Magnesium
Take 400 to 500 mg each evening to relax your nervous system and muscles.

Super Prescription # 5 Valerian root
Take 800 mg of an extract at bedtime. Research has shown it to benefit RLS.

Super Prescription #6 N-acetyl tyrosine
Take 500 mg each evening to increase dopamine levels and reduce restless legs.

Super Prescription #7 Pycnogenol
Take 100 mg at bedtime to improve circulation to the legs and reduce inflammation.

Other Recommendations

Those with RLS should definitely try acupuncture. Studies have shown benefit. While acupuncture may not cure RLS, it can certainly help to reduce symptoms.

REFERENCES

Wang J., B. O'Reilly, et al. 2009. Efficacy of oral iron in patients with restless legs syndrome and a low-normal ferritin: A randomized, double-blind, placebo-controlled study. *Sleep Medicine* 10(9).

Rosacea

Rosacea is an inflammatory skin disorder in which the nose, the cheeks, the forehead, or the chin are chronically reddened and prone to breaking out in acne-like welts. Unlike acne, however, rosacea never produces blackheads or whiteheads, and it rarely appears during adolescence. Instead, rosacea generally sets in during a person's thirties or forties, beginning with a mild pink blush that doesn't go away. If treated early, the condition may never progress any further or may even recede a bit. But in advanced cases, it can cause permanent thickening and redness, especially on the nose. Although women are more likely to have rosacea than men are, men who do have rosacea tend to have more severe cases.

Anything that dilates blood vessels in the face can lead to a flare-up of rosacea. Specific triggers differ from person to person, but the most common are alcohol, hot liquids, coffee, spicy or fatty foods, extreme temperatures, sun exposure, harsh wind, and stress. It's important to minimize the exposure to triggers, because each time the blood vessels expand, they lose some elasticity. Over time, they become incapable of constricting properly and they remain in a dilated state—hence the redness. A person who already has the early flushing of rosacea will find that triggers make his or her face even redder, or that they lead to pimples that may or may not disappear when the trigger is removed.

Although we understand the elements that make rosacea worse, there is no one underlying cause of the disorder. Skin conditions generally point to some kind of digestive problem, and rosacea is no exception. Many rosacea sufferers have been found to have low levels of stomach acid, which prevents proper digestion of trace minerals and possibly the overgrowth of bacteria that aggravates the skin. Sluggish bowels and constipation may have a similar effect on digestion. And whenever pimples or red spots appear, it's likely that the skin is pushing out toxins that an impaired digestive tract is unable to process. Leaky gut syndrome, which is characterized by malabsorption, may be an issue for people with rosacea. Also, B-vitamin deficiencies, especially of B12, are common with this condition. Friendly flora that are involved with detoxification and that prevent the overgrowth of infectious bacteria are often depleted. We have also found that rosacea becomes a problem as the result of a hormone imbalance. Premenopausal and menopausal woman often find that rosacea starts to act up until they get their hormones balanced with natural therapies. On the other hand, synthetic hormone replacements and birth-control-pill use initiate or worsen this condition for some women. Finally, hidden food allergies may cause flushing that is mistaken for rosacea.

Conventional treatment for rosacea involves antibiotics, either oral or topical, which have a minimal effect and which must be taken continuously. While people with severe cases that may lead to disfigurement might want to consider medication, most people will be better off making an effort to avoid their personal triggers and improve their digestion.

SYMPTOMS

- Redness across the nose, the cheeks, the forehead, or the chin
- Red pimples or welts

ROOT CAUSES

- Repeated exposure to rosacea triggers (alcohol, wind, sun, etc.)
- Nutritional deficiencies (especially of B vitamins)
- Low levels of stomach acid
- Dysbiosis (imbalance of the gut bacteria)
- Constipation
- A diet that's high in fat and low in fiber
- Hormone imbalance
- Reaction to synthetic hormones
- Food allergies

Testing Techniques

The following tests help assess possible reasons for rosacea:

Hormone testing (thyroid, DHEA, cortisol, testosterone, IGF-1, estrogen, progesterone)—saliva, blood, or urine

Intestinal permeability—urine

Detoxification profile—urine

Vitamin and mineral analysis (especially B12)—blood

Digestive function and microbe/parasite/candida testing—stool analysis

Food and environmental allergies/sensitivities—blood, electrodermal

---

TREATMENT

Diet

Recommended Food

Eat lots of raw foods. In their natural state, vegetables, fruits, nuts, sprouts, and seeds all possess enzymes that help you convert food into the nutrients that are needed for skin and circulatory health. Green leafy vegetables are especially good for rosacea patients as they're an excellent source of trace minerals.

Drink several glasses of fresh vegetable juice a day. If you have rosacea, it's likely that your digestive system isn't processing food thoroughly, and juices are a potent way to deliver nutrients directly to your bloodstream.

Make sure your diet includes plenty of fiber. If you're eating a couple of servings of raw foods at every meal, you're probably getting almost as much fiber as you need to keep toxins moving through your digestive tract instead of erupting from your skin. Add whole grains and beans to round out your meals.

Essential fatty acids reduce inflammation. Have cold-water fish from a clean source several times a week, and eat flaxseeds (1 to 2 tablespoons, with 10 ounces of water) each day.

A deficiency of B vitamins has been found in many people who have rosacea. Brown rice, oats, wheat germ, nutritional brewer's yeast, and whole-grain bread and crackers are all good sources. If you tend to be anxious, B vitamins will also help you feel calmer.

It's generally inadvisable to take antibiotics for most cosmetic disorders (save them for the more severe infections), but if you feel you must take them, be sure to eat some live unsweetened yogurt or another cultured product every day. Cultured foods replace the "friendly" intestinal bacteria that antibiotics strip away.

Food to Avoid

Avoid food items that make you flush. Spicy food, caffeine, and alcohol are tripwires for most rosacea sufferers. Sugar and iodized salt may also dilate your blood vessels. Learn which foods bother your skin, and eliminate them from your diet.

Be careful of food and drinks that are hot in temperature. Allow hot beverages and soups to cool before you eat them.

Saturated fat has an inflammatory effect on many body systems, including the skin. If you stay away from red meat and fried, greasy foods, you'll also improve your digestion.

Food allergies may mimic the symptoms of rosacea or make an existing problem worse. Read the Food Allergies section on pages 312–317, and follow the elimination diet there.

℞ Super Seven Prescriptions—Rosacea

Super Prescription #1 Gentian root (*Gentiana lutea*)
Gentian root improves overall digestive function. Take 300 mg or 10 to 20 drops five to fifteen minutes before meals. It also works well as part of a bitters digestion formula.

Super Prescription #2 Betaine hydrochloride
Take 1 to 3 capsules with each meal. Reduce the dose if you feel a warming or burning sensation. This supplement improves stomach acidity and digestion, especially of proteins. It also prevents the overgrowth of bacteria in the digestive tract that may influence rosacea.

Super Prescription #3 B-complex vitamins
Take a 50 mg B-complex twice daily. It supplies B vitamins that improve rosacea.

Super Prescription #4 Vitamin B12
Take 400 to 800 mcg sublingually or 1 cc injected by your doctor weekly. This B vitamin works to reduce flare-ups of rosacea.

Studies completed during the early part of the twentieth century found that a significant percentage of people with rosacea had low stomach acid (hypochlorhydria). Supplementation with hydrochloric acid resulted in an improvement of their skin.

A study of ninety-six people with rosacea found that supplementation with six tablets of brewer's yeast plus iron resulted in an improvement of their skin lesions.

> ### Super Prescription #5 Burdock root (*Articum lappa*)
> Take 300 mg or 3 ml three times daily. Burdock has historically been prescribed for rosacea and other chronic skin disorders. It appears to improve detoxification as well as hormone balance.
>
> ### Super Prescription #6 Natural progesterone
> See the Menopause section for proper usage, which depends on where you are in your menopausal transition. This hormone has anti-inflammatory benefits and improves skin conditions if it is deficient and then supplemented correctly.
>
> ### Super Prescription #7 Probiotic
> Take a product containing at least four billion active organisms twice daily, thirty minutes after meals. It supplies friendly bacteria, such as *Lactobacillus acidophilus* and *bifidus*, which improve skin health.

General Recommendations

Milk thistle (*Silybum marianum*) improves liver function and detoxification for optimal skin health. Take 250 mg three times daily of a 80 to 85 percent silymarin extract.

Digestive enzymes help you to digest food more efficiently. Take 1 or 2 capsules of a full-spectrum enzyme product with each meal. Lipase enzymes that digest fat appear to be particularly important for people with this condition.

Black cohosh (*Cimicifuga racemosa*) improves hormone balance for premenopausal and menopausal women affected by rosacea. Take 80 mg of a 2.5 percent triterpene glycoside extract daily.

Green tea (*Camellia sinensis*) contains a rich source of antioxidants and substances that assist detoxification. Drink the organic tea regularly (2 cups or more daily) or take 500 to 1,500 mg of the capsule form.

Essential fatty acids reduce inflammation of the skin. Take 1 to 2 tablespoons of flaxseed oil or 5 grams of fish oil daily, or a formulation that contains a mixture of omega-3, -6, and -9 fatty acids.

Reishi (*Ganoderma lucidum*) extract improves liver function, which is important for healthy skin. Take 800 mg twice daily.

A super-green-food supplement supplies phytonutrients that improve skin health. Take an organic super green food such as chlorella, spirulina, alfalfa, or a mixture of super green foods each day. Take as directed on the container.

Aloe vera gel is soothing and anti-inflammatory. Apply it directly to the affected area. Test it out on a small patch of your skin first, as you may be highly sensitive to many preparations, even gentle herbal ones.

Topical vitamin C (5 percent) and alpha lipoic acid (3 percent) once daily can help to reduce inflammation of the skin.

Homeopathy

Choose the appropriate remedy from the following list, and take 6C three times daily for up to three weeks. Use a combination acne formula or one of the following if it matches your symptoms. Use a 6x, 12x, 6C, 12C, or 30C potency for two weeks. If there is improvement, discontinue using unless symptoms return.

Arsenicum Album is for hot, dry, and flaky skin. The person tends to be anxious and restless, gets cold easily, and prefers warm drinks.

Hepar Sulphuris may provide relief if you have several pus-filled spots that are painful when touched, and if the skin lesions feel better with a warm compress.

Pulsatilla (*Pulsatilla pratensis*) is for rosacea associated with the hormonal changes of puberty, menstrual onset, or menopause. Women tend to be sensitive and weepy. They crave sweets. They feel better in the fresh air and worse in warm rooms.

Sepia is for rosacea associated with the hormonal changes of puberty, menstrual onset, or menopause. Great irritability and fatigue are present. The woman craves chocolate and salty and sour foods. She tends to get chilly easily.

Sulfur is for chronic redness and inflammation that is worsened by the sun, hot baths or showers, and warm climates. The person has a high thirst for cold drinks and prefers a cool climate.

Acupressure

See pages 787–794 for information about pressure points and administering treatment.

- Stomach 36 (St36) improves digestion and the absorption of nutrients.
- Spleen 10 (Sp10) clears excess heat from the blood.
- Stomach 3 (St3) will clear up rosacea blemishes.
- Use Bladder 10 (B10) if rosacea is aggravated by stress.

Bodywork

Reflexology
See pages 804–805 for information about reflexology areas and how to work them.

To cleanse your blood, work the liver and the kidneys.

If you need to reduce stress, work the solar plexus and the diaphragm.

Hydrotherapy
Some people find that a warm foot bath pulls heat away from the face; for others, this treatment simply makes their faces even more inflamed. In no case should you use hot water for the foot bath, nor should you take hot baths, showers, or saunas.

Aromatherapy

Try placing a cool—not cold—compress made with lavender oil on your skin to reduce heat and swelling. Take advantage of the relaxing scent, and breathe deeply.

Stress Reduction

It's helpful if you can minimize stress before it brings on a flare-up (which usually leads to even more stress). As soon as you feel any anxiety, take a moment to breathe deeply. If you have five or ten minutes, try a brief meditation session.

Other Recommendations

- Bright sunlight is one of the most common rosacea triggers. Stay out of the midday sun, and when you do go outside, wear protective clothing and sunscreen. If over-the-counter sunscreens irritate your skin, ask your doctor about a gentle prescription formula.
- Limit the time you spend in cold and windy weather. When you must go outside, cover your face with a soft scarf or even a ski mask made from hypoallergenic material.
- If you want to wear makeup, use gentle, hypoallergenic cosmetics and makeup-removal products.
- If you are taking a synthetic horomone replacement, consult with a holistic doctor for a more natural approach, as these hormones can contribute to your acne rosacea.
- Laser therapy by a dermatologist can be effective.

REFERENCES

Ryle, J. A., et al. 1920. Gastric analysis in acne rosacea. *Lancet* 2:1195–96.

Tulipan, L. 1947. Acne rosacea: A vitamin B complex deficiency. *Archives of Dermatology* 56:589–91.

Sarcopenia

The loss of muscle mass as one ages is a major risk to one's health. Muscle mass is required for strength, mobility, bone density, immunity, temperature regulation, blood sugar control, and balance. Over half of seniors have some degree of significant muscle loss. Most seniors are surprised at the medical impact of losing muscle mass and the connection to failing health and loss of independence.

The medical term for the loss of skeletal muscle mass and strength is age-related sarcopenia. Sarcopenia comes from the Greek word meaning "poverty of the flesh." With our aging population the medical treatment of sarcopenia could become a specialty in itself. In general, as people get older they become more sedentary, and as a result their muscle fibers shrink. In addition, hormonal and other metabolic shifts occur in the body that reduce muscle mass. Inadequate nutrition combined with poor digestion becomes more prevalent in seniors, and all these factors contribute to shrinkage of the muscles and loss of strength.

Sarcopenia increases the risk of mobility disorders, falls and fractures, impaired ability to perform activities of daily living, disabilities, loss of independence, and death.

The number-one concern for seniors when it comes to nutrition is the lack of protein intake. This is particularly true of those in nursing homes, those who are hospitalized, and those who live alone. Studies show that approximately 25 percent of seniors do not consume enough protein.

For reasons not well understood, studies show that sarcopenia is much more common in white men and women than in the black population. There is a gender difference as well, with women at higher risk than men. This is likely due to the fact that women generally have less lean muscle mass to begin with. Then the hormonal changes of menopause make them more susceptible to muscle loss. However, women's muscle mass does respond quickly to hormonal therapy.

In conclusion, sarcopenia is one of the biggest health threats affecting Americans today, especially seniors. Utilize muscle-boosting techniques to live a longer and healthier life.

SYMPTOMS

- Muscle weakness
- Reduced stamina
- Weakened immunity
- Mobility problems

ROOT CAUSES

- Nutritional deficiencies
- Digestive dysfunction (especially low stomach acid)
- Hormone imbalance (particularly low DHEA, low testosterone, low growth hormone, elevated cortisol)
- Cachexia (tissue wasting from diseases like cancer)
- Neurodegenerative disease
- Aging
- Increased oxidative stress
- Weight issues (low body weight and obesity)
- Inactivity
- Genetics
- Race and gender

Testing Techniques

There are different ways to test for sarcopenia. Muscle mass can be measured with diagnostic imaging such as computed tomography (CT scan), magnetic resonance imaging (MRI), or dual energy X-ray absorptiometry (DXA). CT and MRI are the most precise imaging tests since they can differentiate fat from other soft tissues of the body. The problem with these tests is the cost; in addition, the CT scan includes radiation exposure. DXA is a reasonable test as it produces lower radiation and can measure bone density as well as muscle mass. A very good alternative that is cost effective and has no risks of radiation exposure is bioimpedance analysis (BIA). This test is done in a doctor's office or by a licensed personal trainer. It involves the application of sensor-pad electrodes on a hand and foot and sends a small current through the body. No pain is felt. Impedance or resistance to the electrical flow is measured. Electricity flows better in lean tissue than fat tissue. A calculation based on the impedance, person's age, weight, and height gives a pretty accurate assessment of lean muscle mass. This test has been shown to correlate well with MRI testing. One can also analyze muscle strength by using a hand-grip testing device or a leg-extensor machine with added resistance. Physical performance can be tested by having the patient walk or climb steps.

In addition, the following lab tests can assess underlying factors that may contribute to muscle wasting:

Hormone testing (estradiol, progesterone, thyroid, growth hormone, testosterone, cortisol, DHEA, pregnenolone)—blood and urine

Vitamin D—blood

TREATMENT

Diet

Recommended Food

A mixture of plant and animal protein sources can be effective in supplying amino acids for muscle tissue. Some people do well on plant protein sources, but others need an ample amount of animal protein for optimal results. The general recommendation for protein intake for adults is approximately 50 grams daily. Some patients require closer to 100 grams for muscle-mass growth. *Note*: If you have liver or kidney disease consult with your health care professional before altering your diet.

Food to Avoid

Avoid simple sugars and processed foods that are devoid of nutrients.

 Super Seven Prescriptions—Sarcopenia

Super Prescription #1 Whey protein
Blend 25 grams of the powder form in a shake. A number of studies have verified that whey protein is indeed a valid and safe way to provide essential amino acids for muscle growth.

Protein-Rich Foods

Chicken (4 ounces) 35 grams

Turkey (4 ounces) 34.09 grams

Tuna (4 ounces) 33.99 grams
   (*Note*: use low-mercury tuna only)

Beef (4 ounces) 32.33 grams
   (*Note*: use lean, organic beef only)

Salmon (4 ounces) 30.97 grams

Lamb (4 ounces) 30.15 grams

Soybeans (1 cup) 28.63 grams
   (*Note*: fermented soy products are best)

Lentils (1 cup) 17.86 grams

Dried peas (1 cup) 16.35 grams

Kidney beans (1 cup) 15.35 grams

Pumpkin seeds (quarter cup) 9.75 grams

Eggs (1 medium) 6.92 grams

Spinach (1 cup) 5.35 grams

Mustard greens (1 cup) 3.16 grams

Asparagus (1 cup) 2.95 grams

Super Prescription #2 Amino acid formula
Take as directed. Make sure it contains branched-chain essential amino acids, including the ones most critical for your muscles: L-leucine, L-isoleucine, and L-valine.

Super Prescription #3 Creatine monohydrate
Take 5 grams daily. It is used by muscle cells for energy and to hold water inside muscle tissue to enhance muscle mass.

Super Prescription #4 Vitamin D
Take 5,000 IU daily with a meal. Research shows vitamin D deficiency contributes to a loss of muscle mass.

Super Prescription #5 Fish oil
Take 1,000 mg of combined DHEA and EPA. Omega-3-rich fish oil reduces muscles inflammation.

Super Prescription #6 Betaine HCL with pepsin
Take 1 to 3 capsules with each regular meal to improve protein breakdown and absorption.

Super Prescription #7 Magnesium
Take 250 mg twice daily to support muscle health and growth.

A recent study found that supplementing with whey protein and essential amino acids, in combination with restricting calories, resulted in a substantial loss of fat tissue and a minimal loss of muscle tissue in a group of obese seniors. Whey-protein supplementation has also been shown to increase both lean body mass and muscular strength when compared to another cow-milk protein known as casein. Whey protein is a valuable food supplement to help patients lose fat and gain muscle. It is well tolerated by most people. Those who are extremely lactose intolerant (i.e., who cannot digest the milk sugar lactose) can use reduced-lactose formulas.

Other Recommendations

- Follow the steps outlined in this chapter to improve digestion of important nutrients, especially protein.
- We believe that one of the most overlooked reasons why seniors and many other adults suffer from low protein blood levels is poor digestion and absorption. As people age, their ability to break down and absorb protein becomes reduced. One of the key areas of protein digestion is the stomach. Stomach acid (hydrochloric acid) converts pepsinogen, a proenzyme secreted by the stomach cells, into the enzyme pepsin. In turn, pepsin helps to break protein down into individual amino acids, making them easier to absorb in the small intestine. Low levels of hydrochloric acid are responsible for much of the problem with protein digestion and absorption. If protein is insufficiently broken down in the stomach, the intestines have difficulty doing so later. Besides aging and chronic disease another factor contributing to low stomach acid is acid-suppressing medications, used by millions of Americans.
- Once partially digested food exits the stomach and enters the small intestine, enzymes secreted by the pancreas break it down further. Aging, stress, medications, and chronic disease can lead to deficiencies in these enzymes, causing more problems with nutrient breakdown and absorption. Lastly, microbial infections such as yeast and parasites, and the use of common medications such as non steroidal anti-inflammatories for pain reduction, can damage the intestinal lining, further compromising absorption. Fortunately, a good holistic physician can help you with all these issues.
- One of the areas conventional medicine ignores when it comes to sarcopenia is hormone imbalance. We feel it is essential to get a thorough hormone evaluation and treatment by a doctor well versed in bioidentical (natural) hormones. There are many hormones that should be assessed, including testosterone, growth hormone, thyroid, cortisol, DHEA, pregnenolone, and, for women, estrogen and progesterone. We find that many seniors are particularly deficient in testosterone, growth hormone, DHEA, and pregnenolone, all of which contribute to muscle growth.
- Nerve health is important in relation to muscle health. Conditions that negatively affect nerve flow to the muscles ultimately reduce muscle mass. Without nerve stimulation the muscles cannot be activated, which is needed for growth and maintenance. Neurological problems affecting muscle activity

A study reported in the *American Journal of Cardiology* showed that daily amino-acid supplements led to significant increases in muscle after six months and additional muscle after sixteen months.

Creatine is a popular supplement that is composed of three amino acids known as arginine, glycine, and methionine. A 2012 study found that creatine supplementation combined with resistance training improved muscle strength, fat-free mass, and muscle mass in older women compared to those taking a placebo plus exercise.

need to be treated. Natural therapies such as acupuncture, massage, and spinal manipulation can be very helpful.

- Free radicals contribute to muscle damage. A lack of antioxidants in the diet combined with heavy free-radical damage from chronic disease, medications, and other toxins overload the body with these damaging particles. Boosting antioxidants from plant foods and supplementing with super antioxidants such as resveratrol, coenzyme Q10, pine-bark extract, and others should be part of a comprehensive program.
- Maintain a healthy body weight. Studies show that those who are underweight lose muscle mass. This is particularly true of patients who have cachexia (tissue wasting) from a chronic disease such as malnutrition or cancer. Research also shows that obese individuals have a lack of muscle mass.
- Being inactive is a big risk for sarcopenia. Patients who are bedridden can lose up to 9 percent of their lower-extremity muscle mass. We recommend resistance training two to three times weekly to help build muscle. Work with a certified trainer so that all your muscle groups are being enhanced.

REFERENCES

Aguiar, A. F., et al. 2012. Long-term creatine supplementation improves muscular performance during resistance training in older women. *Eur J Appl Physiol* Oct 7.

Alfonso, J., et al. 2010. Sarcopenia: European consensus on definition and diagnosis: report of the European working group on sarcopenia in older people. *Age and Ageing* 39(4):412–23. Accessed December 16, 2012 at http://www.medscape.com/viewarticle/723929_5.

Borst, S. 2004. Interventions for sarcopenia and muscle weakness in older people. *Age and Ageing* 33:6.

Coker, R., et al. 2012. Whey protein and essential amino acids promote the reduction of adipose tissue and increased muscle protein synthesis during caloric restriction-induced weight loss in elderly, obese individuals. *Nutrition Journal* 11:105, doi:10.1186/1475-2891-11-105.

Cribb, P. J., et al. 2006. The effect of whey isolate and resistance training on strength, body composition, and plasma glutamine. *It J Sport Nutr Exerc Metab.*

Dawson-Hughes, B., S. Harris, L. Ceglia. 2008. Alkaline diets favor lean tissue mass in older adults. *American Journal of Clinical Nutrition* 87:662–65.

Elgoweini, M., N. Nour El Din. 2009. Response of vitiligo to narrowband ultraviolet B and oral antioxidants. *J Clin Pharmacol* 49(7):852–55.

Kinney, J. 2004. Nutritional frailty, sarcopenia and falls in the elderly. *Current Opinion in Clinical Nutrition and Metabolic Care* 7:15–20.

Losing muscle is a part of aging, but you can minimize the effects. 2007. *Environmental Nutrition* 30:11.

The World's Healthiest Foods website. Accessed December 16, 2012 at www.whfoods.com.

Seasonal Affective Disorder (SAD)

Seasonal affective disorder (SAD) is characterized by symptoms of depression that develop in the dark winter months and that lift with the onset of spring and summer. Although many of us feel a little less energetic in the winter, people with SAD suffer from more than just a prolonged bad mood. They have a medical condition typified by fatigue, poor concentration, and an intense craving for carbohydrates. They may also feel an overwhelming need for sleep, although the sleep itself is rarely refreshing. This general slowdown of the body, combined with an excessive intake of carbohydrates, may lead to weight gain and a suppressed immune system. Seasonal affective disorder should not be confused with the depression that afflicts some people during the holidays, when unresolved conflicts or problems tend to rise to the surface.

The most compelling theory regarding the cause of SAD has to do with the decreased amount of light that is available in the winter. Depending on the latitude, a winter day in the United States can have fewer than eight hours of sunlight, compared to sixteen hours of sun in the summer. In the last few years, we've learned that there's a reason that people feel more exuberant in the summer: natural sunlight acts as a control mechanism for a substance in our bodies called melatonin. As the sun sets, our pineal glands (located at the base of the brain) sense the decrease in light and begin to secrete the sleep-inducing hormone melatonin. Melatonin secretion can be magnified by increasing our exposure to sunlight during the day. But when we're deprived of sunlight, there's nothing to keep melatonin levels in check, and it takes all our effort just to get out of our warm beds in the morning. In addition, levels of the stress hormone cortisol may rise, contributing to fatigue, insomnia, depression, and decreased immunity. Finally, levels of the neurotransmitter serotonin may drop, contributing to depression. Researchers have found that serotonin production is directly affected by the duration of bright sunlight.

It is unclear why some people are affected by a lack of sunlight more than others. What has been demonstrated time and again, however, is that light therapy is the most effective way to alleviate the symptoms of SAD. If you suffer from winter depression, there's a very good chance that you'll benefit greatly from just a few simple changes: utilizing specific light therapy, installing full-spectrum lights that imitate the effects of the sun, spending time outdoors every day, and arranging your life so that you're near a window as often as possible. Other natural treatments, including dietary changes and some herbal supplements, will round out an effective course of action for lifting the "winter blues."

SYMPTOMS

- Fatigue and lethargy
- Increased desire to sleep
- Fitful, unrestful sleep
- Inability to concentrate
- Cravings for sweets and other carbohydrates
- Weight gain
- Reduced sex drive

ROOT CAUSE

- Lack of natural sunlight

Testing Techniques

The following tests help assess possible causes of SAD:

Hormone testing (thyroid, DHEA, cortisol, testosterone, IGF-1, estrogen, progesterone)—saliva, blood, or urine

Intestinal permeability—urine

Detoxification profile—urine

Vitamin and mineral analysis (especially magnesium, B12, folic acid, B1)—blood

Digestive function and microbe/parasite/candida testing—stool analysis

Food and environmental allergies/sensitivities—blood, electrodermal

Blood sugar balance—blood

Toxic metals—hair or urine analysis

Amino acid analysis—blood or urine

TREATMENT

Diet

Recommended Food

One way to maintain a good mood is to keep your blood sugar levels steady. Vegetables and lean protein will stabilize blood sugar. Make a small meal or a snack of them every few hours to ward off the urge for bread or sweets. When you do eat carbohydrates, make sure they're complex carbohydrates, like oats, brown rice, or whole wheat. These foods are high in fiber, which slows the release of sugars into your bloodstream.

Put turkey, chicken, tuna, or salmon on your daily menu. These foods are high in protein, which you need for energy, and tryptophan, which stimulates the "feel-good" hormone in your brain.

B vitamins act as a tonic on the nervous system. Include brewer's yeast, green leafy vegetables, and live unsweetened yogurt in your meals or snacks.

Brussels sprouts are a perfect food for SAD sufferers. Brussels sprouts are a concentrated source of vitamin C, which fights fatigue and has a stimulating effect on your mood. Unlike citrus fruits, brussels sprouts are also low in sugar. Cooking destroys vitamin C, so eat brussels sprouts raw, perhaps in a salad or served with a dip.

Food to Avoid

Try to resist your cravings for sugar, bread, and other simple carbohydrates. Although these foods may temporarily lift your mood, your blood sugar will soon crash, leaving you feeling even worse than before. And the weight gain that often results from over-indulging in carbohydrates will aggravate your fatigue and leave you susceptible to colds, the flu, and other winter ailments. If you must treat yourself to simple carbohydrates, make sure to have them as part of a complete meal—have an occasional sweet dessert, say, after eating a meal that consists of protein, vegetables, and some whole grains. That way, the sugar won't deliver as potent a punch to your bloodstream.

People with SAD also tend to rely on caffeine to rouse them in the morning and keep them alert during the day. But caffeine works much like sugar does, in that once the rush peaks and declines, you're left feeling exhausted and crabby. Caffeine also depletes your body of several nutrients that are essential for a healthy nervous system. Limit yourself to one cup of coffee or tea a day.

Junk food probably isn't a direct cause of SAD, but it can certainly exacerbate the symptoms: Weight gain, a suppressed immune system, and fatigue have all been linked to the consumption of additives and artificial ingredients. Avoid food that's had all the life processed out of it.

Alcohol is a depressant, so avoid wine, beer, and liquor. If you are so unhappy that you feel as if you need alcohol, talk to a doctor or a therapist. You may have a drinking problem—or you may be headed for one.

℞ Super Seven Prescriptions—Seasonal Affective Disorder

Super Prescription #1 Melatonin
Take 3 to 5 mg before bedtime. Studies show that this nutrient tends to be low in patients with SAD.

Super Prescription #2 Saint-John's-wort (*Hypericum perforatum*)
Take 300 mg of a product standardized to 0.3 percent hypericin three times daily (a total of 900 mg). Saint-John's-wort has been shown to be helpful for SAD, when combined with light therapy.

Super Prescription #3 S-adenosylmethionine (SAMe)
For two weeks, take 200 mg twice daily of an enteric-coated form on an empty stomach. If you notice improvement, stay on this dosage. If there is little improvement, increase to 400 mg two or three times daily. SAMe increases the concentration of brain neurotransmitters that are responsible for your mood. Take a 50 mg B-complex, because B6, folic acid, and B12 are involved with proper SAMe metabolism. *Note*: People with bipolar disorder should use this supplement only with medical supervision.

Super Prescription #4 5-hydroxytryptophan (5-HTP)
Start with 50 mg taken three times daily on an empty stomach. The dosage can be increased to 100 mg three times daily, if necessary. The supplement 5-HTP is a precursor to the neurotransmitter serotonin. Take a 50 mg B-complex, as B6 is required for the proper metabolism of 5-HTP. *Note*: Do not take in conjunction with pharmaceutical antidepressants or antianxiety medications.

Super Prescription #5 L-tryptophan
Take 1,000 mg three times daily between meals. This increases serotonin, which reduces depression.

Super Prescription #6 B-complex vitamins
Take a 50 mg B-complex one or two times daily. B vitamins such as B12, folic acid, and B6 are intricately involved with neurotransmitter metabolism. Sublingual B12 and folic acid supplements are useful for seniors or people with absorption difficulties.

> **Super Prescription #7** *Ginkgo biloba*
> Take 60 to 120 mg twice daily of a standardized product containing 24 percent flavone glycosides and 6 percent terpene lactones. Ginkgo improves blood flow to the brain and enhances neurotransmitter activity.

General Recommendations

Fish oil can be effective because essential fatty acids such as DHA improve neurotransmitter function. Take a product containing a daily combined dosage of 500 to 1,000 mg of EPA and DHA.

DL-phenylalanine (DLPA) is an amino acid used by the brain to manufacture neurotransmitters. Take 500 to 1,000 mg on an empty stomach each morning. It should be avoided by people with anxiety, high blood pressure, or insomnia. Do not take it in combination with pharmaceutical antidepressants or antianxiety medications.

L-tyrosine is an amino acid that also helps depression. Take 100 to 500 twice daily on an empty stomach. Do not take it in combination with pharmaceutical antidepressants or anti anxiety medications.

Ashwagandha (*Withania somniferum*) improves stress-hormone balance and relaxes the nervous system. Take 1,000 mg two or three times daily.

If you are low in the hormone DHEA, work with a doctor to normalize your levels. A good starting dosage is 5 to 15 mg.

Phosphatidylserine improves memory, and studies show that it's helpful for depression. Take up to 300 mg daily.

Vitamin D3 has been found in studies to help improve mood. It is particularly important for people who do not get regular sunlight, especially seniors. Take up to 1,000 IU daily.

Acetyl-L-carnitine has been shown to be helpful for seniors with depression. Take 500 mg three times daily.

Take a high-potency multivitamin to provide a base of nutrients that are involved with brain function.

If you feel tense and on edge, several herbal teas can help you calm down. Peppermint and chamomile have mild relaxing properties, but if you need something a little stronger, try hops (*Humulus lupulus*) or passionflower (*Passiflora incarnata*).

Oatstraw (*Avena sativa*) tea is a good tonic for the nerves. Drink a cup as needed.

For insomnia that accompanies or causes depression, valerian or kava kava tea, taken before bedtime, can be quite helpful.

Homeopathy

Pick the remedy that best matches your symptoms in this section. Take a 6x, 12x, 6C, or 30C potency twice daily for two weeks to see if there are any positive results. After you notice improvement, stop taking the remedy, unless symptoms return. Consultation with a homeopathic practitioner is advised.

Arsenicum Album is for people who are susceptible to depression and who also suffer from anxiety and insecurity. They are often perfectionists who may have severe phobias. Restlessness and insomnia between midnight and 2 A.M. are common.

Aurum Metallicum is for deep depression, in which there are thoughts of suicide. The person feels no joy and is in despair. There is relief from being in the sun. *Note*: Suicidal tendencies should always be discussed with a doctor.

Ignatia (*Ignatia amara*) eases depression that is brought on by grief or emotional trauma and that is characterized by rapid mood swings. Frequent sighing and a sensation of a lump in the throat are characteristics of people who benefit from this remedy.

Kali Phosphoricum is for depression as a result of overwork. Mental fatigue is a common symptom that this remedy will help.

Natrum Muriaticum is for depressed people who do not reveal their emotions and who hold their feelings inside. They feel emotionally reserved and withdrawn. They feel a deep need for the company of others but are then aggravated when people console them. They often have a strong craving for salt and an aversion to sunlight.

Pulsatilla (*Pulsatilla pratensis*) is for people who burst into tears at little or no provocation. They may also be driven to seek constant comfort and reassurance. They are very sensitive and feel better from crying, attention, sweets, and being in the open air. Their symptoms are worse in a warm environment. In women, depression is often worse around the menstrual cycle or with menopause.

Sepia is for women who feel indifferent to their families. They have feelings of depression, fatigue, and irritability, as well as a low sex drive. They feel worse when others console them and better when they exercise. They are usually chilly. They have a strong craving for sweets (chocolate) and salty or sour foods. Depression that is associated with a hormone imbalance, as seen with PMS and menopause, is a strong indication for this remedy.

Staphysagria is for people who have suppressed emotions (such as anger) that contribute to depression. They usually are quiet and do not stand up for themselves, which results in their shame and resentment. Headaches and insomnia are also common.

Acupressure

See pages 787–794 for information about pressure points and administering treatment.
- Lung 1 (Lu1) relieves fatigue and depression. It also improves concentration.
- Other points that stimulate energy are Bladder 23 (B23), Gallbladder 20 (GB20), and Stomach 36 (St36).

Bodywork

Massage
A circulatory massage will get your blood flowing and will increase your energy levels. If you don't have the time or the money for a professional massage, ask a loved one to give you a head massage. This therapy stimulates blood flow to the brain.

Reflexology
See pages 804–805 for information about reflexology areas and how to work them. To improve brain function, work the big toe, which controls the head. Work the solar plexus and the diaphragm to balance the nervous system.

Hydrotherapy
Hot and cold hydrotherapy is an invigorating way to increase circulation and energy.

Aromatherapy

Lemon balm, melissa, and geranium will each rouse your spirits. Use them in any preparation you like.

If you have trouble sleeping, place a lavender-scented sachet under your pillow. This relaxing oil encourages a satisfying rest.

Stress Reduction

General Stress-Reduction Therapies

If you're depressed, you're experiencing powerful and probably continuous levels of stress. It is vital for your emotional and physical health that you find at least one way to control anxiety, fear, or tension. Prayer, counseling, and positive mental imagery are all helpful.

If you sense that your depression is more than you can handle, don't hesitate to seek help from a psychotherapist, a religious adviser, or a support group. It helps a great deal to talk to people who work with others' emotional pain.

Make an effort to stay in contact with beauty. If you have a garden or live near a nice park, spend as much time there as possible. And try to bring some of that beauty indoors: buy yourself a bouquet of flowers, listen to a favorite CD, or hang a water-color of a nature scene on the wall in your office.

Regular exercise has been shown to be effective in improving depression. Try to get some physical activity every day for thirty minutes.

It may sound simplistic, but one quick way to feel better, at least temporarily, is to go dancing. Dancing releases endorphins, powerful hormones that will raise your spirits, and you'll benefit from the touch of other people, not to mention from the pleasure of losing yourself in the music.

Helping others with their problems is a great way to relieve depression.

Other Recommendations

- The very best way to reduce the effects of SAD is to work with a doctor who can help with the proper use of light therapy. This can be done by getting outdoors between 5 and 7 A.M. and being exposed to light or using a bright-light box (especially in northern climates, where the sun doesn't rise until later in the morning during short winter days, and frequent overcast skies dim the sunlight). Several different companies make bright-light boxes. The most important thing to look for is a brightness rating of at least 10,000 lux. (In comparison, at a distance of two feet a standard 60-watt light bulb gives off only 300 lux.) Make sure the light box is equipped with a UV filter to protect the skin and the eyes. Also, use full-spectrum fluorescent lights in your home and workplace.
- Exercise is a proven mood-booster, and exercise in the sunlight does double duty for SAD sufferers. Take frequent walks outside, or participate in outdoor winter sports like ice-skating or cross-country skiing.
- Human beings weren't meant to spend their days in windowless offices. If changing jobs is not an option—and for most of us, it isn't—take your breaks outdoors. When the weather is good, pack a salad or another healthful lunch and dine al fresco. If it's too cold where you live to eat outdoors, then at least

use your breaks to bundle up and take a quick stroll around the block. Even on cloudy, snowy, or rainy days, enough sunlight comes through to make a difference in your melatonin production.

Shingles (Herpes Zoster)

Shingles is a painful condition caused by herpes zoster, the same virus that causes chickenpox. Once you've had chickenpox (and most adults have had the disease at some point in their lives), the virus doesn't leave your body. Instead, it takes up residence in the nerves near the spine, where it lies dormant, usually for the rest of your life. Sometimes, however, herpes zoster is triggered back into activity. This time around, the symptoms are different and more severe. At the beginning of the illness, the area along one branch of nerves, usually one side of your trunk or face, is more sensitive than usual; you may also develop a fever or chills. The sensitive area then becomes acutely painful, and a rash of small blisters develops. After two or three weeks, these clear, water-filled blisters will turn yellow and form scabs. Eventually, they fall off, and sometimes they leave scars.

The nerve pain caused by shingles can be agonizing. You may not be able to bear even the lightest touch, and simple activities like shaving and showering may be out of the question. Even the weight of clothes or bed sheets may be too much. But this pain usually disappears when the blisters drop off. In a few cases, though, the blisters fade but the pain remains for months or even years. This condition, which usually strikes people over fifty, is known as postherpetic neuralgia. No single trigger will always cause herpes zoster to reactivate in the body, but the virus seems to thrive when the immune system is weakened. People undergoing aggressive treatment for cancer or other illnesses are at a greater risk for shingles, as are those who are under extreme emotional stress. Immune-compromising diseases like AIDS or lupus can also leave a body vulnerable to shingles.

Most people will be healthy and pain-free once the disease has run its course. Nevertheless, your doctor should monitor you frequently to make sure the virus doesn't spread to your eyes or your internal organs, where it can have a devastating effect. Sometimes the virus can lead to pneumonia or other secondary infections, which can be deadly to older people or those who suffer from severely compromised immune systems. Between visits to your doctor, you'll find that a wide range of complementary therapies can bolster your immune system and reduce your need for aggressive conventional pain medication.

SYMPTOMS

The symptoms usually appear in the following order:

- Sensitivity in one side of the chest, the back, or the face
- Fever, chills, or other flulike symptoms
- Extreme pain in the sensitive area
- Clear blisters that break out in the affected area
- Blisters that turn yellow and scab over, then fall off

ROOT CAUSES

- Herpes zoster virus
- A weakened immune system

Testing Techniques

The following tests help assess possible causes of chronic shingles:

Immune-system imbalance or disease—blood

Hormone testing (thyroid, DHEA, cortisol, testosterone, IGF-1, estrogen, progesterone)—saliva, blood, or urine

Intestinal permeability—urine

Detoxification profile—urine

Vitamin and mineral analysis—blood

Food and environmental allergies/sensitivities—blood, electrodermal

Blood sugar balance—blood

Toxic metals—hair or urine

Amino acid analysis—blood or urine

TREATMENT

Diet

Recommended Food

During a case of shingles, the nervous system is under attack. Heal the damage by eating foods that are high in B vitamins, including wheat germ, brewer's yeast, eggs, and whole grains.

Eat green, orange, and yellow vegetables at every meal. These foods are packed with vitamins A and C, which will speed your skin's recovery from the inflammation and the blisters. Green leafy vegetables are also good sources of calcium and magnesium, which will help heal your nerve endings.

Food to Avoid

Avoid foods that encourage an overly acidic body system. Do not eat red meat, fried foods, or chocolate, and do not drink carbonated beverages (not even fizzy water) or drinks containing caffeine.

Sugar suppresses the activity of white blood cells, the immune system's foot soldiers in the war on illness. Stay away from refined sugar products, including cookies, cakes, sweet baked goods, and sodas, and eat naturally occurring sugars, such as those found in fruit, in moderation.

℞ Super Seven Prescriptions—Shingles

Super Prescription #1 Homeopathic Rhus Toxicodendron
Take a 30C potency three times daily. This remedy is effective if you have burning pain that feels better from warm applications. The rash is itchy, with

---

blisters. See the Homeopathy section for a complete listing of homeopathic remedies for shingles.

Super Prescription #2 Vitamin B12

Have your doctor give you a 1 cc injection daily for five days and then twice weekly. This helps the body recover more quickly and reduces the pain associated with shingles.

Super Prescription #3 Vitamin C

Take 1,000 mg four times daily for immune support. Reduce the dosage if diarrhea occurs.

Super Prescription #4 Capsaicin cream

Apply a cream with a 0.025 to 0.075 percent capsaicin extract two to four times daily to the affected area. This herbal extract blocks pain. *Note*: When this cream is first applied, you may feel a burning, stinging sensation during the first few days, but the pain will subside.

Super Prescription #5 Olive leaf extract (*Olea europa*)

Take 500 mg four times daily, to benefit from olive leaf's potent antiviral benefits.

Super Prescription #6 Echinacea (*Echinacea purpurea*)

Take 4 ml or 500 mg four times daily for immune support and antiviral effects.

Super Prescription #7 Vitamin E-complex

Take 1,200 to 1,600 IU daily for the treatment of postherpetic neuralgia and 400 IU daily to prevent neuralgia. You can also apply vitamin E oil topically.

In a double-blind study, thirty-two elderly patients with chronic post herpetic neuralgia were treated with either capsaicin cream or a placebo for a six-week period. After six weeks, almost 80 percent of capsaicin-treated patients experienced some relief from their pain.

General Recommendations

Lomatium root (*Lomatium dissectum*) is used for its immune support and antiviral effects. Take 4 ml or 500 mg four times daily.

Saint-John's-wort (*Hypericum perforatum*) has antiviral properties. Take 300 mg or 4 ml of the tincture three times daily.

Licorice root (*Glycyrrhiza glabra*) has antiviral properties. Take 500 mg in capsule form or 4 ml of the tincture three times daily. *Note*: Do not use it if you have high blood pressure.

Cat's claw (*Uña de gato*) works against viruses and inflammation. Take 500 to 1,000 mg two or three times daily, until the inflammation is gone.

Zinc supports the immune system. Take 30 mg daily, along with 2 mg of copper.

Vitamin A supports immune function. Take 50,000 IU daily for two weeks.

A high-potency multivitamin/-mineral provides a base of nutrients for immune support. It should include 200 mcg of selenium, a mineral that helps with viral infections.

Homeopathy

Pick the remedy that best matches your symptoms in this section. For acute shingles pain, take a 30C potency three times daily. For chronic shingles discomfort, take 6x, 12x, 6C, 12C, or 30C twice daily for two weeks to see if there are any positive results. After you notice improvement, stop taking the remedy, unless symptoms return. Consultation with a homeopathic practitioner is advised.

Arsenicum Album is a good remedy when there is a burning, itching pain that is relieved by warm applications. Symptoms are often worse between midnight and 2 A.M. The person is restless, anxious, and chilly.

Apis Mellifica is for people who experience stinging and burning pain that feels better from cold applications and worse from warmth.

Iris Versicolor is indicated when the shingles are accompanied by stomach problems, with burning sensations and nausea. Eruptions tend to appear on the right side of the abdomen.

Mezereum is for people who feel burning that is followed by bright-red eruptions that itch intolerably. The pain is relieved from cold applications and is worse from warmth.

Ranunculus Bulbosus is a specific remedy for when the shingles affect the front or the back of the ribcage.

Rhus Toxicodendron is a great remedy if you have burning pain that feels better from warm applications. The rash is itchy, with blisters.

Sulfur is a good choice for burning pains that feel better from cold applications and worse from warmth. The person is usually very warm and prefers ice-cold drinks.

Variolinum is a remedy that stimulates the immune system to combat the shingles virus more effectively. It can be used in addition to any of the remedies described here for quicker healing.

Acupressure

See pages 787–794 for information about pressure points and administering treatment.

Large Intestine 4 (LI4) is the point for effective relief of general pain. For more specific treatment of this complex condition, it's best to turn to an acupressure professional.

Bodywork

Reflexology
See pages 804–805 for information about reflexology areas and how to work them.
To reduce pain and fight the virus, work the spine in addition to the painful area.
To heal nerves and reduce stress, work the solar plexus and the diaphragm.
Stimulate the lower thoracic area to promote healing of the skin.

Hydrotherapy
Constitutional hydrotherapy stimulates the immune system and relieves pain. See pages 795–796 for directions.

Other Bodywork Recommendations
Acupressure and acupuncture (especially electroacupuncture) have a good track record of successfully treating many painful conditions, including shingles and post herpetic neuralgia. Chinese herbal therapy can be very helpful as well.

Aromatherapy

Tea tree oil is a powerful antiviral agent that will help dry up blisters. Combine it with lavender or bergamot, two oils that have milder antiviral properties but that also reduce pain and stress. You can use a cotton swab to apply the oils directly to the blisters or the painful area, or you can add them to a bath. No matter what preparation you choose, use just a little at first, as tea tree oil is extremely potent and can be irritating in large quantities.

Stress Reduction

General Stress-Reduction Therapies

Constant pain is terribly stressful and can result in further depression of your immune system, so it's essential to find an activity that thoroughly engages your mind and takes you away from your pain, if only for a little while.

Other Recommendations

Seek the consultation of a naturopathic or holistic doctor who can help you with a specific therapy for quicker improvement. Severe cases may also require pharmaceutical therapy.

Intravenous vitamin C and B12 are effective, as are intramuscular injections of B12.

REFERENCES

Bernstein, J. E., et al. 1989. Topical capsaicin treatment of chronic postherpetic neuralgia. *Journal of the American Academy of Dermatology* (2 Pt 1):265–70.

Sinusitis

The sinuses are cavities in the bones around the nose, the cheeks, and the eyes. These cavities are lined with membranes that produce mucus, and when the sinuses are functioning normally, this mucus serves a protective purpose: it warms and moistens incoming air and filters it for germs. When sinuses can't drain properly, however, the mucus accumulates and becomes stagnant, making the area ripe for infection.

Sinusitis, which is the name for an infection of the sinus cavities, can be quite unpleasant and often painful. The mucus buildup leads to clogged nasal passages, thick drainage, and a general feeling of weariness and discomfort. The swollen membranes feel even worse, because they can fill up the tiny sinus cavities and press against the bones of the face. If you are unsure whether your head congestion is sinusitis, bend forward from the waist. If you feel heavy pressure or pain against your cheekbones or your eyes, you probably have sinusitis.

Sinusitis may be either acute or chronic. Acute sinusitis is usually caused by a complication from another respiratory infection, such as a cold, the flu, or bronchitis. Any of these infections can lead to blocked drainage, which in turn causes sinusitis. If the sinus membranes don't have a chance to heal fully, an acute case can easily turn into a chronic one.

Recurring colds and flus—warning signs of a suppressed immune system—may lead to chronic sinusitis, as can other factors that consistently cause an obstruction of the sinus cavities. Repeated exposure to environmental allergens and irritants, such as mold spores or tobacco, is a common cause, as are food allergies or a diet that's high in mucus-forming foods.

Research has shown that chronic sinusitis is most often related to an immune response to a fungal infection in the sinus cavity. This research was first released in 1999 by a Mayo Clinic study, and the results have since been duplicated in subsequent studies. Natural practitioners often treat people who have chronic sinusitis for a systemic fungal infection, and this condition is helped by such an approach.

Sinusitis is an all-too-familiar ailment, but it can often be treated and prevented with simple home care and immune-boosting strategies. If your symptoms don't disappear within a few weeks, however, or if you have intense sinus pain, consult your doctor. In severe and prolonged cases, sinusitis can lead to serious diseases like pneumonia or even meningitis.

SYMPTOMS

- Pressure and pain around the cheekbones and the eyes
- Clogged nasal passages
- Thick, greenish-yellow nasal discharge
- Diminished sense of smell or taste
- Toothache
- Fatigue
- Fever (more often in acute cases; rarely in chronic)

ROOT CAUSES

Anything that blocks the sinus cavities or causes the mucus membranes to swell can lead to sinusitis.

- A respiratory infection
- Environmental allergies, especially hay fever
- Environmental irritants, including tobacco and pollution
- Food allergies or sensitivities, especially to milk
- A diet that's high in mucus-forming foods
- A dental infection
- Any activity that places pressure on the sinuses: swimming, scuba diving, flying in planes
- An immune-system reaction to a fungal infection in the sinus cavity
- Systemic candidiasis

Testing Techniques

The following tests help assess possible reasons for chronic sinusitis:

Nasal swab—check for yeast or bacteria

Immune-system imbalance or disease—blood

Blood pressure

Hormone testing (thyroid, DHEA, cortisol, testosterone, IGF-1, estrogen, progesterone)—saliva, blood, or urine

---

Intestinal permeability—urine

Detoxification profile—urine

Vitamin and mineral analysis (especially magnesium, B12, iron, and CoQ10)—blood

Digestive function and candida testing—stool analysis

Anemia—blood test (CBC, iron, ferritin, % saturation)

Food and environmental allergies/sensitivities—blood, electrodermal

Blood sugar balance—blood

A Mayo Clinic study looked at the ability to test for sinus fungal infections in fifty-four patients who had a history of chronic sinusitis. Researchers found that with one of the testing methods, 100 percent of the patients tested positive for fungus, while another testing method showed that 76 percent had signs of fungus.

TREATMENT

If allergies or recurring colds are the cause of your sinusitis, the following recommendations will help, but you should also see the appropriate section in this book. The suggestions there will help you resolve the root of your problem.

Diet

Recommended Food

During an acute infection, eat lightly. In addition to 1 glass of clean, quality water every two waking hours, drink plenty of herbal teas, vegetable juices, and broths. Chicken soup—especially with lots of vegetables—is still one of the best therapies for any respiratory infection.

Once the worst stage of an infection has passed, focus on foods that produce little or no mucus: whole grains, fresh vegetables and fruits, cold-pressed oils, and raw seeds and nuts.

Several foods will aid mucus drainage and ease the pressure in your sinuses. Add cayenne, garlic, onions, or horseradish to your soups or meals. For a powerful sinus-drainage remedy, eat a small spoonful of crushed horseradish mixed with lemon juice. (You may want to be near a sink or have a towel handy after taking this potent combination.)

Flaxseeds and flaxseed oil will reduce inflammation. Take a teaspoon of oil every day during the infection, or add some flaxseeds to cereals or salads.

If you must take an antibiotic for a sinus infection, be sure to consume a nondairy source of friendly bacteria, such as kefir or sauerkraut.

Food to Avoid

People who suffer from chronic sinusitis must banish all mucus-forming foods from their diet. Dairy products are the worst culprit, but refined flours, chocolate, eggs, and fried and processed food cause high levels of mucus as well. If your case is acute, avoid these products for the duration of your illness. When you feel better, restrict your consumption of them to prevent a recurrence.

Sugar and fruit juices should be reduced or eliminated because they feed yeast, which is often present in people who have chronic sinusitis.

See the Food Allergies section, especially the elimination diet on page 316, to see whether a certain food is triggering your sinus blockage. Examine your reaction to dairy and wheat very closely; these foods often cause coldlike symptoms.

Salt and alcohol both have dehydrating effect on the sinuses and result in further inflammation. Avoid alcohol and severely restrict salt intake.

R Super Seven Prescriptions—Sinusitis

Super Prescription #1 Homeopathic Combination Sinusitis Formula
Take as directed on the container four times daily. These types of formulas contain the most common homeopathic remedies that are used for acute sinusitis.

Super Prescription #2 Grapefruit seed extract
This is available as a nasal spray for sinusitis. Use the spray four times daily for acute sinusitis and twice daily for chronic sinusitis.

Super Prescription #3 Oregano oil (*Origanum vulgare*)
Take 500 mg or 0.5 ml four times daily, or take as directed on the container. Oregano oil has potent antibacterial and antifungal properties.

Super Prescription #4 N-acetylcysteine
Take 500 mg three times daily. This nutrient thins mucus secretions so that the sinuses can drain more effectively.

Super Prescription #5 Colloidal silver
Use it as a nasal spray, or dilute it in a saline solution. Use the spray four times daily for acute sinusitis and twice daily for chronic sinusitis.

Super Prescription #6 Echinacea (*Echinacea purpurea*) and goldenseal (*Hydrastis canadensis*)
Take 5 ml or 500 mg four times daily. This combination of herbs works well for acute sinusitis by enhancing immune function and reducing mucus congestion.

Super Prescription #7 Bromelain
Take 500 mg three times daily between meals. Look for products standardized to 2,000 MCU (milk-clotting units) per 1,000 mg or 1,200 GDU (gelatin-dissolving units) per 1,000 mg. Bromelain has a natural anti-inflammatory effect and has been shown in studies to improve acute sinusitis. Protease-enzyme products also have this benefit.

Victoria had suffered from chronic sinusitis for more than five years. When her sinuses became inflamed, her doctor prescribed a nasal steroid and antibiotics. She sought natural treatment at our clinic. A four-week antifungal program combined with daily doses of natural antihistamines such as quercitin brought tremendous improvement. Now, three years later, her sinuses continue to do well without pharmaceutical treatment.

General Recommendations

Vitamin C has antiallergy and immune-enhancing effects. Take 1,000 mg four times daily. *Note*: Reduce the dosage if diarrhea occurs.

Bioflavonoids are helpful for people with allergies. Take 500 mg three times daily of a mixed bioflavonoid formula.

Grapeseed extract or maritime pine-bark extract reduces inflammation of the sinus. Take up to 300 mg daily for chronic sinusitis.

Garlic (*Allium sativum*) also fights infection and also helps to drain sinuses. Take 250 to 500 mg twice daily.

Elderflower tea is another traditional remedy that thins mucus. It also increases circulation to the sinus area.

Turmeric (*Curcuma longa*) is an anti-inflammatory herb—as well as a cooking spice—that will reduce sinus pressure. Find an extract standardized for 400 to 600 mg of curcumin (the active ingredient in turmeric) and take 400 to 600 mg three times a day, or use 1 to 2 cc of a tincture three times a day.

Homeopathy

Pick the remedy that best matches your symptoms in this section. For acute sinusitis, take a 30C potency four times daily. For chronic sinusitis, take a 6x, 12x, 6C, 12C, or 30C twice daily for two weeks to see if there are any positive results. After you notice improvement, stop taking the remedy, unless symptoms return. Consultation with a homeopathic practitioner is advised.

Belladonna (*Atropa belladonna*) is helpful for the first stage of a sinus infection. The person experiences a high fever and throbbing pain, especially on the right side of the sinus. The pain is made worse by bending the head forward.

Bryonia (*Bryonia alba*) is a remedy for when movement of the head, especially bending the head downward, causes sinus pain. The person has a great thirst and feels irritable.

Hepar Sulphuris is for a blocked, sore nose that's made worse by even the slightest draft. People who benefit from this remedy tend to be irritable while ill.

Kali Bichromium is indicated when there is thick, stringy, yellow and/or green mucus that causes pain at the root of the nose.

Mercurius Solubilis or Vivus is needed for people who are feverish and have pain around the nose and the cheekbones. They salivate excessively and have a thick white- or yellowish-coated tongue. Their nasal discharge is foul smelling and so is their breath.

Pulsatilla (*Pulsatilla pratensis*) is for people with a thick yellow/green mucus discharge. They feel better in the open air or with a window open. Their symptoms are worse in a warm room. They have little thirst.

Silica (*Silicea*) is good remedy for chronic sinusitis where the nasal cavities will not drain. The person feels worse in the cold air, but the sinuses feel better with cold applications.

Acupressure

See pages 787–794 for information about pressure points and administering treatment.
- To relieve sinus congestion and headaches, work Bladder 2 (B2).
- Large Intestine 4 (LI4) eases pain anywhere in the body but is particularly effective at treating pain in the front of the head, including in the sinus cavities.

Bodywork

Massage

To drain mucus and carry it away from the body, get a facial lymphatic drainage massage. You can also try this home technique: Lean over a sink or a towel and gently rub the areas over and below your eye sockets, then extend out from beneath your eye sockets in a straight line across your cheeks. This will allow your sinuses to drain. Hanging your head down over the edge of the bed aids in draining the sinuses.

Reflexology

See pages 804–805 for information about reflexology areas and how to work them. The toes correspond to the sinuses. Work all of them. Work the lymph area to encourage the production of antibodies and to fight infection.

Hydrotherapy

Hot baths, showers, and steams are all relaxing, effective ways to relieve sinus pressure. Add any of the essential oils listed in this entry for extra benefits. Alternating hot (two minutes) and cold (thirty seconds) over the sinus area helps to reduce pain and inflammation of the sinuses.

Aromatherapy

Eucalyptus oil will clear out sinuses quickly. Use it in a massage, a steam inhalation, or a bath, or simply inhale deeply over an open bottle of oil.

Tea tree oil will fight both bacterial and viral infections. It's a powerful oil, so use just a few drops in a bath or a steam. You can also diffuse a little in your bedroom for nighttime sinus relief.

Lavender is a gentle oil that stimulates your immune system and helps you get to sleep. Use it in any preparation you like, or add it to any of the previous oils.

Stress Reduction

General Stress-Reduction Techniques

Stress isn't a direct cause of sinusitis, but constant unresolved tension can leave you less able to fight off infections. Use stress-reduction techniques to create a healthy immune system. You'll relieve stress, and the deep breathing will encourage good airflow through your nasal passages.

Other Recommendations

- Regular exercise will help keep your nasal passages clear. Try to work out daily, but use some common-sense precautions: don't exercise if you have a fever, and don't go outside if seasonal allergies are likely to strike.
- Saline rinses for the sinus are helpful, to reduce the effect of allergens that contribute to sinusitis. Saline nasal sprays are available; look for those that also contain xylitol, a natural extract that prevents bacteria from adhering to the nasal cavity.
- If you have chronic sinusitis, you may well have problems with Candida overgrowth. See the Candidiasis section for more information.
- Nebulized N-acetylcysteine, available with a doctor's prescription, works very well to drain clogged sinuses.

REFERENCES

Taylor, M. J., et al. 2002. Detection of fungal organisms in eosinophilic mucin using a fluorescein-labeled chitin-specific binding protein. *Otolaryngology: Head and Neck Surgery* 127(5):377–83.

Small Intestine Bacterial Overgrowth

Small intestine bacterial overgrowth, or bacterial overgrowth syndrome—also known as SIBO (pronounced *see-bow*)—is the culprit behind a huge number of digestive disorders. In fact, SIBO is associated with 78 percent of IBS cases, 67 percent of celiac disease cases, 88 percent of Crohn's disease cases, and 81 percent of ulcerative colitis cases.

Approximately seventy million Americans are living with a digestive disease such as irritable bowel syndrome (IBS), and 74 percent of Americans experience digestive discomfort such as gas, bloating, diarrhea, or abdominal pain. SIBO is likely involved in a lot of these cases. In addition, SIBO plays a role in up to 44 percent of diabetics, nearly 54 percent of those with hypothyroidism, up to 20 percent of those with fibromyalgia, and up to 41 percent of the obese. It is also known to increase the risk of osteoporosis, restless leg syndrome, chronic fatigue, and interstitial cystitis.

The small intestine is the section of the digestive tract that connects the stomach to the colon. It's a critical area since it's where the body absorbs most of the nutrients from the foods we eat. As with the other areas of the digestive tract (including the mouth), the small intestine contains bacteria—although fewer than you'll find in the colon. Scientists and doctors refer to these healthy and expected bacteria as commensal or native bacteria. SIBO occurs when either these native bacteria *or* nonnative bacteria overgrow in the small intestine, particularly in regions that usually have relatively low levels of bacteria. The resulting fermentation of food leads to gas, bloating, and pain. Inflammation kicks in, and the body becomes less effective at absorbing needed nutrients from food. Malabsorption of nutrients in turn affects energy levels, brain function, muscles and joints, and many other bodily systems.

Gut bacteria involved in SIBO include the categories of methanogens, hydrogen sulfide and hydrogen sulfate producers, and other hydrogen producers.

When things are working correctly the nerves and muscles in the digestive tract rhythmically contract and relax to move food along. Known as peristalsis, the process moves food through the stomach to the small intestine, then through the colon, and finally out the rectum as waste. Contractions occur between meals approximately every one and a half to two hours. This regular function sweeps bacteria through the small intestine, preventing bacterial overgrowth. But in people with a sluggish small intestine, this process doesn't work quite as well. Research has found that people with small intestine–motility problems—for example, many IBS sufferers—are at higher risk for SIBO.

As mentioned, a huge percentage of IBS sufferers (up to 78 percent) *also* have small intestinal bacterial overgrowth. Some experts theorize that SIBO develops in people with IBS as the result of digestive-tract infections, either viral, parasitic, bacterial, or worm-driven. The infectious agent releases a toxin that damages the cells of the gut that are involved in muscle contraction. With the muscles in the small intestine unable to expand and contract effectively, the stage is set for bacteria to overgrow.

SIBO sufferers may also experience fungal overgrowth in the small intestine. The symptoms of fungal overgrowth (usually from *Candida albicans*) in the digestive tract are very similar to those of bacterial overgrowth. A low-sugar diet, combined with antifungal herbs and supplements or antifungal medications, can help drive down fungal infections in the gut.

SYMPTOMS

- Bloating after meals
- Diarrhea, constipation, or both
- Bad breath and/or a fishy body odor
- Generalized abdominal

discomfort (usually mild)
- General body discomfort including fatigue, joint and muscle pain, brain fog

ROOT CAUSES

- Constipation
- People who have shorter bowels as the result of surgery
- Diseases that can infect the intestinal muscles, including Parkinson's disease, type 2 diabetes, chronic kidney disease, hypothyroidism, or scleroderma

- Digestive diseases, including diverticulitis, Crohn's disease, celiac disease
- Antibiotic and steroid medications
- Low stomach acid
- Chemotherapy and radiation

Testing Techniques

Lactulose hydrogen breath test—The test begins with the patient breathing into a container to provide a sample baseline breath. Next he or she swallows lactulose, a synthetic sugar that's not broken down until it reaches the colon. When bacteria in the small intestine act on the lactulose, hydrogen and methane gases are produced. These gases are then absorbed into the bloodstream and carried to the lungs, where they're released through the breath. Air samples are collected over the next one and a half to two hours. The laboratory compares the baseline sample to the rest of the samples. In someone with SIBO, the hydrogen and methane gases will increase over time as the lactulose is fermented by the overgrown bacteria in the small intestine. The breath test does a good job of identifying many SIBO sufferers, but it doesn't always work. Your doctor may still elect to treat you based on your symptoms.

Lab markers that suggest SIBO:

Elevated D-lactic acid levels—urine or blood

Elevated 4-hydroxyphenylacetic acid—urine

TREATMENT

Diet

Food, naturally, plays a large part in the bacterial balance of your belly. When battling SIBO you should eliminate any foods that can aggravate your condition and add foods that are healing to the gut. The most well-studied gut-friendly diet is known as the low-FODMAP diet (low fermentable oligosaccharide, disaccharide, monosaccharide, and polyols).

Short-chain carbohydrates are poorly absorbed in the small intestine. The goal of the low-FODMAP diet is to cut back on, or eliminate, these readily fermentable foods, reducing both SIBO and IBS symptoms. SIBO sufferers should avoid the following high FODMAPs:

Fructose (fruits, honey, high-fructose corn syrup [HFCS], etc.)

Lactose (dairy)

Fructans (wheat, garlic, onion, inulin, etc.)

Galactans (legumes such as beans, lentils, soybeans, etc.)

Polyols (sweeteners containing isomalt, mannitol, sorbitol, xylitol, etc.)

Stone fruits (avocadoes, apricots, cherries, nectarines, peaches, plums, etc.)

Avoid caffeine and be aware of any medications that hinder the movement of foods through your gut (motility), including opioid medications such as hydrocodone (e.g., Vicodin), oxycodone (e.g., OxyContin, Percocet), morphine (e.g., Kadian, Avinza), and codeine.

Acid-suppressing medications for acid reflux and other digestive ailments can also put you at higher risk for SIBO. Common brand names include Nexium, Prevacid, Prilosec, Protonix, and Aciphex.

In addition to reducing FODMAPs, increasing the amount of water and fiber you're getting will help foods move through your body more efficiently. Healthy bacteria thrive on fiber, so consuming more of it will also improve your gut-flora balance. Psyllium, chia seeds, or ground flaxseeds taken with 60 ounces of water or more a day will help bowel movements.

℞ Super Seven Prescriptions—Small Intestine Bacterial Overgrowth

Super Prescription #1 Berberine
Take 500 mg three times a day before meals. This extract from various herbs such as barberry has antibacterial properties that kill SIBO-related bacteria.

Super Prescription #2 Betaine hydrochloride
Take one or more capsules with each meal to improve stomach acid levels, which make it more difficult for bacterial overgrowth. It also helps with digestion and absorption.

Super Prescription #3 Enteric-coated peppermint oil
Take 0.2 ml three times daily for three weeks. Research has shown benefit for symptoms as well as improvement in lab results.

Super Prescription #4 Probiotics
Take twenty billion to one hundred billion organisms daily. For some individuals with SIBO, probiotics help to treat the bacterial imbalance. For others it works better to use probiotics after antimicrobial therapy, to prevent recurrence.

A study of 104 people aged eighteen to sixty-five who were diagnosed with SIBO were given either antibiotic therapy (rifaximin, 400 mg three times daily) or thirty days of a combination herbal formula. Researchers found the herbal therapy to be just as effective as standard antibiotic treatment for SIBO.

Super Prescription #5 Gentian root or Swedish bitters
Take as directed on the label. These herbs improve stomach acid levels, which make it more difficult for bacterial overgrowth. They also help with digestion and absorption.

Super Prescription #6   Colloidal silver
Take as directed on the label. Colloidal silver has antibacterial properties.

Super Prescription #7 Garlic
Take 500 mg with each meal to lower levels of pathogenic bacteria.

General Recommendations

Formulas containing essential oils that are specific for SIBO are available. They can be very effective. Use under the guidance of a holistic doctor.

Dietary supplements that heal the small intestine lining—such as glutamine, aloe vera, deglycyrrhizinated licorice (DGL), and N-acetyl glucosamine—are also useful after antimicrobial therapy is completed.

Other Recommendations

- Your doctor might choose to use antibiotics to treat your case. The antibiotics that are most commonly used to treat SIBO include rifaximin (550 mg three times per day), neomycin (500 mg twice daily), and Cipro (250 mg twice daily) for seven to fourteen days. If you do start on a course of antibiotics don't forget to take probiotics both during and after the treatment to prevent further bacterial imbalance and fungal overgrowth.
- Chiropractic, acupuncture, and massage can help keep food moving through your system efficiently.
- Intravenous nutrient therapy helps increase nutrient levels while the SIBO is being treated. It can alleviate a lot of symptoms, such as fatigue, and also help the body heal more effectively.

REFERENCES

Chedid, V., S. Dhalla, J. O. Clarke, et al. 2014. Herbal therapy is equivalent to rifaximin for the treatment of small intestinal bacterial overgrowth. *Global Adv Health Med* 3(3):16–24.

Stanford Healthcare website. Accessed November 2, 2014 at http://stanford-healthcare.org/content/dam/SHC/for-patients-component/programs-services/clinical-nutrition-services/docs/pdf-lowfodmapdiet.pdf.

Sore Throat

Throat pain and painful swallowing are classic symptoms of a sore throat, medically known as pharyngitis. This condition is one of the most common reasons why people visit the doctor. Many people are concerned that they have a bacterial infection such as strep, but the vast majority of cases are viral. This means that antibiotics are usually not required and would not be effective.

A sore throat often signals a cold or the onset of the flu. Fever, fatigue, headache, runny nose, swollen neck glands, and earaches can also accompany a sore throat.

Natural remedies will not only reduce throat pain but also enhance the immune system to eradicate the underlying infection. Again, the vast majority of our patients are treated successfully with natural medicine and not antibiotics.

You should seek immediate medical attention if you have pus patches on your throat, extreme difficulty swallowing, extreme throat pain, throat pain that does not improve in five days, vomiting, blood in phlegm, a skin rash that accompanies a sore throat (a sign of meningitis or strep throat), excessive drooling in a young child, weakness or signs of dehydration, swollen tonsils, exposure to someone with strep throat, or high fever (over 103 degrees F for adults or 101 degrees F for babies).

Be aware that recurring or chronic sore throats may be caused by allergens (mainly environmental, such as pollens, molds, and animal dander), pollution (including tobacco smoke), acid reflux, strain of the throat muscles, and dryness.

SYMPTOMS

- Throat pain when swallowing, talking, or breathing
- Scratchy, dry, swollen throat
- Swollen lymph nodes in the neck

ROOT CAUSES

- Viral infection (including common cold viruses)
- Allergies
- Pollution
- Bacterial infection (including strep throat)
- Strain of the throat muscles
- Dryness

Testing Techniques

The following tests help assess possible reasons for a sore throat:
Physical exam of throat and mouth
Throat culture or rapid strep test
Allergy testing

TREATMENT

Diet

Recommended Food

Increase your intake of fluids such as water, herbal teas (especially ginger, cinnamon, and peppermint), soups, and broths. Drink 80 ounces of water daily. Chicken soup and miso are often soothing. Warm water mixed with honey and lemon can relieve both the pain and any coughing that may be present with a sore throat.

Food to Avoid

Dehydrating substances such as alcohol and caffeine should be avoided. Restrict sugar products because they suppress the immune system. Fruit juices should be highly diluted because of their sugar content. Avoid dairy products, which tend to increase mucus production.

Rx **Super Seven Prescriptions—Sore Throat**

Super Prescription #1 Licorice root
Take 1 ml of the tincture form in 2 ounces of water four times daily. This herb reduces inflammation of the throat and has immune-enhancing properties.

Super Prescription #2 Echinacea (*Echinacea purpurea*) and goldenseal (*Hydrastis canadensis*)
Take 500 mg of the capsule or 2 to 4 ml of the tincture four times daily. This combination of herbs enhances immune function and has antiviral and antibacterial properties. It's especially good if mucus is present.

Super Prescription #3 Lomatium dissectum
Take 500 mg or 2 to 4 ml of the tincture four times daily. Lomatium has strong antiviral effects.

Super Prescription #4 Slippery elm
Suck on slippery elm lozenges throughout the day or take 2 ml of the tincture form four times daily.

Super Prescription #5 Colloidal silver
Take ½ to 1 teaspoon four times daily. Colloidal silver has antiviral and antibacterial properties.

Super Prescription #6 Oregano oil
Take 5 to 10 drops of the liquid form in 2 ounces of water or 300 mg in capsule form four times daily.

Super Prescription #7 Pelargonium sidoides
Children should take ½ to 1 teaspoon and adults should take 1½ teaspoons three times daily. It has been shown to shorten the duration and intensity of a sore throat.

General Recommendations

Andrographis paniculata has been shown to fight the common cold and sore throats. Take 100 mg twice daily of a standardized extract.

Vitamin C enhances immune function and benefits those with allergies. Take 500 to 1,000 mg three times daily.

Vitamin A improves immune function. Take 25,000 to 50,000 IU daily for five days. Do not use if pregnant or nursing.

Garlic has antimicrobial effects. Take 300 to 600 mg or 2 ml three times daily.

Thyme extract optimizes immunity. Take 1 or 2 capsules twice daily or as directed on the container.

Zinc lozenges (zinc gluconate, zinc gluconate-glycine, or zinc acetate) fight the common cold and soothe sore throats. Take 15 to 25 mg every two waking hours for five days.

Homeopathy

At the first signs of a sore throat, take 2 pellets of a 30C potency four times daily for three days of the remedy that best matches your symptoms in this section. If you notice improvement, stop taking the remedy unless the symptoms return. If your symptoms do not abate within twenty-four hours, pick another remedy.

Aconitum Napellus is used for the sudden onset of a sore throat, especially when it occurs after exposure to cold weather. It should be used when the throat is dry, red, and hot. Other symptoms include a red face as well as anxiety and restlessness.

Apis Mellifica should be used when a person has red and swollen tonsils and throat. The uvula (the tissue in the middle of the throat) is often swollen and there may be a stinging or burning pain that feels better when drinking cold liquids or eating ice and that feels worse when drinking warm liquids.

Belladonna should be used at the first stage of a sore throat when high fever, flushed face, and burning throat pain occur. The throat pain tends to be more right-sided, and it may be difficult to swallow.

Ferrum Phosphoricum should be used for a mild sore throat and fever when a person does not feel very sick.

Hepar Sulphuris is for a sore throat with pus or a sensation of a stick or a splinter in the throat. The sore throat is irritable and feels better with warm drinks.

Lachesis Muta is for throat pain that is worse on the left side or that begins on the left side and moves to the right. A person with this kind of throat pain does not want anything touching the throat, and there is a sensation of constriction or of having a lump in the throat.

Lycopodium should be used for a sore throat that is worse on the right side or that begins on the right side and moves to the left. The throat feels better with warm drinks or food.

Mercurius Solubilis or Vivus is for a raw, burning sore throat accompanied by pus and swollen glands, especially on the right side. Increased salivation and swollen glands are often present. This may be accompanied by a heavily coated tongue and bad breath. The person is feverish and may sweat at night.

Phytolacca should be used for a sore throat with swollen lymph nodes in the neck. There may be radiating pain to the ears during swallowing, and the throat feels better with cold drinks and worse with warm drinks.

Sulphur should be used for a burning sore throat that feels better from ice-cold drinks. The person has high thirst and sweats easily.

Bodywork

Reflexology
See pages 804–805 for areas corresponding to the throat (under the big toe, in the crease).

Hydrotherapy
Alternate a hot hand towel (one minute) with a wrung-out cold hand towel (five minutes). This brings immune cells to the throat area and reduces inflammation.

Aromatherapy

The oils of lemon and frankincense boost the body's natural defenses and promote healthy respiratory function. You can gargle with these oils or use them in a warm compress over the throat.

Other Recommendations

- Gargle with warm salt water three times daily. Use ½ teaspoon of salt in a full glass of warm water.
- Humidify the air to prevent the throat membranes from drying out.
- Avoid pollution, including smoke.

REFERENCES

Bereznoy V. V., et al. 2003. Efficacy of extract of Pelargonium sidoides in children with acute non-group A beta-hemolytic streptococcus tonsillopharyngitis: A randomized, double-blind, placebo-controlled trial. *Alternative Therapies in Health and Medicine* 9:68–79.

Mossad, S. B., et al. 1996. Zinc gluconate lozenges for treating the common cold. A randomized, double-blind, placebo-controlled study. *Annals of Internal Medicine* 125:81–88.

Thamlikitkul, V., et al. 1991. Efficacy of Andrographis paniculata, Nees for pharyngotonsillitis in adults. *Journal of the Medical Association of Thailand* 74:437–42.

Sprains and Strains

Although most of us will experience a sprain or a strain at some point in our lives, very few people know the difference between the two kinds of injuries. A strain is what's commonly referred to as a "pulled muscle." As its name implies, a strain occurs when a muscle is overstressed by too much weight or by overuse. The injured muscle fibers may go into spasm, form knots, or swell up. If you have a strained muscle, you may feel a sharp pain when you try to use it, or you may experience a dull throb in the affected area. When muscles knot or spasm, the pain can be constant and severe. The worst symptoms of a strain will usually subside after a week, but they may leave behind an ache that lingers as long as a month.

Sprains, contrary to what most people believe, are not the result of muscle injury. In a sprain, the damage is done to a ligament, which is a band of fibrous connective tissue that holds bones together at the joints. When a ligament is overstressed, it may tear or stretch out of its normal position. You may even hear a snapping or popping sound at the time of injury. Not surprisingly, sprains cause immediate, acute pain. Once the first shock of pain passes, it is replaced by swelling and extreme soreness and sensitivity. In most cases, putting weight on the affected joint is out of the question. With proper treatment, the swelling goes away after about a week, but you may have pain for several weeks longer. The joint will usually feel stiff for months to come.

Most strains and sprains respond well to rest and home care, but you should be alert for signs that your injury needs a doctor's attention. If the pain is unbearable and if you can't move the joint, you may have a broken or fractured bone. Instead of going to bed, visit a doctor's office or the emergency room. Other red flags are discolored joints or severe swelling that doesn't go down after a few days.

Although sprains and strains are quite common, you can reduce your chances of injuring a muscle or a ligament. First, get some exercise on a regular basis. People who don't use their muscles and bones regularly are far more prone to damaging them. Second, always warm up your muscles before engaging in an activity. Stretch gently and ease into the movement. Finally, use common sense: don't lift objects that are too heavy for you, and don't participate in activities that are painful.

SYMPTOMS OF STRAINS

- Acute pain when the muscle is in use
- A dull throb at other times
- Muscle spasms or knots
- Swelling

SYMPTOMS OF SPRAINS

- Severe pain at time of injury, subsiding into soreness
- Joint discoloration (indicative of a serious sprain)
- Swelling

ROOT CAUSES

- Overstressing muscles or ligaments, usually through lifting, exercise, or by accident
- Imbalance in oppositional muscles
- Nutritional deficiencies, making one more susceptible to injury

---

Testing Techniques

The following tests help assess possible reasons for the slow repair of sprains/strains:

Intestinal permeability—urine

Detoxification profile—urine

Vitamin and mineral analysis (especially magnesium, vitamin C, iron)— blood

---

TREATMENT

Diet

You might not think of diet as an important part of healing an injury, but good nutritional choices in the weeks following a sprain or a strain can speed your recovery and reduce your pain.

Recommended Food

You need lean protein to rebuild strong, elastic muscles and ligaments. Eat reasonable amounts of high-quality chicken, turkey, and fish, and incorporate beans into your meals.

An injury can result in the formation of free radicals, the unbalanced molecules that are thought to be responsible for many diseases. Combat free radicals with the antioxidants found in deeply colored fruits and vegetables.

Vitamin C will help to reduce swelling and repair tissues. Eat citrus fruits as a light dessert.

Food to Avoid

You may be housebound and depressed following a sprain or a strain, but resist the temptation to console yourself with junk food. Fast food, processed food, fried food, and food that's high in salt and sugar will only make inflammation and swelling worse.

ouble-blind trials have shown that proteolytic enzymes, such as bromelain, papain, and trypsin/chymotrypsin, speed the recovery of athletic injuries.

℞ Super Seven Prescriptions—Sprains and Strains

Super Prescription #1 Bromelain
Take 500 mg three times daily between meals. Look for products standardized to 2,000 MCU (milk-clotting units) per 1,000 mg or 1,200 GDU (gelatin-dissolving units) per 1,000 mg. Bromelain has a natural anti-inflammatory effect. Protease-enzyme products also have this benefit (chymotrypsin, trypsin, fungal-derived protease).

Super Prescription #2 Methylsulfonylmethane (MSM)
Take 1,000 mg three to four times daily. This supplement has potent anti-inflammatory effects and is a natural source of the mineral sulfur, which promotes ligament and tendon health.

Super Prescription #3 Vitamin C
Take 1,000 mg two or three times daily. Vitamin C is required for the formation of connective tissue and has anti-inflammatory benefits.

Super Prescription #4 DMSO
Consult with a doctor to use this pain-relieving substance topically for pain relief.

Super Prescription #5 Boswellia (*Boswellia serrata*)
Take 1,200 to 1,500 mg of standardized extract containing 60 to 65 percent boswellic acids two or three times daily. This herb has a strong anti-inflammatory effect.

Super Prescription #6 Arnica (*Arnica montana)* oil
Apply to the injured site twice daily. This herbal oil reduces pain, bruising, and swelling. Do not use on broken skin.

Super Prescription #7 Essential fatty acids
Take 1 to 2 tablespoons of flaxseed oil or 5 grams of fish oil daily, or take a formulation that contains a mixture of omega-3, -6, and -9 fatty acids. Essential fatty acids reduce inflammation and promote tissue healing.

General Recommendations

A high-potency multivitamin/-mineral supplies a host of vitamins and minerals required for ligament and tendon healing. Take as directed on the container.

A cool compress made with comfrey will ease pain and swelling.

White willow bark (*Salix alba*) is a natural pain reliever that doesn't have the side effects of aspirin and other over-the-counter drugs. Find an extract standardized for salicin content, and take 30 to 60 mg twice a day. If you prefer to use a tincture, take 1 to 2 cc three times daily.

Silica (*Silicea*) extract is important for connective-tissue healing. Take 500 mg three times daily. Glucosamine sulfate provides the raw materials known as glycosaminoglycans that are required by the body to manufacture ligaments and tendons. Take 1,500 mg daily. Collagen supplies substances that are required for ligament and tendon healing. Take as directed on the container.

Emergency Care for Sprains and Strains

When you suspect that you've experienced a strain or a sprain, it helps to take quick action. The following simple techniques, if used immediately after the injury, will promote faster healing and can greatly reduce the amount and the duration of pain.

1. If you experience severe pain, significant swelling, or discoloration at the site, get to a doctor as soon as possible. Be especially careful with injuries to the wrist or the ankle; these body parts are relatively delicate and vulnerable to fractures.

2. To reduce swelling and pain, apply an ice pack or a cold compress to the injured area. In a pinch, you can place some ice cubes in a plastic bag and then wrap the package up in a clean towel. You can even use a box of frozen vegetables. Just be sure that the ice doesn't touch your skin directly; otherwise, you'll have a sprain or a strain and frostbite. Keep the cold pack on for twenty minutes, then take a ten-minute break before reapplying.

3. To the extent possible, elevate the injured area so that it's higher than your heart. This allows blood to flow away from the site and decreases swelling.

4. Continue elevation and cold applications for the next day or two, and then alternate cold and warm applications. You no longer need to apply cold as often as in the first hour and a half after the injury; simply apply it intermittently as needed. If the swelling has not gone down significantly after this time, see a doctor.

Homeopathy

Pick the remedy that best matches your symptoms in this section. For acute sprain/ strains, take a 30C potency four times daily. For chronic sprains/strains that have not healed, take a 6x, 12x, 6C, 12C, or 30C twice daily for two weeks to see if there are any positive results. After you notice improvement, stop taking the remedy, unless symptoms return. Consultation with a homeopathic practitioner is advised.

Arnica (*Arnica montana*) is helpful at the beginning of an injury, when there is bruising and swelling.

Bryonia Alba should be used when there is pain from any movement. The person feels irritable from the pain.

Calcarea Fluorica is indicated for chronic sprains and strains that do not heal, or for people who are susceptible to getting these types of injuries due to weak ligaments or tendons.

Ledum Palustre is for sprained ankles or knees that are swollen and that feel better with ice applications.

Rhus Toxicodendron should be used for injuries that cause stiffness, especially during the first movement, but that loosen up later in the day. The injury feels better from warm applications.

Ruta (*Ruta graveolens*) is for overused ligaments and sprains that result in swelling and a lame feeling in the joint.

Acupressure

See pages 787–794 for information about pressure points and administering treatment.
- To relieve pain and relax your muscles, use Gallbladder 20 (GB20).
- Kidney 3 (K3) will reduce pain in either ankle.
- If you've strained your lower back, use Bladder 60 (B60).

Bodywork

Reflexology
See pages 804–805 for information about reflexology areas and how to work them.

Work the area that corresponds to the injured body part. Obviously, you should not practice reflexology on a hand or a foot that has been injured.

Hydrotherapy
Once the swelling has gone down, you can soak the injured part in warm water to relieve pain.

Other Bodywork Recommendations
Avoid putting weight on an injured joint or muscle, but do keep mobile. After the swelling is down and any acute pain has passed, try to work the body part through its range of motion. You'll help prevent stiffness.

Cold laser therapy from a practitioner stimulates healing of the ligaments, tendons, and cartilage.

Aromatherapy

After the swelling has subsided, try a combination of eucalyptus, peppermint, and lavender to stimulate a nourishing flow of blood to the area and reduce pain. You can use these oils in a warm bath or a compress.

REFERENCES

Blonstein, J. L. 1967. Oral enzyme tablets in the treatment of boxing injuries. *Practitioner* 198:547.

Buck, J. E., and N. Phillips. 1970. Trial of Chymoral in professional footballers. *British Journal of Clinical Practice* 24:375–77.

Deitrick, R. E. 1965. Oral proteolytic enzymes in the treatment of athletic injuries: A double-blind study. *Pennsylvania Medical Journal* 35–37.

Holt, H. T. 1969. Carica papaya as ancillary therapy for athletic injuries. *Current Therapeutics Research* 11:621–24.

Rathgeber, W. F. 1971. The use of proteolytic enzymes (Chymoral) in sporting injuries. *South African Medical Journal* 45:181–83.

Tsomides, J., and R. I. Goldberg. 1969. Controlled evaluation of oral chymotrypsin-trypsin treatment of injuries to the head and face. *Clinical Medicine* 76(11):40.

Stroke

Like all parts of the body, the brain needs a continuous supply of oxygen to function properly. When that oxygen supply is cut off, brain tissues begin to die within minutes, never to regenerate. This tissue death is what happens during a stroke. A stroke occurs when blood carrying oxygen and other nutrients to the brain is blocked or interrupted; the extent of the damage to the brain usually depends upon the length of the interruption and the speed with which treatment is received. As most of us know, strokes are extremely serious and often fatal. They are the third leading cause of death in the United States, behind only heart disease and cancer.

An overwhelming percentage of strokes are caused by arteriosclerosis, a condition in which fatty deposits buildup inside the arterial walls and obstruct blood flow. An artery leading to the brain may become so thick with plaque that the passage of blood is effectively blocked. The blood supply may also be shut off if a clot lodges itself in an artery that's already damaged and narrow. In a few cases, a cerebral blood vessel will actually rupture. High blood pressure gives a person a major predisposition to strokes, which damage the arteries and may cause a rupture; it, too, can often be managed with proper diet, exercise, supplementation, and stress management (see Blood Pressure, High).

Although we've been conditioned to think of strokes as tragic but unpreventable accidents that occur in old age, the truth is that arteriosclerosis is often a condition caused or made more probable by controllable lifestyle factors. Although arteries do tend to weaken as we get older, poor diet and lack of exercise, along with uncontrolled stress, are reasons that plaque builds up in the arteries in the first place. Genetic cardiovascular risk factors also play a role for many people. See the Cardiovascular Disease section for a more in-depth discussion of these risk factors.

A few other factors also increase the risk for stroke. If you have an irregular heartbeat or a damaged heart valve or have suffered a recent heart attack, you should be especially vigilant about your health and should be monitored regularly by a doctor. Women who take oral contraceptives and those who smoke also have a greater chance of developing blood clots, as do women on certain types of synthetic hormone replacement.

If you have a stroke, you have a significantly greater chance of surviving and even fully recovering if you receive medical treatment within three hours after the symptoms begin—the earlier, the better. Call an ambulance or get to an emergency room immediately if you experience any of the following symptoms: weakness or numbness along one side of the body; difficulty talking or understanding speech; blurred vision; confusion; a sudden, intense headache; unexplained dizziness or loss of balance; or loss of consciousness. These symptoms may come on suddenly, within a matter of seconds or minutes, or they may develop over the course of a day or two. If you have arteriosclerosis or are over fifty, you should be aware of these stroke warning signs so that you know when to get help, should it ever be necessary.

It's difficult to say exactly what the consequences of a stroke will be. The damage largely depends upon which brain tissues are deprived of oxygen and how long the interruption of blood flow lasts. If the blood flow is suspended for only a few seconds, you may experience visual and speech problems, weakness, trembling, or confusion, but it's likely that you'll soon return to normal. People who survive longer periods of oxygen deprivation may suffer lasting damage to their vision, speech, coordination, or movement, although physical therapy may restore some or even total functioning.

SYMPTOMS

- Paralysis or numbness on one side of the face or the body
- Dizziness
- A sudden, severe headache
- Blurred vision or blindness
- Confusion
- Impaired speech
- Loss of balance
- An inability to understand others' speech
- Loss of consciousness

ROOT CAUSES

- Poor diet
- Obesity
- Genetic cardiovascular risk factors (elevated fibrinogen, homocysteine, etc.)
- Blood that clots too easily
- Irregular heartbeat
- Damaged heart valve
- High blood pressure
- Oral contraceptives (especially in women over thirty-five)
- Smoking
- Diabetes
- Synthetic hormone replacement

Testing Techniques

The following tests help to assess your stroke risk:

Cardiovascular risk factors (cholesterol, homocysteine, fibrinogen, etc.)— blood (see the Cardiovascular Disease section for more information)

Blood pressure

Hormone testing (thyroid, DHEA, cortisol, testosterone, IGF-1, estrogen, progesterone)—saliva, blood, or urine

Vitamin and mineral analysis (especially magnesium, vitamin E, potassium, CoQ10)—blood

Essential fatty acid balance—blood

Blood sugar balance—blood

Toxic metals—hair or urine

TREATMENT

If you experience any of the symptoms listed previously, get medical help immediately. The following treatments will assist in the recovery from strokes or will prevent future strokes from occurring, but they cannot substitute for emergency care by doctors.

If you have arteriosclerosis, see the Cardiovascular Disease section for further suggestions. For high blood pressure, see Blood Pressure, High.

Diet

Recommended Food

Follow a diet consisting of whole, natural foods, including fresh fruits and vegetables, whole grains, beans, legumes, fish, nuts, and seeds. This eating plan, which is high in nutrients and fiber, will reduce your risk of forming blood clots. The antioxidants in these foods will also counteract free-radical damage, making you less likely to develop arteriosclerosis.

Fish are high in essential fatty acids and decrease your risk of stroke. They contain "good" fats that improve circulation and act as natural blood thinners. The Nurses' Health Study found a significant decrease in the risk of thrombotic stroke among women who ate fish at least two times per week, when compared with the risk in women who ate fish less than once per month. Although you should eat a wide variety of fruits and vegetables, try to have two servings of those that are blue-red or purple in color at least twice a day. Purple grapes, berries, red cabbage, and eggplant are all high in anthocyanidins, a substance that lowers the risk of stroke and heart disease.

Potassium helps to reduce blood pressure and thereby decreases stroke risk. Good sources include leafy green vegetables, tomatoes, potatoes, and citrus fruits.

Consume green and white tea, which contains powerful antioxidants.

Drink 1.7 ounces of pomegranate juice daily to prevent plaque buildup in the carotid arteries.

Studies show that increased dietary calcium intake reduces the risk of stroke. Consume foods high in calcium (see Osteoporosis).

Food to Avoid

A diet that's high in saturated fat and trans-fatty acids is thought to be a leading cause of both arteriosclerosis and high blood pressure. Eliminate red meat, butter, fried and greasy food, and all junk food from your diet. You must also avoid margarine and shortening, as well as products made with these items. This includes many sweet baked goods. Vegetable oils should not be used for frying. The exception is canola oil. Avocado and macadamia nut oils are good for frying.

Although we don't tend to think of sugar as a cause of heart disease, high amounts of it will increase the inflammation in artery walls. Decrease the amount of simple sugars in the diet, such as those from white breads, pastas, candy, and soda pop.

Sodium can send blood pressure levels soaring in many people. Don't use table salt, and avoid processed food, which is the leading source of sodium in the American diet.

A review of studies in the *Journal of the American Medical Association* looked at the relationship between fruit and vegetable intake and the risk of ischemic stroke. This review included 75,596 women, ages thirty-four to fifty-nine years, in the Nurses' Health Study and 38,683 men, ages forty to seventy-five years, in the Health Professionals' Follow-Up Study. An increment of one serving per day of fruits or vegetables was associated with a 6 percent lower risk of ischemic stroke. Researchers found that cruciferous and green leafy vegetables, as well as citrus fruit and juice, were most helpful in decreasing ischemic stroke risk.

A meta-analysis published in *Stroke* found that treatment with citicholine in the first twenty-four hours after a moderate to severe stroke increased the probability of complete recovery at three months.

℞ Super Seven Prescriptions—Stroke

Super Prescription #1 Citicholine
Take 2,000 mg daily within twenty-four hours of a stroke.

Super Prescription #2 Nattokinase
Take 2,000 FU daily on an empty stomach. This enzyme acts as a natural blood thinner. *Caution*: Do not take with aspirin or other blood thinners.

Super Prescription #3 Fish oil
Take a daily dosage of a fish oil product containing 1,000 mg of EPA and 500 mg of DHA. Fish oil reduces inflammation in the arteries and lowers cholesterol and triglyceride levels.

Super Prescription #4 Garlic (*Allium sativum*)
Take 300 to 500 mg of aged garlic twice daily. It reduces cholesterol levels and increases HDL cholesterol.

Super Prescription #5 Vitamin E
Take 400 IU daily of a mixed complex. It prevents cholesterol oxidation and is a natural blood thinner.

Super Prescription #6 Green tea (*Camellia sinensis*) extract
Take 500 to 1,500 mg of the capsule form. Look for a product standardized to between 80 and 90 percent polyphenols and between 35 and 55 percent epigallocatechin gallate. Green tea contains a rich source of antioxidants and substances that assist detoxification.

Super Prescription #7 *Ginkgo biloba*
Take 180 to 240 mg daily of a 24 percent flavone glycoside extract. Ginkgo has blood-thinning and antioxidant properties.

General Recommendations

Take a high-potency multivitamin as directed on the container. It contains a variety of antioxidants, as well as minerals that are associated with reducing the risk of stroke.

Pantetheine is a metabolite of vitamin B5 that has been shown in studies to reduce total and LDL cholesterol, as well to increase HDL. It can be particularly effective for people with diabetes. Take 600 to 900 mg daily.

Soy protein has been shown in studies to reduce total and LDL cholesterol and to increase HDL. Take 25 to 50 grams daily.

Reishi (*Ganoderma lucidum*) is a mushroom extract that reduces cholesterol. Take 800 mg two or three times daily.

Vitamin E prevents LDL oxidation. Take 400 to 800 IU of a mixed blend daily.

Vitamin C reduces total cholesterol and LDL levels and acts to prevent their oxidation.

A full B-complex is as important as folic acid, B6, and B12 for stroke prevention. Take 50 mg of B-complex daily.

Alpha GPC has been shown to help improve recovery, including cognitive and behavioral functions. Take 400 mg three times daily. Intramuscular injections are also available from a doctor.

Homeopathy

If you experience the symptoms of a stroke, you must get medical assistance at once. The following remedies may be helpful as part of a comprehensive stroke-recovery protocol. Pick the remedy that best matches your symptoms in this section. Take a 6x, 12x, 6C, 12C, or 30C potency twice daily for two weeks to see if there are any positive results. After you notice improvement, stop taking the remedy, unless symptoms return. Consultation with a homeopathic practitioner is advised.

Aconitum Napellus will help calm someone who's panicked and afraid of dying while waiting for medical attention. Take a 30C potency or whatever potency is available.

Baryta Carbonica is a good remedy when there is mental weakness after a stroke and weakness on one side of the body. The person has childish characteristics as a result of the stroke.

Causticum is indicated for paralysis of the muscles of speech, paralysis of the bladder, and numbness of the hands and the feet. It is a specific remedy for right-sided paralysis.

Gelsemium Sempervirens is helpful for aftereffects of a stroke, characterized by muscle weakness and trembling, numbness of the face and the tongue, and the eyelids remaining half opened.

Lachesis Mutas is for left-sided paralysis after a stroke and for paralysis of the throat and the tongue.

Acupressure

- Gallbladder 20 and 21 (GB20 and GB21) stimulate circulation, especially to the head.
- Use Liver 3 (Lv3) to induce a sense of peacefulness and calm.

Bodywork

Massage
Have frequent circulatory massages to increase your energy and sense of well-being.

Reflexology

See pages 804–805 for information about reflexology areas and how to work them.

Work the spine to stimulate any damaged nerves and promote good circulation.

People who've suffered a stroke often have some numbness or paralysis on one side of their bodies. Reflexology can encourage the healing process. If your left side is damaged, work the big toe on the right foot. If the stroke has affected your right side, work the big toe on the left foot. In addition, you should massage the regions that correspond to any affected body parts.

Other Bodywork Recommendations
Acupuncture can be very helpful in speeding recovery and as a complement to physical therapy. Acupuncture treatments should begin as soon as possible after one has suffered a stroke.

Aromatherapy

Mix a few drops of juniper with a carrier oil, and use in a massage to help break down toxins in the blood and carry them out of the body. You can also add juniper to a bath.

Black pepper, ginger, and rosemary all stimulate circulation. Again, you can use them in a massage or a bath.

If you feel fatigued, geranium, jasmine, neroli, bergamot, and rose can give a lift to your energy levels and your mood. These oils can also aid in stress reduction. Use them in any preparation you like.

Stress Reduction

General Stress-Reduction Therapies

Stress-reduction techniques, which include exercise, prayer, yoga, and positive mental imagery, should be incorporated as part of stroke recovery.

Other Recommendations

- Hyperbaric oxygen therapy may help you to recover from a stroke, as it improves oxygen flow to the brain. Consult with a doctor who is trained in this therapy.
- As with other circulatory conditions, exercise is an important factor in both recovery from and prevention of a stroke. You don't have to climb mountains— a daily walk or swim will suffice. Try to exercise in the early-morning sunshine, which will lift your spirits.
- Stop smoking. This habit increases the risk of high blood pressure and arteriosclerosis, the two most frequent causes of stroke.
- If you have diabetes, you're at risk for circulatory diseases like strokes and heart problems. You must eat well, exercise, manage stress, and work closely with an experienced doctor. For more information, see Diabetes.
- People who are overweight are more vulnerable to strokes than the rest of the population is. The diet and exercise guidelines here should help you lose weight, but if you want further suggestions, see Obesity.

REFERENCES

Davalos, A., et al. 2002. Oral citicoline in acute ischemic stroke: An individual patient data pooling analysis of clinical trials. *Stroke* 33:2850–57.

Joshipura, K. J., et al. 1999. Fruit and vegetable intake in relation to risk of ischemic stroke. *Journal of the American Medical Association* 282(13):1233–39.

Skerrett, P. J., and C. H. Hennekens. 2003. Consumption of fish and fish oils and decreased risk of stroke. *Preventative Cardiology* 6(1):38–41.

Substance Abuse (Drug and Alcohol Addiction)

Substance abuse is a dependency—whether psychological, physical, or both—on drugs (including prescription medications and alcohol). No one knows why some people develop such a dependency while others don't, but evidence indicates that genetics, environment, and individual psychology all have roles to play in the illness.

Drugs and alcohol can cause severe damage to almost every system in the body. Both of them have a toxic effect on the liver, an organ whose functioning is crucial to many bodily systems. Obviously, brain damage is always a concern. Aside from the very real possibility of a fatal overdose—the likelihood of which increases if drugs and alcohol are mixed—abusing drugs can create several life-threatening conditions.

The free radicals in these substances are carcinogenic, and addicts experience a high rate of breast, mouth, esophageal, and liver cancers. Cocaine and heroin can severely damage the heart. Shared needles can lead to AIDS and hepatitis transmission. Drugs can also cause mental disorders, such as anxiety, panic, and depression; kidney failure from excessive urine production (this is especially a problem for alcoholics); stroke and impotence, as a result of a depressed central nervous system; and a host of other disorders that result from a suppressed immune system. Substance abuse is the leading cause of traffic fatalities and plays a significant role in homicides, suicides, spousal and child abuse, and other violent acts.

Effective treatment begins when an addict makes the decision to give up drugs or alcohol. The process, however, rarely ends there. Many people suffer from withdrawal symptoms, which include heart problems, sweats, tremors, dehydration, seizures, and hallucinations. It is often a good idea to have medical supervision during this period. In addition, most serious users will need to address the psychological components of their addiction and may benefit from therapy or from a support group such as Narcotics Anonymous or Alcoholics Anonymous. Spiritual support is also strongly advised.

Biochemical imbalances can predispose one to drug dependency. For example, people who are prone to biochemical depression may use alcohol or drugs as a crutch. People with alcoholism often have a blood sugar imbalance and candidiasis (see the Candidiasis section for more information), which increase their alcohol cravings. Other nutrient deficiencies may worsen their susceptibility to becoming addicted.

Complementary therapies for drug dependency and withdrawal focus on balancing the body's systems and address underlying emotional, mental, and spiritual disorders. Detoxification using natural therapies improves the person's vitality.

SYMPTOMS: HOW DO YOU KNOW IF IT'S A PROBLEM?

If you're trying to determine whether you or someone you know has a problem with drugs, it's important to realize that addiction can take many forms and that there is no one pattern of abuse. Usually, an addiction develops over time, as occasional social drinking or drug use progresses into heavy use and then to total dependency, but some people find themselves addicted from their first drink, puff, or hit. Some alcoholics drink only wine, beer, or certain kinds of hard liquor; others will drink anything that contains a trace of alcohol, including mouthwash and perfume. The frequency of use also varies. Some addicts will use small amounts of substances throughout the day (alcoholics may spike coffee, juice, tea, or other beverages with liquor), while others may stay sober for long periods in between binges. The personalities of people who abuse substances also comprise a wide range, from the stereotypical violent, angry, sloppy addict to one who maintains a composed and polished front. Substance abuse can occur at any age and in either sex.

One general rule does seem to apply: if you require drugs or alcohol not just to release tension but to feel "normal," then you are in a late stage of addiction and need to seek help as soon as possible.

ROOT CAUSES

It's unclear why some people are more prone to addiction than others are. Following are some of the leading possibilities:

- A genetic tendency toward addiction
- Psychological problems, including depression
- Environmental factors, such as
- the general availability of drugs and social pressure
- Nutritional deficiencies
- A blood sugar imbalance (alcoholism)

Testing Techniques

The following tests help assess possible reasons for substance-abuse tendencies:

Vitamin and mineral analysis (especially magnesium, B vitamins, chromium)—blood

Digestive function and microbe/parasite/candida testing—stool analysis

Food and environmental allergies/sensitivities—blood, electrodermal

Blood sugar balance—blood

Amino acid balance—blood or urine

TREATMENT

Diet

Recommended Food

You need to rebuild your damaged body systems. Start by eating well-rounded meals of natural foods. A variety of fresh fruits and vegetables, whole grains, beans, nuts, seeds, and lean animal protein will help you feel balanced and energetic again.

If you haven't been eating much as a result of your addiction, you may find it difficult to sit down to three large meals a day. Instead, plan several smaller snacks. This strategy will also keep your blood sugar levels even and help you avoid cravings.

Drink a glass of clean, quality water every two waking hours. You'll be surprised at how much better you feel when you're properly hydrated, and you'll be less tempted to fill up on junk food. Water also helps flush the accumulated toxins out of your system.

You may experience some trouble sleeping without the aid of drugs or alcohol. If that's the case, try eating a snack of turkey or chicken on whole-grain crackers before you go to bed. These foods are all good sources of tryptophan, a chemical that activates the sleep-inducing neurotransmitter serotonin. For additional suggestions, see Insomnia.

Complete abstention from solid food is not recommended if you are going through withdrawal, as balanced nutrition will help curb your cravings. Once you've been sober for a while, however, you should go on supervised detoxification protocols to eliminate all the poisons you've consumed via drugs or alcohol. You can (and should) drink plenty of juices, herbal teas, and broths while detoxifying. It will take at least four months of good eating and monthly fasts to fully detoxify your body.

If you haven't been eating lots of fiber—and few substance abusers do—you may be severely constipated. Following the previously described eating plan will help, but it's also important to get the toxic matter out of your bowels. If you are having problems, see the Constipation section.

Food to Avoid

As you're trying to kick the habit, you may instinctively reach for sugary treats or caffeinated beverages. Avoid this temptation, as caffeine and refined sugar will only increase your cravings for drugs.

Obviously, alcohol use is out of the question, even if you haven't formerly had a problem with alcohol.

℞ Super Seven Prescriptions—Substance Abuse

Super Prescription #1 High-potency multivitamin/ -mineral
Take as directed on the container. It supplies a combination of vitamins and minerals that assists detoxification and improves your mood.

Super Prescription #2 Milk thistle (*Silybum marianum*)
Take 250 mg three times daily of a product standardized to 80 to 85 percent silymarin extract. Milk thistle supports liver detoxification and has been shown to reduce elevated liver enzymes.

Super Prescription #3 B-complex
Take 50 mg twice daily. Many of the B vitamins are required for detoxification, as well as for mood and energy support.

Super Prescription #4 Homeopathic Nux Vomica
Take a 30C potency twice daily for up to two weeks. It reduces withdrawal symptoms of irritability, nausea, constipation, and fatigue.

Super Prescription #5 Chromium
Take 200 mcg two or three times daily. It reduces sugar (and possibly alcohol) cravings.

Super Prescription #6 L-glutamine
Take 500 mg three times daily on an empty stomach. It improves mood and energy levels.

Super Prescription #7 5-hydroxytryptophan (5-HTP)
Take 100 mg three times daily on an empty stomach. It reduces the depression and the anxiety that come on during withdrawal symptoms. Taken before bedtime, it also promotes restful sleep. *Note*: Do not take this if you are on a pharmaceutical antidepressant or antianxiety medication.

General Recommendations

DL-phenylalanine helps fight depression and low energy. Take 500 mg three times daily on an empty stomach.

If you suffer from mild or moderate depression, take Saint-John's-wort (*Hypericum perforatum*). It will lift your mood and help you face your daily challenges. It will also bolster your weakened immune system. Use 300 mg three times daily of a 0.3 percent hypericin extract. Do not take Saint-John's-wort if you are already on medication for depression or anxiety.

Super-green-food supplements, such as spirulina, chlorella, or a blend of greens, promote healthful detoxification. Take as directed on the container.

If you need some help getting to sleep, drink a cup of valerian (*Valeriana officinalis*) tea before going to bed.

Many people who are trying to kick a drug or alcohol habit feel nervous and anxious. Passionflower (*Passiflora incarnata*) is a gentle yet effective herb to use. Take 3 ml of the tincture form or 500 mg of the capsule version three times daily. Hops (*Humulus lupulus*), kava (*Piper methysticum*), oatstraw (*Avena sativa*), and valerian (*Valeriana officinalis*) are other good herbal options. (See the Anxiety section.)

Reishi (*Ganoderma lucidum*) extract improves liver and immune-system function. It also helps with concentration and focus. Take 800 mg twice daily.

Calcium and magnesium relax the nervous system; they are especially good if you experience twitches and cramps. Take 500 mg of calcium and 250 mg of magnesium twice daily.

People with alcoholism may benefit from supplementing niacin. Take 500 mg twice daily of the flush-free version.

N-acetylcysteine increases levels of glutathione, an important antioxidant. Take 300 mg three times daily.

Vitamin C is important for detoxification, and it increases glutathione levels. Take 1,000 mg three times daily.

Vitamin B1 (thiamine) is particularly important for people with alcoholism, to prevent cognitive dysfunction, memory impairment, and visual changes. Take up to 200 mg daily. For severe deficiencies, intravenous or injection forms given by a doctor are required.

Eleutherococcus/Siberian ginseng works to help the body adapt to mental and physical stress by improving adrenal-gland function. Take 600 to 900 mg of a standardized product daily.

Kudzu (*Pueraria lobata*) may help to decrease craving and consumption. Take as directed on the label.

Homeopathy

Pick the remedy that best matches your symptoms in this section. Take a 6x, 12x, 6C, 12C, or 30C potency twice daily for two weeks to see if there are any positive results. After you notice improvement, stop taking the remedy, unless symptoms return. Consultation with a homeopathic practitioner is advised.

Arsenicum Album is indicated when one feels tremendous restlessness, fatigue, and anxiety. There may be burning pains that feel better from warmth. Symptoms are worse between midnight and 2 A.M.

A study was completed that included 507 people with alcoholism, who were treated with 3 grams or more of niacin daily for five years. Results suggested that a majority benefited from supplementation, by experiencing symptom reduction and fewer relapses.

Ignatia Amara is for hysteria and emotional breakdown. The person has constantly changing mood and symptoms, cries but wants to be left alone, has a sensation of a lump in the throat, is anxious, and has twitches and spasms.

Lachesis is for people with addictions who get violent. They have intense feelings of jealousy, paranoia, and suspiciousness. They tend to be warm and feel worse from heat. There is an intolerance of anything touching the throat.

Lycopodium (*Lycopodium clavatum*) is indicated for people with an alcohol or drug addiction. They are irritable and have low self-esteem. They are chilly and feel better from warmth. They usually have a strong craving for sweets and often have digestive problems, such as gas and bloating.

Nux Vomica is good for emotional withdrawal symptoms that include irritability and anger, as well as physical symptoms of nausea, constipation, chilliness, and fatigue. There is great sensitivity to sound, light, odors, and touch.

Sulphur is a good remedy for people who crave alcohol and go on binges. They tend to feel warm and feel better from cool air and cold drinks. There is a craving for spicy foods. Skin rashes are common.

Acupressure

See pages 787–794 for information about pressure points and administering treatment.

- Stomach 36 (St36) improves your ability to absorb nutrients and gives you an overall sense of well-being.
- Spleen 10 (Sp10) will speed up the detoxification process.
- For anxiety or depression, work Lung 1 (Lu1).
- If you are fatigued, use Gallbladder 20 (GB20).

Bodywork

Massage
A lymphatic massage will break down toxins that have been stored in fatty deposits.

Reflexology
See pages 804–805 for information about reflexology areas and how to work them. To encourage the release of toxins, give extra attention to the liver and the kidneys.

Hydrotherapy
Constitutional hydrotherapy supports detoxification. See pages 795–796 for directions.

Other Bodywork Recommendations
Acupuncture has a strong history of successfully treating addictions of all kinds. Consult a licensed practitioner who has experience in treating this problem.

Aromatherapy

Juniper breaks up poisons and speeds their exit from the body. Mix some with a carrier oil and use it in a lymphatic massage, or add a few drops to a hot bath.

Lavender, bergamot, and chamomile are antidepressants. Use them in any way you like to lift a case of the blues.

If you find that you're hungry all the time, inhale bergamot to suppress the appetite and reduce stress.

Stress Reduction

General Stress-Reduction Therapies

Substance abuse is often an unproductive way of coping with stress or emotional pain. If you are to remain sober, then you must find another, more healthful way to manage stress. Read about various techniques in the Exercise and Stress Reduction chapter and experiment until you find one or two that you like enough to use regularly.

Other Recommendations

- If you have problems with alcohol, be aware that some everyday products contain small amounts that may throw your good intentions off track. Avoid mouthwash, and read the labels on cold and flu medicines.
- Many people who abuse stimulants are actually trying to jump-start an underactive thyroid. For more information about testing yourself for this problem, see Hypothyroidism.
- If you've been abusing heroin, barbiturates, tranquilizers, or other depressants, you should be under medical supervision during your withdrawal period, which may last anywhere from a few weeks to a number of months. It's too dangerous for you to quit cold turkey; instead, you should check yourself into a respected program that allows you to gradually and safely reduce your dependence on the drug.
- People who have been taking hallucinogens also need help as they pass through the acute stage of withdrawal. A health-care professional should be present to help them handle the uncontrollable, frightening, and sometimes violent thoughts that can occur during this time.
- Join a support group for your addiction. Also, spiritual support through a local house of worship is recommended.

REFERENCES

Smith, R. F. 1974. A five-year trial of massive nicotinic acid therapy of alcoholics in Michigan. *Journal of Orthomolecular Psychiatry* 3:327–31.

Surgery Preparation and Recovery

Surgery can afford many benefits, including pain reduction, greater mobility, tumor removal, cosmetic improvements, and others. But for many Americans the risks and complications of surgery can be problematic. The Centers for Disease Control and Prevention reports that fifty-one million inpatient surgeries and at least thirty-five million outpatient surgeries take place every year. Yet little instruction is given to most surgery patients regarding proper nutrition and supplementation to prepare the body for surgery and an efficient recovery.

The goal of a good preoperative nutrition plan is to boost levels of antioxidants, healthful fatty acids, phytonutrients, amino acids, vitamins, minerals, and other important nutrients that optimize tissue healing. By following such a plan, a patient can reduce the length and cost of hospitalization, improve immunity to reduce the risk of infection, improve the likelihood of survival, reduce the risk of complications, and improve quality of life.

Studies show that up to 65 percent of people admitted to hospitals are malnourished, and the majority of patients experience nutritional depletion during hospital admission. This nutrient depletion worsens during the course of a hospital stay. Poor nutritional status leads to changes in the body's composition, loss of muscle mass and function, impaired organ function, and ultimately impaired immune function. The body requires good nutrition to work properly. This is even more critical for those who undergo surgery of the digestive tract, where absorption of nutrients can be impaired.

The first phase of surgery is known as the preoperative period. Those who do not need emergency surgery and are able to schedule surgery in advance are at an advantage as they have time to improve their nutritional status. The consequences of malnutrition for those scheduled for surgery was recognized as far back as the 1930s. A 1936 article in the *Journal of the American Medical Association* found a direct relationship between preoperative weight loss and operative mortality rate, independent of factors such as age, impaired cardiorespiratory function, and type of surgery. For many, the preoperative period is a time of anxiety and stress. Concerns about success of the surgery, complications, pain, and restrictions from activity and work may cause worry. There are a variety of natural products that can prevent and treat anxiety, depression, and general worry during this time.

The second phase is known as the postoperative or recovery period. This is the time immediately following the procedure, when the body heals from surgery. Again, proper nutrition is essential for tissue healing and for the prevention of secondary infections. Research has shown that nutrient deficiencies are a major factor in the development of postoperative complications and poor outcome. Those given orally administered supplements have been shown to have fewer infections, fewer days in intensive care, fewer overall hospital days, and improved wound healing compared to those who receive the typical substandard nutrition offered by hospitals. Research shows that nutritional needs in the postoperative period are higher than at almost any other period in the adult life.

SYMPTOMS

- Anxiety
- Pain
- Insomnia
- Constipation
- Secondary infections
- Bed sores

ROOT CAUSES

- Nutritional deficiencies that make healing and recovery from surgery more difficult

---

Testing Techniques

Vitamin and mineral analysis—blood
Protein and amino acid levels—blood, urine
Omega-fatty-acid balance—blood

TREATMENT

Diet

Supporting immunity with good nutrition is very important. Approximately one in twenty-five hospital patients has at least one health care–associated infection.

Recommended Food

A modified Mediterranean diet that is low in refined grain products and rich in vegetables, fruits, nuts, seeds, legumes, and fresh fish is recommended.

Prior to and after surgery, protein intake is key. Low levels both complicate tissue healing and compromise immunity. Consuming half your body weight in grams of protein each day for the two weeks or longer preceding surgery can be helpful. For example, if you weigh two hundred pounds then aim to consume approximately 100 grams of protein per day. If you have existing liver or kidney disease, check with your doctor before consuming this much protein.

Research has shown one surprising habit that can decrease your hospital stay—chewing gum! Controlled trials have shown that chewing gum after surgery improves bowel-function recovery and decreases the length of hospital stay. The action of chewing activates peristalsis (gut motility). And since constipation is a common complication of inactivity and of pain medications and antibiotics, it is important to counter this problem, especially for those undergoing digestive-tract surgery. We recommend a gum that does not contain artificial sweeteners.

Most of your immune power begins in the digestive tract. It is positively affected by the healthy bacteria provided by probiotics and by cultured foods such as miso, sauerkraut, and tempeh, which supercharge the immune system and act as shields against intruders that may take up residence in the digestive tract.

Food to Avoid

Before and after surgery make sure to avoid sugars and refined carbohydrates that suppress immunity and interfere with tissue healing. Also restrict foods that have a blood-thinning effect, such as garlic and ginger.

℞ Super Seven Prescriptions—Surgery Preparation and Recovery

Super Prescription #1 Homeopathic Arnica Montana

Take two pellets of a 200C potency immediately after surgery and again every eight hours for two to three days. Another option is to take a 30C potency immediately after surgery and every four hours for two to three days. It is helpful in reducing tissue swelling, bruising, and pain. It does not interfere with pain medications or antibiotics. It is also helpful for those recovering from plastic surgery.

Super Prescription #2 Multivitamin/-mineral

A high-potency multivitamin and -mineral formula should be a daily supplement to provide a base of nutrients that promote immunity and tissue health.

Super Prescription # 3 Vitamin C

Take 1,000 mg two to three times daily after surgery to promote tissue healing.

Super Prescription # 4 Probiotic

Take at least twenty billion organisms for two weeks preoperatively and for at least eight weeks postoperatively for good immune function and digestive health.

Super Prescription # 5 Whey protein

Take 25 grams blended into a shake every day postoperatively for tissue healing. The other option would be to take an amino acid blend that supplies all the essential amino acids.

Super Prescription # 6 Glutathione

Take 250 mg to 500 mg twice daily to support detoxification from surgery medications and to improve immunity.

Super Prescription #7 Bromelain or proteolytic enzymes

Take 500 mg three times daily on an empty stomach after surgery to reduce inflammation. If you are on blood-thinning medication consult with your doctor before using.

General Recommendations

GABA is an amino acid that is quite effective for reducing the anxiety that often flares up preoperatively. A typical dose would be 200 to 300 mg two to three times daily.

Ashwagandha helps replenish the energy and immunity that are depleted from the stress of surgery. Take 250 mg of an extract twice daily.

Melatonin helps with insomnia related to pre- and postsurgery stress. Take 1 to 3 mg one hour before bedtime.

Milk thistle promotes liver detoxification from the medications used with surgery. Take 250 mg to 500 mg three times daily.

B-complex supports recovery and energy levels after surgery. Take 50 to 100 mg daily.

Glutamine supports muscle and gut recovery. Take 2,500 mg twice daily on an empty stomach.

Zinc at a dose of 25 mg is important to help with wound healing.

Vitamin A helps with skin and digestive-tract healing. A typical dose is 5,000 IU daily.

Omega-3 fatty acids reduce tissue inflammation. Take 1,000 mg of EPA and DHA for a good starting dosage after surgery.

Vitamin E can help with tissue healing, reduce inflammation, and possibly prevent excess scarring. Take 400 IU of a mixed vitamin-E complex.

A greens formula that contains organic super foods such as wheatgrass, chlorella, spirulina, and barley grass promotes bowel regularity, which is often a problem postsurgery due to anesthesia, pain medications, lack of fibrous food, and reduced body movement. Some of these super green foods also contain RNA (ribonucleic acid), which is involved in the formation of protein and in wound healing.

Colloidal silver gel is for skin infections that occur after surgery.

MSM reduces inflammation and soreness after surgery. Take 1,000 mg three times daily.

Coenzyme Q10 (CoQ10) is important for those undergoing heart surgery. One of the major causes of death after a heart operation is low cardiac output. This means the heart muscle is not effectively pumping blood throughout the coronary arteries and the rest of the body. Studies have shown that CoQ10 is quite remarkable in preventing both reduced cardiac output and arrhythmias. It also has been shown to preserve the structure of heart muscle, shorten hospital recovery time, and reduce length of hospital stay following heart surgery. The recommended CoQ10 dosage is 100 mg twice daily.

Homeopathy

Pick the remedy that best matches your symptoms in this section. Take a 6x, 12x, 6C, 12C, or 30C potency twice daily for two weeks to see if there are any positive results. After you notice improvement, stop taking the remedy, unless symptoms return. Consultation with a homeopathic practitioner is advised.

Calcarea Fluorica is for connective tissue that is damaged from surgery.

Hypericum Perforatum is specific for those who have had trauma to nerves from surgery. Examples would include surgery of the mouth, teeth, or spine.

Nux Vomica is for constipation or a bad reaction to anesthesia.

Silica is for scar tissue that forms after surgery.

Other Recommendations

- Take steps to avoid hospital infections, which are a major concern. They can cause complications during a patient's recovery from surgery and can also develop into deadly superinfections. Organisms such as MRSA and *Clostridium difficile* are opportunistic microbes that are best prevented with good hygiene and an immune system that is functioning optimally. This is why probiotics and other immune-supportive supplements should be started preoperatively and continued postoperatively. Fungal organisms are also present in hospitals. When a patient receives antibiotics with surgery, an environment is provided for these parasitic organisms to flourish, potentially causing infection and damaging the small intestine, where most of our nutrient absorption takes place. Again, ensuring that your system has adequate good bacteria by supplementing with probiotics helps guard against this problem. For patients that end up on antibiotic therapy for prolonged periods of time, the use of antifungal herbs and antifungal medications is often helpful.
- Most surgeons are unaware that anesthesia and pain medications damage the digestive tract and contribute to increased intestinal permeability, also known as leaky gut syndrome. In leaky gut, the normal mechanisms that control what passes into the bloodstream from the intestines don't work, allowing larger particles through. The result is compromised immunity and healing. Proper diet and the supplements recommended in this chapter will guard against this problem.
- Exercise regularly leading up to surgery. Physical activity improves circulation, muscle mass, heart and lung function, and immunity, and prepares the body for healing after surgery.
- You should discuss with your surgeon which medications should be discontinued prior to surgery and for how long. It's especially important to discontinue antiplatelet medications like aspirin and blood-thinning medications such as Coumadin, Xarelto, and Plavix.

Forty people scheduled for coronary-artery bypass surgery were given either a placebo or 150 mg of CoQ10 daily for seven days before their operation. The number of arrhythmias and blood markers of heart damage during the postoperative period were significantly less for those who supplemented CoQ10. Another similarly designed study found that those given CoQ10 had significantly less medication, fewer blood transfusions, and a 31 percent decrease in average hospital stay.

- Your surgeon will also request that you be off all supplements that have a blood-thinning effect, such as ginkgo, cayenne, fish oil, vitamin E (more than 400 IU), garlic, nattokinase, bromelain, and others. However, question any doctor that tells you that you need to be off all supplements for a week or longer before surgery. This is not accurate. In our opinion, probiotics, beta glucans, multivitamins, and other supplements that are not strong blood thinners do not need to be avoided for long periods of time before surgery.

- One of the serious complications of the postoperative period is bedsores, also known as pressure sores or pressure ulcers. These occur on pressure points of the body when the patient is unable to move. The constant pressure on a specific location causes a reduction in blood flow to the area, which in turn prevents oxygen, immune cells, and nutrients from getting to the affected tissue. Inflammation, tissue damage, and cell death are the results. Moisture from sweating as well as urinary and fecal incontinence increase the risk for bedsores. Changes in position at least every two hours are necessary—with the help of an assistant if needed. Poor nutritional status is a known major risk factor for bedsores. Research has shown that both oral and intravenous nutrients significantly reduce the incidence of bedsores by approximately 26 percent. Nutrients most often studied include vitamin C, zinc, and the amino acid arginine. Typical doses include vitamin C at 500 to 3,000 mg, arginine at 3,000 to 9,000 mg, Pycnogenol at 100 mg, and zinc at 30 mg.

- We also recommend the use of natural topical healing agents. Manuka honey, which is available at health food stores and online, has antibacterial properties and stimulates tissue healing for mild to moderate bedsores. Put one to two teaspoons on a piece of sterile gauze. Fasten the gauze with skin tape to the affected sore. Change the bandage every twelve hours. In combination with proper repositioning of the body, manuka honey can heal mild to moderate bedsores within two to three weeks. For additional treatment support for bedsores, consider oxygen therapies such as intravenous ozone therapy and hyperbaric oxygen. These therapies deliver oxygen to stimulate tissue healing and eliminate infections associated with bedsores.

- An increasingly popular treatment for those recovering from surgery is acupuncture. Normative in the East, acupuncture is becoming more accepted by mainstream medicine for its role in reducing pain and inflammation.

- Lastly, once the postoperative recovery period is complete, work with a holistic doctor to detoxify from all the medications used during and after surgery. Several excellent treatments have already been described in this chapter. The use of saunas, massage, hydrotherapy, intravenous nutrients—especially glutathione and detoxification-specific supplements—will help the body to regenerate.

REFERENCES

CDC website. Accessed June 6, 2015 at http://www.cdc.gov/nchs/fastats/inpatient -surgery.htm.

CDC website. Accessed June 6, 2015 at http://www.cdc.gov/media/pressrel/2009 /r090128.htm.

Deren, M., et al. 2014. Assessment and treatment of malnutrition in orthopaedic surgery. *JBJS Reviews* 2(9).

McWhirter, J. P., C. R. Pennington. 1994. The incidence and recognition of malnutrition in hospital. *BMJ* 308:945–8.

Ward, N. 2003. Nutrition support to patients undergoing gastrointestinal surgery. *Nutrition Journal* 2:18.

CDC website, Accessed June 6, 2015 at http://www.cdc.gov/HAI/surveillance/.

Kouba, E. J., et al. 2007. Gum chewing stimulates bowel motility in patients undergoing radical cystectomy with urinary diversion. *Urology* 70:1053–56.

Schuster, R. et al. 2006. Gum chewing reduces ileus after elective open sigmoid colectomy. *Arch Surg* 141:174–76.

Chello, M., et al. 1994. Protection by coenzyme Q10 form myocardial reprofusion injury during coronary artery bypass grafting. *Ann Thorac Surg* 58:1427–32.

Makhija, N., et al. 2008. The role of coenzyme Q10 in patients undergoing coronary artery bypass graft surgery. *J Cardiothorac Casc Anesth* 22:832–39.

Giner, M., et al. 1996. In 1995 a correlation between malnutrition and poor outcome in critically ill patients still exists. *Nutrition* 12:23–29.

Crowe, T., and C. Brockbank. 2009. Nutrition therapy in the prevention and treatment of pressure ulcers. *Wounds Practice and Research* 17(2).

Syndrome X

Syndrome X refers to a group of health problems that may include high blood pressure, overweight, and abnormal blood fats (cholesterol or triglycerides) and always includes a metabolic disorder known as insulin resistance. Insulin resistance is the resistance of one's cells to the blood sugar–transporting hormone insulin, which results in poor glucose metabolism. Excessive production of insulin leads to obesity, increased blood pressure, and high blood fats (triglycerides). Other terms that are sometimes used by doctors to describe syndrome X include metabolic syndrome, glucose intolerance, insulin resistance, and prediabetes.

Syndrome X was so named because researchers in the past did not fully understand the condition, and "X" represents the unknown. Today syndrome X is a recognized condition and is well understood as a metabolic disorder. People who have untreated syndrome X are more prone to inflammatory disorders, such as cardiovascular disease, cancer, diabetes, and other chronic illnesses.

The modern American diet of refined carbohydrates, low fiber, a deficiency of essential fatty acids, and other nutritional deficiencies, combined with a lack of exercise, sets the stage for insulin resistance. Once insulin resistance has occurred, the cluster of symptoms known to accompany syndrome X—such as a weight problem or obesity, high blood pressure, high cholesterol, and high triglycerides—becomes evident. If you have two or more of these symptoms, many experts believe that you have syndrome X.

People with syndrome X often have an apple-shaped body, as insulin promotes fat storage around the belly.

Syndrome X is best prevented and treated through nutrition, nutritional supplements, exercise, and other natural methods. As a matter of fact, we find that once a patient has been identified as having syndrome X and follows our specific natural protocol, there is often a dramatic reduction in weight, blood lipids, and blood pressure, as well as an improved energy level.

SIGNS AND SYMPTOMS

- Insulin resistance and glucose intolerance (as diagnosed by blood testing)
- High blood pressure
- Abnormal blood lipids (high total cholesterol and triglycerides, and low HDL cholesterol)
- Excess fat around the belly or the chest

ROOT CAUSES

- Heredity
- Unhealthful diet
- Chronic stress and the resulting stress-hormone imbalance
- Nutritional deficiencies, especially of chromium, B vitamins, zinc, vanadium
- Obesity
- Lack of exercise

Testing Techniques

The following tests help assess possible reasons for syndrome X and insulin resistance:

Hormone testing (thyroid, DHEA, cortisol, testosterone, IGF-1, estrogen, progesterone)—saliva, blood, or urine

Intestinal permeability—urine

Vitamin and mineral analysis (especially magnesium, chromium, vanadium, zinc, B vitamins)—blood

Digestive function and microbe/parasite/candida testing—stool analysis

Food and environmental allergies/sensitivities—blood, electrodermal

---

TREATMENT

Diet

The most important therapy for syndrome X and insulin resistance is a healthful diet. The following dietary suggestions will help regulate your levels of sugar and also reduce your risk of complications such as cardiovascular disease.

Recommended Food

Follow a diet that's high in fiber (vegetables, nuts, seeds, whole grains). Water-soluble fiber, as found in oat bran, beans, nuts, seeds, and apples, helps to balance blood sugar. Ground flaxseeds should be consumed daily. Consume 1 teaspoon with each meal or ¼ cup daily. Make sure to drink plenty of clean, quality water when you start taking flax-seeds (10 ounces per tablespoon). A daily total of 35 to 50 mg of fiber is a great goal.

Consume vegetable protein (legumes, nuts, seeds, peas) or lean animal protein (turkey, chicken, fish) with each meal and most snacks. Protein drinks that have low sugar levels can be consumed. Protein helps smooth out blood sugar levels. Many people with diabetes find benefit by increasing the relative amount of protein in the diet.

Focus on quality fats. Fish such as salmon is excellent, as are nuts and seeds. Use olive and flaxseed oil with your salads.

Instead of eating three large meals, have several smaller meals throughout the day to keep your insulin and blood sugar levels steady. Or have three main meals, with healthful snacks in between. Do not go longer than three hours without eating.

A chromium deficiency contributes to blood sugar problems, so eat plenty of brewer's yeast, wheat germ, whole grains, cheese, soy products, onions, and garlic. Onions and garlic will also help lower blood sugar levels and protect against heart disease.

Enjoy plenty of berries, plums, and grapes, which contain phytochemicals that protect your vision.

Focus on foods with a low glycemic index and load value. See the Diabetes entry on pages 241–249 for more information.

Food to Avoid

Stay away from simple sugars. Obvious foods to avoid are candy, cookies, sodas, and other sweets.

White, refined bread also spikes blood sugar levels. Whole-grain breads, cereals, and pastas are better choices, although you need to read the labels because they may contain an overabundance of carbohydrates. Brown rice, barley, oats, spelt, and kamut are complex carbohydrates that are good choices.

Eliminate alcohol and caffeine from your diet, as they can spike blood sugar levels and thus insulin for some people.

Cut back on your consumption of saturated fat. Found in red meat and dairy products, it has been shown to increase the risk of diabetes and heart disease.

Avoid artificial sweeteners. Instead use diabetic-safe and more healthful natural sweeteners such as stevia or xylitol.

Stay away from oils and foods that contain trans-fatty acids. Margarine, deep-fried foods, and most packaged foods, such as cookies, crackers, and pastries, contain hydrogenated oils. These land mines of trans-fatty acids promote insulin resistance.

Avoid high glycemic–load foods.

℞ Super Seven Prescriptions—Syndrome X

Super Prescription #1 Chromium
Take a daily total of up to 1,000 mcg. Chromium improves glucose tolerance and balances blood sugar levels.

Super Prescription #2 Gymnema sylvestre
Take 400 mg of a 25 percent gymneic acid extract daily. Gymnema lowers blood sugar levels.

Super Prescription #3 Alpha lipoic acid
Take 300 to 1,200 mg daily. Alpha lipoic acid improves insulin sensitivity.

Super Prescription #4 Vanadyl sulfate
Take 100 to 300 mg daily. It improves glucose tolerance in people with insulin resistance. Higher dosages should be used under the supervision of a doctor.

Super Prescription #5 Biotin
Take 9 to 16 mg daily. Biotin is involved with proper glucose metabolism.

In a study of 180 men and women with type 2 diabetes, twice daily the participants were given a placebo, 100 mcg of chromium picolinate, or 500 mcg of chromium picolinate. Insulin values decreased significantly in both groups that received supplemental chromium after two and four months.

Super Prescription #6 High-potency multivitamin

It supplies many of the nutrients involved with blood sugar metabolism. Take as directed on the container.

Super Prescription #7 Essential fatty acids

Take a formulation that contains a mixture of omega-3, -6, and -9 fatty acids. Flaxseed or fish oil, combined with evening primrose oil, is common. Take as directed on the container. This supplement provides essential fatty acids that are needed for proper insulin function.

General Recommendations

An antioxidant formula supplies additional antioxidants, which are generally required in higher amounts in people with insulin resistance. Take as directed on the container.

B-complex vitamins are involved in blood sugar metabolism. Take a 50 mg B-complex daily.

Zinc is required for proper insulin production and function. Take a total of 30 mg daily.

Vitamin C helps prevent oxidative damage, which is more common with this condition. Take 1,000 mg two or three times daily.

Magnesium is involved with insulin production and utilization. Take a daily total of 500 to 750 mg. Reduce the dosage if loose stools occur.

Vitamin E-complex improves glucose regulation and prevents cholesterol oxidation. Take 800 to 1,200 IU daily of a formula containing tocotrienols and tocopherols.

Milk thistle has been shown to improve blood sugar levels. Take 600 mg of silymarin extract daily.

Banaba leaf has been shown in both animal and human studies to lower blood sugar levels. Take 16 mg three times daily.

Adrenal extract supports adrenal-gland function, which is also important for blood sugar regulation. Take 500 mg twice daily on an empty stomach or as directed on the container.

DHEA is often low in people who have insulin resistance. If tests show that you have low levels, take 5 to 25 mg daily under a doctor's supervision.

Psyllium will reduce blood sugar levels. It is a good source of fiber. Take up to 5 grams daily.

Asian ginseng (*Panax ginseng*) has been shown in a study to help improve blood sugar levels. Take 200 mg daily.

Bitter melon (*Momordica charantia*) can help balance blood sugar levels. Take 5 ml twice daily of the tincture or 200 mg three times daily of a standardized extract.

Garlic (*Allium sativum*) is an important herb for stabilizing blood sugar. It also helps reduce one's risk of heart disease and other circulatory disorders by improving blood flow, lowering elevated blood pressure, and reducing levels of "bad" cholesterol. Take 300 to 450 mg twice daily.

Fenugreek (*Trigonella foenum-graecum*) is another herb that stabilizes blood sugar. Take a product with an equivalent dosage of 15 to 50 grams daily.

Policosanol is a good supplement to use for elevated cholesterol levels. Take 10 mg with the evening meal.

Take 125 to 250 mg daily of resveratrol to support healthy glucose metabolism.

Soluble fiber supplements reduce glucose levels. Take as directed on the label.

Homeopathy

Consultation with a homeopathic practitioner is advised to individualize homeopathic treatment.

Acupressure

See an acupressurist for a specific treatment based on your symptoms.

Bodywork

Massage

Diabetics and people with unhealthy blood sugar levels often suffer from poor circulation. A massage is a relaxing way to improve blood flow. Regular massaging of the feet may be especially beneficial to help ward off foot ulcers.

Reflexology

See pages 804–805 for information about reflexology areas and how to work them.

Work the points that correspond to the pancreas, the liver, and the thyroid, pituitary, and adrenal glands. You will probably have to massage these points every day for several months to see an effect.

Aromatherapy

Have fun trying the many different relaxing oils. Refer to pages 771–781 for more information on aromatherapy oils; you may want to start with bergamot, jasmine, lavender, rose, sandalwood, or ylang-ylang. Use them in a massage, a bath, lotions, or any of the other methods listed in the Aromatherapy chapter.

Stress Reduction

General Stress-Reduction Therapies

Insulin resistance puts additional stress on almost every part of your body and every area of your life. Keep up your emotional health by experimenting with the stress-reduction techniques discussed in the Exercise and Stress Reduction chapter. When you find one or two you like, practice them on a regular basis.

Other Recommendations

- Don't smoke or expose yourself to secondhand smoke. If you have insulin resistance, you are vulnerable to heart and kidney damage, both of which are linked to smoking. You may also have circulation problems, and smoking impairs blood flow.
- If you are overweight, it is imperative that you lose weight safely. Read the Obesity entry on pages 489–497.
- Exercise regularly to maintain optimal blood sugar levels. Walking after meals is effective for some people.

REFERENCES

Anderson, R. A., et al. 1997. Elevated intakes of supplemental chromium improve glucose and insulin variables in individuals with type 2 diabetes. *Diabetes* 46(11):1786–91.

TMJ (Temporomandibular Joint) Syndrome

The temporomandibular joint connects the jawbone to the skull. When it is functioning properly, the bones of the joint allow the mouth to open smoothly and easily. Sometimes, however, there is a misalignment of the teeth or the jaw. In more serious cases, the cartilage that protects the joint wears down. Without cartilage to act as a cushion, the bones rub against each other.

TMJ can be caused by anything that places unusual pressure on the joint. A blow to the jawbone, habitual gum chewing, and poor orthodontic work are all possible factors. But by far the most frequent cause of TMJ is frequent grinding or clenching of the teeth. This seemingly benign habit is usually brought on by stress that causes muscles in the jaw to tighten. Another common underlying cause of TMJ is a structural misalignment of the jaw or the teeth (called malocclusion by doctors and dentists); sometimes the cranial or facial bones are involved. Imbalanced musculature and spinal alignment in other areas of the body can be an underlying root cause of TMJ syndrome. Finally, deficiencies of nutrients such as magnesium can make this problem worse, because muscles tend to spasm and tighten more easily.

No matter what the cause, TMJ is at best uncomfortable and at worst almost unbearably painful. The first sign of a problem may be difficulty opening the mouth all the way or perhaps a popping or clicking sound when yawning or chewing. As the disorder progresses, the jaw muscles will begin to feel tender. This tenderness may develop into an ache or a sharp pain, which can spread to the neck, the ears, or the face.

A note of caution: Despite what some doctors or dentists may tell you, TMJ syndrome is real. But there have been many reports of unscrupulous professionals touting "miracle" cures for TMJ in the form of expensive and invasive treatments, including surgery. Before you undergo any aggressive measures, try the gentle home care and relaxation therapies suggested here. Chances are that they'll bring you substantial, if not total, relief. If you try these therapies and still have a great deal of pain, consult with a reputable, qualified specialist—and as always, ask for a full explanation of any procedure before you agree to it. Many naturopathic, osteopathic, or chiropractic physicians can help people with TMJ syndrome, using nonsurgical techniques. Acupuncture can also be quite helpful, as can stress-reduction techniques.

SYMPTOMS

- Clicking, popping, or grating noises when chewing or opening the mouth
- Difficulty opening the mouth all the way
- Stiffness, tenderness, or pain in the jaw
- Neck pain
- Earache
- Facial pain
- An asymmetrical appearance to the face
- Dizziness
- Ringing in the ears

ROOT CAUSES

- Grinding or clenching the teeth (usually the result of stress or a blood sugar imbalance)
- Misalignment of the teeth or the jaw
- Poor orthodontia or dental work

625

- Injuries to the jaw
- Postural problems
- Frequent gum-chewing
- Prolonged thumb-sucking

- Muscle and spinal alignment imbalance
- Nutritional deficiencies (e.g., magnesium, calcium)

Testing Techniques

The following tests help assess possible reasons for TMJ syndrome:

Spinal and posture assessment—visual exam and X-ray

Vitamin and mineral analysis (especially magnesium, calcium)—blood

Food and environmental allergies/sensitivities—blood, electrodermal

Blood sugar balance—blood

TREATMENT

Diet

Recommended Food

If your TMJ syndrome is acute, eat foods that require less chewing or that are easier to chew. Examples include soups, stews, steamed or cooked vegetables, and protein shakes.

Focus on foods that will stabilize your blood sugar levels. Vegetables, beans, whole grains, nuts and seeds, soy products, and fish should be the mainstays of your diet.

Instead of eating three large meals, plan on five or six smaller ones through the day. You'll keep your blood sugar in balance and won't be tempted to snack on sweet treats.

Food to Avoid

Avoid sugary foods like candy, chocolate, sodas, and most baked goods. They disturb blood sugar levels and contribute to stress.

Stay away from caffeine, which causes muscles to tighten. Tea and coffee are obvious sources of caffeine, but chocolate, some pain relievers, and over-the-counter cold medications have high amounts as well.

Alcohol has been linked to teeth-grinding. Although a drink or two may seem like a good way to relax, herbal teas are a much wiser choice for people with TMJ.

Don't chew anything that's hard on your jaw. Gum, caramels, bagels, animal meats, and hard or gooey candy are off-limits.

℞ Super Seven Prescriptions—TMJ Syndrome

Super Prescription #1 Magnesium
Take 250 mg two or three times daily. This mineral relaxes the nervous system and the musculature around the jaw. *Note*: Reduce the dosage if loose stools occur.

Super Prescription #2 Calcium
Take 500 mg twice daily. It works synergistically with magnesium to relax tight muscles.

Super Prescription #3 Kava (*Piper methysticum*)

Take a standardized product containing 70 mg of kavalactones three times daily. Kava relaxes the nervous system and tight muscles. It is also very good for stress and anxiety. *Note*: Do not take with alcohol or any psychiatric medication.

Super Prescription #4 Methylsulfonylmethane (MSM)

Take 1,000 mg three times daily. MSM reduces muscle spasms and inflammation.

Super Prescription #5 Homeopathic Magnesia Phosphorica

Take 3 pellets of the 6x potency three times daily. This remedy relaxes tight muscles.

Super Prescription #6 B-complex

Take a 50 mg complex twice daily to reduce the effects of stress.

Super Prescription #7 *Valeriana officinalis*

Take 3 ml or 300 mg three times daily to reduce the effects of stress and relax tight muscles.

General Recommendations

Glucosamine sulfate builds cartilage. Take 1,500 mg daily if you have cartilage deterioration in the TMJ.

Homeopathy

Pick the remedy that best matches your symptoms in this section. For acute TMJ pain, take a 30C potency four times daily. For chronic TMJ pain, take a 6x, 12x, 6C, 12C, or 30C twice daily for two weeks to see if there are any positive results. After you notice improvement, stop taking the remedy, unless symptoms return. Consultation with a homeopathic practitioner is advised.

Arnica (*Arnica montana*) is the classic homeopathic remedy for deep, bruising pain. It is especially helpful for TMJ pain that occurs immediately after an injury.

Hypericum Perforatum is indicated when there is a shooting, radiating nerve pain in the jaw area.

Ignatia (*Ignatia amara*) is for someone who is highly sensitive to stress that results in tight jaw muscles and TMJ pain. It is specific for TMJ syndrome that occurs after emotional grief or a trauma.

Kali Phosphoricum reduces the effects of stress and nerve pain.

Magnesia Phosphorica is a good general remedy for tight muscles that spasm and that feel better with warm applications.

Rhus Toxicodendron is for a stiff jaw that loosens up during the day and then stiffens up again in the evening. The jaw feels better with warm applications.

Acupressure

See pages 787–794 for information about pressure points and administering treatment.

- Large Intestine 4 (LI4) is a point that will relieve pain and relax the muscles of the head and the jaw.

- Another point for pain located anywhere on the neck and head is Gallbladder 20 (GB20).
- If you clench or grind your teeth at night, devote a few minutes before bedtime to working Lung 1 (Lu1). Breathe deeply, and try to clear your mind of obsessive thoughts.
- Pericardium 6 (P6) will ease panic or anxiety. Because it's located on the wrist, you can easily work this point whenever you feel your jaw tense up, even if you're in public.

Bodywork

Because it gently relaxes muscles and eases stress, bodywork offers some of the most effective treatments for TMJ. Experiment until you find the ones that work best for you.

Massage
A massage of the neck, the shoulders, the scalp, the jaw, and the muscles inside the mouth can do wonders. See a professional for an initial treatment, and then ask a loved one to practice home massage for daily maintenance.

A light facial massage can help you relax and develop a greater awareness of your jaw muscles.

Reflexology
See pages 804–805 for information about reflexology areas and how to work them.

Work the areas corresponding to the jaws, the neck, the ears, and the solar plexus.

Hydrotherapy
For immediate relief of pain, lie down with a warm compress held against your jaw. Add any of the essential oils suggested under Aromatherapy in this section for a stronger relaxing effect.

Other Bodywork Recommendations
A chiropractic adjustment can often relieve pain and bring the bones back into proper alignment. Consult a practitioner who has experience in working with TMJ patients. Naturopathic doctors and osteopathic doctors are also good choices.

Craniosacral therapy is a gentle way to align facial and cranial bones that contribute to TMJ.

Aromatherapy

Marjoram, black pepper, and rosemary have a warming and relaxing effect on clenched muscles. For best relief, add a few drops of oil to a warm compress.

Experiment with several of the relaxing oils until you find a few you like. Lavender, jasmine, rose, and bergamot are always good choices. Use them in any preparation you like, but don't rely on just one for a prolonged period of time, as you might become immune to its calming effects.

Stress Reduction

General Stress-Reduction Therapies
Many TMJ sufferers report good results from biofeedback, which teaches awareness of the bones and the muscles in the jaw.

If you suffer from a high degree of stress, you may want to supplement biofeedback with another technique, such as meditation or yoga.

Other Recommendations

- Try to retrain your jaw posture. Every few minutes, stop to ask yourself whether your jaw is clenched; if it is, relax it. Proper jaw position is slightly relaxed, with your lips closed.
- Check your other postural habits. Do you tend to cradle the telephone between your jaw and shoulder? Do you slump forward at your desk? Try to sit up straight, as a general rule, and if you must speak on the phone for long periods, use a speaker phone or a headset.
- Clenching and grinding can be hard habits to break. If, despite your own attempts at relaxation and retraining, you still tense your jaw muscles, ask your dentist about a bite guard. He or she can fit one to your mouth, and you can wear it at night to prevent unconscious jaw damage.

Thrush. See Candidiasis

Tinnitus

Tinnitus refers to ringing or other noise in the ears. It is very common, affecting approximately one in five people. It is classified not as a disease or a disorder but as a symptom related to another condition, such as ear injury or aging.

Severe cases can greatly decrease one's quality of life, although the condition isn't usually caused by a serious health problem.

Conventional therapies focus on noise-suppression techniques, such as white-noise machines that produce environmental sounds (e.g., ocean waves) that can help one to fall asleep. Other options are hearing aids that produce low-level noise to mask or suppress tinnitus, antidepressants, or antianxiety medications.

Natural therapies are focused on providing the nutrients that may be deficient and that make one susceptible to tinnitus and on supplementing with natural agents that improve inner-ear blood flow.

SYMPTOMS

Tinnitus noise can range from a low- to a high-pitched sound. It can be constant or intermittent.

- Ringing
- Buzzing
- Whistling
- Roaring
- Hissing
- Clicking

ROOT CAUSES

The conventional causes are the following:

- Noise damage
- Earwax

- Age-related hearing loss
- Inner-ear bone abnormalities
- Stress
- TMJ disorder
- Tumor of the cranial nerve (usually one-sided tinnitus) or the head and neck
- Head injury

- Atherosclerosis
- Hypertension
- Ménière's disease
- Medications such as high-dose aspirin, antibiotics, cancer medications, diuretics, or malaria drugs

Holistic doctors also believe that a lack of inner-ear circulation, food sensitivities, and adrenal-gland dysfunction may contribute to this condition.

Testing Techniques

Hearing and diagnostic images of the ears and the brain are done to identify the root causes. Additional holistic testing may include the following:

Food-sensitivity testing—blood, electrodermal

Hormone balance—blood, saliva, or urine

Nutrient deficiencies such as zinc—blood

TREATMENT

Diet

Recommended Food
Eat a whole-foods diet that focuses on live, unprocessed foods.

Food to Avoid
Caffeine-containing foods may worsen tinnitus, so they should be avoided. Also avoid known food sensitivities.

Studies on the effectiveness of *Ginkgo biloba* have been mixed. Two smaller trials found that ginkgo extract at a dosage of 120 mg per day was effective at relieving the symptoms of tinnitus.

℞ Super Seven Prescriptions—Tinnitus

Super Prescription #1 *Ginkgo biloba*
Take 120 mg twice daily of a 24 percent extract. This improves circulation through the inner ear.

Super Prescription #2 Homeopathic Tinnitus Combination Formula
Take as directed on the label for the relief of symptoms.

Super Prescription #3 Pycnogenol
Take 150 mg daily to help inner-ear circulation and tinnitus.

Super Prescription #4 Coenzyme Q10
Take 100 mg three times daily. This may be helpful for those low in CoQ10.

> ### Super Prescription #5 Magnesium
> Take 250 mg twice daily to support normal hearing.
>
> ### Super Prescription #6 Vitamin B12
> Take 1,000 mcg daily to support healthy nerves.
>
> ### Super Prescription #7 B-complex
> Take 50 mg of B-complex daily to support healthy nerves.

General Recommendations

Work with a holistic doctor to try different natural approaches depending on your testing and health history.

Homeopathy

See a qualified practitioner for individual therapy.

Bodywork

Reflexology
Work the areas of the foot that correspond to the ears.

Other Recommendations

- Acupuncture and Chinese herbal therapy may benefit this condition.
- Cold-laser therapy to the ear region may benefit tinnitus.
- Avoid products with nicotine, which impairs circulation.

REFERENCES

Meyer, B. 1988. A multicenter randomized double-blind study of Ginkgo biloba extract versus placebo in the treatment of tinnitus. In *Rokan (Ginkgo Biloba): Recent Results in Pharmacology and Clinic*, ed. E. W. Funfgeld. New York: Springer-Verlag, 245–50.

Morgenstern, C., and E. Biermann. 1997. Ginkgo biloba special extract EGb 761 in the treatment of tinnitus aurium: Results of a randomized, double-blind, placebo controlled study. *Fortschritte der Medizin* 115:7–11.

Toenail Fungus

Toenail fungus, known medically as onychomycosis or tinea unguium, is a fungal, yeast, or mold infection that invades the nail bed. It accounts for half of all nail disorders. Up to 13 percent of the North American population has toenail fungus, which causes disfiguration of the nails as they become thickened and discolored. Discoloration results in shades ranging from white to brownish-yellow to greenish-brown to black. Occasionally, in more severe cases, the condition is painful due to the thickened nail pushing against the inside of the shoe. For many people the resulting appearance is a source of embarrassment.

SYMPTOMS

Symptoms range from mild discoloration to pain and discomfort of the affected area.

ROOT CAUSES

- Genetics
- Poor immunity
- Poor hygiene
- Trauma to the area
- Poor circulation
- Shoes with poor ventilation
- Moist environment caused by humidity or physical activity
- System-wide fungal overgrowth
- Use of steroids or antibiotics

Testing Techniques

Culture of the organism(s) present at the affected area

TREATMENT

Diet

Recommended Food

Eat a diet rich in vegetables, nuts, seeds, and cold-water fish. Foods such as carrots, oregano, garlic, and onions have antifungal properties.

Food to Avoid

Restrict all forms of simple sugar, which suppress immunity and feed yeast.

℞ Super Seven Prescriptions—Toenail Fungus

Super Prescription #1 Tea tree oil
Apply topical tea tree oil to affected nail twice daily for two months or longer.

Super Prescription #2 Garlic
Take 500 mg of garlic extract twice daily and apply garlic oil to affected toenail twice daily.

Super Prescription #3 Oregano
Take 250 to 500 mg of oregano oil capsules three times daily and apply oregano oil to affected toenail twice daily.

Super Prescription #4 Probiotics
Take twenty billion organisms or more daily to improve flora balance systemically.

Super Prescription #5 Caprylic acid
Take 500 mg three times daily for its antifungal properties.

Super Prescription #6 Pycnogenol
Take 100 mg twice daily to improve circulation to the extremities, which helps immune cells get to the affected area more efficiently.

> **Super Prescription #7 Essential oil blend**
> Apply essential oil blend that is suitable for skin applications. Use as directed.

One study looked at the combination of tea tree oil and an antifungal medication known as butenafine hydrochloride. A randomized, double-blind, placebo-controlled study examined the clinical efficacy and tolerability of 2 percent butenafine hydrochloride and 5 percent *Melaleuca alternifolia* (tea tree) oil incorporated into a cream base to manage toenail onychomycosis.

Sixty outpatients (thirty-nine male, twenty-one female) aged 18 to 80 years (mean 29.6) with six to thirty-six months duration of disease were randomized to two groups (forty active therapy, twenty placebo). After sixteen weeks, 80 percent of patients using the medicated cream were cured, as opposed to none in the placebo group. Four patients in the active treatment group experienced subjective mild inflammation without discontinuing treatment. During follow-up, no relapse occurred in cured patients and no improvement was seen in medication-resistant and placebo participants.

Other Recommendations

- Conventional therapy involves the topical application of antifungal medications and/or the use of oral antifungal medications. The problem with topical applications is that the treatment often does not penetrate the nail deeply enough to fully cure the problem. Oral medications such as Lamisil (terbinafine), Diflucan (fluconazole), and Sporanox (itracanozole) are commonly used over a three-month period and require proper monitoring. A better way to use antifungal medications is to apply them locally over the area in a specialized compounded cream. A compounded cream is made by a compounding pharmacy from several components. The treatment used for toenail fungus normally includes the carrier agent DMSO, which drives medications deeper into the nail bed for a more therapeutic effect. The same approach can be used with natural antifungal agents such as tea tree oil.
- A natural treatment used by dermatologists is the use of laser to kill the microbes causing the nail fungus. The treatment works by sending a series of tiny, painless pulses of energy into the nail. The laser pulses generate enough heat to kill the fungus; most patients feel no side effects or only a slight warming sensation—and rarely burning pain. The treatment takes five to ten minutes (depending on the size and thickness of the nail), but the benefits are long-term. The nail with the dead fungus will grow out slowly over six to twelve months as it's replaced with the new, fungus-free nail. The treatment can be used for both fingernails and toenails. If you have even just one toenail with fungus, it's best to treat all the nails of the same foot since all the toes have been exposed to the fungus contained in your shoe and you want to avoid a reinfection. Furthermore, sometimes nails can have a minimal or early infection despite looking mostly normal.
- For a home remedy, mix one cup of household bleach with ten cups of warm water. Soak the toes of the affected foot for three minutes, and then thoroughly

rinse off the bleach solution. Do this twice weekly, with three days between treatments. Most cases resolve in two to three months. The more severe the case, the longer the treatment takes. Keep the nails as short as possible, so the bleach is more likely to come in contact with the infected areas. We should note that boosting the strength of the bleach-and-water mixture beyond the one-to-ten ratio will not increase the effectiveness of the treatment and will irritate the skin. Nor is it wise to increase the frequency or duration of treatments. Do not use this treatment if you have an open wound near the infection site.

Healthy-Nail Tips from the American Academy of Dermatology

- Keep your nails clean and dry to help prevent bacteria from collecting under them.
- Cut your fingernails and toenails straight across and rounded slightly in the center. This keeps them strong and will help you avoid ingrown toenails.
- If your toenails are thick and difficult to cut, soak your feet in warm salt water (one teaspoon of salt per pint of water) for five to ten minutes, and then apply urea or lactic acid cream. This will soften the nails, making them easier to trim.
- Wear proper-fitting shoes and alternate shoes on a regular basis. Tight shoes can cause ingrown toenails.
- Don't try to self-treat ingrown toenails, especially if they are infected. See a dermatologist.
- Don't bite your fingernails. You can transfer infections between your fingers and mouth. Also, nail biting can damage the skin around your fingers, allowing infections to enter.
- Nail problems are more common if you have diabetes or poor circulation. At the first sign of a problem, see a dermatologist.

REFERENCES

American Academy of Dermatology website. Accessed May 25, 2015 at http://www.aad.org/media-resources/stats-and-facts/prevention-and-care/nails.

Syed, T. A., et al. 1999. Treatment of toenail onychomycosis with 2% butenafine and 5% Melaleuca alternifolia (tea tree) oil in cream. *Trop Med Int Health* 4(4):284–7.

Ulcers

Peptic ulcers most frequently affect the stomach and the duodenum, which is the upper part of the small intestine. Both the stomach and the duodenum process high quantities of gastric juices. These juices have to be strong in order to break food down into digestible particles; in fact, they're composed largely of hydrochloric acid, a substance that can dissolve not just last night's dinner but body tissues as well. To protect the stomach and duodenum walls against damage from gastric acid, both organs are coated with a protective mucus layer. In addition, bicarbonate ions are secreted by the lining of the stomach and the duodenum. Under normal conditions, this mucus layer and the alkalinizing bicarbonate ions prevent the acid from eating away at the digestive-tract lining. But when the lining is too weak and there is decreased bicarbonate secretion, some of the stomach tissues may be eroded. An eroded spot is called a peptic ulcer.

Most people know that stress increases the output of gastric acid. If you have an ulcer, reducing the levels of tension and anxiety in your life will go a long way toward healing the physical wound. But many other factors can cause or contribute to ulcers as well. Some drugs are notorious for increasing acid production—most notably, aspirin and the class of medications called nonsteroidal anti-inflammatory drugs (NSAIDs, for short). People who take aspirin or NSAIDs like ibuprofen on a regular basis are at a high risk for getting stomach ulcers. Smokers develop ulcers much more often than nonsmokers do. And as with every digestive disorder, a poor diet, especially one that includes spicy foods, citrus fruits, soda pop, caffeine, and alcohol, is frequently at the root of the problem. Food allergies or sensitivities can cause problems as well. One must also consider that low antioxidant status appears to predispose one to ulcers.

The bacteria *Helicobacter pylori* has been strongly linked to ulcer formation. Studies show that some people with ulcers have this bacterium in the affected organ, and elimination of *H. pylori* often helps with healing. Antibiotic therapy, as well as natural therapies, can be very effective for this infection. Make sure to supplement with probiotics to replace the helpful bacteria that antibiotics destroy. These good bacteria also play a role in preventing *H. pylori* infection.

Conventional therapy generally focuses on antacid medications, which suppress stomach-acid formation. For severe or acute ulcer problems, such as a bleeding ulcer, these medications can be very effective and warranted. However, for many people these medications are prescribed on a long-term basis and do not treat the cause of the ulcer. In addition, long-term use can contribute to digestive problems in other areas of the digestive tract, as hydrochloric acid is required for protein digestion and the liquefaction of foods. Without proper digestion in the stomach, there is additional stress on the rest of the digestive organs. Also keep in mind that stomach acid is a natural barrier to bacteria such as *H. pylori* and other microbes. Suppression of stomach acid in the long term theoretically makes you more prone to an infection in the digestive tract. Finally, the body requires stomach acid to absorb minerals, so long-term acid suppression makes one prone to mineral deficiency.

Ulcers are a common complaint, but that doesn't mean they should be ignored. Without treatment, the pain and the burning will only get worse. In fact, the eroded area may grow larger and deeper until it begins to bleed. The ulcer may even perforate the stomach or intestinal wall. Bleeding or perforating ulcers should be treated as medical emergencies; if left unattended, they can be fatal.

SYMPTOMS

- Burning or gnawing pain in the upper abdomen that usually occurs when the stomach is empty or about an hour after eating or sometimes at night
- Loss of appetite
- Increased appetite (sometimes food actually soothes the ulcer)
- Nausea
- Vomiting

ROOT CAUSES

- Stress
- Smoking
- Medications, including aspirin and nonsteroidal anti-inflammatory drugs
- Alcohol use
- Infection with *H. pylori* (you are more susceptible if you have low stomach acid and not enough friendly flora)
- Dietary factors, including food allergies

Caution: If your stools or vomit are dark or bloody, or if you have intense abdominal pain that doesn't go away, you may have a bleeding or perforating ulcer. Consult a doctor immediately.

Testing Techniques

The following tests help assess possible reasons for ulcers:

  H. pylori—blood, stool, breath

  Digestive function and microbe/parasite/candida testing—stool analysis

  Antioxidant status—blood, urine

  Food and environmental allergies/sensitivities—blood, electrodermal

---

Know Your NSAIDs

Nonsteroidal anti-inflammatory drugs—NSAIDs, for short—are some of the most commonly used medications in the world. Millions of people are dependent upon them for relief of back pain, headache, arthritis, and other conditions. Unfortunately, these drugs also increase the amount of gastric acid and can lead to peptic ulcers.

Following are some common and brand names for NSAIDs. If you've been regularly using any NSAID for a prolonged amount of time, you may be at risk for peptic ulcers. Consider switching to an herbal preparation for effects that are just as potent but far gentler to your body.

If a doctor has prescribed an NSAID for you, consult with him or her before changing your regimen.

Popular NSAIDs include

- Advil
- Clinoril
- Feldene
- Ibuprofen
- Nalfon
- Nuprin
- Orudis
- Oruvail
- Relafen
- Tolectin
- Voltaren

TREATMENT

Diet

Recommended Food

Although you may not feel like eating, good nutrition is essential for healing ulcers. Eat several small meals a day to avoid placing a heavy burden on your digestive system.

Eat plenty of fiber. Although the smooth foods of the famous "bland diet" were once thought safest for ulcer patients, increased fiber intake has been shown to repair ulcers. Focus on sources of soluble fiber, such as oats.

Vitamin K has been shown to repair damage from gastric juices. Eat several servings of green leafy vegetables a day, and drink lots of green juices.

Studies have shown that cabbage juice has remarkable healing powers for ulcers. Drink a quart of cabbage juice daily. It may be diluted with water or carrot juice.

Cultured products will provide the friendly bacteria that fight *H. pylori*. Drink kefir or eat some live cultured yogurt every day.

Zinc is healing to the digestive tract. Good sources include pumpkin seeds and whole grains.

Consume garlic with your meals; test tube studies show it has anti–*Helicobacter pylori* properties.

Food to Avoid

Avoid sugar, spicy foods, citrus fruits and juices, coffee, black tea, and alcohol. They all contribute to high levels of gastric acid or are irritating to the stomach lining.

Consult the Food Allergies section, and use the elimination diet to determine whether a food allergy is causing or aggravating your ulcer. Although a reaction to any food can conceivably cause an ulcer, milk allergies are strongly linked to gastric problems.

Doctors once prescribed milk as a remedy for ulcers, but that practice has largely stopped. We now know that milk actually encourages stomach acid to form. In addition, many cases of ulcers are linked to a milk allergy.

℞ Super Seven Prescriptions—Ulcers

Super Prescription #1 Licorice root (DGL, *Glycyrrhiza glabra*)

Chew 500 to 1,000 mg twenty minutes before meals or between meals, three times daily. DGL (deglycyrrhizinated licorice) stimulates the regeneration of the mucus layer and has anti-inflammatory effects. Preliminary research shows an inhibiting effect on the growth of *H. pylori*.

Super Prescription #2 Mastic gum (*Pistachia lentiscus*)

Take 500 mg three times daily. This supplement comes from the mastic tree and has been shown in test tube studies to destroy *H. pylori* and in human studies to be effective in healing ulcers.

Super Prescription #3 Aloe vera

Drink ¼ cup three times daily. Aloe promotes healing of the lining of the intestinal tract and has antimicrobial benefits.

In a single-blind study of 100 people with peptic ulcers, participants took DGL (760 mg three times daily) or the pharmaceutical Tagamet (cimetidine). Researchers found that both groups showed equal healing of ulcers after six and twelve weeks. Another study of 874 people found DGL as effective as antacids and the anti-ulcer medication Tagamet.

One double-blind trial compared 1 gram of mastic gum per day with a placebo in the treatment of thirty-eight people with duodenal ulcer. After only two weeks of treatment, symptoms improved significantly in 80 percent of those receiving mastic gum. Endoscopic (visual exam with a scope) examination verified healing in 70 percent of the mastic group but in only 22 percent of the placebo group.

Super Prescription #4 Homeopathic Nux Vomica

Take a 30C potency three times daily. This is the most common remedy for ulcers. See Homeopathy in this section for other helpful remedies.

Super Prescription #5 Probiotic

Take a product containing at least four billion active organisms twice daily, thirty minutes after meals. It supplies friendly bacteria, such as *Lactobacillus acidophilus* and *bifidus*, which prevent infection and aid digestion. It is particularly important to take if you are using antibiotics.

Super Prescription #6 Zinc carnosine

Take 75 mg twice daily to heal the linings of the stomach and intestines. This nutrient also fights *H. pylori* bacteria.

Super Prescription #7 Chamomile (*Matricaria chamomilla*)

Drink a fresh cup of tea four times daily. Animal studies show that it has anti-ulcer activity, and it also relaxes the nervous system.

General Recommendations

Slippery elm has a soothing and healing effect on the lining of the digestive tract. Take 3 ml or 500 mg in capsule form or suck on a lozenge three times daily between meals.

Vitamin A stimulates the healthy growth of intestinal cells and improves immune function. Take 25,000 IU daily, with a doctor's supervision. *Note*: Pregnant women or women planning for pregnancy should avoid doses above 5,000 IU.

Vitamin C acts as an antioxidant in the stomach lining and has been shown to retard *H. pylori* growth. Take 500 to 1,000 mg three times daily. Make sure to use a nonacidic vitamin C. Reduce your dosage if loose stools occur.

Essential fatty acids have been shown to help heal gastric and duodenal ulcers. Take 4,000 mg of fish oil or 1 tablespoon of flaxseed oil daily. Also, take 400 IU of vitamin E to prevent oxidation of these essential fatty acids.

L-glutamine promotes healthy intestinal cells. Take 1,000 mg three times daily on an empty stomach.

Homeopathy

Pick the remedy that best matches your symptoms in this section. For relief of acute ulcer pain, take a 30C potency every fifteen minutes, up to four doses. For chronic ulcer problems, take a 6x, 12x, 6C, 12C, or 30C twice daily for two weeks to see if there are any positive results. After you notice improvement, stop taking the remedy, unless symptoms return. Consultation with a homeopathic practitioner is advised.

Arsenicum Album is helpful for a burning sensation in the stomach that is alleviated by drinking milk or frequently sipping warm water and sitting up. The person feels anxious and restless.

Lycopodium (*Lycopodium clavatum*) is for gas and bloating, as well as for stomach pain. Symptoms are usually brought on by anxiety and a lack of confidence. The person feels worse when wearing tight clothes and better when sipping warm drinks. There may be a sour taste in the mouth. Symptoms are often worse in the late afternoon and the evening.

Nux Vomica is for people with heartburn and reflux that occur from stress, spicy foods, and alcohol. They are generally chilly, irritable, and oversensitive to stimuli (noise, light). Constipation is often a problem as well.

Pulsatilla (*Pulsatilla pratensis*) is helpful if your ulcer feels worse after you eat rich and fatty foods. Your symptoms feel worse in a warm room and better with fresh air. You also tend to feel tearful when ill, and you greatly desire comfort.

Phosphorus helps when you have a burning pain in the stomach that feels better from cold drinks. However, soon after drinking, you feel nauseous and may vomit.

Sulfur is for burning pain and belching, accompanied by diarrhea. You tend to be very warm and get relief from ice-cold drinks.

Acupressure

See pages 787–794 for information about pressure points and administering treatment.
- To strengthen your entire gastrointestinal tract, work Stomach 36 (St36).
- Another point that benefits the digestive system is Spleen 16 (Sp16). Work it on a daily basis to relieve the pain of ulcers and to restore your appetite for healthful food.

Bodywork

Massage
The primary benefit that massage offers the ulcer sufferer is stress relief.

Reflexology
See pages 804–805 for information about reflexology areas and how to work them.

Work the areas corresponding to the stomach, the duodenum, the diaphragm, and the solar plexus.

Acupuncture
See a qualified practitioner for acupuncture and Chinese herbal therapy.

Hydrotherapy
Constitutional hydrotherapy is an excellent treatment that focuses blood flow back to the stomach to promote healing. See pages 795–796 for directions.

Aromatherapy

Lavender, ginger, and clary sage will calm gastric upset. Try them in a massage or add them to a bath or a warm compress.

Many oils have potent stress-relieving properties. Refer to pages 771–781 for more information on aromatherapy oils; you may want to start with one or more of the following: lavender, rose, bergamot, and jasmine. Find a few that you like, and rotate them so that you don't become immune to their effects. You can use these oils in any preparation.

Side effects from the use of antibiotics are quite common. One study found that people supplementing probiotics while on antibiotic therapy (three antibiotics concurrently) had a significant reduction in diarrhea, nausea, and taste disturbance, as compared to those taking a placebo with their antibiotics.

Stress Reduction

General Stress-Reduction Techniques
General stress-reduction techniques, such as deep breathing, prayer, yoga, and positive mental imagery, are helpful for recovery.

Other Recommendations

- Tobacco smoke causes ulcers. Don't smoke or expose yourself to secondhand smoke.
- Do not take any NSAIDs or aspirin if you have a history of ulcers. If your doctor has prescribed these for you, check with him or her about a less-irritating alternative, or, better yet, work with a holistic doctor for a natural alternative.

REFERENCES

Al-Habbal, M. J., Z. Al-Habbal, and F. U. Huwez. 1984. A double-blind controlled clinical trial of mastic and placebo in the treatment of duodenal ulcer. *Clinical Experimental Pharmacology and Physiology* 11(5):541–44.

Armuzzi, A., F. et al. 2001. The effect of oral administration of *Lactobacillus GG* on antibiotic-associated gastrointestinal side effects during *Helicobacter pylori* eradication therapy. *Alimentary Pharmacology and Therapeutics* 15(2):163–69.

Kassir, Z. A. 1985. Endoscopic controlled trial of four drug regimens in the treatment of chronic duodenal ulceration. *Irish Medical Journal* 78(6):153–56.

Morgan, A. C., et al. 1982. Comparison between cimetidine and Caved-S in the treatment of gastric ulceration, and subsequent maintenance therapy. *Gut* 23:545–51.

Underactive Thyroid. See Hypothyroidism

Urinary Incontinence

Urinary incontinence or the inability to control urination is a troublesome condition for 60 percent of women and 15 percent of males over the age of sixty-five. For those living in long-term facilities the rate is between 50 and 84 percent. Overall this accounts for up to thirteen million people in the United States. It has also been estimated that most women with this condition do not seek medical treatment due to embarrassment.

The body forms urine as a waste product when the kidneys filter the blood. The bladder acts as a storage unit for the urine until a person is ready to urinate. The inability to control the urination results in the involuntary loss of urine. This results in obvious hygiene and social problems. There are two major body systems involved in controlling urination. This includes, of course, the urinary system, which for this condition would mainly be the bladder. The second would be the nervous system, which controls nerve impulses to the bladder. A problem with either system can result in incontinence.

There are different types of urinary incontinence. The most common type in younger and middle-aged women is stress incontinence. It occurs when one is physically active, which leads to an increase in pressure in the abdominal muscles. This in turn puts pressure on the bladder and the urethra (tube that carries urine from the bladder to outside the body). Stress incontinence can occur when the urethra moves too much due to muscular and structural problems with the pelvis. This is why treatments such as spinal manipulation and soft-tissue techniques that affect the structure of the pelvis and its muscles can help incontinence. Another cause can be weakness in or damage to the muscle that closes off the urethra to prevent urine from leaving the bladder. Stress incontinence is very common during pregnancy, after childbirth, and with menopause. It is also more common in female athletes.

Another type is known as urge incontinence, also referred to as an overactive bladder. It occurs when a person cannot hold their urine long enough to get to the bathroom in time. It is more common in the elderly and in those who have had a stroke or who have Alzheimer's, diabetes, Parkinson's disease, multiple sclerosis, or prostate enlargement. This type of incontinence is related to problems in the bladder muscle and/or nervous system. As mentioned, it is more common in men with prostate enlargement, which can be improved by the use of natural therapies that help reduce prostate swelling.

There are also other, less common types of urinary incontinence. One example is overflow incontinence, in which the bladder fails to empty completely, resulting in dribbling of urine. Another type is functional incontinence, caused by physical or mental impairment that prevents one from getting to the restroom on time. The causes of functional incontinence range from conditions like severe arthritis, in which the patient is unable to move quickly, to intellectual disability. People can have a combination of different types of incontinence. Advancing age may be a contributing factor. As people age, the muscles of the urethra and bladder lose tone and strength, which makes it more difficult to control urination. Finally, being overweight puts pressure on pelvic muscles and the bladder, which ultimately weakens them.

It is important to find out what is causing incontinence as it may be a symptom of a more serious condition. Of course, having this problem can restrict a person's daily activities and limit social interactions. A sufferer of incontinence will be more prone to rashes, skin infections, sores, and urinary tract infections from skin that is constantly wet. A proper diagnosis is important. Your doctor can help you identify the root problem(s) of your incontinence. Consider seeing a urologist, a specialist who can diagnose the cause of your incontinence based on your symptoms and with testing.

This chapter outlines a variety of conventional and holistic methods for treating urinary incontinence.

TREATMENT

Diet

Recommended Food
Consuming a healthy diet that is rich in anti-inflammatory and nutrient-dense foods is advised. A good option is the Mediterranean diet.

Pumpkin seed oil is one of nature's greatest allies in the treatment of urinary incontinence. European literature cites pumpkin seeds as an effective treatment for urinary problems as far back as the 1500s. Native American Indians used pumpkin seed for urinary disorders. Also, German health authorities have approved pumpkin seeds as a treatment for irritable bladder and urinary symptoms related to prostate enlargement.

A 2014 study was conducted on men and women aged forty-one to eighty years with urinary incontinence. The men in the study did not have benign prostate enlargement. Scores rating symptoms were remarkably reduced in subjects given pumpkin seed oil. In another study of fifty women aged thirty-five to eighty-four years with incontinence, subjects supplemented pumpkin seed extract combined with soy extract. There was a 67 percent decrease in stress-induced incontinent episodes. Other research has shown that the same combination reduced nighttime urinations by 60 percent.

Food to Avoid

Avoids caffeine-containing products as they stimulate the excretion of urine. Examples include coffee, tea, hot chocolate, chocolate milk, and colas.

Some studies demonstrate that carbonated beverages, citrus-fruit drinks, and acidic juices may worsen symptoms.

Another possible aggravator of urinary incontinence is artificial sweeteners.

For some people spicy foods worsen incontinence, as do various fruits and juices.

Keep a diet diary and see if you find any foods that worsen your symptoms, and then avoid or limit them. Or visit a holistic doctor, who can test your food sensitivities.

℞ Super Seven Prescriptions—Urinary Incontinence

Super Prescription #1 Pumpkin seed oil
Take 750 mg of an extract daily or as directed on the label. A variety of studies have demonstrated improvement for urinary incontinence.

Super Prescription #2 Vinpocetine
Take 10 mg three times daily to improve symptoms of urinary incontinence.

Super Prescription #3 Horsetail (*Equisetum arvense*)
Take 300 mg two to three times daily. Historically this herb has been prescribed by herbalists and naturopathic doctors for improved bladder control.

Super Prescription #4 Magnesium
Take 250 mg twice daily to relax the bladder muscle.

Super Prescription #5 Homeopathic Combination Urinary Incontinence Formula
Take as directed on the label. Contains a variety of common homeopathic remedies used for urinary incontinence.

Super Prescription #6 Soy isoflavone extract
Take 150 mg twice daily to support bladder-muscle health.

Super Prescription #7 Passionflower
Take 300 mg or 30 drops of the tincture twice daily for urinary incontinence worsened by stress and worry.

Homeopathy

Pick the remedy that best matches your symptoms in this section. Take a 6x, 12x, 6C, 12C, or 30C potency twice daily for two weeks to see if there are any positive results. After you notice improvement, stop taking the remedy, unless symptoms return. Consultation with a homeopathic practitioner is advised.

Causticum is for stress incontinence associated with difficulty urinating. Symptoms are worse with coughing, sneezing, or laughing.

Natrum muriaticum is for stress incontinence associated emotional stress.

Sepia is for stress incontinence associated with menopause and hormonal changes.

Other Recommendations

- Conventional therapy has some good, noninvasive options. One remedy involves bladder training, in which an individual delays urination after feeling the urge to go. The patient starts by waiting an extra few minutes, gradually lengthening the time between trips to the bathroom.

- More effective are exercises for the pelvic-floor muscles, also known as Kegel exercises. These exercises are helpful for those with stress incontinence and sometimes for those with urge incontinence. To perform Kegel exercises, the individual tightens the muscles involved in stopping the flow of urine. Hold the muscle contraction for five to ten seconds, relax for five to ten seconds, and repeat the sequence several times daily. Another technique women can use to strengthen the pelvic-floor muscles to help with stress incontinence involves the use of vaginal weights. These small, cone-shaped weights are inserted into the vagina and held in place by tightening the muscles around the vagina. Sessions usually last between fifteen and thirty minutes and are done twice daily. As one improves, heavier weights are used. Best results occur when Kegel exercises and vaginal-weight exercises are both used. For premenopausal women the rate of improvement or cure is very high with these techniques.

- The next level of nondrug and nonsurgical conventional treatment is biofeedback. It involves an electronic device and a computer to help the user identify which muscles are contracting. This is done by inserting a special tampon-shaped sensor in the vagina or rectum; a different sensor is placed on the abdomen. The user contracts and relaxes the pelvic-floor muscles when the technician tells him or her to do so. The electrical signals generated by the muscle contractions are viewed on a computer screen so the patient can make sure they are contracting and improving the tone of the specific muscles causing problems. This type of treatment is effective for both stress incontinence and urge incontinence. Up to 87 percent of users will note improvement. It is also affective for men who have urinary incontinence after prostate surgery.

- A more aggressive type of biofeedback for incontinence involves electrical stimulation of the pelvic and urinary muscles. It is particularly helpful for women with stress incontinence and very weak or damaged pelvic-floor muscles. It also helps both men and women with urge incontinence caused by diseases of the nervous system. Electro-acupuncture, in which the individual receives acupuncture simultaneously with electrical stimulation of the needles, is very effective. When done by a competent acupuncturist it can be even more beneficial than regular electrical stimulation.

- Many seniors end up taking medications for their incontinence. One common drug is oxybutinin (Ditropan). It acts to reduce spasms of the bladder and urinary tract. It is used for an overactive bladder, urine leakage, and increased nighttime urination. Various side effects can include drowsiness, dizziness, dry mouth, and blurred vision. It should not be used for those with uncontrolled glaucoma, those unable to urinate, or those with intestinal disorders such as a history of digestive-tract blockage. Other medications prescribed for incontinence include tricyclic antidepressants such as imipramine and amitriptyline, as well as anticholinergic drugs such as tolterodine (Detrol).

- Lastly, conventional medicine offers a variety of different surgeries for

When the production of nitric oxide levels is low there is increased bladder activity and reduced bladder volume. Pumpkin seed oil increases nitric oxide synthesis. The other known reason for its benefit is its hormonal effects. Pumpkin seed oil has a tissue-building effect on the pelvic floor muscles. It does this by inhibiting the aromatase enzyme which makes more active testosterone available to the pelvic muscles, allowing them to strengthen.

A study in the *World Journal of Urology* demonstrated evidence that supplementing vinpocetine at a dosage of 10 mg taken three times daily for two weeks can reduce daytime and nighttime frequency of urination in people with urinary incontinence. For approximately 58 percent of the participants there were improvements in urinary symptoms or testing parameters.

incontinence. The type of surgery depends on the structural problem associated with the incontinence. In some cases surgery is required due to extreme problems with the structure of the pelvic floor and bladder. In some women the bladder prolapses so severely that it droops into the vagina. This condition is more common after menopause, when the muscles of the vagina and pelvis weaken as a result of lower estrogen levels. The use of bioidentical estrogen as well as certain homeopathic and herbal remedies can help these women in the earlier stages.

- The use of bladder slings to treat urinary incontinence in women is fairly common. The sling is made of surgical mesh and usually inserted through two small abdominal incisions and one vaginal incision. It supports the bladder from prolapsing or falling down into the vagina. Unfortunately, we have seen a number of women who underwent this procedure and had serious complications. The most serious tend to be synthetic slings or meshes that produce symptoms ranging from a worsening of urination to infection to pelvic pain. Correcting these issues can require multiple surgeries and medical treatments. Research has shown that about one in five procedures will end up with a complication. If you require surgery, make sure to obtain more than one opinion, and look into getting the most indicated and up-to-date surgery for your specific case.

- Bioidentical hormones are particularly helpful for middle-aged women suffering from urinary incontinence, especially stress incontinence. Most important are the hormones estrogen and testosterone. The use of bioidentical estrogen and testosterone as a vaginal suppository or cream has helped many of our female patients. These hormones strengthen the muscles of the bladder and pelvis. They are particularly helpful if a woman also experiences vaginal dryness and thinning.

- Men can be helped by testosterone therapy. Research has shown that transdermal testosterone replacement in men aged thirty-eight to seventy-three years improves bladder function and capacity.

- Besides estrogen and testoterone, correcting other hormone deficiencies may help urinary incontinence. Consult with a doctor who is knowledgeable in bioidentical hormone replacement.

REFERENCES

Friederich, M., C. Theurer, G. Schiebel-Schlosser. 2000. Prosta Fink Forte capsules in the treatment of benign prostatic hyperplasia. Multicentric surveillance study in 2245 patients. *Forsch Komplementarmed Klass Naturheilkd* 7:200–04.

Nishimura, M., et al. 2014. Pumpkin seed oil extracted from Cucurbita maxima improves urinary disorder in Human overactive bladder. *J Tradit Complement Med* 4(1):72–74.

Truss, M. C. 2000. Initial clinical experience with the selective phosphodiesterase-I isoenzyme inhibitor vinpocetine in the treatment of urge incontinence and low compliance bladder. *World J Urol* 18(6):439–43.

Yanagisawa, E. 2003. Study of effectiveness of mixed processed food containing Cucurbita pepo seed extract and soybean seed extract on stress urinary incontinence in women. *Jpn J Med Pharm Sci* 14(3):313–22.

Uterine Fibroids. See Fibroids, Uterine

Vaginitis

Vaginitis is an inflammation of the mucus membrane that lines the vagina. The symptoms usually include burning or itching and may extend to abnormal vaginal discharge, painful urination, and pain during sexual intercourse. The vast majority of women will experience vaginitis at some point during their lives, and the unpleasant symptoms usually send women to their doctors for treatment.

Vaginitis is commonly caused by an overgrowth of yeast (*Candida albicans*). A physician can make a diagnosis after a microscopic examination and a culture of the vaginal secretion. Other common conditions can mimic vaginal yeast infections. These include bacterial vaginosis (BV); the symptoms of this bacterial infection can include an abnormal grayish-white vaginal discharge and a foul-smelling vaginal odor. Another common cause is trichomonad vaginitis. This is a sexually transmitted disease caused by a one-celled microorganism called *Trichomonas vaginalis*. Symptoms include a foul-smelling, yellowish-green vaginal discharge and itching. Symptoms worsen during menstruation.

This section focuses on yeast-related vaginitis. It is important to see your doctor to discover the cause of your vaginitis, because certain infections can be quite serious.

Women who experience chronic yeast infections often have a common history of being on repeated courses of antibiotics. While antibiotics may destroy harmful bacteria, they also have the potential to wipe out helpful normal flora in the vagina, as well as in the urinary and digestive tracts. Good bacteria, such as *Lactobacillus acidophilus*, play an important role as part of the local immune system in the vaginal area. They function to prevent the overgrowth of yeast and other opportunistic organisms that can cause infection. In addition, these good acidophilus species help to maintain an acidic pH in the vagina, which makes it less likely that an overgrowth of yeast will occur. These good bacteria also produce hydrogen peroxide, which is a natural antimicrobial agent that kills bacteria and fungus. Acidophilus supplements, either taken internally or applied directly into the vagina (insert at night and cover with a pad), are an effective means to prevent and treat yeast infections. This remedy is best done under the supervision of a doctor. In addition, it's helpful to eat yogurt that is rich in friendly bacteria. A 1992 study found that women who consumed 8 ounces of yogurt daily had a three times lower incidence of vaginal yeast infections, as compared to women who did not eat the yogurt.

A key dietary factor that will help prevent reoccurring vaginal yeast infections is to reduce consumption of simple sugars. Yeast thrives on sugar, and too much of it has a suppressive effect on the immune system. Finally, be aware that food sensitivities can aggravate yeast infections for some women.

The immune system is constantly on the lookout for opportunistic organisms such as the yeast *Candida albicans*. When functioning optimally, it keeps unhealthful organisms in check. High stress, poor nutrition, and other factors can impair immune function, allowing for the overgrowth of candida. Many conventional doctors argue that only people with severe immune-suppressive diseases, such as HIV/AIDS, have immune systems that are weak enough to allow for the overgrowth of yeast. This appears to be untrue, and a surprising number of seemingly healthy persons suffer from a weakened immune system linked to systemic candidiasis.

Hormone balance is important in preventing vaginal yeast infections. These infections commonly occur one week prior to the beginning of a woman's menstrual flow. This is a sign that hormone balance plays a key role in the susceptibility to vaginal yeast infections. It is not unusual for women who experience PMS to also have problems with yeast overgrowth. Imbalanced estrogen and progesterone levels lead to an unfavorable vaginal pH. Typically, many of these cases are caused by what doctors call estrogen dominance. The normal increase of progesterone does not occur during ovulation, and as a result, the relative balance of estrogen is too high. We have also found that many women resolve their chronic susceptibility to vaginal infections once they discontinue use of the birth-control pill. It is a well-known fact that this medication increases the incidence of yeast infections.

In summary, natural approaches are your best bet to resolve chronic cases of vaginal yeast infections. They can also be effective for relieving acute cases when used under the supervision of a medical professional. If you are pregnant, do not start any therapy unless instructed to do so by your doctor.

SYMPTOMS

Vaginal:

- Itch
- Soreness
- Burning
- Cottage cheese–like discharge
- Pain during intercourse

ROOT CAUSES

- Antibiotics
- Poor diet (especially too many simple sugars)
- Pregnancy
- Stress
- Birth-control pills
- Sexually transmitted diseases
- Tight clothing
- Excessive douching
- Poor hygiene
- Food allergies or sensitivities
- Candidiasis (systemic)
- A suppressed immune system
- Diabetes
- HIV
- A hormone imbalance
- Flora imbalance

Testing Techniques

The following tests help assess possible reasons for reoccurring vaginal yeast infections:

Immune-system imbalance or disease—blood

Hormone testing (thyroid, DHEA, cortisol, testosterone, IGF-1, estrogen, progesterone)—saliva, blood, or urine

Digestive function and microbe/parasite/candida/flora testing—stool analysis

Food and environmental allergies/sensitivities—blood, electrodermal

Blood sugar balance—blood

TREATMENT

Diet

Recommended Food

Fortify your immune system by eating a diet that's focused on natural, whole foods.

One of the best dietary strategies for restoring the natural balance of vaginal flora is to eat a cup of unsweetened live yogurt every day. Make sure the yogurt contains *L. acidophilus* and other friendly flora.

Garlic and onions can be consumed liberally for their antifungal properties. Flaxseeds also fight yeast infections. Take 1 to 2 tablespoons daily, along with 10 ounces of water.

Women with vaginitis often suffer from dehydration. Drink a glass of clean, quality water every two waking hours.

Food to Avoid

If you have vaginitis, you have two reasons to avoid sugar. For one, many of the organisms that cause vaginal infections, such as *Candida albicans*, feed on sugar. Second, sugar depresses the immune system, making it difficult to recover from your current infection and leaving you vulnerable to repeated cases of vaginitis. Do not eat any refined sugars, and restrict your intake of simple sugars from fruits, honey, molasses, and other natural sources.

Avoid foods that are high in yeast or mold, especially alcohol, aged cheese, dried fruit, nuts, and nut butters. You must also stay away from fermented foods, including vinegar, pickles, tempeh, and soy sauce.

Food allergies may be the cause of recurring vaginitis. Read the Food Allergies section and follow the elimination diet there. If your symptoms disappear when you stop eating a certain food, eliminate that product from your diet.

℞ Super Seven Prescriptions—Vaginitis

Super Prescription #1 *Lactobacillus acidophilus*

Insert 1 capsule intravaginally each evening, and cover with a pad overnight. Repeat for seven consecutive days for acute infections. Also, take a probiotic supplement (with friendly bacteria such as *Lactobacillus acidophilus*) orally that contains at least four billion organisms twice daily, thirty minutes after meals. These friendly bacteria fight yeast overgrowth.

Super Prescription #2 Homeopathic Combination Vaginitis Formula

Take as directed on the container. It contains the most common homeopathic remedies used for vaginal yeast infections.

Super Prescription #3 Boric acid

Insert a 600 mg capsule intravaginally each morning and evening for seven days for acute infections (cover with a pad). For a chronic infection, repeat for a total of two to four weeks. Vitamin E oil can be used on the external genitalia to prevent burning and discomfort. *Note*: Do not ingest boric acid orally.

A study of women who had recurrent vaginal yeast infections looked at the effects of daily ingestion of yogurt that contained *Lactobacillus acidophilus*. Women who consumed 8 ounces of yogurt daily for six months had a threefold decrease in infections and in vaginal candida colonization.

In a study, one hundred women with chronic vaginal yeast infections who were unresponsive to prolonged conventional therapy were treated with 600 mg of boric acid suppositories twice daily for two or four weeks. As a result, 98 percent of the women who were unresponsive to common antifungal treatments were cured.

Super Prescription #4 Echinacea (*Echinacea purpurea*)

Take 3 ml or 500 mg four times daily for immune support.

Super Prescription #5 Vitamin C

Take 1,000 mg two to three times daily for immune support.

Super Prescription #6 Oregon-grape root (*Mahonia aquifolium*) or goldenseal (*Hydrastis canadensis*)

Take 3 ml or 500 mg four times daily for immune support.

Super Prescription #7 Oregano oil (*Origanum vulgare*)

Take 500 mg of the capsule form or 0.5 ml of the liquid twice daily or as directed on the container. Oregano oil has potent antifungal effects and is very important for women who have repeated vaginal yeast infections due to systemic candidiasis.

Echinacea (*Echinacea purpurea*) has been shown to enhance immune function and have antifungal properties. A German study looked at the effect of oral echinacea supplementation on women who had a history of reoccurring vaginal yeast infections. Of the sixty women taking echinacea, only ten had recurrences of yeast infections.

General Recommendations

Pau d'arco (*Tabebuia avellanedae*) has antifungal properties. Take 100 mg or 0.5 to 1.0 cc three times daily.

Garlic (*Allium sativum*) counteracts yeast infections and improves the immune system's defenses. Use several drops of garlic oil in a douche. For extra strength, you can also take garlic orally. Take 300 to 450 mg twice a day.

Vitex (chasteberry) is effective for women with hormone imbalance who experience repeated, cyclical vaginal yeast infections. Take 180 to 240 mg of a 0.6 percent standardized extract daily. *Note*: It should not be taken in conjunction with the birth-control pill.

Homeopathy

Pick the remedy that best matches your symptoms in this section. For an acute vaginal yeast infection, take a 30C potency four times daily. For a chronic vaginal yeast infection, take a 6x, 12x, 6C, 12C, or 30C potency twice daily for two weeks to see if there are any positive results. After you notice improvement, stop taking the remedy, unless symptoms return. Consultation with a homeopathic practitioner is advised.

Borax is a remedy to use when you have a vaginal discharge that resembles egg whites or a white paste and have a feeling that warm water is flowing out. Vaginitis that responds to borax often appears midway between the menstrual periods.

Calcarea Carbonica is a good choice when a woman experiences burning and vaginal itching before and/or after the menstrual period. Women who require this remedy are usually chilly, are overweight, and crave sweets, milk, and eggs. They become fatigued and overwhelmed easily.

Kali Bichromium is useful when the discharge is thick yellow and makes the external genitalia itch and burn.

Kreosotum is the most common remedy for acute vaginal yeast infections. There is a burning discharge with a putrid odor, along with great itching. The discharge is worse before menses or during pregnancy.

Natrum Muriaticum is used when the burning discharge resembles an egg white. There is often vaginal dryness along with the discharge. The woman craves salt and tends to be reserved. She feels worse in the sun and in warm rooms.

Pulsatilla (*Pulsatilla pratensis*) is indicated when there is a creamy-white or yellowish discharge. Symptoms often change throughout the day. The woman feels better in the open air. She has a strong craving for sweets and a desire for company.

Sepia is helpful when the vaginal discharge is yellow and itchy or white and offensive-smelling. A woman who requires this remedy often feels run down and irritable and wants to be left alone. She may feel a bearing-down sensation in the pelvic area.

Sulfur is used when the discharge is yellowish and offensive smelling, with great burning and itching. The woman's symptoms may worsen from warmth and bathing.

Acupressure

See pages 787–794 for information about pressure points and administering treatment.
- If you have a vaginal discharge, use Conception Vessel 4 and 6 (CV4 and CV6).
- Work Lung 1 (Lu1) to ease stress.

Bodywork

Reflexology

See pages 804–805 or information about reflexology areas and how to work them.

Work all the female-reproductive areas to stimulate blood flow and encourage healing.

To stimulate the immune system, especially the production of antibodies, work the lymph and the spleen.

Hydrotherapy

Add several cups of organic apple cider vinegar to your bath, and soak for fifteen to thirty minutes. Allow the water to flow into your vagina.

Aromatherapy

Tea tree oil, a natural antiseptic, is a highly potent remedy for vaginitis. You can use the oil in a douche or in a compress two times a day, as needed, until the inflammation is under control. Tea tree oil is sometimes irritating, so start off by using just two or three drops of oil; if you don't have a reaction, you can try a few drops more.

To relieve tension, use lavender, rose, geranium, bergamot, or jasmine in a bath, a diffuser, or whatever preparation suits you best.

Stress Reduction

General Stress-Reduction Techniques

Some women who have a history of sexual abuse experience chronic vaginitis. Besides the recommendations in this section, seek counseling and spiritual support.

Other Recommendations

- Avoid sexual intercourse during the course of treatment to prevent irritation and reinfection. For some chronic cases of yeast-related vaginitis, the male partner needs to be on an antifungal protocol (see the Candidiasis section).
- Wear loose cotton clothing that allows your genitals to breathe. Avoid tight jeans and pantyhose with nylon crotches.

- If you go swimming, change out of your wet bathing suit quickly. Otherwise, you'll create a breeding ground for bacteria.

REFERENCES

Coeugniet, E., and R. Kuhnast. 1986. Recurrent candidiasis: Adjuvant immunotherapy with different formulations of Echinacin®. *Therapiewoche* 36:3352–58.

Hilton, E., H. D. Isenberg, P. Alperstein, et al. 1992. Ingestion of yogurt containing Lactobacillus acidophilus as prophylaxis for candidal vaginitis. *Annals of Internal Medicine* 116:353–57.

Jovanovic, R., et al. 1991. Antifungal agents vs. boric acid for treating chronic mycotic vulvovaginitis. *Journal of Reproductive Medicine* 36(8):593–97.

Varicose Veins

Two primary kinds of blood vessels exist in the circulatory system. Arteries are one kind; they deliver blood away from the heart to the rest of the body. Veins are the second type of blood vessel, and their function is to conduct blood back to the heart. Of the two kinds of vessels, veins have the more difficult task. Unlike the arteries, they cannot rely upon the heart's direct pumping motion to propel the blood to its destination. Instead, the pumping action comes from the contracting and relaxing effect of muscles surrounding the veins. Luckily, however, the veins are equipped with a series of valves that help keep the blood flowing in one direction only: toward the heart.

When one of these valves malfunctions, or when a vein wall is somehow weakened, the blood cannot continue to flow properly. Instead, it pools and accumulates within the veins, which are burdened by the excess blood. They grow weaker, and they begin to stretch and bulge. These enlarged, raised blood vessels are called varicose veins. They usually appear on the legs—especially on the thigh or the back of the calf— where the veins have to fight strong gravitational pressure as they push blood back up to the heart. Varicose veins can also appear in other parts of the body, including the anus, where they are called hemorrhoids. (For more information about anal varicose veins, see Hemorrhoids.)

Varicose veins may be tender and painful and may cause the legs to feel tight and swollen, but in general, they do not pose a health risk. They are also quite common: about 50 percent of middle-aged Americans have some varicose veins. In many people, the condition is brought on by a genetic weakness in a vein wall or valve, but it can also be caused by anything that puts excess pressure on the veins. A diet that's high in fat and low in fiber can stress the veins (by contributing to constipation), as can inactivity, obesity, and long periods of sitting or standing. Many women develop varicose veins during pregnancy, when the legs are burdened with a great deal of extra pressure. We often see women with hormone imbalances who have problems with varicose veins, particularly women taking a synthetic hormone replacement.

Although no one has a cure for varicose veins, home treatment is quite effective at reducing the pain and the swelling. Home therapies can also strengthen the vein walls and prevent the condition from growing worse. Of particular importance is a group of herbs known as venotonics. This class of herbs improves the tone of the venous wall. Horse chestnut (*Aesculus hippocastanum*) and butcher's broom (*Ruscus aculeatus*) are two prime examples and are discussed in this section. We find that the natural therapies in this section often prevent a further progression of varicose veins and in some cases even promote a mild improvement. In most cases, patients find that their circulation improves. Sometimes, however, professional care is in order. In rare cases, varicose veins deep in the leg can lead to a more serious circulatory disorder, such as phlebitis or a blood clot that can travel to the lungs, resulting in a life-threatening pulmonary embolism. If you have an intense pain deep in your legs, or if you experience persistent swelling in one or both legs, consult your doctor.

SYMPTOMS

- Swollen, raised veins that may be tender and painful
- Bruising in the affected area
- Itchy skin near the varicose veins
- Heavy, tight, swollen, or fatigued legs
- Ulceration over the varicose veins

ROOT CAUSES

- A genetic weakness in the vein or in a vein's valve
- A diet that's low in fiber and high in fatty and refined food
- Obesity
- Inactivity
- Long periods of sitting or standing
- Liver disease
- A hormone imbalance
- Nutritional deficiencies

Testing Techniques

The following tests help assess possible reasons for varicose veins:

Blood pressure

Hormone testing (thyroid, DHEA, cortisol, testosterone, IGF-1, estrogen, progesterone)—saliva, blood, or urine

Vitamin and mineral analysis (especially vitamins C, E)—blood

Digestive function and microbe/parasite/candida testing—stool analysis

Food and environmental allergies/sensitivities—blood, electrodermal

---

TREATMENT

Diet

The low-fiber Western diet leads to constipation. Straining during bowel movements puts intense pressure on the veins of the lower body; over time, it can cause veins to weaken and enlarge. Therapies that encourage regular elimination are an important part of the treatment for varicose veins.

Recommended Food

A high-fiber diet is your best weapon against varicose veins. Reduce your risk of constipation by eating plenty of fresh vegetables and fruits, whole grains, and nuts and seeds.

Consume 1 to 2 tablespoons of ground flaxseeds, along with 10 ounces of water, daily to obtain healthful fiber.

Certain kinds of flavonoids will strengthen the walls of the veins and improve their elasticity. Berries that have a bluish-red color—cherries, blueberries, and blackberries, for example—are rich in the flavonoids you need, so enjoy them often as snacks or dessert. Buckwheat, as a food and in tea form, is a good source of a flavonoid called rutin, which increases the strength of capillaries. Use it in whole-grain pancakes or breads.

To improve circulation, flavor your meals with garlic, onions, ginger, or cayenne pepper.

Vitamin E is good for the circulation and also helps prevent blood clots. Wheat germ is an excellent source, as are soybeans and leafy greens.

Food to Avoid

Saturated fats, along with hydrogenated or partially hydrogenated oils, slow down your circulation and worsen the inflammation of the blood vessels. Avoid them.

Sugar and other refined carbohydrates can lead to weight gain and constipation. Dramatically reduce your intake of sweets and refined foods.

Caffeine and alcohol are dehydrating, and they worsen varicose veins.

℞ Super Seven Prescriptions—Varicose Veins

> **Super Prescription #1 Horse chestnut (*Aesculus hippocastanum*)**
> Take a standardized extract that contains 100 mg of aescin daily. This herb strengthens vein walls and valves and also improves circulation and reduces swelling.
>
> **Super Prescription #2 Butcher's broom (*Ruscus aculeatus*)**
> Take a standardized extract that gives you 200 to 300 mg of ruscogenins daily. Ruscogenins are constituents within this herb that are believed to reduce inflammation of veins.
>
> **Super Prescription #3 Grapeseed extract or maritime pine bark extract**
> Take 200 to 300 mg daily. These supplements contain proanthocyanidins, constituents that improve circulation and strengthen the integrity of the vein wall.
>
> **Super Prescription #4 Bioflavonoid complex**
> Take 1,000 mg two or three times daily. Various flavonoids, such as rutin and hesperidin, have been shown to be effective as accessory nutrients in treating varicose veins.
>
> **Super Prescription #5 Bilberry (*Vaccinium myrtillus*)**
> Take a standardized extract containing 25 percent anthocyanosides at 160 mg twice daily. Bilberry improves the circulation and strengthens capillary walls.

In one study of 240 people, horse-chestnut extract was found to be as effective as conventional methods that used specialized compression stockings and diuretic therapy. Preliminary studies have shown that horse-chestnut extract reduces the formation of enzymes that contribute to varicose veins.

Super Prescription #6 Vitamin E

Take 400 IU of a mixed complex twice daily. Vitamin E acts as a natural blood thinner to promote blood flow and reduce inflammation of the veins.

Super Prescription #7 Witch hazel (*Hammamelis virginiana*)

Apply as a gel or a cream to external hemorrhoids, or add 1 ounce to a sitz bath daily. Witch hazel has an astringent effect on external varicose veins.

General Recommendations

Gotu kola (*Centella asiatica*) is an herb that improves blood flow and strengthens the integrity of the vein walls. Take a product that provides 60 mg of triterpenic acids daily. A high-potency multivitamin provides a base of nutrients for healthy veins. Take as directed on the container.

Vitamin C is important for healthy vein walls and strengthens the rectal tissue. Take 500 mg two or three times daily.

Bromelain reduces inflammation of the veins and may help prevent blood clots. Take 500 mg three times daily, between meals. Look for products standardized to 2,000 MCU (milk-clotting units) per 1,000 mg or 1,200 GDU (gelatin-dissolving units) per 1,000 mg. Protease-enzyme products also have this benefit.

Essential fatty acids are important for reducing the inflammation of blood vessels. Take 400 mg of fish oil or 1 tablespoon of flaxseed oil daily, along with 1,000 mg of evening primrose oil (*Oenothera biennis*).

A greens drink that contains a blend of super green foods, such as chlorella, spirulina, and so on, provides fiber and improves liver function. Take as directed on the container.

Ginkgo biloba is a popular treatment for all circulatory disorders. Find an extract standardized to 24 percent flavone glycosides and take 60 to 120 mg twice daily.

Dandelion root (*Taraxacum officinale*) promotes bile flow and improved regularity. Take 300 mg or 2 ml of tincture three times daily.

Psyllium is a good fiber supplement and has been shown to reduce the pain and the bleeding associated with hemorrhoids. Take 5 to 7 grams daily, along with 10 ounces of water.

Homeopathy

Pick the remedy that best matches your symptoms in this section. Take a 6x, 12x, 6C, 12C, or 30C potency twice daily for two weeks to see if there are any positive results. After you notice improvement, stop taking the remedy, unless symptoms return. Consultation with a homeopathic practitioner is advised.

Aesculus Hippocastanum is for distended, purple veins that cause hot, sticking pains. Symptoms are worse when walking and in the cold.

Arnica (*Arnica montana*) is for veins that look and feel bruised. The veins are swollen and painful to touch.

Bellis Perennis is for varicosities that occur during pregnancy and make it difficult to walk. There is a deep bruising pain.

Carbo Vegetabilis is a good remedy when one experiences mottled skin with distended veins. One's legs feel heavy, weak, and chilly, yet have burning pains. The symptoms are worse from warmth and lying down and feel better from elevating the feet.

Hamamelis is for varicose veins of the thighs and the legs, in which there is a feeling of heaviness and bruising, with signs of swelling. The veins can become itchy. Symptoms are worse from touch, jarring, and pressure and feel better from motion.

Lachesis is for a blue-red swelling of varicose veins. The veins may bleed easily. The person tends to be hot and intolerant to heat. Symptoms often come on with menopause or pregnancy.

Pulsatilla (*Pulsatilla pratensis*) is for swollen veins in the legs that are bluish and have stinging pain. The symptoms are worse in the heat and feel better in the fresh air. Pulsatilla is a common remedy for varicose veins that occur during pregnancy.

Sepia is for purplish, congested veins that have lost their elasticity. The problem comes on with pregnancy or during menopause. The woman is prone to constipation and being chilly. She has a craving for sour, salty, and chocolate foods. The symptoms are better from exercise and warmth.

Acupressure

See pages 787–794 for information about pressure points and administering treatment.
- To encourage bowel movements, work Conception Vessel 6 (CV6) and Large Intestine 4 (LI4).
- Large Intestine 11 (LI11) strengthens the colon. If you tend to be constipated, work this point on a daily basis.
- To improve circulation to your legs, work Gallbladder 34 (GB34).

Bodywork

Reflexology
See pages 804–805 for information about reflexology areas and how to work them.
Work the areas corresponding to the colon, the liver, and the endocrine glands.

Hydrotherapy
Hot and cold hydrotherapy is a gentle but highly effective way to stimulate circulation and reduce inflammation in the legs. You can alternate hot and cold baths, if you like, or use a shower nozzle to spray your legs directly.

A wet compress is another gentle treatment for varicose veins. Apply it directly to the affected area. For added benefit, you can make the compress with any of the essential oils listed under Aromatherapy in this section or with witch hazel, which has a toning effect.

Other Bodywork Recommendations
Try to find ten minutes a day to lie down with your feet elevated. You'll encourage the blood to flow in its proper direction, and you'll reduce the pressure and the swelling.

Aromatherapy

To stimulate circulation and tone the legs, use rosemary, geranium, black pepper, or ginger. Don't massage the oil into the weakened veins; instead, add the oils to a bath or a wet compress.

Other Recommendations

- Exercise is one of the best ways to improve varicose veins. Bicycling is highly recommended, as it works the legs without putting a great deal of pressure on them.
- Avoid long periods of standing and sitting, if you can. Take frequent breaks to walk around or to put your feet up.
- Elevate the foot of your mattress so that it's five to eight inches higher than the head. When you sleep, your blood will flow to your heart more easily, instead of pooling in your veins.
- Support hose will take pressure off your veins and improve circulation. To get the maximum results, lie down with your legs raised before putting on the hose, so that you aren't trapping blood in the lower half of your body.
- If you're obese, you can significantly reduce varicose veins by losing weight. The dietary suggestions in this section will give you a start; if you'd like further help, see Obesity.
- Don't wear tight clothes that restrict your circulation. Tight pants, garters, and poorly fitting pantyhose will make the condition worse.

REFERENCES

Diehm, C., et al. 1996. Comparison of leg compression stocking and oral horse chestnut seed extract therapy in patients with chronic venous insufficiency. *Lancet* 347:292–94.

Kreysel, H. W., H. P. Nissen, and E. Enghofer. 1983. A possible role of lysosomal enzymes in the pathogenesis of varicosis and the reduction in their serum activity by Venostasin. *Vasa* 12:377–82.

Vertigo

Vertigo is the sensation that your environment is spinning or that the inside of your head is spinning. This chapter focuses on benign paroxysmal positional vertigo (BPPV), a very common cause of vertigo. It is conservatively estimated that incidences of BPPV number sixty-four cases per one hundred thousand people per year. Women are affected twice as often as men. It also occurs more often in the elderly, although it can occur at any age.

With this condition, one experiences brief episodes of dizziness that can vary in severity. The position of the head triggers these episodes. Fortunately, most cases are not related to a serious health problem.

SYMPTOMS

- Dizziness
- Unsteadiness
- Sensation that you or the environment is spinning or moving
- Light-headedness
- Unsteadiness
- Loss of balance
- Blurred vision
- Nausea
- Vomiting

ROOT CAUSES

- Displacement of calcium carbonate particles into the semicircular canals of the inner ear (vestibular labyrinth), which leads to confusing messages to the brain and triggers vertigo

- Viral infection
- Head trauma
- Surgical damage to the inner ear

Testing Techniques

Consult with a doctor for a diagnosis. The doctor will review your history and administer the Hallpike test. This test involves hanging the head in a certain position after turning the head to the side. After a few seconds, vertigo occurs and usually resolves within thirty to sixty seconds. Other tests are those that measure inner-ear disease, such as electronystagmography (ENG) or videonystagmography (VNG). A magnetic resonance imaging (MRI) test may be done to look for a tumor on the nerves of the ear.

TREATMENT

Diet

Diet does not appear to be a big factor with BPPV. However, it may be helpful to consume a healthier diet for a better recovery.

Recommended Food

Consume live foods that are healing to the body. Fresh vegetable juice may be helpful for some people.

Food to Avoid

Avoid artificial sweeteners, colorings, and flavorings that may irritate the nervous system. Avoid alcohol and caffeine, which may worsen dizziness.

℞ Super Seven Prescriptions—Vertigo

A double-blind crossover placebo trial found that 1 gram of ginger root reduced the symptoms of vertigo better than a placebo did.

Super Prescription #1 Homeopathic Cocculus
Take 2 pellets of a 30C potency three times daily for two days to see if your vertigo dissipates. If there is no improvement, try another therapy.

Super Prescription #2 Ginger root (*Zingiber officinale*)
Take 500 mg twice daily in capsule or tablet form. An alternative form is tea, at a dosage of 1 cup twice daily.

Super Prescription #3 *Ginkgo biloba*
Take 60 mg two or three times daily. Studies have shown it to help treat vertigo symptoms.

Super Prescription #4 Vinpocetine

Take 15 mg daily. This has been shown to reduce the symptoms of vertigo.

Super Prescription #5 Cayenne

Take 300 mg twice daily. It improves circulation and may reduce the symptoms.

Super Prescription #6 Coenzyme Q10

Take 100 mg daily. Some patients report that it reduces vertigo symptoms.

Super Prescription #7 Turmeric

Take 500 mg twice daily to reduce inflammation and promote circulation.

A randomized, double-blind study published in the *Journal of Alternative and Complementary Medicine* demonstrated that a homeopathic product containing Cocculus (called Vertigoheel or Cocculus Compositum) was as effective as a leading conventional drug in the treatment of vertigo. A total of 105 patients with vertigo of various origins were given either the homeopathic formula or a conventional drug for vertigo (betahistine). Both the homeopathic and the conventional treatments showed a clinically relevant ability to reduce the frequency, duration, and intensity of vertigo attacks.

General Recommendations

Work with a holistic doctor to try different natural approaches depending on your testing and health history.

Homeopathy

Pick the remedy that best matches your symptoms in this section. Take a 6x, 12x, 6C, 12C, or 30C potency twice daily for three days to see if there is any improvement. If you notice improvement, stop taking the remedy unless the symptoms return. Consultation with a homeopathic practitioner is advised.

Borax should be used for those who experience vertigo from tilting the head downward.

Nux Vomica is for vertigo accompanied by great nausea and vomiting. People with these symptoms often feel better lying down.

Tabacum is for vertigo characterized by nausea and a cold, clammy feeling.

Bodywork

Reflexology

Work on points that correspond to the ear. See pages 804–805 for a diagram of the foot points.

Other Recommendations

- Chiropractic, acupuncture, and craniosacral therapy can all be very effective for this condition. See a qualified practitioner.

- If you feel dizzy, sit down or lie down immediately.
- If you are unstable while walking, use a cane to avoid a fall.

REFERENCES

Grøntved, A., et al. 1986. Vertigo-reducing effect of ginger root: A controlled clinical study. *Journal for Oto-Rhino-Laryngology and Its Related Specialties* 48:282–86.

Issing, W., et al. 2005. The homeopathic preparation vertigoheel versus ginkgo biloba in the treatment of vertigo in an elderly population: A double-blinded, randomized, controlled clinical trial. *Journal of Alternative and Complementary Medicine* 11:155–60.

Vitiligo

Vitiligo is an acquired pigment disorder of the skin and mucus membranes. Patches of depigmented skin appear and are typically chalk-white or milk-white in color with a clear border. Vitiligo can affect any part of the skin, including the hair, inside the mouth, and the eyes. The condition tends to be more noticeable in people with darker skin. The disorder affects up to 2 percent of the world population; the average age at onset is twenty years. Approximately 30 percent of cases have a familial history.

Depending on the type of vitiligo you have, the discolored patches may cover:

- Many parts of your body. With this most common type, called generalized vitiligo, the discolored patches often progress similarly on corresponding body parts (symmetrically).
- Only one side or part of your body. This type, called segmental vitiligo, tends to occur at a younger age, progress for a year or two, then stop.
- One or only a few areas of your body. This type is called localized (focal) vitiligo.

The exact cause of vitiligo is unknown, although both genetic and nongenetic factors appear to be involved. One theory is that the body's own immune cells attack and destroy the cells that produce melanin, called melanocytes. Vitiligo is more common in people who have autoimmune conditions such as Hashimoto's thyroiditis, Graves' disease, diabetes, inflammatory bowel disease, or psoriasis. Another common theory is that increased oxidative stress overwhelms the body's antioxidant systems, making them unable to prevent damage to melanocytes. Nerve damage and simple genetics are other potential causes for the condition.

Topical corticosteroids are often used early on in the disease, but they can lead to skin thinning or the appearance of lines and streaks on the skin. Medicinal ointments containing calcineurin inhibitors, drugs that suppress the body's immune response, are also sometimes prescribed. Examples include tacrolimus and pimecrolimus. Calcineurin inhibitors can cause skin irritation, reduce a person's ability to fight infections such as herpes, and may even be linked to skin cancer or lymphoma.

The diagnosis is made based on the appearance of the skin, although a biopsy may be helpful in differentiating it from other skin conditions.

SYMPTOMS

- Skin discoloration
- Premature whitening or graying of the hair on the scalp, eyelashes, eyebrows, or beard (usually before age thirty-five)
- Loss of color in the tissues that line the inside of the mouth and nose (mucus membranes)
- Loss of or change in color of the inner layer of the eyeball (retina)
- Discolored patches around the armpits, navel, genitals, and rectum

ROOT CAUSES

- Autoimmunity
- Family history (heredity)
- Oxidative stress
- A trigger event, such as sunburn, stress, or exposure to industrial chemicals
- Adrenal burnout

Testing Techniques

Food sensitivities—blood

Antioxidant status—blood

Autoimmune markers—blood

Digestive health—stool analysis

Hormone analysis (especially stress hormones)—blood, saliva, urine

---

TREATMENT

Diet

Recommended food

Increase your antioxidant levels by eating more antioxidant-rich foods. Antioxidants work to neutralize the free-radical damage that may be promoting vitiligo. You should aim to eat seven to ten servings of fruits and vegetables a day. Blending or juicing can help you easily reach the recommended number of servings. And while you are at it, try to eat more carotenoid-rich foods such as carrots, winter squash, pumpkin, tomatoes, tangerines, collard, kale, red peppers, watermelon, cantaloupe, and spinach to help prevent ultraviolet damage from the sun.

Food to Avoid

Avoid those foods that worsen autoimmunity and inflammation. This includes trans fats and excessive red meat.

℞ Super Seven Prescriptions—Vitiligo

Super Prescription #1 Combo nutrient and UV treatment
Take alpha lipoic acid (50 mg), vitamin C (50 mg), vitamin E (20 mg), cysteine (50 mg), and polyunsaturated fatty acids (12 percent) combined

with ultraviolet B phototherapy. This combination has been shown to be effective.

Super Prescription #2 *Ginkgo biloba*

Take 60 mg twice daily of a ginkgo extract. Research has shown benefit for vitiligo.

Super Prescription #3 Khella or *Ammi visnaga*

Take 160 mg of khellin daily to reduce vitiligo lesions.

Super Prescription #4 Vitamin B12

Take at least 100 mcg of B12 daily. Injections of B12 may be more effective. Also, research has shown that when B12 is combined with folate and sunlight, noticeable results are achieved.

Super Prescription #5 Betaine hydrochloride with pepsin

Take one to three capsules with each meal to enhance absorption of nutrients to help with immune-system balancing.

Super Prescription #6 Vitamin C

Take 1,000 mg three times daily as an aid in skin healing and reduced inflammation.

Super Prescription #7 Alpha lipoic acid

Take 300 mg twice daily to offset the oxidative stress that may be involved with vitiligo.

Certain supplements may help improve vitiligo. In one study, alpha lipoic acid (50 mg), vitamin C (50 mg), vitamin E (20 mg), cysteine (50 mg), and polyunsaturated fatty acids (12 percent) were combined with ultraviolet B phototherapy. The combo, taken twice a day for six months, increased repigmentation by 75 percent compared to just 18 percent in the placebo group.

A trial published in the journal *BMC Complementary and Alternative Medicine* found that 60 mg of a standardized *Ginkgo biloba* extract taken twice a day for twelve weeks was associated with a significant improvement in vitiligo. This may be due to ginkgo's antioxidant properties.

General Recommendations

There are several natural options for treating vitiligo. One holistic approach that can be very effective is to support adrenal function. Your adrenal glands produce stress hormones such as pregnenolone, DHEA, and cortisol. An imbalance in these hormones from chronic mental or physical stress could be at the root of the autoimmune problems that lead to melanocyte destruction.

Other Recommendations

There are several conventional therapies used for treating vitiligo. Ultraviolet B (UVB) phototherapy or light therapy uses a specialized medical light machine to deliver ultraviolet B wavelengths of light to the skin. This has been shown to be effective in about 70 percent of cases in which small areas of the skin are affected. This therapy typically needs to be used relatively early in the progression of the disease. A specific wavelength of UVB can also be delivered using a laser. UVB laser therapy is generally well tolerated, but it can be costly and take several dozen sessions to complete treatment. Note that research shows that UVB is often even more effective when combined with vitamin E therapy.

Consider Chinese herbal therapy, Ayurvedic therapy, and homeopathy since these therapies have a long history of treating chronic skin conditions such as vitiligo. Consult with a qualified practitioner.

REFERENCES

Abdel-Fattah, A., et al. 1982. An approach to the treatment of vitiligo by khellin. *Dermatologica* 165:136–40.

Dell'Anna, M. L., et al. 2007. Antioxidants and narrow band-UVB in the treatment of vitiligo: a double-blind placebo controlled trial. *Clin Exp Dermatol* 32(6):631–36.

Juhlin L., M. J. Olsson. 1997. Improvement of vitiligo after oral treatment with vitamin B12 and folic acid and the importance of sun exposure. *Acta Derm Venereol* 77:460–62.

Szczurko, O., et al. 2011. Ginkgo biloba for the treatment of vitiligo vulgaris: an open label pilot clinical trial. *BMC Complement Altern Med* 11:21.

Khella has been used medicinally in Egypt. In a double-blind study published in the journal *Dermatologica,* thirty people with vitiligo were given khellin, the active component in khella, while being regularly exposed to natural sunlight for four months. Of those taking the khellin, five (16.6 percent) repigmented 90 to 100 percent; seven (23.3 percent) repigmented 50 to 60 percent; eleven (36.6 percent) repigmented 25 percent or less; and seven (23.3 percent) showed no response. None of those taking the placebo had any improvement at all.

Warts

These small bumpy mounds of overgrown skin usually appear on fingers, hands, knees, elbows, or toes. Warts are usually brown or fleshy colored and have rough, dry surfaces. Although anyone at any age can develop warts, they seem to strike more often during childhood and adolescence. They tend to recur and spread. Warts are caused by a host of viruses and can be spread to other parts of the body or to other people through direct contact. Experts have identified at least seventy different types of the human papillomavirus (HPV) that are known to infect the skin and leave warts.

Warts are usually identified by their location. A few of the more dominant ones are:

- Common warts: This type tends to surface on the skin of the hands and the fingers. These warts usually don't hurt and are caused by HPV types 2 and 4.
- Plantar warts: This type usually appears on the soles of the feet and tends to grow down into the skin, instead of creating mounds. Caused by HPV type 1, plantar warts are painful and attack blood vessels that are embedded deeply in the skin.
- Plane warts: These are small, flat, and flesh-colored warts that grow in clusters.
- Venereal warts: This type (known medically as condyloma acuminata or genital warts) affects the genital and anal areas. These moist, fleshy mounds of skin feature surfaces that resemble cauliflower. At least four different types of HPV cause this type of wart, which is spread through sexual contact.

Children's and many adult cases of warts often disappear over time without treatment.

The conventional treatment for warts is a topically applied acid (salicylic acid) to slowly peel away the skin. Cryosurgery involves freezing the wart with liquid nitrogen, which destroys the wart cells. The last resort is to surgically remove a wart. This may be done for stubborn plantar warts that cause foot pain while one is walking or standing.

Natural therapy generally focuses on enhancing immune function to eradicate or suppress the virus that causes wart development.

Note: Venereal warts need to be treated by a doctor.

Testing Techniques

The following tests help assess possible reasons for warts:

      Immune-system imbalance or disease—blood

      Intestinal permeability—urine

      Detoxification profile—urine

      Vitamin and mineral analysis—blood

      Food and environmental allergies/sensitivities—blood, electrodermal

---

TREATMENT

Diet

Recommended Food
Eat a variety of whole, nutritious foods for optimal immune health.

Food to Avoid
Avoid simple sugars, which can reduce the effectiveness of the immune system against the virus that causes the warts.

℞ Super Seven Prescriptions—Warts

Super Prescription #1 Homeopathy
Pick the remedy that matches your warts in the Homeopathy section. We find that homeopathy is the most effective treatment, but it requires an individualized remedy to be effective.

Super Prescription #2 Thuja (*Thuja occidentalis*)
Apply one drop of thuja oil to the wart(s) twice daily for four weeks. Thuja has a caustic effect on the wart and also has antiviral properties.

Super Prescription #3 Olive leaf extract (*Olea europa*)
Take 500 mg twice daily. Olive leaf has antiviral properties.

Super Prescription #4 Garlic (*Allium sativum*) oil
Apply one drop of garlic oil to the wart(s) twice daily for four weeks. Garlic oil has antiviral properties.

Super Prescription #5 Echinacea (*Echinacea purpurea*)
Take 2 ml or 300 mg twice daily. Echinacea enhances immune function and has antiviral properties.

Super Prescription #6 Selenium
Take 200 mcg daily. A selenium deficiency makes it easier for viruses to replicate.

A study in the *International Journal of Dermatology* found that applying liquid garlic extract topically to warts on the hands twice daily resulted in wart resolution in one to two weeks.

Super Prescription #7 Vitamin E

Take 400 IU daily. Vitamin E is important for immune function and to combat viral infections.

General Recommendations

Take a high-potency multivitamin for general immune support. Take as directed on the container.

Homeopathy

Pick the remedy that best matches your symptoms in this section. Take a 6x, 12x, 6C, 12C, or 30C potency twice daily for two weeks to see if there are any positive results. After you notice improvement, stop taking the remedy, unless symptoms return. Consultation with a homeopathic practitioner is advised.

Antimonium Crudum is specific for hard, flat warts that are often located on the tips of the fingers or the toes (plantar warts) and under or around the nails.

Causticum should be used for large, fleshy, and soft warts that bleed easily. They are often located on the hands, the arms, and the face.

Dulcamara is indicated for large, smooth warts found on the back of the hand or on the palm.

Nitric Acid is a good choice for cauliflower-looking warts that bleed easily and are painful. They are often found on or near the genital area, the mouth, and the anus.

Thuja (*Thuja occidentalis*) is used for extensive crops of warts (usually large) that tend to come back after being burned off or surgically removed. It is also used for warts that have formed after one has a vaccination.

Bodywork

Visualization and Hypnosis

Visualize your warts falling off. Some studies have shown this technique to be effective.

Hypnosis is another alternative treatment that is successful for some people with warts. The emerging field of psychoneuroimmunology demonstrates the powerful connection between the mind, the nervous system, and the immune system. The immune system can eradicate the virus that causes warts when it is working properly.

Aromatherapy

Place 1 drop of lemon and 1 drop of tea tree (*Melaleuca alternifolia*) oil on a Q-tip and dab onto the wart(s). Cover with a Band-Aid. Repeat daily for two to three weeks.

Other Recommendations

Tape a new piece of banana peel to the wart with adhesive tape every day (plantar wart) for two to four weeks. It contains a substance that kills warts.

Topical ozone therapy from a holistic doctor can be effective.

One six-week controlled trial found that hypnosis sessions twice weekly resulted in greater wart disappearance than did medication, placebo, or no treatment.

REFERENCES

Dehghani, F., et al. 2005. Healing effect of garlic extract on warts and corns. *International Journal of Dermatology* 44:612–15.

Spanes, N. P., V. Williams, and M. I. Gwynn. 1990. Effects of hypnotic, placebo, and salicylic acid treatments on wart progression. *Psychosomatic Medicine* 52:109–14.

Yeast Infection. See Candidiasis

PART TWO

The Essentials of Natural Medicine

Diet and Nutrition

A nutritious diet is essential to good health and vitality. Few "health experts" would disagree with this statement, since history and medical science have proven it to be true. The concept is so simple that many people forget that food provides the fuel and the building blocks that allow the body to function. This section of the book will guide you on what foods you should eat and why they are healthful. In addition, we will help you learn about the foods that contribute to disease so that you don't let them inhibit your vitality.

Modern Poisons

A century ago, our meals were prepared from fresh, whole foods. Generally, food crops were grown on local land that was considered a valuable commodity. People took time to prepare their food and enjoy the intrinsic flavors and aromas. Today, the combination of technology and globalization has turned much of our food supply into semisynthetic, genetically engineered, nutrient-lacking packaged goods. Take a look at your local supermarket. Most of the food you see is stuffed into boxes or other packages. It contains preservatives that ensure a long shelf life. Many North Americans tend to be overfed, yet simultaneously malnourished. What a paradox!

Tips for Adopting a Healthful Diet

- Learn as much as you can about nutrition. This book and many others are loaded with sound, effective advice on optimal nutrition.
- Influence your children positively by being a role model for how to eat nutritiously. Kids learn more by watching than from listening to us preach to them. Follow the same recommendations yourself that you instruct your children to follow. You will find that this is a powerful way to develop healthful eating habits in your children.
- Be enthusiastic about eating healthfully. Enthusiasm begins with the belief that you really can make a difference in the quality of your health and vitality.
- Be patient. In a society where junk food is the norm, it takes time to adapt to a healthful diet.
- Take action. You can immediately affect how your children feel by controlling what goes in their mouths. Also, you can play a major role in preventing diet-related illnesses, such as obesity, diabetes, cancer, fatigue, anemia, and most other chronic diseases.

Back to Eden

Nature produces a variety of foods designed by our Creator that are perfectly compatible with the human body. History shows that the further we get away from these naturally occurring foods, the worse our health becomes. Some of the most interesting research in this regard was done by Dr. Weston Price, a dentist with a passion for anthropology and health. He traveled the world to study primitive cultures and their dietary habits. He found that people who consumed a traditional diet, consisting of plant foods they could collect and animals they could catch (especially fish), had superior health and longevity. More recent research has shown that a whole-foods, Mediterranean-style diet confers tremendous disease-prevention benefits, including prevention of heart disease, diabetes, and cancer. More than ever, health-conscious people in America are choosing to eat fresh, organic whole foods. This great trend, we predict, will gain momentum as nutritional research continues to demonstrate the multitude of health benefits that accrue from eating natural foods.

Avoiding the SAD Diet

The rates of obesity, diabetes, cancer, heart disease, and many other chronic diseases continue to skyrocket, due in large part to the standard American diet (SAD). The obvious solution is not to eat what most Americans are consuming, if you want to be healthy.

The standard American diet is high in refined carbohydrates (a technical term for, basically, sugar), saturated fatty acids and trans-fatty acids (the types of fats that are linked to disease), and animal protein. Most commercial foods are loaded with artificial sweeteners, dyes, and preservatives. Meals commonly consist of fast food or frozen foods, or they are skipped altogether. Meals do not usually include plant foods, such as fruits, vegetables, legumes, whole grains, nuts, and seeds. Instead of water, people drink coffee, alcohol, soda, or sweetened fruit juice. Pesticides, herbicides, and other toxic chemicals are present in the food supply (even in the leading brands of baby food). From childhood through the adult years, people have abandoned their basic instincts to eat nutritious food and have succumbed to television commercials that promote fake foods. For example, the *Journal of the American Dietetic Association* reported on a study of preschool children in which researchers found that the most commonly eaten foods were fruit drinks, carbonated beverages, 2 percent milk, and French fries. Vegetables dominated the lists of children's least-favorite foods.

Beyond the Food Pyramid

Thankfully, USDA's latest way of picturing food groups is a step in the right direction. The USDA calls it MyPlate and, as the name suggests, it's a drawing of a plate divided roughly into four quarters. It's much simpler visually and easy to understand, but in our opinion it still needs improvement.

The good news is that half the plate represents fruits and vegetables. The bad news is that the grain portion—a little more than one-fourth of the plate—is far too much for most people who are generally sedentary. Another problem is that there's a glass next to the plate representing milk or some other type of dairy food. The dairy industry is very powerful, so of course it had to be included.

This is how we would make the plate better: The vegetable and protein sections should be the largest ones, with protein coming from both animal and plant sources. Fruit, which has been cultivated for a high sugar content, should be less than one-quarter of the plate.

And what of the grains? This part of the plate should be much smaller for most people. That's because refined grains (and sugars) are the main culprits in today's epidemics of obesity and diabetes. Nonetheless, physically active people need the extra carbs provided by whole grains. And instead of a glass representing milk or other dairy products, we would suggest a glass of still or sparkling water, with a wedge of lemon or lime for flavoring. So, our plate would be 50 percent vegetables, 20 percent fruit, 25 percent protein, and 5 percent nongluten grains.

Our suggestion would be to make your plate, whether at home or in a restaurant, look a lot like our recommendations. It's easy to do—in a restaurant, just ask for extra veggies. I'd add one other important point that's hard to show in an illustration: if your plate is brimming with food, save some for another meal.

Macronutrients: The Essentials of Good Health

Macronutrients make up the basis of our foods and provide us with energy. These include carbohydrates, proteins, and fats.

CARBOHYDRATES

A carbohydrate is a compound that contains carbon and water molecules. Actually, individual sugar molecules joined together make up carbohydrates. The simplest of sugar molecules are glucose, fructose (fruit sugar), and galactose (a milk sugar). These are known as monosaccharides, as they each contain one sugar molecule. Within the category of carbohydrates are simple and complex carbohydrates. Examples of simple carbohydrates include table sugar, honey, and fruit sugars.

As you read in the description of the standard American diet, most people consume far too many simple carbohydrates. Although the body ultimately breaks carbohydrates down into glucose (the simplest of sugars), most simple carbohydrates, such as candy, potato chips, soda, and refined flours (white breads, crackers, chips, cookies, muffins), have little to no fiber, vitamins, minerals, or phytonutrients. These carbohydrates are often called empty calories. When consumed in excess, especially on an empty stomach, they lead to immune-system suppression, mood swings, attention problems, and weight gain (fat deposition). Many of these effects are due in large part to the spike in blood sugar that results after they are eaten. As a result, the hormone insulin is released to help transport blood sugar to the cells. As a by-product of this, the pancreas (which produces insulin) is overtaxed, immune cells are weakened, and the body stores fat. Too high a percentage of simple carbohydrates in the diet predisposes people to develop obesity, diabetes, cavities, and heart disease. The question then arises: what about fruits, because most of them contain simple carbohydrates? Research has shown that many types of fruit are good to eat, when consumed in moderation. As it turns out, fruits contain a great deal of fructose. This simple sugar does not cause a rapid rise in glucose and insulin levels because fructose must first be converted into glucose by the liver, to be available for the body to use. Fructose has a much more stable effect on blood sugar levels than do other common sugars, such as sucrose, maltose (found in rice syrup and malt), dextrose, and honey. Certain fruits, such as apples, contain fiber that helps to normalize blood sugar levels.

Glycemic Index

Glycemic index (GI) has become a popular term; it is more meaningful than the label "simple carbohydrate." GI refers to the rise in your blood sugar after you ingest a specific food. This numerical value is compared to the GI of glucose at a value of 100. It is recommended that people with obesity, diabetes, and insulin resistance eat foods that have lower glycemic values. For example, a Coca-Cola soft drink has a glycemic index of 63, whereas as a serving of kidney beans has a value of 23.

A GI of 70 or more is considered high.

A GI of 56 to 69 is considered medium.

A GI of less than 55 is considered low.

Glycemic Load

Recently, doctors and researchers have placed more value on the glycemic load (GL) value of foods. The glycemic load takes into account the amount of carbohydrate in one serving of a particular food. The glycemic index tells us how quickly a carbohydrate turns into blood sugar, but it neglects to take into account the amount of carbohydrate in a serving, which is important. The higher the glycemic load value, the higher the blood sugar level and the resulting stress on insulin levels. This value is derived by multiplying the amount of carbohydrate contained in a specified serving size of the food by the glycemic index value of that food, and then dividing by 100. For example, an apple has a GI of 40, compared to that of glucose, which is the baseline at 100, but the amount of carbohydrate available in a typical apple is 16 grams. The GL is calculated by multiplying the 16 grams of available carbohydrates times 40 and then divided by 100, to arrive at a decimal number of approximately 6. Compare this to a serving of Rice Krispies, which has a glycemic index of 82 and 26 grams of available carbohydrate, giving it a glycemic load of 21. A serving of macaroni and cheese has a glycemic load of 32.

A GL of 20 or more is considered high.

A GL of 11 to 19 is considered medium.

A GL of 10 or less is considered low.

One study found a 50 percent reduction in people's white blood cell activity (good immune cells) for two hours after they ingested a sugar solution. Studies have found that this negative effect can last for five hours or more.

Complex carbohydrates should be the dominant type of carbohydrates in the diet. They provide a longer-lasting energy source, help us to feel fuller, maintain our blood sugar balance, contain fiber that helps us with elimination, and contain more vitamins, minerals, and phytonutrients than simple carbohydrates do. Examples of complex carbohydrates include whole grains (such as whole wheat pasta, whole grain breads and cereals, and oatmeal), beans, brown rice, peas, and most root vegetables.

Consuming carbohydrates along with protein, fiber, and fat (good fats) helps to smooth out their effect on blood sugar levels. This is another reason why a balance of all the nutrients is so important.

PROTEINS

Protein is found in both plant and animal foods. The body uses protein as a fuel source and to form or repair tissues, organs, and muscles. Protein consists of enzymes and hormones and is found in every cell of the body. Amino acids are the individual building blocks of protein. There are approximately twenty different amino acids. Ten of the amino acids are known as "essential amino acids," which means that our bodies cannot manufacture them, so it is essential that we consume them in our diets. The remaining ten nonessential amino acids can be manufactured in the body.

Debate continues among nutritionists about whether humans should consume animal protein as compared to plant protein. We must remember that humans are omnivores, and that our digestive tracts (including our teeth) were designed to handle both animal and plant foods.

Animal protein contains complete proteins, which means that it contains all of the essential amino acids. It has a higher biological value, meaning that animal proteins are more digestible and easily utilized by the body. However, certain types of animal meat, especially the red meats, tend to be much higher in saturated fats. Another concern is that contaminants, such as hormones, antibiotics, and microbes (parasites, bacteria, virus), may be found in animal products. This is why it is so important to buy organic meat products and cook them properly. Also, our fish supply has become increasingly contaminated with toxins, including heavy metals such as mercury.

Plants also contain protein that is vital to our health. One advantage of eating plants, aside from their protein content, is their fiber content. In addition, they are a valuable source of phytonutrients, in which researchers continue to discover a host of health benefits. Keep in mind that most plants are an incomplete protein source. However, this is not a problem, because a variety of combined plant foods provides all the essential amino acids. It is important to consume organic fruits and vegetables to limit the amount of pesticides and herbicides your body is exposed to. People with insulin resistance or diabetes may fare better by not having a completely vegetarian diet and often benefit from eating animal foods. Also, people who have celiac disease or a gluten intolerance must avoid most types of grains.

Quality protein sources include soy, eggs, poultry, legumes, fish, nuts, and occasional amounts of red meat. For infants, breast milk is the best source of protein.

FATS

Most people fear fat, because they associate it with obesity. However, to be healthy, humans require fat in the diet. The key is to eat the right kind of fats and to reduce or avoid harmful fats. Fat is required to produce energy; for healthy brain development and function; for normal growth and development; to absorb fat-soluble vitamins; for healthy skin, nails, and hair; for a healthy immune system; and for many other vital functions. All fats are composed of carbon, hydrogen, and oxygen molecules. The differences between fats come down to the number of carbon atoms in each type of fat and the way they are arranged. There are three main categories of fats:

Monounsaturated fat refers to fatty acids that have one double bond. The double bond affects the function of the fatty acids and makes the fat useful for certain cell functions. Monounsaturated fatty acids are healthful and are found in foods such as avocados and olive oil.

Polyunsaturated fats comprise all of the essential fatty acids. Essential fatty acids must be obtained through the diet, as the body cannot manufacture them. Polyunsaturated fatty acids contain more than one double bond. Good sources are fish such as salmon and mackerel, as well as flaxseeds and flaxseed oil, walnuts, soybeans, and certain other plant foods. See the next section for more information on essential fatty acids.

The term *saturated fats* means that all the carbon molecules are filled (saturated) with hydrogen molecules. This makes the fats solid to semisolid at room temperature. Examples of foods that are high in saturated fats include red meat, pork, and dairy products. Lard is another one. Some oils, such as palm and coconut oil, contain high amounts of saturated fats. There is a role for saturated fats in the body. For example, they are one component of brain cells. However, most people tend to go overboard with foods that contain saturated fats.

Fats to Avoid

Read ingredient labels closely to determine which foods contain hydrogenated or partially hydrogenated fats. These "synthetic fats" cause oxidation and cell damage. Common food sources include margarine, cookies, crackers, salad dressings, and many commercial baked items. Alternative foods that do not contain these harmful fatty acids are available.

Essential Fatty Acids

It is important that you not only consume foods with essential fatty acids but also maintain a proper balance of these good fats. As mentioned earlier, the body cannot manufacture essential fatty acids. They are so vital to life, humans cannot live without them. Two types of fatty acids are considered essential. They are alpha linolenic acid (ALA), of the omega-3 family, and linoleic acid (LA), from the omega-6 family.

The Three Families of Fatty Acids

Most of the research in regard to fatty acids has been done with omega-3 and omega-6 fatty acids. A third type, known as omega-9 fatty acids, is also important, but not much is yet known about all of its roles. The numbering of fatty acids (e.g., omega-3) is in reference to the first double bond location. Following is a summary of the omega families:

Omega-3 Fatty Acids
Alpha linolenic acid (ALA)
Eicosapentaenoic acid (EPA)
Docosahexanoic acid (DHA)

Omega-6 Fatty Acids
Linoleic acid (LA)
Gamma linolenic acid (GLA)
Arachidonic acid (AA)

Omega-9 Fatty Acids
Oleic acid

The Two Essential Fatty Acids

All the fatty acids are important. The body requires about twenty fatty acids to function properly. However, unlike the other fatty acids, alpha linolenic acid and linoleic acid cannot be manufactured by the body and must be obtained from the diet.

Alpha linolenic acid. ALA is a member of the omega-3 fatty acid family. You have probably heard of it in regard to the health benefits of eating fish and flaxseeds. Other examples of foods that contain ALA include walnuts, green leafy vegetables, and canola oil.

Linoleic acid. LA is a member of the omega-6 family. This fatty acid is found in foods such as sunflower, safflower, corn, and sesame, borage, and evening primrose oils.

What Are Essential Fatty Acids Used For?

Essential fatty acids are part of the cell membranes. They are needed for cells to carry out their normal functions. Here is a sample of the roles that essential fatty acids play:

Brain and retina development	Proper circulation
Balanced mood	Kidney function
Hormone synthesis	Nerve transmission
Regulation of pain and inflammation	Energy production
Immune function	Skin, nail, and hair health

Physical signs of essential fatty acid deficiency or imbalance include:

Dry skin, cracked skin	Frequent urination
Dry eyes	Soft nails, nails that break easily
Dandruff	Dry, listless hair
Poor wound healing	"Chicken skin" on the back of the arms
Irritability	Excessive thirst

Conditions associated with fatty acid deficiency or imbalance include:

Arthritis	Hair loss
Diabetes	Hypertension
Asthma	Cancer
Eczema	Lupus
Attention-deficit disorder	Depression
Fatigue	Memory problems
Cardiovascular disease (heart attack, stroke)	Dry skin
	Schizophrenia

The Importance of Fatty Acid Balance

Think of a scale, with the omega-3 fatty acids on one side and the omega-6 fatty acids on the other. To maintain a balance, each side must be equal. The problem with most children's diets in our modern society is that this scale is tipped in favor of the omega-6 fatty acids. This imbalance can lead to a whole host of problems, including behavioral changes, decreased immunity, cardiovascular problems, joint problems, skin problems, and a variety of other medical conditions. Researchers have stated that the Western diet contains anywhere from fourteen to twenty times more omega-6 fatty acids than omega-3s.

Dr. Ronald Rudin, an expert in essential fatty acids, estimates that over the last seventy-five years, our omega-3 fatty acid consumption has decreased by 80 percent. Following are some major reasons why this imbalance has occurred:

- Decreased consumption of foods that are rich in omega-3 fatty acid (fish, flaxseeds, whole grains)
- Refining of grains
- Increased sugar intake (interferes with fatty acid metabolism)
- Increased intake of trans-fatty acids (fast foods and margarine)
- Increased hydrogenation of oils
- Nutritional deficiencies (certain minerals, such as B6, are needed for fatty acid metabolism)
- Increased use of pharmaceutical medications (these may deplete nutrients and fatty acids)
- Infant formulas are not balanced with essential fatty acids
- Digestive problems

Harmful Fats

Saturated fats, described earlier, make up one category of unhealthful fats (see page 672). Hydrogenated fats and trans-fatty acids refer to the unsaturated fatty acid molecules from vegetable oils that have had hydrogen molecules added. This results in unnatural fats that are now semisolid or solid. Trans-fatty acids are found in margarine, salad dressings, commercial breads, cookies, and crackers. They should be avoided, due to their harmful effects on the body. They have no known beneficial function. As a spread or for baking, butter is a better option than margarine is. Oils such as canola and olive oil should be used for frying.

Fatty Acids Worthy of Description

DHA (docosahexanoic acid) is an omega-3 long-chained fatty acid that's found in high concentrations in breast milk and fish. Humans have the ability to make DHA from the essential fatty acid ALA, but the efficiency of this process varies, depending on the individual. DHA plays a pivotal role in the development of a baby's brain and retinas. It also plays an important role in joint health and cognitive function. Sources of DHA include fish, especially cold-water fish, such as salmon, mackerel, herring, and tuna. Other good sources include eggs and some types of algae.

EPA (eicosapentaenoic acid) is an omega-3 fatty acid that helps to regulate inflammation, the immune system, blood clotting, and circulation (including to the brain). It is also found in DHA-rich fish.

GLA (gamma linoleic acid) is a member of the omega-6 family. It has a powerful effect on the functions of the brain, on joint health, and on hormone balance. Sources include borage oil, evening primrose oil, and black currant seed oil.

AA (arachidonic acid) is first found in the mother's breast milk, where it helps with her infant's brain development. At approximately one year of age, an infant can make its own AA. Many animal products, such as beef and turkey, contain AA, so a deficiency is rare in our society. Too much AA can act as a precursor to inflammatory conditions in the body. Linoleic acid can also be converted into AA. Sources include animal fat, peanuts, and some algae.

Gotta Get Your Fiber

One key to a healthful diet is making sure that you get enough fiber on a daily basis. Plant foods are the only source of fiber. There are two types of fiber. Soluble fiber means that the fiber dissolves in water. An example would be the fiber contained in oat bran or dried beans and peas. This type of fiber helps to slow the absorption of glucose from the intestines into the bloodstream and thus improves the blood sugar balance. It also helps to lower cholesterol. Insoluble fiber does not dissolve in water, and it helps to bind water and bulk up the stools to allow for efficient bowel movements. It also helps to bind excess fats and toxins in the digestive tract, to be excreted out with the stools. Populations that consume a lot of fiber have less risk of developing colon and other cancers. Fiber also provides a sense of fullness without containing empty calories. It is recommended you get at least 25 grams of total fiber a day.

FIBER CHART

Constipation, straining at a bowel movement, abdominal pain, or hard stools can all be signs that you are not getting enough fiber. People with sensitive digestive systems (who are prone to bloating, gas, cramps, etc.) often do better by starting with steamed or cooked vegetables, such as broccoli, carrots, and cauliflower. Over time, they can convert to larger quantities of raw vegetables. Also, enzyme supplements are helpful for people who have trouble digesting raw vegetables. By including five or more servings of fruits and vegetables a day in your diet, you will obtain enough fiber. Essentially, try to get in a good source(s) of fiber with every meal.

Fiber Chart	Serving Size	Soluble Fiber (grams)	Insoluble Fiber (grams)	Total Fiber (grams)
Fruits				
Apples	1 apple	0.4	2.6	3.0
Banana	1 banana	0.5	1.3	1.8
Blueberries	½ cup	0.2	1.9	2.1
Blackberries	½ cup	0.4	4.5	4.9
Grapes	10 grapes	trace	0.5	0.5
Grapefruit	½ grapefruit	0.1	0.3	0.4
Honeydew Melon	½ cup	0.1	0.4	0.5
Peach	1 peach	0.6	1.1	1.7
Raisins	¼ cup	0.2	1.4	1.6

	Serving Size	Soluble Fiber (grams)	Insoluble Fiber (grams)	Total Fiber (grams)
Vegetables				
Artichoke (fresh, cooked)	1 medium	3.5	2.9	6.4
Beans (black, dry, cooked)	½ cup	0.1	2.7	2.8
Broccoli	½ cup	1.6	1.0	2.6
Brussels sprouts (frozen, cooked)	½ cup	0.4	2.8	3.2
Lettuce	½ cup	0.2	0.3	0.5
Spinach (canned, cooked, or raw)	½ cup cooked or canned			
	2 cups raw	0.3	2.0	2.3
Vegetable soup (canned)	1 cup	0.6	1.6	2.2
Grains				
Bread (white or Italian)	1 slice	0.2	0.6	0.8
Bread, rye	1 slice	0.2	0.5	0.7
Bread, whole wheat	1 slice	0.3	2.2	2.5
Cereal, Total cornflakes	1 cup	trace	0.8	0.9
Cereal, Rice Krispies	1 cup	0.1	0.4	0.5
Cereal, Special K	1 cup	0.1	0.7	0.8
Cookies, oatmeal	1 large	0.3	0.6	0.9
Cookies, plain sugar	1 cookie	0.1	0.1	0.2
Crackers, Ritz	4 crackers	0.1	0.2	0.3

Water

Drink before You Think

Do not wait until you have the sensation of feeling thirsty to start drinking water. By the time you feel thirsty, you are likely to be mildly dehydrated. Regular water intake throughout the day is encouraged.

An adequate water intake is very important for both children and adults. Most of our body consists of water, making it a crucial substance that enables all the cells, the organs, and the tissues of the body to work properly. This includes the brain. Mild dehydration can interfere with concentration and cause headaches. Most people do not consume enough water on a daily basis. Infants should consume 1.5 ounces of water per pound of body weight daily. Infants who are breastfed do not need to drink water, as they get plenty in the breast milk. Children should drink an average of 40 ounces a day. Adults should drink 48 to 60 ounces a day. A warm climate, exercise, soft drinks, and high-sodium foods lead to dehydration. Also, a person may need more water to help recover from an illness.

The other consideration in regard to water is quality. Tap water in North American homes is laced with chemicals. Chlorine is a good disinfectant but should not be consumed, as it destroys the good bacteria in the digestive tract and is linked to bladder and rectal cancer. It can be removed with a filtration system and with a charcoal filter in the showerhead. Fluoride is contained in the municipal water supply, depending on which area of the country you live in. Fluoridation of the water supply is a controversial topic; fluoridation is a serious health hazard. Pesticides, heavy metals (e.g., lead), and other contaminants are found in the water supply. Parasites and bacteria are in higher-than-acceptable concentrations in some areas of this country's water.

We consider reverse osmosis, carbon-filtered, and distilled water to be clean, quality water. Have your drinking water tested by a certified water-testing company in your area. You can also contact the Environmental Protection Agency Safe Drinking Water Hotline (1-800-426-4791 or www.epa.gov) to get more information about water safety standards and testing.

Whole Foods Diet

Your diet should focus on whole foods that are unprocessed and as fresh as possible. Although it's difficult to have a diet that is 100 percent whole foods, shoot for this as a goal when you prepare meals. Whole foods diets are much richer in nutrients and enzymes than diets that include mostly packaged, processed foods.

Examples of whole foods include whole grain breads and cereals; fruits; vegetables; fresh fish, poultry, and meats; and nuts and seeds. Essentially, foods that have not been processed are whole foods—just the way nature intended them to be. We should mention that a number of people are gluten sensitive. Examples of carbohydrate options for those with gluten sensitivity or allergy include brown rice, tapioca, quinoa, buckwheat,

Variety in the Diet

A healthful diet includes a wide a variety of foods. Every food has a different nutritional profile. By eating as many different healthful foods as possible, you expand the amount and the types of nutrients you take in. In addition, your taste and desire for a wide variety of foods will increase after you experience so many different flavors, textures, and so on. Furthermore, a varied diet prevents food sensitivities from developing; thus you will avoid present and future problems (see the Food Sensitivities section for more information). Try to eat fruits and vegetables in every color of the rainbow: green, yellow, red, and so on. They all contain different phytonutrients, which are so valuable for preventing serious illnesses.

Why Organic Foods Are Best

Over one billion pounds of pesticides and herbicides are sprayed on US crops each year. Yes, it is realistic to assume that you are ingesting these potential toxins.

According to the Environmental Protection Agency, "Adverse effects of pesticide exposure range from mild symptoms of dizziness and nausea to serious, long-term neurological, developmental and reproductive disorders. Americans use more than a billion pounds of pesticides each year to combat pests on farm crops, in homes, places of business, schools, parks, hospitals, and other public places. For the first time, the EPA is calling for hundreds of additional studies on pesticides to better understand their effects on children, specifically on developmental neurotoxicity and acute and subchronic neurotoxicity. In addition, the EPA has developed new tests and risk assessment methods to target the factors unique to infants and children."

The long-term effects of pesticide and herbicide exposure are unclear, but a scary picture is beginning to emerge. Population studies on adults suggest a link with certain types of cancers and neurological diseases. As parents and doctors, we do not want to wait until "absolute" scientific evidence links these chemicals to various diseases. Pesticides that had been considered safe and were used for decades are now being banned. For example, methyl parathion, a type of organophosphate, was recently banned from being sprayed on apples.

GO ORGANIC

Foods are one of the few environmental substances that we can specifically control in regard to our health. It's hard to control the air we breathe outdoors unless we move to a different area. But we can control the safety of our food, to a certain extent, and it starts when we buy organic.

Organic means foods that have not been sprayed with synthetic chemicals and have been grown in safe soil. Look for foods that are labeled "certified organically grown." Organic foods may not be totally pesticide-free, due to cross contamination from other crops and circumstances beyond anyone's control. A 1997 Consumer Reports study of one hundred pounds of organic and nonorganic food (randomly selected from grocery stores around the country) found that 25 percent of the organic samples had traces of pesticides, while 77 percent of the nonorganic food did. Yes, organic foods cost more, but your health is worth it. Be wary of the following fruits and vegetables, as they contain some of the highest amounts of toxic pesticides:

Peaches	Raspberries
Grapes	Winter squash
Apples	Spinach
Strawberries	Green beans
Pears	Potatoes

Baby food is contaminated with pesticides and chemicals as well. Fortunately, well-known baby food brands are now selling organic. The next-best thing to buying certified organic food is to buy fruits and vegetables at local farmer markets. Get to know local farmers who do not use pesticides on their crops. You can also purchase poultry and meat products made from chickens, sheep, and cattle that consumed nonpesticide feed and are free of added hormones and antibiotics. Organic milk is now available as well.

Clean Your Fruits and Vegetables

All foods, whether organic or not, should be cleaned thoroughly to rinse off bacteria as well as pesticides. The problem with soft foods, such as pears, is that pesticides saturate into the core of the fruit. We recommend washing your fruits and vegetables with dish detergent or special soaps that dissolve pesticides.

Organic Is More Nutritious than Other Food

One study compared the amounts of healthful and toxic minerals in organically and conventionally grown foods. Following are the results, which highly favor organically grown foods.

Healthful Minerals

Rubidium—28% higher in conventionally grown (not a desirable mineral)

Potassium—125% higher in organically grown

Selenium—390% higher in organically grown

Silicon—86% higher in organically grown

Boron—70% higher in organically grown

Sodium—159% higher in organically grown

Calcium—63% higher in organically grown

Strontium—133% higher in organically grown

Chromium—78% higher in organically grown

Sulfur—20% higher in organically grown

Cobalt—same in both groups

Vanadium—8% higher in organically grown

Copper—48% higher in organically grown

Zinc—60% higher in organically grown

Iodine—73% higher in organically grown

Iron—59% higher in organically grown

Lithium—118% higher in organically grown

Magnesium—138% higher in organically grown

Molybdenum—68% higher in organically grown

Nickel—66% higher in organically grown

Phosphorous—91% higher in organically grown

Toxic Minerals

Aluminum—40% higher in conventionally grown

Cadmium—5% higher in organically grown

Lead—29% higher in conventionally grown

Mercury—25% higher in conventionally grown

Fish

As we mentioned, fish is an excellent source of protein and essential fatty acids. Unfortunately, certain species of fish are known to contain dangerous levels of mercury and other toxins. The boxed text on the next page lists fish that are deemed to be safe from mercury and those that are considered borderline or unsafe. The quality and the safety of fish depend on the area where you live. You can check the status of the contamination of fish in your area at the website of the EPA, www.epa.gov, or contact your local or state department of health.

Don't Skip Meals

It is important that you eat regular meals. This will help you to maintain regular blood sugar levels. Regular meals improve concentration, mood, and energy levels. Snacks between meals are important for people who are very active or are prone to blood sugar problems, such as hypoglycemia, insulin resistance, diabetes, and obesity.

Bring Your Lunch to School and Work

Well-known fast-food chains infiltrate many schools. Although fast foods pose no problem if you have them only on occasion (once a week), your child should not eat them for lunch on a regular basis. They are loaded with harmful trans-fatty and saturated acids, artificial preservatives and sweeteners, and sugars. Many adults eat out at lunchtime. It is more economical and healthful to bring your own lunch. When you do eat out, choose reputable, more healthful restaurants.

Tips for Eating Out

You can enjoy eating out and still get a relatively healthful meal. Following are some tips:

- Tell the waiter that you do not want a dessert menu or sample at the end of the meal.
- Choose fruit juice, milk, or water over soda.
- Choose fruit instead of french fries as a side dish.
- Avoid fried foods.
- Order a salad with the dressing on the side (so that you can use a small amount instead of the heaping that usually drenches the salad).
- Give your children menu options that do not include fried foods.

Acid/Alkaline Levels

Our bodily fluids' pH registers on a scale of 0.0 to 14.0. Seven is neither acid nor alkaline. The higher the number over 7, the more alkaline it is. Anything 0 to 7.0 is increasingly acidic, and it increases at an exponential rate—with 5 on the scale being 10 times more acidic than 6, and so on—as the number drops. Alkalis offset acids, and acids neutralize alkalis. Different elements in the body have different pH values. For example, urine is normally mildly acidic, but the blood has a mildly alkaline pH and works to maintain a narrow blood plasma level pH of 7.4 (a range between 7.35 and 7.45). Having a slightly alkaline blood pH is best. But odds are that your body is constantly battling a trend towards acidity. If your pH leans toward being acidic the body works to restore balance as best as possible.

A blood pH that tends toward acidity increases the risk of several diseases. Research has shown it increases the risk of osteoporosis, weak muscles, physical frailty, falls, fractures, breast cancer, hormone problems, diabetes, hypertension, and heart disease.

Your blood pH is related to the acidic or alkaline metabolic *effect* of food, not whether a specific food happens to be acidic. Your kidneys monitor the amount of potassium, bicarbonate, sodium, and chloride in food. If a meal is high in potassium and bicarbonate, which promotes an alkaline pH, the kidneys do not need to buffer the acidity. However, when you consume foods that are loaded with acidifying salt, high in sodium and chloride, then your kidneys send signals to your bones to release calcium and magnesium and to your muscles to break down and release ammonia to the buffer acid.

The diet of our ancient ancestors was higher in potassium than sodium and higher in bicarbonate than chloride. Our processed diet is way too high in sodium and chloride from salt. In addition, excess amounts of red meat, grains, and sugars promote acidity. The key is to consume a diet rich in the fruits and vegetables that have high levels of potassium and bicarbonate. This is especially true of leafy green vegetables. Super green foods such as wheat grass, chlorella, and spirulina are good sources. Juicing with dominantly vegetables and some fruits promotes optimal blood and tissue pH. Also make sure to drink plenty of water to dilute acidifying foods.

Phytonutrients

A major area of interest in nutritional science concerns the therapeutic benefits of phytonutrients, also known as phytochemicals. These naturally occurring substances give plants their characteristic flavor, color, aroma, and resistance to disease. When consumed, they also help people resist disease. Thousands of phytonutrients have been identified in fruits, vegetables, grains, seeds, algae, and nuts. They have tremendous benefits for people by helping to prevent illnesses such as cancer and cardiovascular disease. For example, two phytochemicals found in cruciferous vegetables (such as broccoli and cauliflower), known as indole-3 carbinol and sulforaphane, help the body to metabolize toxins and are associated with preventing certain types of cancers. Flavonoids, found in citrus fruits, protect us against heart disease, stroke, and cancer. Many phytochemicals are powerful antioxidants that protect against cell damage and environmental pollutants. Others help cells to detoxify more efficiently. For example, green vegetables are high in chlorophyll, a potent detoxifying phytochemical. We need all the support that nature has to offer in our modern but toxic world.

Bottom line: You are what you eat. People who grow up eating whole food diets, including abundant amounts of plant foods, stand a better chance of avoiding cancer, heart disease, and other maladies. Many health benefits of phytochemicals are yet to be discovered.

Be Wary of Artificial Sweeteners

The regular use of artificial sweeteners is a hidden health risk to everyone who consumes them. Aspartame, also known as Equal and NutraSweet, is a popular artificial sweetener found around the globe in the little blue packets atop the tables in most restaurants. It's also commonly used in diet soda, instant tea, sugarless candy and chewing gum, and over-the-counter drugs such as cough syrups and liquid pain relievers. It is considered a "general purpose sweetener" by the FDA. According to the Calorie Control Council this synthetic sweetener is found in more than six thousand products and is ingested by over two hundred million people around the world.

A study was conducted by Brigham and Women's Hospital and Harvard Medical School that assessed the relation between regular and diet soft drink consumption and risks of lymphoma and leukemia in 77,218 women and 47,801 men over a twenty-two-year period. Every two years, participants were given a detailed dietary questionnaire, and their diets were reassessed every four years. Researchers found that one diet soda a day increased subjects' risk of leukemia, multiple myeloma, and non-Hodgkin's lymphomas.

Sucralose, known by the retail name Splenda, is a common artificial sweetener in the United States. No long-term human studies have ever been conducted on Splenda. The studies done on animals are not reassuring. They show effects that include reduced growth rate, enlargement of the liver and brain, decreased red blood cell count, and increased risk of cataracts. Admittedly, the quantities of sucralose fed to the study animals were very high—yet still there is a great need for clinical studies on humans.

The other one to mention is saccharin, also known as Sweet'N Low and Necta Sweet. Saccharin has been a controversial artificial sweetener since its creation in the early 1900s. Some users report reactions to saccharin, including itching, hives, headache, nausea, and diarrhea. Studies done in the late 1970s and the 1980s showed that high doses could cause bladder cancer in male rats.

Dr. Swithers, a professor of behavioral neuroscience at Purdue University, published a review of studies warning that people who consume sugar substitutes "may... be at increased risk of excessive weight gain, metabolic syndrome, type 2 diabetes, and cardiovascular disease." Researchers took notice recently when a French study suggested that women who drink large amounts of diet soda are at increased risk for type 2 diabetes.

We advise readers to avoid artificial sweeteners such as acesulfame, aspartame, neotame, saccharin, and sucralose. Instead try natural sweeteners such as honey, stevia, erythritol, and lo han.

AVOID GMOs

In our world of modern technology there can be a price to pay with experimentation. Such is the case with GMO (genetically modified organisms) foods, also referred to as geneticially engineered foods. Millions of people consume genetically engineered foods daily in the United States without knowing what type of potential harm they may be causing to their body. The use of GMOs introduces foreign genes into the food supply. Based on an extensive amount of research, there are concerns about their toxicity, allergic potential, immune-damaging effects, cancer risk, and contribution to antibiotic resistance. Some of the most commonly genetically engineered foods are corn and soy; in fact, most corn and soy has been genetically modified. As of yet there have been no labeling laws established to identify GMO foods.

We have only seen the tip of the iceberg when it comes to the potential health and environmental problems created by GMOs. Shopping at holistic food stores and growing your own plant foods are the best ways to avoid GMOs. And when you're shopping for supplements, look for GMO-free versions, which are becoming increasingly available.

References

Bernstein, J., S. Alpert, K. Nauss, and R. Suskind. 1977. Depression of lymphocyte transformation following glucose ingestion. *American Journal of Clinical Nutrition* 30:613.

Brüngger, M., H. N. Hulter, R. Krapf. 1997. Effect of chronic metabolic acidosis on the growth hormone/IGF-1 endocrine axis: new cause of growth hormone insensitivity in humans. *Kidney Int* 51:216–21.

Brüngger, M., H. N. Hulter, R. Krapf. 1997. Effect of chronic metabolic acidosis on thyroid hormone homeostasis in humans. *American Journal of Physiology* 272:F648–53.

Buclin, T., et al. 2001. Diet acids and alkalis influence calcium retention in bone. *Osteoporos International* 12(6):493–9.

Calorie Control Council website Aspartame Information Center. Accessed November 25, 2012 at http://www.aspartame.org.

Fagherazzi, G., et al. 2013. Consumption of artificially and sugar-sweetened beverages and incident type 2 diabetes in the Etude Epidémiologique auprès des femmes de la Mutuelle Générale de l'Education Nationale–European Prospective Investigation into Cancer and Nutrition cohort *Am J Clin Nutr* March.

Franch, H. A., W. E. Mitch. 1998. Catabolism in uremia: the impact of metabolic acidosis. *Journal of the American Society of Nephrology* 9:S78–81.

Macdonald, H. M., et al. 2005. Low dietary potassium intakes and high dietary estimates of net endogenous acid production are associated with low bone mineral density in premenopausal women and increased markers of bone resorption in postmenopausal women. *American Journal of Clinical Nutrition* 81(4):923–33.

Marlett, J., and T. Cheung. 1997. Database and quick methods of assessing typical dietary fiber intakes using data for 228 commonly consumed foods. *Journal of the American Dietetic Association* 97:1139–47.

Medscape Today News. Accessed online August 8, 2013 at http://www.medscape.com/viewarticle/807615?nlid=31982_1049&src=wnl_edit_dail&uac=130325DZ.

Reddy, S. T., et al. 2002. Effect of low-carbohydrate high-protein diets on acid-base balance, stone-forming propensity, and calcium metabolism. *American Journal of Kidney Diseases* 40(2):265–74.

Ringsdorf, W., E. Cheraskin, and R. Ramsay. 1976. Sucrose, neutrophilic phagocytosis, and resistance to disease. *Dental Survey* 52:46–48.

Rudin, D. O., and C. Felix. 1987. *The Omega 3 Phenomenon*. New York: Rawlinson Associates.

Schernhammer, E. S., et al. 2012. Consumption of artificial sweetener– and sugar-containing soda and risk of lymphoma and leukemia in men and women. *American Journal of Clinical Nutrition* 96:1419–28.

Sebastian, A., Frassetto L. A., Morris R. C. 2007. "The Acid-Base Effects of the Contemporary Western Diet: An Evolutionary Perspective," in *Seldin and Giebisch's The Kidney: Physiology & Pathophysiology* (4th ed.). Ed. Alpern and Hebert. Waltham, MA: Academic Press. 1621–44.

Skinner, J. D., et al. 1999. Longitudinal study of nutrient and food intakes of white preschool children aged 24 to 60 months. *Journal of the American Dietetic Association* 99(12):1514–21.

Smith, B. 1993. Organic foods versus supermarket foods. Element levels. *Journal of Applied Nutrition* 45:35–39.

Fasting

Fasting has been used for thousands of years as a medical therapy to help the body detoxify and rejuvenate from all kinds of health problems. It is defined as voluntarily not eating food for various lengths of time. Many of the world's oldest systems of health relied upon fasting for healing and as a way to prevent disease. The father of Western medicine, Hippocrates, found that fasting helped the body to heal itself, and he extolled its tremendous healing potential in his writings. Most world religions have used fasting as a way to improve physical and spiritual clarity. The Bible makes frequent references to the benefits of fasting, combined with prayer. Currently, fasting is becoming a more accepted method of detoxification for health practitioners throughout North America.

How Does Fasting Work?

The primary way in which fasting is beneficial is by simply giving the body time to rest. Specifically, the digestive organs are given a break from digesting food. A tremendous amount of energy is required for digestion, and the body can use this "saved" energy for healing and regeneration. In addition, a time of fasting prevents more toxic substances from entering the body and simultaneously allows for the expulsion of toxins. This is particularly true for the liver, which has to break down and metabolize all the toxic substances that enter the body. In addition, the immune system is also given a break from dealing with toxins from our food and water supply, as well as from our environment.

During the first day of a fast, the body burns stored sugar, known as glycogen. After this, the body begins to burn fat for fuel. There is one exception, though, and this occurs with the brain, which requires blood sugar. During the second day of a fast, some muscle tissue may be broken down into amino acids, which are converted by the liver into glucose to feed the brain. During the second to third day of fasting, the body goes into what is called ketosis. During this state, the liver converts stored fat into chemicals called ketones, which can be used by the brain, the heart, and the muscles for energy. Generally, during this period of time, people lose their hunger pains and have increased energy and a heightened sense of awareness, which often includes clarity of the mind and the spirit. People may lose up to two pounds a day during this stage. As fat is increasingly burned for fuel, stored toxins (such as pesticides and other chemicals) are released into the bloodstream, to be metabolized by the liver and the kidneys. (Bear in mind, however, we do not advocate fasting as a weight-loss protocol.)

Length of a Fast

The length of a fast really depends on a person's health. The healthier one is, the longer one can fast. Many practitioners recommend two- to three-day fasts with each change of the season. More commonly, a spring fast is recommended to cleanse the body of toxins that accumulated during the dormant winter season. Some people enjoy preventative fasts of one day per week.

The most basic fast is the water fast, in which you consume only water for a specified amount of time. This is the most aggressive type of fast and is best used by people in good health or those who are experienced in fasting. If you are trying it for the first time, it is recommended that you start with just one day. You should consume at least 80 ounces of clean, quality water daily. People who are more experienced at fasting may drink only water for up to five days.

Juice fasts are also very popular. They are not as intense as a water fast because the naturally occurring sugars from vegetable and fruit juices prevent ketosis from occurring. Common juices include carrot, lemon, apple, beet, celery, and various greens, such as wheatgrass, spirulina, barley grass, and other super green foods. You should consume approximately 64 ounces of fresh juices daily. This type of fasting is indicated for people who are fasting for the first time or for those who cannot take time out of their schedules for a more intense fast.

Getting Started

It is important to start and stop a fast properly. The best way to start is to gradually decrease the amount of food consumed three days before the fast. Also, you should avoid heavier foods, such as dairy products and meats. The day before the fast, your diet should consist of easily digested foods, such as light salads, fresh soups, fruits, and herbal teas.

A Good Ending

The end of the fast should be similar to the days before you began the fast. You should transition to light foods for a few days and then gradually incorporate heavier foods. Remember to keep drinking plenty of water, because detoxification will still be occurring.

Safety

A fast lasting longer than three days should be supervised by a medical doctor or a naturopathic physician. People with blood-sugar problems, such as hypoglycemia or diabetes, should consult with a doctor before starting any fast. This is also true of any other systemic disease you may have.

It is not uncommon for people to experience symptoms of detoxification during a fast. These can include fatigue, headache, bad breath, nausea, skin rash, or feeling as if they have the flu or a cold. These symptoms should clear up as the fast progresses beyond the second or third day.

It is important to get plenty of rest during a fast. Exercise should be very light, as should mental activities. In all, you should choose a fast that is most suitable to your particular needs and health. Fasting truly is nature's way of cleansing and regenerating the body.

Nutritional Supplements

Nutritional supplements have become regular items in the households of most Americans. For decades, people have intuitively known that deficiencies of nutrients contribute to poor vitality and disease. Holistic doctors such as ourselves have seen the difference that nutritional supplements can make in the prevention and the treatment of most health conditions.

To the detriment of the public, most conventional doctors in the past have had little support for the use of these nontoxic nutrients. Fortunately, times are changing. Two decades ago, the prestigious *Journal of the American Medical Association* (JAMA) advised that there was no evidence that healthy people would benefit from taking multivitamins. In June 2002, JAMA published an article that was a complete turnaround on the use of nutritional supplements. The authors of the study concluded that vitamin deficiency was an apparent cause of chronic diseases. Considering that only 20 percent of the population consumes the recommended minimum servings of fruits and vegetables each day, nutritional deficiencies are undoubtedly a widespread problem. Added to this is the fact that pharmaceutical medications, pollution, high stress levels, nutrient-depleted soils, and refined and packaged foods all contribute to nutritional deficiencies.

This chapter and the protocols in this book go well beyond general recommendations for nutritional supplements. We have provided not only the minimal doses people should strive for (such as the RDA) but also the optimal dosages to prevent diseases and deficiencies. In the conditions sections, we give the therapeutic amounts for each nutritional supplement, as well as the exact type to use to optimize your results.

Vitamins and Minerals

WHAT ARE VITAMINS?

A vitamin is an organic substance that is essential (i.e., vital) for life. Most vitamins cannot be synthesized in the body and so must be obtained from the diet or supplements. Vitamins fall into two main groups. Fat-soluble vitamins require a certain amount of fat to be absorbed. They are also stored longer in the body. Common examples of fat-soluble vitamins include vitamins A, D, K, and E. The second major group of vitamins is termed water-soluble. Vitamins in this group do not need fat to be absorbed and are excreted out of the body much more readily than fat-soluble vitamins are. Vitamins C and B are water-soluble.

WHAT ARE MINERALS?

Minerals are inorganic substances that are important components of tissues and fluids. They are necessary for the proper functioning of vitamins, enzymes, hormones, and other metabolic activities in the body. Minerals compose 4 percent of the body's weight. Most minerals, such as calcium, phosphorous, and magnesium, are found in the bones. Some minerals are required in minute amounts; these are called trace minerals. Chromium is an example of a trace mineral, because it is required in micrograms (1/100th of a milligram), as opposed to minerals like calcium, which are required in milligrams.

DOSAGE RECOMMENDATIONS

The Dietary Reference Intakes (DRI) are issued by the Food and Nutrition Board of the National Academy of Science. The Dietary Reference Intakes refer to four nutrient reference values that can be used to assess diet, as well as for other purposes. The DRIs are a replacement for the well-known RDAs (Recommended Dietary Allowances) of the United States, which have been published since 1941 by the National Academy of Sciences, and the RNIs (Recommended Nutrient Intakes) of Canada. These values are the collaborative work of the Standing Committee on the Scientific Evaluation of Dietary Reference Intakes of the Food and Nutrition Board, the Institute of Medicine, the National Academy of Sciences, and Health Canada. Unlike the RDAs, which establish the minimal amounts of nutrients required to protect against possible deficiencies, the new DRIs are designed to reflect a more modern understanding of nutrient requirements, to optimize health in people and groups of people.

The DRIs are comprised of four reference values. These include the RDA and three other values:

Recommended Daily Allowance (RDA): The average daily dietary intake level that is sufficient to meet the nutrient requirement of nearly all (97 to 98 percent) healthy individuals in a group. In other words, the RDA is the amount of vitamins and minerals that a healthy person requires to stay healthy. These amounts will prevent obvious vitamin deficiencies, such as scurvy and rickets. However, these values are really quite conservative, and most nutritionally trained doctors like ourselves feel that they are generally too low for optimal health.

Adequate Intake (AI): A value based on observed or experimentally determined approximations of nutrient intake by a group (or groups) of healthy people. Used when an RDA cannot be determined.

Tolerable Upper Intake Level (UL): The highest level of daily nutrient intake that is likely to pose no risk of adverse health effects to almost all individuals in the general population. As intake increases above UL, the risk of adverse effects increases.

Estimated Average Requirement (EAR): A nutrient intake value that is estimated to meet the requirement of half the healthy individuals in a group.

Note: In our discussion of each vitamin and mineral we have included our own adult Optimal Intake reference ranges. The Optimal Intake references are our estimates of the dosages of vitamins and minerals that provide the best chance of bringing about optimal health and not just the prevention of disease.

VITAMINS IN DETAIL

Dietary Reference Intakes (DRIs): Recommended Dietary Allowances and Adequate Intakes, Vitamins
Food and Nutrition Board, Institute of Medicine, National Academies

Life Stage Group	Vitamin A (µg/d)[a]	Vitamin C (mg/d)	Vitamin D (µg/d)[b,c]	Vitamin E (mg/d)[d]	Vitamin K (µg/d)	Thiamin (mg/d)	Riboflavin (mg/d)	Niacin (mg/d)[e]	Vitamin B6 (mg/d)	Folate (µg/d)[f]	Vitamin B12 (µg/d)	Pantothenic Acid (mg/d)	Biotin (µg/d)	Choline (mg/d)[g]
Infants														
0 to 6 mo	400*	40*	10	4*	2.0*	0.2*	0.3*	2*	0.1*	65*	0.4*	1.7*	5*	125*
6 to 12 mo	500*	50*	10	5*	2.5*	0.3*	0.4*	4*	0.3*	80*	0.5*	1.8*	6*	150*
Children														
1–3 y	**300**	**15**	**15**	**6**	30*	**0.5**	**0.5**	**6**	**0.5**	**150**	**0.9**	2*	8*	200*
4–8 y	**400**	**25**	**15**	**7**	55*	**0.6**	**0.6**	**8**	**0.6**	**200**	**1.2**	3*	12*	250*
Males														
9–13 y	**600**	**45**	**15**	**11**	60*	**0.9**	**0.9**	**12**	**1.0**	**300**	**1.8**	4*	20*	375*
14–18 y	**900**	**75**	**15**	**15**	75*	**1.2**	**1.3**	**16**	**1.3**	**400**	**2.4**	5*	25*	550*
19–30 y	**900**	**90**	**15**	**15**	120*	**1.2**	**1.3**	**16**	**1.3**	**400**	**2.4**	5*	30*	550*
31–50 y	**900**	**90**	**15**	**15**	120*	**1.2**	**1.3**	**16**	**1.3**	**400**	**2.4**	5*	30*	550*
51–70 y	**900**	**90**	**15**	**15**	120*	**1.2**	**1.3**	**16**	**1.7**	**400**	**2.4**[h]	5*	30*	550*
>70 y	**900**	**90**	**20**	**15**	120*	**1.2**	**1.3**	**16**	**1.7**	**400**	**2.4**[h]	5*	30*	550*
Females														
9–13 y	**600**	**45**	**15**	**11**	60*	**0.9**	**0.9**	**12**	**1.0**	**300**	**1.8**	4*	20*	375*
14–18 y	**700**	**65**	**15**	**15**	75*	**1.0**	**1.0**	**14**	**1.2**	**400**[i]	**2.4**	5*	25*	400*
19–30 y	**700**	**75**	**15**	**15**	90*	**1.1**	**1.1**	**14**	**1.3**	**400**[i]	**2.4**	5*	30*	425*
31–50 y	**700**	**75**	**15**	**15**	90*	**1.1**	**1.1**	**14**	**1.3**	**400**[i]	**2.4**	5*	30*	425*
51–70 y	**700**	**75**	**15**	**15**	90*	**1.1**	**1.1**	**14**	**1.5**	**400**	**2.4**[h]	5*	30*	425*
>70 y	**700**	**75**	**20**	**15**	90*	**1.1**	**1.1**	**14**	**1.5**	**400**	**2.4**[h]	5*	30*	425*
Pregnancy														
14–18 y	**750**	**80**	**15**	**15**	75*	**1.4**	**1.4**	**18**	**1.9**	**600**[i]	**2.6**	6*	30*	450*
19–30 y	**770**	**85**	**15**	**15**	90*	**1.4**	**1.4**	**18**	**1.9**	**600**[i]	**2.6**	6*	30*	450*
31–50 y	**770**	**85**	**15**	**15**	90*	**1.4**	**1.4**	**18**	**1.9**	**600**[i]	**2.6**	6*	30*	450*
Lactation														
14–18 y	**1,200**	**115**	**15**	**19**	75*	**1.4**	**1.6**	**17**	**2.0**	**500**	**2.8**	7*	35*	550*
19–30 y	**1,300**	**120**	**15**	**19**	90*	**1.4**	**1.6**	**17**	**2.0**	**500**	**2.8**	7*	35*	550*
31–50 y	**1,300**	**120**	**15**	**19**	90*	**1.4**	**1.6**	**17**	**2.0**	**500**	**2.8**	7*	35*	550*

NOTE: This table (taken from the DRI reports, see www.nap.edu) presents Recommended Dietary Allowances (RDAs) in **bold type** and Adequate Intakes (AIs) in ordinary type followed by an asterisk (*). An RDA is the average daily dietary intake level; sufficient to meet the nutrient requirements of nearly all (97-98 percent) healthy individuals in a group. It is calculated from an Estimated Average Requirement (EAR). If sufficient scientific evidence is not available to establish an EAR, and thus calculate an RDA, an AI is usually developed. For healthy breastfed infants, an AI is the mean intake. The AI for other life stage and gender groups is believed to cover the needs of all healthy individuals in the groups, but lack of data or uncertainty in the data prevent being able to specify with confidence the percentage of individuals covered by this intake.

[a] As retinol activity equivalents (RAEs). 1 RAE = 1 µg retinol, 12 µg β-carotene, 24 µg α-carotene, or 24 µg β-cryptoxanthin. The RAE for dietary provitamin A carotenoids is two-fold greater than retinol equivalents (RE), whereas the RAE for preformed vitamin A is the same as RE.

[b] As cholecalciferol. 1 µg cholecalciferol = 40 IU vitamin D.

[c] Under the assumption of minimal sunlight.

[d] As α-Tocopherol. α-Tocopherol includes *RRR*-α-tocopherol, the only form of α-tocopherol that occurs naturally in foods, and the *2R*-stereoisomeric forms of α-tocopherol (*RRR*-, *RSR*-, *RRS*-, and *RSS*-α-tocopherol) that occur in fortified foods and supplements. It does not include the *2S*-stereoisomeric forms of α-tocopherol (*SRR*-, *SSR*-, *SRS*-, and *SSS*-α-tocopherol), also found in fortified foods and supplements.

[e] As niacin equivalents (NE). 1 mg of niacin = 60 mg of tryptophan; 0–6 months = preformed niacin (not NE).

[f] As dietary folate equivalents (DFE). 1 DFE = 1 µg food folate = 0.6 µg of folic acid from fortified food or as a supplement consumed with food = 0.5 µg of a supplement taken on an empty stomach.

[g] Although AIs have been set for choline, there are few data to assess whether a dietary supply of choline is needed at all stages of the life cycle, and it may be that the choline requirement can be met by endogenous synthesis at some of these stages.

[h] Because 10 to 30 percent of older people may malabsorb food-bound B₁₂, it is advisable for those older than 50 years to meet their RDA mainly by consuming foods fortified with B₁₂ or a supplement containing B₁₂.

[i] In view of evidence linking folate intake with neural tube defects in the fetus, it is recommended that all women capable of becoming pregnant consume 400 µg from supplements or fortified foods in addition to intake of food folate from a varied diet.

Vitamin A (Retinol, Retinal)

DRIs:

0 to 6 months: 1,332 IU/d

6 to 12 months: 1,665 IU/d

1–3 years: 1,000 IU/d (2,000 IU upper limit)

4–8 years: 1,300 IU/d (3,000 IU upper limit)

9–13 years: 2,000 IU/d (5,666 IU upper limit)

14–18 years: 1,000 IU/d (9,333 IU upper limit)

Adult male: 3,000 IU/d (10,000 IU upper limit)

Adult female: 2,300 IU/d (10,000 IU upper limit)

Pregnancy: 2,564 IU/d

Lactation: 4,330 IU/d

Note: One RE (retinol equivalent) = 3.33 IU (International Units)

Function: Vision; growth and development; strengthens immune system—especially respiratory tract and mucus membranes; antioxidant.

Sources: Liver, chili peppers, carrots, vitamin A–fortified milk, butter, sweet potatoes, parsley, kale, spinach, mangoes, broccoli, squash.

Optimal Intake: Adult men: 5,000 IU (1,000 RE)

Adult women: 2,500 IU (500 RE)

Deficiency Signs: Night blindness, infectious disease susceptibility, follicular hyperkeratosis (bumps on the skin—mainly, the back of the upper arm, the shoulders, the neck, the buttocks, and the lower abdomen), faulty tooth and bone formation, impaired growth.

Toxicity: Overdoses of vitamin A can produce symptoms of vomiting, joint pain, abdominal pain, bone abnormalities, cracking, dry skin, headache, irritability, and fatigue. Symptoms disappear after supplementation has been discontinued. Pregnant women or those with liver disease should avoid vitamin A supplementation dosages above 2,500 IU (500 RE).

Carotenoids (Carotenes)

Examples of carotenoids include beta carotene, alpha carotene, gamma carotene, beta zeacarotene, cryptoxanthin, lycopene, zeaxanthin, lutein, canthaxanthin, crocetin, capsanthin.

DRIs: None established.

Function: There are over six hundred identified carotenoids. Approximately fifty act as precursors to vitamin A. Carotenoids are potent antioxidants, help with immune function, and are involved with the growth and the repair of tissues.

Sources: Yellow vegetables (carrots, pumpkins, squash, sweet potatoes); green vegetables (broccoli, peas, collard greens, endive, kale, lettuce, peppers, spinach, turnip greens); fruits (apricots, cantaloupe, papaya, peaches, watermelon, cherries, tomatoes).

Optimal Intake: 5,000 to 25,000 IU of mixed carotenoids.

Deficiency Signs: Increased susceptibility to developing certain cancers and cardiovascular disease.

Toxicity: Relatively nontoxic. Too high an intake can lead to carotenemia (yellowing of skin), which disappears after reduction of carotenoid intake.

Vitamin D (Vitamin D2-Ergocalciferol, Vitamin D3-Cholecalciferol)

DRIs:

0 to 12 months: 400 IU/d

1–70 years: 600 IU/d

70+ years: 800 IU/d

Pregnancy: 600 IU/d

Lactation: 600 IU/d

D2—derived from plant sources

D3—derived from animal sources

Function: It promotes calcium and phosphorous absorption from intestines, increases calcium deposition into bones, mobilizes calcium and phosphorous from bones. It prevents certain cancers and is required for proper thyroid function.

Sources: Cod liver oil, cold-water fish (salmon, herring, sardines, mackerel), milk (fortified with vitamin D), egg yolk, small amounts in dark-green leafy vegetables and mushrooms. Sunlight is converted into vitamin D.

Optimal Intake: 2,000 to 5,000 IU.

Deficiency Signs: Rickets—softening of the skull bones, bowing of the legs, spinal curvature, a contracted pelvis, abnormal enlargement of the head, and an increased joint space; delayed tooth eruption; osteoporosis.

Toxicity: Nausea, anorexia, weakness, headache, digestive disturbance, kidney damage, calcification of soft tissues, and hypercalcemia.

Vitamin K (Phylloquinone, Menaquinone)

DRIs:

0 to 6 months: 2 mcg/d

6 to 12 months: 2.5 mcg/d

1–3 years: 30 mcg/d

4–8 years: 55 mcg/d

9–13 years: 60 mcg/d

14–18 years: 75 mcg/d

Adult male: 120 mcg/d

Adult female: 90 mcg/d

Pregnancy: 90 mcg/d

Lactation: 90 mcg/d

Phylloquinone—K1, derived from plants

Menaquinone—K2, derived from gut bacteria

Menadione—K3, derived synthetically

Function: Blood clotting, bone formation, antioxidant.

Sources: Dark-green leafy vegetables, parsley, broccoli, cabbage, spinach, soy, egg yolks, liver, legumes, and synthesized by intestinal bacteria.

Optimal Intake: 50 to 500 mcg.

Deficiency Signs: Blood-clotting problems, osteoporosis, menstrual cramps.

Toxicity: Hemolytic anemia.

Natural vitamin E has been shown to have significantly greater bioavailability than synthetic vitamin E. Make sure to look for natural forms of vitamin E, listed as d-alpha-tocopherol, as opposed to synthetic, which is listed as dl-alpha-tocopherol.

Vitamin E-Complex (Tocopherol, Tocotrienols)

DRIs:

0 to 6 months: 4 IU/d

6 to 12 months: 5 IU/d

1–3 years: 6 IU/d

4–8 years: 7 IU/d

9–13 years: 11 IU/d

14–18 years: 15 IU/d

Adults: 15 IU/d

Pregnancy: 15 IU/d

Lactation: 19 IU/d

Includes alpha, beta, and gamma tocopherol, as well as tocotrienols. Most supplements refer to alpha-tocopherol.

Function: Antioxidant, immunity, wound healing, red blood cell formation, estrogen metabolism, nerve health.

Sources: Vegetable oils, seeds, nuts, brown rice, and whole grains.

Optimal Intake: 400 IU.

Deficiency Signs: Severe deficiency is rare. Dry skin, hemolytic anemia of newborns, muscle and neurological disorders.

Vitamin B1 (Thiamin)

DRIs:

0 to 6 months: 0.2 mg/d

6 to 12 months: 0.3 mg/d

1–3 years: 0.5 mg/d

4–8 years: 0.6 mg/d

9–13 years: 0.9 mg/d

14 years–adult male: 1.2 mg/d

14 years–adult female: 1.1 mg/d

Pregnant or lactating: 1.4 mg/d

Function: Energy metabolism (carbohydrate metabolism), neurological activity, brain and heart function.

Sources: Pork, beef, liver, brewer's yeast, whole grains, brown rice, legumes.

Optimal Intake: 5 to 10 mg.

Deficiency Signs: Beriberi, a condition characterized by fatigue, anorexia, weight loss, gastrointestinal disorders, fluid retention, weakness, heart abnormalities, stunted growth, cyanosis, convulsions, poor memory.

Toxicity: None reported.

Vitamin B2 (Riboflavin)

DRIs:

0 to 6 months: 0.3 mg/d

6 to 12 months: 0.4 mg/d

1–3 years: 0.5 mg/d

4–8 years: 0.6 mg/d

9–13 years: 0.9 mg/d

14 years–18 female: 1 mg/d

14 years–adult male: 1.3 mg/d

19 years–adult female: 1.1 mg/d

Pregnancy: 1.4 mg/d

Lactation: 1.6 mg/d

Function: Energy production, fatty acid and amino acid synthesis.

Sources: Organ meats such as liver, milk products, whole grains, green leafy vegetables, eggs, mushrooms, broccoli, asparagus, fish.

Optimal Intake: 10 to 15 mg.

Deficiency Signs: Cracking at the corners of the mouth, inflamed tongue, reddening of the eyes, vision problems, dermatitis, nerve damage, decreased neurotransmitter production, malformations and retarded growth in children and infants.

Toxicity: None reported.

Vitamin B3 (Niacin)

DRIs:

0 to 6 months: 2 mg/d

6 to 12 months: 4 mg/d

1–3 years: 6 mg/d

4–8 years: 8 mg/d

9–13 years: 12 mg/d

14 years–adult male: 16 mg/d

14 years–adult female: 14 mg/d

Pregnancy: 18 mg/d

Lactation: 17 mg/d

Function: Energy production, formation of steroid compounds, red blood cell formation, cognitive function and mood.

Sources: Organ meats, peanuts, fish, yeast, poultry, legumes, milk, eggs, whole grains, orange juice.

Optimal Intake: 50 to 100 mg.

Deficiency Signs: Pellagra, a condition characterized by dermatitis, diarrhea, dementia; depression, schizophrenia, weakness, lassitude, anorexia.

Toxicity: Large doses can cause dilation of the blood vessels and flushing of the skin. Time-released niacin products may result in liver enzyme elevation.

Vitamin B5 (Pantothenic Acid)

DRIs:

0 to 6 months: 1.7 mg/d

6 to 12 months: 1.8 mg/d

1–3 years: 2 mg/d

4–8 years: 3 mg/d

9–13 years: 4 mg/d

14 years–adult: 5 mg/d

Pregnancy: 6 mg/d

Lactation: 7 mg/d

Function: Metabolism of carbohydrates, proteins, and fats for energy production; production of adrenal hormones and red blood cells.

Sources: Organ meats, fish, chicken, eggs, cheese, whole grains, avocados, cauliflower, sweet potatoes, oranges, strawberries, yeast, legumes.

Optimal Intake: 50 to 100 mg.

Deficiency Signs: Numbness and shooting pains in the feet; fatigue.

Toxicity: None reported.

Vitamin B6 (Pyridoxine)

DRIs:

0 to 6 months: 0.1 mg/d

6 to 12 months: 0.3 mg/d

1–3 years: 0.5 mg/d

4–8 years: 0.6 mg/d

9–13 years: 1 mg/d

14–30 years, male: 1.3 mg/d

51 years +, male: 1.7 mg/d

14–18 years, female: 1.2 mg/d

19–50 years, female: 1.3 mg/d

51+ years, female: 1.5 mg/d

Pregnancy: 1.9 mg/d

Lactation: 2 mg/d

Function: Formation of body proteins, neurotransmitters, red blood cells; immunity.

Sources: Meats, poultry, egg yolk, soy, peanuts, bananas, potatoes, whole grains, cauliflower.

Optimal Intake: 10 to 25 mg.

Deficiency Signs: Mood abnormalities, sleep problems, anemia, impairment of nerve function, eczema, cracking of the lips and the tongue, premenstrual syndrome, depression.

Toxicity: Very high dosages can cause nerve symptoms—numbness and tingling.

Folate (Folic acid, Methylfolate)

DRIs:

0 to 6 months: 65 mcg/d

6 to 12 months: 80 mcg/d

1–3 years: 150 mcg/d

4–8 years: 200 mcg/d

9–13 years: 300 mcg/d

14 years–adult: 400 mcg/d

Pregnancy: 600 mcg/d

Lactation: 500 mcg/d

Function: Prevents neural tube defects (must be taken by the mother in early pregnancy). Methyl donor is required for many processes in the body (reduces homocysteine levels). Cardiovascular health. Red blood cell production. Skin and nail health.

Sources: Dark-green vegetables—spinach, kale, broccoli, asparagus—as well as organ meats, kidney beans, beets, yeast, orange juice, whole grains.

Optimal Intake: 400 to 800 mcg.

Deficiency Signs: Macrocytic anemia, fatigue, irritability, weakness, weight loss, anorexia, dyspnea, sore tongue, palpitations, forgetfulness, digestive upset, diarrhea.

The risk of bearing a child with a common birth defect known as a neural tube defect is reduced by 60 percent if a 400 mcg folic acid supplement is taken daily by the mother one month prior to conception and through the first trimester. It also decreases the risk of limb and urinary defects. The optimal form of folate is L-5 methyl tetrahydrofolate.

Intresting Facts: Even though folic acid is added to many foods, folic acid deficiency is the most common vitamin deficiency in the world. The activated, natural form of folic acid is available in supplement form. It is known as L-5 methyl tetrahydrofolate.

Toxicity: None.

Vitamin B12 (Cobalamin)

DRIs:

0 to 6 months: 0.4 mcg/d

6 to 12 months: 0.5 mcg/d

1–3 years: 0.9 mcg/d

4–8 years: 1.2 mcg/d

9–13 years: 1.8 mcg/d

14 years–adult 2.4 mcg/d

Pregnancy: 2.6 mcg/d

Lactation: 2.8 mcg/d

Function: Synthesis of DNA, red blood cells; nerve development.

Sources: Gut bacteria synthesis, organ meats, clams, oysters, soy, milk products, cheese, chlorella, spirulina.

Optimal Intake: 50 to 200 mcg.

Deficiency Signs: Macrocytic anemia; glossitis; spinal cord degeneration; digestive upset; fatigue; mental abnormalities, including irritability, depression.

Toxicity: None reported.

Biotin

DRIs:

0 to 6 months: 5 mcg/d

6 to 12 months: 6 mcg/d

1–3 years: 8 mcg/d

4–8 years: 12 mcg/d

9–13 years: 20 mcg/d

14–18 years: 25 mcg/d

Adults: 30 mcg/d

Pregnancy: 30 mcg/d

Lactation: 35 mcg/d

Function: Metabolism of fats, proteins, and carbohydrates; nail and hair growth.

Sources: Gut bacterial synthesis, organ meats, cheese, soybeans, eggs, mushrooms, whole wheat, peanuts.

Optimal Intake: 300 mcg.

Deficiency Signs: Seborrheic dermatitis (cradle cap) and hair loss in infants; brittle nails and hair.

Toxicity: None reported.

Vitamin C (Ascorbic Acid)

DRIs:

0 to 6 months: 40 mg/d

6 to 12 months: 50 mg/d

1–3 years: 15 mg/d

4–8 years: 25 mg/d

9–13 years: 45 mg/d

14–18 years, male: 75 mg/d

14–18 years, female: 65 mg/d

Adult male: 90 mg/d

Adult female: 75 mg/d

Pregnancy: 80–85 mg/d

Lactation: 115–120 mg/d

Function: Antioxidant, immunity, collagen formation, bone development, cancer prevention and treatment, gum health, hormone and amino acid synthesis, adrenal-gland hormones, wound healing.

Sources: Citrus fruits, tomatoes, green peppers, dark-green leafy vegetables, broccoli, cantaloupe, strawberries, brussels sprouts, potatoes, asparagus.

Optimal Intake: 500 to 1,500 mg.

Deficiency Signs: Scurvy (rare in North America), signs of which include bleeding gums, poor wound healing, joint tenderness and swelling, recurrent infections, and profuse bruising.

Toxicity: The first symptom of too much vitamin C is generally diarrhea, which disappears when the dosage is reduced.

Choline

DRIs:

0 to 6 months: 125 mg/d

6 to 12 months: 150 mg/d

1–3 years: 200 mg/d

4–8 years: 250 mg/d

9–13 years: 375 mg/d

14–70+ years, male: 550 mg/d

14–18 years, female: 400 mg/d

19–70+ years, female: 425 mg/d

Pregnancy: 450 mcg/d

Lactation: 550 mcg/d

Function: Required to manufacture the neurotransmitter acetylcholine; metabolism of fats. Choline isn't technically considered a vitamin, but it is an essential micronutrient, and it's usually grouped with the vitamins because it works in concert with many of them.

Sources: Grains, legumes, egg yolks, and soy.

Optimal Intake: 500 mg.

Deficiency Signs: Potential liver and kidney dysfunction.

Toxicity: Rare, but symptoms of fishy breath, sweating, salivation, low blood pressure, and liver toxicity.

MINERALS IN DETAIL

Calcium

DRIs:

0 to 6 months: 200 mg/d

An 8-ounce glass of milk contains 300 mg of calcium. The absorption of calcium from milk is 25 to 30 percent. Therefore, about 75 mg of calcium are actually absorbed. Calcium-enriched plant milks are readily available. Examples include coconut, hempseed, rice, almond, hazelnut, and cashew.

6 to 12 months: 260 mg/d

1–3 years: 700 mg/d

4–8 years: 1,000 mg/d

9–18 years: 1,300 mg/d

18–30 years: 1,000 mg/d

31–50 years: 1,000 mg/d

51–70 years, male: 1,000 mg/d

70 years and older, male: 1,200 mg

51 years and older, female: 1,200 mg

Pregnancy: 1,000 mg/d

Lactation: 1,000 mg/d

Function: Bone and tooth formation, muscle contraction, heartbeat, blood clotting, and nerve impulse.

Sources: Kelp, cheese, collards, kale, turnip greens, almonds, yogurt, milk, broccoli, and soy.

Optimal Intake: 1,000 to 1,500 mg.

Deficiency Signs: Bone deformity (rickets), growth retardation, insomnia, muscle and leg cramps.

Toxicity: Normally, there are no toxic effects with large doses. Some researchers believe that people with a tendency to develop kidney stones should avoid high doses of calcium, although this has not been proven.

Magnesium

DRIs:

0 to 6 months: 30 mg/d

6 to 12 months: 75 mg/d

1–3 years: 80 mg/d

4–8 years: 130 mg/d

9–13 years: 240 mg/d

14–18 years, male: 410 mg/d

14–18 years, female: 360 mg/d

19–30 years, male: 400 mg/d

31 years and older, male: 420 mg/d

19–30 years, female: 310 mg/d

31 years and older, female: 320 mg/d

Pregnancy: 350–360 mg/d

Lactation: 310–320/d

Function: Bone and teeth formation, energy production, glucose metabolism, muscle and nerve impulses.

Sources: Whole grains, nuts, legumes, soy, green leafy vegetables.

Optimal Intake: 400 to 600 mg.

Deficiency Signs: Weakness, confusion, mood changes, muscle spasms/tremors, nausea, poor coordination, heart disturbances, insomnia, susceptibility to kidney stones.

Toxicity: People with kidney disease or on heart medications should not supplement magnesium unless instructed to do so by their doctor. Diarrhea is usually the first symptom of too much magnesium.

Phosphorus
DRIs:
0 to 6 months: 100 mg/d
6 to 12 months: 275 mg/d
1–3 years: 460 mg/d
4–8 years: 500 mg/d
9–18 years: 1,250 mg/d
18–70+ years: 700 mg/d
Pregnancy: 700 mg/d
Lactation: 700 mg/d

Function: Growth, bone production, energy production, kidney function.

Sources: Meats, fish, eggs, poultry, milk products.

Optimal Intake: 800 to 1,200 mg.

Deficiency Signs: Deficiency is very rare. Symptoms may include muscle cramps, bone abnormalities, and dizziness.

Toxicity: Too much phosphorus in the form of phosphoric acid leads to urinary calcium excretion.

Potassium
DRIs:
0 to 6 months: 0.4 g/d
6 to 12 months: 0.7 g/d
1–3 years: 3 g/d
4–8 years: 3.8 g/d
9–13 years: 4.5 g/d
14–70+ years: 4.7 g/d
Pregnancy: 4.7 g/d
Lactation: 5.1 g/d

Function: Nerve transmission, water balance, acid-base balance, heart function, kidney function, adrenal function.

Sources: Fruits and vegetables, especially apples, bananas, carrots, oranges, potatoes, tomatoes, cantaloupe, peaches, plums, strawberries; and meat, milk, fish.

Optimal Intake: 2,000 to 3,000 mg.

Deficiency Signs: Muscle wasting, weakness, and spasm; fatigue, mood changes, heart disturbances, nerve problems.

Toxicity: Impaired heart and kidney function; people with heart or kidney conditions or on blood pressure medication should not take potassium unless instructed to do so by a physician.

Sodium
DRIs:
0 to 6 months: 0.12 g/d
6 to 12 months: 0.37 g/d
1–3 years: 1 g/d
4–8 years: 1.2 g/d
9–70+ years: 1.5 g/d
Pregnancy: 1.5 g/d
Lactation: 1.5 g/d

Function: Acid-base balance, muscle contraction, nerve impulse, amino acid absorption.

Sources: Naturally occurring in meats, milk products, water, eggs, poultry, and fish; abundant in canned foods and other commercially processed foods.

Optimal Intake: 2,000 mg.

Deficiency Signs: Deficiency is very uncommon, except in the case of dehydration through profuse sweating or diarrhea. Symptoms can include muscle weakness and cramping, low blood pressure, muscle twitching, mental confusion, anorexia, and fainting.

Toxicity: High blood pressure, especially when potassium intake is low.

Manganese

DRIs:

0 to 6 months: 0.003 mg/d

6 to 12 months: 0.6 mg/d

1–3 years: 1.2 mg/d

4–8 years: 1.5 mg/d

9–13 years, male: 1.9 mg/d

9–13 years, female: 1.6 mg/d

14–18 years, male: 2.2 mg/d

14–18 years, female: 1.6 mg/d

19–70+ years, male: 2.3 mg/d

19–70+ years, female:1.8 mg/d

Pregnancy: 2 mg/d

Lactation: 2.6 mg/d

Function: Required for enzyme systems involved with energy production, blood sugar control, fatty acid synthesis, thyroid hormone function, connective tissue and bone formation, sprains and strains.

Sources: Liver, kidney, whole grains, nuts, spinach, green leafy vegetables.

Optimal Intake: 5 to 10 mg.

Deficiency Signs: No symptoms have been observed in humans. Animal studies show growth problems.

Toxicity: Too much manganese can interfere with iron absorption and can cause iron deficiency.

Chromium

DRIs:

0 to 6 months: 0.2 mg/d

6 to 12 months: 5.5 mg/d

1–3 years: 11 mg/d

4–8 years: 15 mg/d

9–13 years, male: 25 mg/d

9–13 years, female: 21 mg/d

14–18 years, male: 35 mg/d

14–18 years, female: 24 mg/d

19–70+ years, male: 30 mg/d

19–70+ years, female:25 mg/d

Pregnancy: 29 mg/d

Lactation: 44 mg/d

Function: Blood sugar control.

Sources: Whole grains, meats, potatoes, liver, brewer's yeast.

Optimal Intake: 200 mcg.

Deficiency Signs: Elevated blood sugar levels.

Toxicity: Chromium appears to be safe, with no major toxic side effects reported.

Copper

DRIs:

0 to 6 months: 0.2 mcg/d

6 to 12 months: 5.5 mcg/d

1–3 years: 11 mcg/d

4–8 years: 15 mcg/d

9–13 years, male: 25 mcg/d

9–13 years, female: 21 mcg/d

14–50 years, male: 35 mcg/d

14–18 years, female: 24 mcg/d

51 years and older, male: 30 mcg/d

19–50 years, female: 25 mcg/d

51 years and older, female: 20 mcg/d

Pregnancy: 30 mcg/d

Lactation: 45 mcg/d

Function: Collagen formation, red blood cell formation, bone formation, energy production, mental function, many other enzyme systems.

Sources: Whole grains, shellfish, nuts, eggs, poultry, organ meats, peas, dark-green leafy vegetables, legumes.

Deficiency Signs: Rare, but could include low immune function, poor collagen and connective tissue strength, bone and joint abnormalities, anemia.

Optimal Intake: 2 to 3 mg.

Toxicity: Nausea, vomiting, and dizziness.

Iron

DRIs:

0 to 6 months: 0.27 mg/d

6 to 12 months: 11 mg/d

1–3 years: 7 mg/d

4–8 years: 11 mg/d

9–13 years: 8 mg/d

14–18 years, male: 11 mg/d

14–18 years, female: 15 mg/d

19–50 years, male: 8 mg/d

19–50 years, female: 18 mg/d

51–70+ years: 8 mg/d

Pregnancy: 27 mg/d

Lactation: 9 mg/d

Function: Hemoglobin production to supply oxygen to cells, collagen synthesis, normal immune function.

Sources: Liver and organ meats, beef, legumes, dark-green leafy vegetables, kelp, blackstrap molasses.

Optimal Intake: Men—10 mg; women with a normal cycle or no cycle—10 mg; women with a heavy cycle—20 mg.

Deficiency Signs: Iron deficiency is characterized by fatigue, paleness, poor memory and concentration, developmental delays and behavioral disturbances, chronic colds, and weakened immunity, as well as a craving for indigestible materials (e.g., pencils, dirt, ice).

Iron sulfate, the most widely prescribed form of supplemental iron, can be constipating and irritating to the digestive tract. We recommend other forms, such as iron citrate, iron glycinate, and other types of chelated iron.

Toxicity: Too much iron is associated with an increased risk for developing heart disease and cancer. Acute iron poisoning in children can result in damage to the intestinal tract, liver failure, nausea and vomiting, shock, and death.

Selenium

DRIs:
0 to 6 months: 15 mcg/d
6 to 12 months: 20 mcg/d
1–3 years: 20 mcg/d
4–8 years: 30 mcg/d
9–13 years: 40 mcg/d
14 years–adult: 55 mcg/d
Pregnancy: 60 mcg/d
Lactation: 70 mcg/d

Function: Antioxidant, cancer prevention, immunity, thyroid function, development of the fetus during pregnancy.

Sources: Liver, kidney, meats, seafood. Grains and vegetables are good sources, but selenium content depends on the level in the soil where they are grown.

Optimal Intake: 200 mcg.

Deficiency Signs: Selenium deficiency is associated with an increased risk for heart disease, cancer, and poor immune function.

Toxicity: Teeth abnormalities, depression, nausea, and vomiting.

Iodine

DRIs:
0 to 6 months: 110 mcg/d
6 to 12 months: 130 mcg/d
1–8 years: 90 mcg/d
9–13 years: 120 mcg/d
14–70+ years: 150 mcg/d
Pregnancy: 220 mcg/d
Lactation: 290 mcg/d

Function: Required to manufacture the thyroid hormone.

Sources: Iodized salt and water; seafood; seaweeds, such as kelp.

Optimal Intake: 250 mcg.

Deficiency Signs: Goiter (enlargement of thyroid gland), fatigue, depression.

Toxicity: Too much iodine can interfere with thyroid activity (hypothyroid) and may cause acne eruptions.

Molybdenum

DRIs:
0 to 6 months: 2 mcg/d
6 to 12 months: 3 mcg/d
1–3 years: 17 mcg/d
4–8 years: 22 mcg/d
9–13 years: 34 mcg/d
14–18 years: 43 mcg/d
19–70+ years: 45 mcg
Pregnancy: 50 mcg/d
Lactation: 50 mcg/d

Function: Active in enzyme systems involved with the metabolism of alcohol, uric acid, and sulfur.

S ilicon has been shown in published studies to help bone, hair, and nail development.

Sources: Meats, whole-grain breads, legumes, leafy vegetables, organ meats, and brewer's yeast.

Optimal Intake: 200 mcg.

Deficiency Signs: None known, but the inability to detoxify sulfites (preservatives in foods) is reported.

Toxicity: None reported.

Silicon

DRIs: None given.

Function: Bone, cartilage, and ligament formation; skin elasticity.

Sources: Unrefined grains, cereals, and root vegetables.

Optimal Intake: 50 mg.

Deficiency Signs: None known, but brittle hair and nails are suspected.

Toxicity: Miners who were exposed to large dosages of silicon over a prolonged period of time have developed silicosis—a fibrotic formation of the lungs. The amounts found in foods and multivitamins appear to be very safe.

Vanadium

DRIs: None given.

Function: Blood sugar balance, bone and teeth development.

Sources: Shellfish, mushrooms, black pepper, and buckwheat.

Optimal Intake: 50 mg (as vanadyl sulfate form).

Deficiency Signs: None known, but blood sugar imbalances are suspected.

Toxicity: Little is known, but very high amounts may lead to cramps and diarrhea.

Zinc

DRIs:

0 to 6 months: 2 mg/d

6 to 12 months: 3 mg/d

1–3 years: 3 mg/d

4–8 years: 5 mg/d

9–13 years, female: 8 mg/d

14–18 years, female: 9 mg/d

19–70+ years, female: 8mg/d

14–70+ years, male: 11 mg/d

Pregnancy: 11 mg/d

Lactation: 12 mg/d

Function: Involved in over two hundred enzymatic reactions; required to manufacture many hormones; immunity; skin healing; growth; vision; blood sugar metabolism; antioxidant support; reproductive development and fertility.

Sources: Oysters, herring, shellfish, red meat, whole grains, legumes, and nuts.

Optimal Intake: 15 to 30 mg.

Deficiency Signs: Hair loss, poor wound healing, poor immune function, diarrhea, skin conditions (acne), mental disturbance, white spots on the nails.

Toxicity: Rare. Very high dosage (above 150 mg) can lead to immune-system suppression, digestive upset, or anemia.

Other Recommended Supplements

Alpha Lipoic Acid

Function: Antioxidant; energy production; potentiates the effects of vitamins C and E.

Sources: Liver, yeast, potatoes, spinach, red meat.

Optimal Intake: 50 to 100 mg.

Deficiency Signs: No specific symptoms given, but people with diabetes and diabetic neuropathy tend to benefit from supplementation.

Toxicity: None known.

Inositol

Function: Component of cell membranes; used to treat depression and to prevent complications of diabetes.

Sources: Citrus fruit, whole grains, nuts, seeds, and legumes.

Optimal Intake: 250 mg.

Deficiency Signs: None known.

Toxicity: None known.

Coenzyme Q10

Function: Antioxidant, heart activity, energy production.

Sources: Meat, seafood.

Optimal Intake: 30 to 100 mg.

Deficiency Signs: Gum disease, heart failure, fatigue, hypertension, atherosclerosis.

Toxicity: None known.

L-Carnitine

Function: Energy production, heart function, triglyceride metabolism.

Sources: Meat, dairy products.

Optimal Intake: 250 to 500 mg.

Deficiency Signs: Loss of muscle tone, recurrent infections, brain swelling, heart irregularities, high triglycerides, fatigue, and failure to thrive.

Toxicity: None.

CITATIONS

http://www.nal.usda.gov/fnic/DRI/DRI_Tables/recommended_intakes_individuals.pdf
http://lpi.oregonstate.edu/mic/vitamins/vitamin-A
https://www.consumerlab.com/RDAs/

Selecting Vitamins and Minerals

Make sure to purchase vitamins and minerals that are free of artificial sweeteners and preservatives or fillers. Work with a knowledgeable nutritional professional to select the highest-quality supplements. Most nutrients are available in tablet, capsule, powder, and liquid forms. Multivitamins should be taken with a meal for optimal absorption and to prevent digestive upset. If you are taking pharmaceutical medications, check with a holistic doctor to see which nutrients are known to be depleted by the drug(s) you are taking. Also, check to see if there are any possible adverse reactions between your medications and supplements.

Nutritional Supplement Guide

The following section lists common nutritional supplements you will find on the shelves of most health food stores, pharmacies, and grocery stores. These are in addition to the ones listed in the preceding section. We have included a brief description of each supplement, conditions that it is indicated for, precautions, and dosage recommendations. For information on vitamin, mineral, herbal, and homeopathic supplements, please see their corresponding sections.

Acetylcarnitine

Description: Acetylcarnitine is a modified form of the amino acid–like substance L-carnitine. The acetyl group allows this nutrient to be readily absorbed across the blood–brain barrier and is used to make the brain neurotransmitter acetylcholine. L-carnitine is used to transport fatty acids into the cell mitochondria for energy production. Acetylcarnitine allows for energy production within brain cells. This supplement is mainly used to enhance cognitive function. Studies have found that it delays the progression of early-stage Alzheimer's disease.

Indications:

Age-related cognitive decline	Down syndrome
Alzheimer's disease	Infertility (male)
Amenorrhea	Peripheral neuropathy
Depression	

Precautions: Side effects are uncommon, although skin rash, body odor, and digestive upset have been reported.

Dosage: Take 1,500 to 3,000 mg daily.

Acidophilus

Description: *Lactobacillus acidophilus* is known as a probiotic. It is a beneficial bacterium that inhabits several areas of the body, including the mouth, the throat, the lungs, the digestive tract, the urinary tract, and the vagina. Acidophilus produces substances called bacteriocins, which act as natural antibiotics to destroy harmful microorganisms or keep them in check. It also helps break down undigested fiber from fruits, vegetables, and milk sugar (lactose). It is involved in the manufacturing of vitamins and amino acids. Finally, acidophilus helps with the proper detoxification of hormones and other substances. Many supplements combine it with *Bifidobacterium*.

Indications:

Cancer prevention	Inflammatory bowel disease
Candidiasis	Irritable bowel disease
Canker sores	Lactose intolerance
Constipation	Leaky gut syndrome
Eczema	Traveler's diarrhea
Food allergies	Vaginitis
Immune support	

Precautions: People with candida overgrowth may notice die-off symptoms, including nausea, diarrhea, bloating, and so on, when they first begin acidophilus supplementation. If you use antibiotics, take acidophilus at least two hours before or after taking the antibiotics.

Dosage: Adults should take a product containing at least four billion active organisms twice a day, thirty minutes after a meal.

Activated Charcoal

Description: Activated charcoal is used to reduce digestive flatulence and also to absorb harmful toxins, including infectious agents that cause diarrhea.

Indications: Diarrhea   Toxin absorption
                   Flatulence

Precautions: Take it with a large glass of water, two hours before or after taking other medications and supplements.

Dosage: Take 500 to 1,000 mg three times daily for up to three days.

Adrenal Extract

Description: Adrenal extracts are supplements derived from bovine adrenal glands or the adrenal cortex. They may contain minute amounts of naturally occurring corticosteroids. Many researchers believe that the nutritional profile, including RNA and polypeptides, supports human adrenal-gland function. In the human body, the adrenal glands are located on top of each kidney. The adrenal glands are responsible for producing stress hormones such as cortisol, to control the effects of stress and inflammation. Fatigue is the most common reason to take adrenal-extract supplements.

Indications: Allergies   Fatigue
                   Arthritis   Lower back pain
                   Autoimmune conditions

Precautions: Sensitive individuals may experience anxiety, irritability, headache, or insomnia.

Dosage: Take 1 or 2 capsules or tablets two to three times daily on an empty stomach.

Alanine

Description: Alanine is a nonessential amino acid that helps to build protein. It is used as a nutritional supplement to reduce the symptoms of prostate enlargement.

Indications: Prostate enlargement

Precautions: People with liver or kidney disease should not supplement amino acids unless under the direction of a health care professional.

Dosage: Men with prostate enlargement can supplement 390 to 780 mg per day, along with the amino acids glycine and glutamic acid at the same dosages.

Amino Acids

Description: Amino acids are the individual building blocks of protein. There are approximately twenty different amino acids. Ten of the amino acids are known as "essential amino acids," which means that our body cannot manufacture them, so it is essential that we consume them in our diets. The remaining ten nonessential amino acids can be manufactured in the body.

Indications: Amino acid supplements are used for a variety of conditions, as mentioned throughout this book. Individual amino acids are described in this section.

Precautions: People with liver or kidney disease should not supplement amino acids unless under the direction of a health care professional.

Dosage: Generally, take 250 to 500 mg three times daily, between meals.

Andrographis

Description: This Asian herb's components have been shown to have antioxidant, antiviral, antibacterial, and anti-inflammatory properties.

Indications: Common cold   Sinusitis
                   Influenza   Tonsillitis
                   Sore throat

Precautions: None known.

Arginine

Description: Arginine is one of the better-studied amino acids and has been shown to be helpful for several conditions.

Indications:

Angina	Infertility
Congestive heart failure	Interstitial cystitis
High blood pressure	Surgical recovery
HIV	Wound healing
Impotence	

Precautions: People with liver or kidney disease should not supplement amino acids unless under the direction of a health-care professional. Arginine should not be used by people with oral or genital herpes.

Dosage: Dosage recommendations vary, depending on the condition. Most conditions require anywhere from 3 to 20 grams daily.

Bee Pollen

Description: Bee pollen is the pollen produced by flowering plants, which clings to bees as they gather nectar. Bee pollen contains many vitamins and minerals, as well as flavonoids such as rutin and quercitin. It is thought that the minute amounts of pollens desensitize a person against allergies to the same pollens.

Indications:

Allergies (mainly hay fever)	Fatigue
Arthritis	Immune support

Precautions: People who are allergic to bee stings should avoid bee pollen. To make sure you are not allergic to a bee pollen product, first try a minute amount on the skin or the tip of the tongue before beginning a regular dosage.

Dosage: Take 500 to 1,000 mg daily.

Bentonite

Description: Bentonite is a type of clay that is used internally and externally to absorb toxic substances. It is often a component of "colon cleansing" protocols.

Indications: Colon cleansing   Ingestion of toxic substances

Precautions: Take it three hours before or after taking any medication or supplement. It is best used short term, and you must drink 8 to 16 ounces of water with each teaspoonful to prevent constipation or bowel obstruction.

Dosage: Take 1 teaspoonful daily or as directed by a health care practitioner.

Beta Glucan

Description: Beta glucans are polysaccharides that are extracted from the cell walls of medicinal mushrooms, oats, barley, and baker's yeast. The structure and the activity of various beta glucans differ, depending on the source.

Indications:

Blood sugar balance	Immune support
High cholesterol	

Precautions: Immune-enhancing beta glucan products should be avoided by people who are on immunosuppressant medications.

Dosage: Dosage recommendations vary greatly, depending on the product. Follow the label recommendations.

Beta-Sitosterol

Description: Beta-sitosterol is a plant sterol that is used as a supplement to lower cholesterol and reduce the symptoms of prostate enlargement.

Indications: High cholesterol   Prostate enlargement

Precautions: This supplement appears to be very safe, with no known precautions.

Dosage: Doses of up to 10 grams are used for high cholesterol, and up to 130 mg daily are used for prostate enlargement.

Betaine Hydrochloride

Description: This hydrochloric acid (HCl) supplement is derived from sugar beets. It is used to increase stomach-acid levels for people who have an HCl deficiency.

Indications: Acne   Asthma

Anemia   Candidiasis

Arthritis   Fatigue

Food sensitivities   Irritable bowel syndrome

Gallstones   Vitiligo

Inflammatory bowel disease

Precautions: People with a history of heartburn, gastritis, or reflux should use caution.

Dosage: Take 1 or more capsules with each meal. Reduce the dosage if you feel a warming or burning sensation in your stomach.

Boric Acid

Description: Boric acid is a substance that's mainly used for the treatment of vaginal yeast infections. It is available in suppository or powder form. It has also been shown to shorten the duration of cold sores when applied topically.

Indications: Cold sores   Vaginal yeast infections

Precautions: Boric acid should never be ingested internally, especially by children. It should also never be applied topically to the skin of infants and children. Do not use boric acid on open wounds.

Dosage: Boric acid suppositories are used intravaginally by inserting 1 or 2 capsules (300–500 mg each) nightly, for up to two weeks.

Bovine Cartilage

Description: This is cartilage extracted from cow trachea. This connective tissue contains collagen, mucopolysaccharides, calcium, sulfur, and proteins. It is mainly used for arthritis, although some doctors prescribe it for cancer as it is thought to inhibit tumor growth. More research is needed to confirm any benefit for these uses.

Indications: Arthritis   Cancer

Precautions: There are no good data on precautions or concerns with supplementing bovine cartilage.

Dosage: A typical dosage is 1,000 to 3,000 mg three times daily.

Branched-Chain Amino Acids

Description: The three branched-chain amino acids include L-isoleucine, L-leucine, and L-valine. They are referred to as branched-chain because of their chemical structure. They are essential amino acids, meaning that the body cannot manufacture them, so they must be present in the diet. They play a key role in maintaining and building muscle tissue.

Indications: Athletic training and performance   Phenylketonuria

Liver cirrhosis   Tardive dyskinesia

Precautions: People with Lou Gehrig's disease, amylotrophic lateral sclerosis (ALS), should avoid supplementation unless instructed to do so by a health care professional. People with liver or kidney disease should not supplement amino acids unless under the direction of a health care professional.

Dosage: The typical daily dosage is 50 mg per 2.2 pounds of body weight.

Brewer's Yeast

Description: Brewer's yeast is made from the dried, pulverized cells of a type of fungus known as *Saccharomyces cerevisiae*. It is rich in B vitamins, chromium, amino acids, and selenium. Real brewer's yeast has a bitter taste.

Indications: Diabetes   Fatigue
                 Diarrhea   High cholesterol

Precautions: Brewer's yeast is a safe supplement to use, although occasional reports of allergic reaction occur. Caution should be used for people on diabetic drugs, as the chromium in brewer's yeast may lower the requirements for these medications.

Dosage: Take 1 to 2 tablespoons daily.

Carnitine

Description: L-carnitine is an amino acid–like substance that is responsible for transporting fatty acids into the mitochondria (energy factories) of cells to produce energy. L-carnitine is manufactured from the amino acids in the body. The richest food source is red meat. It has also been shown to have several benefits for cardiovascular system problems, such as congestive heart failure and high triglycerides.

Indications: Angina   Heart attack recovery
                 Anorexia   High cholesterol
                 Arrhythmias   HIV
                 Athletic performance   Intermittent claudication
                 Cardiomyopathy   Kidney disease
                 Chronic fatigue syndrome   Liver disease
                 Congestive heart failure   Male infertility
                 Diabetes   Premature infants
                 Down syndrome

Precautions: There is no toxicity with L-carnitine, but it should not be taken along with the drug pentylenetetrazol.

Dosage: Take 1,000 to 3,000 mg daily.

Carnosine

Description: This antioxidant substance is composed of the amino acids histidine and alanine. It occurs naturally in the body, especially in muscle, the brain, and the heart, as well as in food. Nerves and muscle cells contain high levels of carnosine. A zinc-carnosine complex has been shown to be effective against *Helicobacter pylori* infection.

Indications: Antioxidant support   Peptic ulcer (zinc–L-carnosine
                 Diabetes   form)
                 Hepatitis C (zinc–L-carnosine   Wound healing
                    form)

Precautions: No side effects have been reported.

Dosage: A dosage of 150 mg (zinc–carnosine complex) twice daily is recommended for the treatment of *Helicobacter pylori* infection. Otherwise, up to 1,500 mg of carnosine can be used daily as an antioxidant.

Cetyl Myristoleate (CMO)

Description: CMO is a fatty acid substance that occurs in certain animals and is used as an anti-inflammatory supplement for arthritis.

Indications: Rheumatoid arthritis and osteoarthritis

Precautions: Too high a dosage may cause diarrhea. The safety of CMO has not been established for pregnant women and nursing mothers.

Dosage: Take 500 mg daily.

Chlorella

Description: Chlorella is a blue-green algae whole-food supplement. It contains more than twenty different vitamins and minerals and is a rich source of amino acids, iron, and chlorophyll. It is commonly used as a daily detoxification supplement.

Indications:

Athlete's support	Constipation
Bad breath	Detoxification
Fatigue	Skin conditions (rashes, etc.)
Heavy-metal toxicity	

Precautions: No side effects are known.

Dosage: Take 1,000 to 3,000 mg daily.

Chlorophyll

Description: Chlorophyll is the pigment that gives plants their green color. It is regarded as a phytonutrient that has antioxidant, detoxifying, blood building, and anti-inflammatory properties.

Indications:

Anemia	Constipation
Bad breath	

Precautions: No side effects are known.

Dosage: Take 100 to 300 mg daily.

Chondroitin Sulfate

Description: Chondroitin sulfate is a nutritional supplement made from cow's cartilage. It consists of glycosaminoglycans, substances that form cartilage. This supplement is mainly used for osteoarthritis.

Indications: Osteoarthritis   Sprains/strains

Precautions: Very high dosages may cause nausea.

Dosage: The dosage used to treat osteoarthritis is 1,200 mg daily.

Collagen

Description: Collagen is the gluelike substance that keeps connective tissue together. It is involved in the formation of tendons, ligaments, cartilage, hair, and eyes.

Indications: Arthritis   Unhealthy skin, hair, and nails
Eye floaters

Precautions: None known.

Dosage: Depends on the type of collagen. For UC-II, a well-studied form, take 40 mg daily.

Colloidal Silver

Description: Colloidal silver refers to silver particles that are suspended in a water solution. Historically, silver was used topically to treat infections and has become more popular again in recent years with holistic doctors. This trace-mineral supplement appears to have potent antibacterial effects.

Indications: Bacterial infections   Conjunctivitis
                   Burns

Precautions: Colloidal silver products appear to vary greatly in quality and potency. They are best taken on a short-term basis, unless used under the guidance of a doctor. Long-term use of high dosages has been reported to result in a condition known as argyria. This permanent condition is characterized by gray or bluish-gray skin.

Dosage: Take 1 teaspoon daily for up to two weeks. Concentrations vary from 1 part per million to 100 parts per million.

Colostrum

Description: Colostrum is the component of breast milk that is formed during the first forty-eight hours after birth. Supplemental colostrum is generally derived from bovine (cow) colostrum. It is rich in antibodies (immunoglobulins) and various growth factors.

Indications: Immune support

Precautions: No side effects are known.

Dosage: Take 1,000 to 5,000 mg daily.

Conjugated Linoleic Acid (CLA)

Description: CLA is a varied form of the essential fatty acid linoleic acid. It is found in the red meat of cattle that are fed natural grasses. It is also found in eggs, poultry, and safflower and corn oil. CLA is mainly used as a supplement to reduce body fat. Animal and test tube studies have demonstrated its anticancer properties, but these results have yet to be proven in human studies.

Indications: Cancer prevention   Weight loss

Precautions: There are occasional reports of digestive upset.

Dosage: Take 1,000 mg two or three times daily.

Creatine

Description: Creatine is a naturally occurring substance in the body and in foods. It is made up of three amino acids—arginine, glycine, and methionine. Creatine is used by the body's muscle cells to create energy and maintain muscle mass.

Indications: Athletic support   Maintaining muscle mass
                  Congestive heart failure
                     in seniors

Precautions: Diarrhea and muscle cramping are the most common side effects. People with liver or kidney disease should check with their doctors before using creatine.

Dosage: Take 2 to 5 grams daily.

Cysteine

Description: Cysteine is a nonessential amino acid that contains the mineral sulfur. It is a component of the antioxidant glutathione and is required for the synthesis of the amino acid taurine. It plays an important role in detoxification and healthy immune-system function.

Indications: Antioxidant support   HIV

Precautions: Do not use it if you are prone to developing cysteine-related kidney stones. People with liver or kidney disease should not supplement amino acids unless under the direction of a health care professional.

Dosage: Take 500 to 1,500 mg daily.

D-Glucarate

Description: D-glucarate is the supplemental form of glucaric acid, a phytonutrient found in fruits and vegetables. D-glucarate is used by the liver to detoxify hormones and carcinogenic agents. This phytonutrient inhibits an enzyme known as beta glucuronidase, which increases toxic hormones that may be reabsorbed into circulation.

Indications: Cancer prevention   Fibrocystic breast syndrome
                  Detoxification   PMS

Precautions: There are no known side effects.

Dosage: Take 400 mg daily.

DHEA (Dehydroepiandrosterone)

Description: The hormone DHEA is currently available over the counter. It is the most abundant hormone produced by the adrenal glands. It has several functions, including but not limited to: supporting the body's reaction to stress; controlling inflammation; and enhancing the libido, cognitive function, immune modulation, and metabolism. DHEA is a precursor hormone to testosterone and androstenedione.

Indications: Allergies   Alzheimer's disease
                  Autoimmunity   Chronic fatigue syndrome
                  Depression   Diabetes
                  Erectile dysfunction   Heart disease prevention
                  Immune support   Inflammation
                  Lupus   Menopause
                  Osteoporosis   Poor memory
                  Prednisone withdrawal

Precautions: Too high a dosage may cause facial-hair growth and acne breakout. Pregnant women and breast-feeding mothers should avoid using DHEA. People with an existing cancer should also avoid it.

Dosage: A starting dosage for women with low levels is 5 to 15 mg and for men 15 to 25 mg.

DMAE (2-Dimethylaminoethanol)

Description: DMAE is a substance that has a chemical composition similar to that of choline. DMAE is used to improve mental alertness and reduce age-related cognitive decline. It has also become popular as a topical agent for skin wrinkles.

Indications: Age-related cognitive decline   Wrinkles
                  Alzheimer's disease

Precautions: DMAE is believed to be nontoxic.

Dosage: Take 100 to 400 mg daily.

Enzymes

Description: Enzymes are protein molecules that are found in every cell. They are required for the life-sustaining enzymatic reactions that occur in the body. Digestive enzymes help to break down food, while metabolic enzymes are involved in energy production, detoxification, immunity, and several other activities. Raw and lightly cooked foods provide enzymes, but there is debate as to whether they really increase the body's endogenous supply. Supplemental enzymes can be taken for a variety of health benefits. There are three main types of supplemental enzymes. Plant enzymes are derived from plants. The most common examples are bromelain from pineapple stems and papain from unripe papayas. Both help you to digest proteins, and bromelain has anti-inflammatory effects when taken on an empty stomach.

Microbial or fungal enzymes (also sometimes labeled as plant enzymes) are derived from the fermentation of fungus. The enzymes are then purified and available for therapeutic use. These types of enzymes can be used as digestive aids. Protease enzymes break down protein, lipase enzymes are for fats, amylase is for carbohydrates, and many others are available to break down other food components. Similar to bromelain, microbial-derived protease enzymes have blood-thinning and anti-inflammatory effects when taken between meals. These types of enzymes tend to have the best stability of the three categories of enzymes.

The third category is animal enzymes. These enzymes are typically derived from animal organs. For example, pancreatic enzymes are usually derived from a sheep or pig pancreas.

Indications:

Arthritis (protease enzymes taken between meals)	Colic
	Digestive disorders (most kinds)
Autoimmune conditions	Food sensitivities
Cancer	Infections
Candidiasis	Sports injuries
Celiac disease	

Precautions: Side effects are uncommon. Protease enzymes are known to aggravate some users who have an active ulcer or gastritis. People taking blood-thinning medications should check with their doctors before using enzymes. People with chronic candidiasis may experience yeast die-off symptoms, such as nausea, diarrhea, bloating, and so on, when they first begin enzyme supplementation.

Dosage: For digestive support, take 1 or 2 digestive-enzyme complexes with each meal. Individual enzymes may be taken between meals for therapeutic effects. Take as directed by a health care professional.

Evening Primrose Oil (EPO)

Description: Evening primrose oil is rich in an omega-6 fatty acid known as GLA (gamma linolenic acid). GLA has been shown to have anti-inflammatory effects and is required for proper brain function.

Indications:

Arthritis	Eczema
Attention-deficit disorder	Multiple sclerosis
Fibrocystic breast syndrome	Peripheral neuropathy
Diabetes	PMS
Dry skin	

Precautions: Digestive upset and headaches are rare side effects. People with epilepsy should use EPO only under the guidance of a doctor. Evening primrose oil is best taken in conjunction with omega-3 fatty acids, such as fish, flaxseed, or perilla oil.

Fish Oil

Description: Fish oil is the richest source of the omega-3 fatty acids DHA (docosa-hexanoic acid) and EPA (eicosapentaenoic acid). Both DHA and EPA have anti-inflammatory effects. DHA plays an important role in brain function and joint health. EPA regulates inflammation, the immune system, blood clotting, and circulation.

Indications:

Arthritis	Diabetes
Asthma	High blood pressure
Attention-deficit disorder	High cholesterol and triglycerides
Bipolar disorder	Inflammatory bowel disease
Cancer	Lupus
Cardiovascular disease	Osteoporosis
Chronic obstructive pulmonary disease	Preeclampsia
	Pregnancy
Depression	Schizophrenia

Precautions: Digestive upset (especially reflux and burping) may occur if the fish oil product is not enteric coated. Fish oil has a mild blood-thinning effect, so consult with your doctor before supplementation if you are on a blood-thinning medication. Some people may have a rise in LDL cholesterol. This can be prevented with garlic supplementation.

Dosage: Take 3 to 5 grams total of EPA and DHA together for therapeutic purposes. Otherwise, take 1 to 2 grams total EPA and DHA together for preventative purposes. For high blood pressure, take a formula that has higher levels of DHA than EPA.

Flaxseed Oil

Description: Flaxseed oil is a rich source of alpha linolenic acid, an omega-3 fatty acid. Alpha linolenic acid is converted into DHA (docosahexanoic acid) and EPA (eicosapentaenoic acid). It is used to reduce inflammation; to promote healthy circulation and healthy skin, hair, and nails; and to improve constipation. It is not as well studied as fish oil.

Indications:

Arthritis	Diabetes
Asthma	High blood pressure
Attention-deficit disorder	High cholesterol and triglycerides
Bipolar disorder	Inflammatory bowel disease
Cancer	Lupus
Cardiovascular disease	Osteoporosis
Chronic obstructive pulmonary disease	Preeclampsia
Constipation	Pregnancy
Depression	Schizophrenia

Precautions: Too much flaxseed oil can cause diarrhea. Men with prostate cancer should avoid supplementation with flaxseed oil and use ground seeds instead. Flaxseed oil has a mild blood-thinning effect, so consult with your doctor before supplementation if you are on blood-thinning medication.

Dosage: Take 1 to 2 tablespoons or 8 to 12 capsules daily.

FOS (Fructooligosaccharides)

Description: FOS refers to short chains of fructose molecules that are incompletely digested by humans. They serve as food or as a probiotic for healthy bacteria such as *Lactobacillus acidophilus* and *Bifidobacterium bifidus*.

Indications: Diabetes   High cholesterol

                     Digestive disorders   Immunity

Precautions: High doses may cause diarrhea. Initial use may increase gas and flatulence, due to alterations in gut flora.

Dosage: Take 2,000 to 3,000 mg daily.

GABA (Gamma-Amino Butyric Acid)

Description: GABA is an amino acid–like substance that has a calming effect on the nervous system. It is naturally produced in the brain from the amino acid glutamate. Nutrition-oriented doctors use it as a calming agent for epilepsy and anxiety.

Indications: ADHD   Epilepsy

                     Anxiety   Muscle tightness

Precautions: GABA should not be combined with pharmaceutical psychiatric or anticonvulsant medications. It is best used under the guidance of a nutrition-oriented doctor.

Dosage: Take 250 to 500 mg three times daily.

Glandulars

Description: Glandulars refer to nutritional supplements made from animal tissue or animal-tissue extracts. Research has found that amino acids, enzymes, and other nutrients from glandular supplements are absorbed into the bloodstream. In addition, minute quantities of hormones are likely present in many glandular products. It is thought that glandular supplements work by supplying minute amounts of hormones and specific nutrition to improve the functioning of the targeted gland. Preparations are available for most glands, such as thyroid, pancreas, adrenals, thymus, and many others. Most products are derived from cow or sheep organs.

Indications: Support for any underfunctioning or imbalanced gland

Precautions: A small percentage of users experience digestive upset. Look for organic products to minimize the likelihood of using a contaminated product.

Dosage: The typical adult dosage is 1 or 2 capsules or tablets two or three times daily between meals. Take as directed on the label, as product potencies vary.

Glucosamine

Description: Glucosamine occurs naturally in the body and is involved in the manufacturing of cartilage. Supplemental glucosamine is mainly derived from the chitin (shell) of shellfish, such as crabs, shrimps, and lobsters. Glucosamine has been shown to support cartilage formation and reduce arthritic pain. The two forms of supplemental glucosamine are glucosamine sulfate and glucosamine hydrochloride. Most of the research to date has been done on the sulfate form.

Indications: Osteoarthritis   Sprains/strains

Precautions: Digestive upset, including diarrhea. Persons who are allergic to shellfish don't normally have a problem as the allergic reaction is usually to the protein found in the meat of shrimp and crab. People who are allergic to sulfa drugs do not need to be concerned as the source of the drugs is different from the mineral sulfur that is part of glucosamine sulfate.

Dosage: Take 1,500 mg daily.

Glutamic Acid

Description: Glutamic acid is an amino acid that is suited to build protein and has been studied for the symptoms of prostate enlargement.

Indications: Prostate enlargement

Precautions: People with liver or kidney disease should not supplement amino acids unless under the direction of a health care professional.

Dosage: Men with prostate enlargement can supplement 390 to 780 mg per day, along with the amino acids glycine and alanine at the same dosages.

Glutamine

Description: Glutamine is the most abundant and metabolically active amino acid in the body. It also serves as an energy source, because it can be converted to glucose, especially for the cells of the intestinal tract.

Indications:

Alcohol withdrawal	HIV
Athletic performance	Surgical recovery
Gastritis	Ulcers

Precautions: People with liver or kidney disease should not supplement amino acids unless under the direction of a health care professional.

Dosage: Take 1,500 to 3,000 mg daily.

Glutathione

Description: Glutathione is a powerful antioxidant that protects cell DNA from damage, helps repair cell DNA, supports liver and kidney detoxification, improves cell energy production, and supports immunity.

Indications:

Aging	Liver diseases (hepatitis, fatty liver, elevated liver enzymes—especially GGT)
Cardiovascular diseases (hypertension, myocardial infarction, cholesterol oxidation)	Pulmonary disease (COPD, asthma, and acute respiratory-distress syndrome)
Chronic age-related diseases (cataracts, macular degeneration, hearing impairment, and glaucoma)	Neurodegenerative disorders (Alzheimer's, Parkinson's, and Huntington's diseases, Amyotrophic lateral sclerosis, Friedreich's ataxia)
Complementary cancer support	
Cystic fibrosis	
Detoxification	
Immune diseases (HIV, autoimmune diseases)	

Glycine

Description: Glycine is an amino acid that is used to build proteins, reduce prostate enlargement symptoms, improve cognitive function, and aid in liver detoxification.

Indications:

Detoxification	Schizophrenia
Prostate enlargement	

Precautions: People with liver or kidney disease should not supplement amino acids unless under the direction of a health care professional.

Dosage: Men with prostate enlargement can supplement 390 to 780 mg per day, along with the amino acids glutamic acid and alanine at the same dosages.

Grapefruit Seed Extract

Description: Grapefruit seed extract is, as the name implies, the extract of grapefruit seeds. This supplement is mainly used for the treatment of infections, particularly fungal and bacterial infections. It is also available as a nasal spray to treat sinusitis.

Indications: Infections   Sinusitis
                    Irritable bowel syndrome (related to candida overgrowth)

Precautions: The internal use of this supplement should be avoided by pregnant women and breast-feeding mothers.

Dosage: Take 10 to 20 drops or 200 mg three times daily.

Grapeseed Extract

Description: Grapeseed extract is, as the name implies, the extract of grapeseeds. This supplement contains a class of flavonoids known as proanthocyanidins. Grapeseed is mainly used as an antioxidant and to improve the stability of collagen and elastin, two substances that are important for healthy skin, joints, ligaments, tendons, and blood vessels. It is also used to improve microcirculation throughout the body.

Indications: Antioxidant support   Retinopathy
                    Bruising   Varicose veins
                    Macular degeneration

Precautions: No side effects have been reported.

Dosage: Take 50 to 300 mg daily.

Green Tea

Description: This tea or supplemental extract is derived from the leaves of *Camella sinensis*, the same plant that is used to make white and black tea. The leaves are lightly steamed and less processed than those of black tea, which accounts for green tea's high antioxidant properties. It has been found to afford very potent antioxidant activity, and it improves detoxification. Green tea is commonly available in liquid, tablet, and capsule form.

Indications: Cancer   Gingivitis
                    Cardiovascular disease   High cholesterol
                    Detoxification   Tooth decay
                    Digestive health   Weight management

Precautions: Green tea that has not had the caffeine removed may cause irritability, insomnia, nervousness, and a fast heartbeat. However, these side effects are less common with green tea than with black tea, since it contains an amino acid known as L-theanine, which has a calming effect on the nervous system.

Dosage: Drink up to 10 cups of green tea daily, although 2 to 3 cups daily will provide good antioxidant protection. The supplement form should be standardized to 80 to 90 percent polyphenols and 35 to 55 percent epigallocatechin gallate, the potent antioxidant in green tea.

Histidine

Description: Histidine is an amino acid that is considered nonessential in humans but may be essential in some children.

Indications: Rheumatoid arthritis

Precautions: People with liver or kidney disease should not supplement amino acids unless under the direction of a health care professional.

Dosage: Take 250 to 500 mg three times daily between meals.

Huperzine A

Description: Huperzine A is a substance that is extracted from club moss (*Lycopodium serratum*). It has been shown to have some benefit for people with Alzheimer's disease and age-related cognitive decline. Huperzine A prevents the breakdown of the neurotransmitter acetylcholine.

Indications: Age-related cognitive decline   Alzheimer's disease

Precautions: Do not use it if you are currently taking a pharmaceutical medication for Alzheimer's disease.

Dosage: Take 100 to 200 mcg two or three times daily.

Hydroxycitric Acid (HCA)

Description: Hydroxycitric acid is a compound found in the fruit known as *Garcinia cambogia*. Animal but not human studies have found that HCA suppresses appetite and causes weight loss.

Indications: Weight loss

Precautions: No side effects are known.

Dosage: Take 500 to 1,000 mg three times daily before meals.

5-Hydroxytryptophan (5-HTP)

Description: The supplement 5-HTP is an amino acid–like substance used as a precursor to make the neurotransmitter serotonin. Serotonin is important for balanced mood, sleep, pain control, and other important functions of the body. This supplement is extracted from the seeds of the African plant *Griffonia simplicifolia*.

Indications: Anxiety   Insomnia
                  Depression   Migraine headaches
                  Fibromyalgia   Seasonal affective disorder
                  Food cravings (carbohydrates)   Weight loss

Precautions: Large amounts may cause digestive upset, headaches, or sleepiness. It should not be taken in conjunction with pharmaceutical antidepressant, antianxiety, or other psychiatric medications.

Dosage: Take 50 to 100 mg three times daily on an empty stomach.

Indole-3-Carbinol

Description: Indole-3-carbinol is a phytonutrient found in cruciferous vegetables, such as broccoli, cauliflower, brussels sprouts, cabbage, and kale. Preliminary research has demonstrated anticancer properties. It also supports healthy estrogen metabolism. Studies have shown that it stopped or reduced the formation of precancerous lesions in the respiratory tract and in the cervix of the uterus.

Indications: Cancer prevention   Estrogen metabolism
                  Cervical dysplasia

Precautions: There are no known side effects.

Dosage: Take 400 mg daily.

Ipriflavone

Description: Ipriflavone is a synthetic copy of a soy flavonoid known as daidzein. It is used as a supplement for the maintenance and the enhancement of bone density. Animal and human studies have shown that when combined with calcium and other minerals, it stimulates bone building by increasing the cells that form bone (osteoblasts) and reducing the activity of cells that break down bone (osteoclasts).

Indications: Hyperparathyroidism   Osteoporosis
                Kidney failure (to maintain   Otosclerosis
                    bone density)   Paget's disease

Precautions: Digestive upset is the most common side effect, which can be ameliorated by taking ipriflavone with food. One study found that lymphocyte count decreased in 29 out of 132 women who were supplementing ipriflavone. This reduction was not regarded as clinically significant, but it is recommended to have your doctor monitor these white blood cells.

Dosage: Take 600 mg daily.

Kelp

Description: Kelp is a type of sea vegetable that's rich in iron and several minerals. It is used as a supplement to support thyroid function.

Indications: Goiter   Hypothyroid

Precautions: People with any type of thyroid disease should check with their doctors before supplementing kelp.

Dosage: Take 2 to 4 capsules daily, or take as directed on the label or as advised by a health care professional.

L-Theanine

Description: L-theanine is an amino acid found in green tea. It has a calming and relaxing effect on the body.

Indications: Anxiety   Insomnia

Precautions: No side effects have been reported. If you are taking pharmaceutical antianxiety medications, talk with your doctor before using this supplement.

Dosage: Take 200 to 400 mg daily.

Lutein

Description: Lutein is a member of the carotenoid family. It has antioxidant activity and is known to be a key component of the macula, an area of the retina that is responsible for vision. It is mainly used as a supplement to prevent and treat macular degeneration.

Indications: Cataracts   Macular degeneration

Precautions: No side effects have been reported.

Dosage: Take 15 mg daily if you have macular degeneration and up to 5 mg daily as a preventative dosage.

Lycopene

Description: Lycopene is a member of the carotenoid family. It has received much attention because studies have shown that it has a protective effect against prostate and other cancers. Studies have also shown that lycopene enhances immune function and protects against heart disease. Tomatoes, watermelon, and pink grapefruit are all good food sources of lycopene.

Indications: Asthma   Immune support
               Atherosclerosis prevention   Macular degeneration
               Cancer prevention   Prostate cancer

Precautions: No side effects have been reported.

Dosage: Take 5 to 10 mg daily, as a good preventative dosage against cancer. Men with prostate cancer should supplement 30 mg daily.

Lysine

Description: Lysine is an essential amino acid that must be obtained in one's diet, as the body cannot manufacture enough of it (gut bacteria synthesize small amounts of lysine). It is found in chicken, cottage cheese, avocados, and wheat germ. It is involved in the growth of children and in bone formation. It is most commonly used as a supplement to prevent and treat herpes outbreaks.

Indications: Cold sores   Osteoporosis
               Genital herpes   Shingles

Precautions: High dosages may cause digestive upset.

Dosage: Take 1,500 to 3,000 mg for the treatment of acute herpes outbreaks and 500 to 1,000 mg to prevent herpes outbreaks.

Malic Acid

Description: Malic acid is a naturally occurring substance that is found in fruits and vegetables, especially in apples. It helps with the production of ATP within cells for energy production. Some holistic doctors use it as a therapy, along with magnesium, for fibromyalgia and aluminum detoxification.

Indications: Aluminum detoxification   Fibromyalgia

Precautions: There are no known side effects.

Dosage: Take 1,200 to 2,400 mg daily.

Medium-Chain Triglycerides (MCTs)

Description: Medium-chain triglycerides are fatty acids that are found in coconut and palm oil, as well as in butter. They are used by athletes for training and may have mild weight-loss properties. Some nutritionists claim that they support thyroid function. MCTs have been shown to have a mild blood glucose–lowering effect.

Indications: Athletic training   Hypothyroidism
               Diabetes

Precautions: Digestive upset is known to occur for some users. They should be used under a doctor's care if you have diabetes or liver disease.

Dosage: The typical dosage is 15 to 30 grams, although athletes often use 50 grams or more.

Melatonin

Description: Melatonin is a natural hormone produced in the brain's pineal gland that regulates the body's biological clock and sleep cycles. Melatonin is produced in response to darkness. This hormone has been shown to be helpful for insomnia, seasonal affective disorder, and other mood disturbances. It has potent antioxidant properties and also protects against radiation damage.

Indications:	Aging	Jet lag
	Cancer (breast and prostate)	Radiation exposure
	Cluster headaches	Seasonal affective disorder
	Insomnia	Tardive dyskinesia

Precautions: Pregnant women or nursing mothers should avoid supplementing melatonin unless instructed to do so by their physicians. People with cancer should also consult with their doctors before supplementing melatonin. Children should not supplement melatonin unless instructed to do so by their doctors. People on steroid medications should avoid taking melatonin unless their doctors feel it is appropriate.

Dosage: Take 0.5 to 3 mg as a starting dosage for insomnia and jet lag.

Methionine

Description: This essential amino acid is necessary for growth, detoxification, and normal metabolism.

Indications:	Detoxification support	Pancreatitis
	HIV	Parkinson's disease

Precautions: B vitamins, especially B6, folic acid, and B12, should be supplemented along with methionine to prevent the buildup of homocysteine, a risk factor for cardiovascular disease. People with liver or kidney disease should not supplement amino acids unless under the direction of a health care professional.

Dosage: Take 500 mg one or two times daily.

MSM (Methylsulfonylmethane)

Description: MSM is a naturally occurring component in the body and is found in many foods, especially green vegetables. It is a good source of the mineral sulfur. MSM is used as a supplement primarily to reduce pain and inflammation.

Indications:	Allergies	Hair and nail health
	Arthritis	Headaches
	Asthma	Heartburn
	Autoimmune diseases	Muscle spasms
	Fibromyalgia	Sports injuries

Precautions: Rare reports of digestive upset, such as diarrhea, cramping, and stomach upset, occur with too high a dosage. Otherwise, MSM is nontoxic. People on blood-thinning medications should check with their doctors before using MSM, as it has mild blood-thinning effects.

Dosage: Take 500 to 2,000 mg for preventative purposes and up to 10,000 mg daily for severe pain and inflammatory disorders.

N-Acetylcysteine

Description: This is a varied form of the amino acid acetylcysteine. It is commonly used to increase the levels of glutathione in the body, for detoxification, and as a mucus thinner.

Indications:	Angina	Cystic fibrosis
	Antioxidant support (via glutathione production)	Flu prevention
		Gastritis
	Bronchitis	HIV
	Chronic obstructive pulmonary disease	Pneumonia
		Postnasal drip

Precautions: Long-term use may deplete zinc and copper levels. Nausea, vomiting, headache, dizziness, and abdominal pain have been reported with supplementation. People with liver or kidney disease should not supplement amino acids unless under the direction of a health care professional.

Dosage: Take 500 to 1,500 mg daily.

NADH (Nicotinamide Adenine Dinucleotide)

Description: NADH is the coenzyme form of vitamin B3 (niacin), which plays a role in cellular energy production. Preliminary research has shown NADH to be helpful for chronic fatigue syndrome and depression. It may also hold promise in reducing the symptoms of Alzheimer's disease and Parkinson's disease, although these uses have not been proven.

Indications:
- Alzheimer's disease
- Chronic fatigue syndrome
- Depression
- Fibromyalgia
- Parkinson's disease

Precautions: NADH appears to be nontoxic.

Dosage: Take 5 to 10 mg daily on an empty stomach.

Ornithine

Description: This amino acid is used in the body for tissue regeneration.

Indications:
- Athletic training
- Liver cirrhosis
- Wound healing

Precautions: High doses, above 10 grams, may cause digestive upset. People with liver or kidney disease should not supplement amino acids unless under the direction of a health-care professional.

Dosage: Take 5 to 20 grams daily.

Pectin

Description: Pectin is a soluble fiber derived from apples, grapefruit, and other citrus fruits.

Indications:
- Diabetes
- High cholesterol

Precautions: Pectin supplements may cause digestive upset.

Dosage: Dosages of up to 15 grams a day are used.

Perilla Oil

Description: Perilla oil is an extract of the Asian beefsteak plant. It is a rich source of alpha linolenic acid. As with other essential fatty acid supplements like flaxseed oil, perilla oil helps to reduce inflammation, improve circulation, and enhance brain function and has several other uses.

Indications:
- Allergies
- Cancer prevention
- Cardiovascular disease prevention
- Inflammatory bowel disease
- Arthritis
- Memory and concentration
- Neurological health

Precautions: Perilla has mild blood-thinning effects. Consult with your doctor before supplementing if you are taking a blood-thinning medication.

Dosage: Take 6,000 mg daily.

Phenylalanine

Description: This amino acid serves to build protein and acts as a precursor to L-tyrosine, L-dopa, norepinephrine, and epinephrine. L-phenylalanine occurs naturally in foods. The supplemental form, D-phenylalanine (DPA), is not naturally occurring in the body but can be converted into phenylethylamine to elevate mood and decrease pain. Also, a common supplement form that combines L-phenylalanine (LPA) and D-phenylalanine (DPA) is known as DLPA (DL-phenylalanine).

Indications for DPA:

Depression	Pain
Lower back pain	Parkinson's disease
Osteoarthritis	Rheumatoid arthritis

Indications for DLPA: Alcohol withdrawal   Depression

Precautions: People with phenylketonuria and tardive dyskinesia must not supplement phenylalanine. Rare instances of heartburn, nausea, and headaches have been reported. People with liver or kidney disease should not supplement amino acids unless under the direction of a health care professional.

Dosage: DLPA is usually taken at a dosage of 500 mg, two to three times daily between meals. LPA is used in dosages of up to 3,500 mg daily.

Phosphatidylcholine (PC)

Description: Phosphatidylcholine is an extract from lecithin that supplies a form of choline, which is used as a building block for cell walls and the neurotransmitter acetylcholine. Lecithin contains anywhere from 10 to 20 percent phosphatidylcholine. PC is important for proper brain and neurological function and supports healthy liver detoxification.

Indications:

Alzheimer's disease	High cholesterol
Bipolar disorder	Liver cirrhosis and detoxification
Hepatitis	Neurological disorders

Precautions: Digestive upset, such as diarrhea or nausea, may occur with high dosages.
Dosage: Take 1,500 to 9,000 mg daily.

Phosphatidylserine (PS)

Description: PS is a type of phospholipid extracted from soy that is used to build and maintain healthy cell membranes. It is used as a supplement to improve memory and depression, as well as to balance stress hormones. It is one of the few substances known to slow down early-stage Alzheimer's disease.

Indications:

Age-associated memory impairment	Dementia
Alzheimer's disease	Depression
Attention-deficit/hyperactivity disorder	Stress hormone imbalance
Brain injury	

Precautions: There are no known side effects.
Dosage: Take 100 to 500 mg daily, although most studies used 300 mg.

Pine Bark Extract (Pycnogenol)

Description: This is an extract from the bark of the maritime pine tree. It has anti-inflammatory, circulation-enhancing, and antioxidant properties. Numerous published studies demonstrate its efficacy.

Indications:

Arthritis	Fertility
Asthma	High blood pressure
Attention-deficit/hyperactivity disorder	High cholesterol
Blood-clot prevention	Menstrual pain
Chemotherapy side-effect prevention	Perimenopause
	Pregnancy

Diabetes	Retinopathy
Diabetic ulcers	Skin protection and
Endometriosis	rejuvenation
Exercise endurance	Varicose veins

Precautions: This has blood-thinning properties, so do not use if you are on blood thinners.

Dosage: Take 100 to 200 mg daily.

Pregnenolone

Description: Pregnenolone is a steroidal hormone produced in large part by the adrenal glands. It is a precursor hormone that the body uses to manufacture DHEA and progesterone. It is commonly used by holistic doctors for arthritis and autoimmune conditions such as lupus.

Indications:	Arthritis (especially	Lupus erythematosus
	rheumatoid form)	Poor memory
	Depression	Psoriasis

Precautions: Pregnenolone should be avoided by people who have seizure disorders or a history of hormone-related cancers.

Dosage: Take 10 to 50 mg daily.

Progesterone

Description: Progesterone is a hormone that's found in both men and women. For women, it is involved in regulating the menstrual cycle and reproductive function. Progesterone is mainly produced and secreted by the ovaries during ovulation. It is also manufactured by the adrenal glands, the brain, and the placenta in pregnant women. Natural progesterone cream is a popular supplement for the treatment of PMS, menopausal symptoms, endometriosis, and several other conditions.

Indications:	Autoimmune conditions	Menopausal symptoms
	Endometriosis	Osteoporosis
	Fibrocystic breasts	Ovarian cysts
	Infertility (female)	PMS
	Irregular menses	Uterine fibroids

Precautions: Natural progesterone cream has a good safety record. Women with a history of cancer should consult with a doctor before using it. Women using the birth-control pill or synthetic progestin should avoid it.

Dosage: The dosage depends on the condition being treated. Menopausal women generally apply a quarter teaspoon (20 mg) to the skin one or two times daily.

Propolis

Description: Propolis is "bee glue," the resinous substance that is formed when bees gather propolis from the buds and the bark of trees. The worker bees, with their salivary secretions and wax flakes, use it to seal the chambers and the entrance of the beehive. Propolis has antimicrobial, antioxidant, and anti-inflammatory properties.

Indications:	Gingivitis	Peptic ulcers
	Herpes	Periodontal disease
	Infections	Ulcerative colitis
	Mouth ulcers	Wound healing
	Parasites	

Precautions: There are rare reports of allergic reactions, such as skin itching and redness.

Dosage: Take 500 to 1,000 mg of the capsule form or 1 to 3 ml of the tincture form, or use it topically as a cream or a spray.

Psyllium

Description: Psyllium is a fiber supplement. Psyllium seed husks are popular for the treatment of constipation. Psyllium has also been shown to lower cholesterol levels.

Indications:	Constipation	Hemorrhoids
	Diabetes	High cholesterol
	Diarrhea	Irritable bowel syndrome
	Diverticulitis	

Precautions: Psyllium should be taken two to three hours before or after taking any medications or supplements as it may hinder absorption.

Dosage: Take 5 grams three times daily, with at least 8 ounces of water.

Pyruvate

Description: Pyruvate is a by-product of carbohydrate and protein metabolism in the body. It is available as a supplement and is mainly used for weight loss. It has also been shown to have antioxidant effects and may improve one's exercise endurance.

Indications:	Antioxidant support	Weight loss
	Athletic support	

Precautions: High dosages may cause digestive upset.

Dosage: Take 5 to 30 grams daily for weight loss.

Red Yeast Rice

Description: Red yeast rice, the fermented product of rice on which red yeast (*Monascus purpureus*) is grown, is a supplement that's used to lower cholesterol. Historically, red yeast rice was described in ancient Chinese texts as an aid to improve circulation. Human studies have shown it to effectively reduce cholesterol levels.

Indications: High cholesterol

Precautions: Mild digestive upset may occur. It should be avoided by pregnant women and breast-feeding mothers, people with liver disease, and those on pharmaceutical cholesterol-lowering medications. It is recommended that coenzyme Q10 (10–200 mg daily) be supplemented while you take red yeast rice extract, as some researchers theorize that it may cause a deficiency of this nutrient.

Dosage: The dosage used in studies was 1.2 to 2.4 grams of red yeast rice standardized to 10 to 13.5 mg of monacolins. However, FDA regulations do not allow supplement manufacturers to list the concentration of monacolins in their products.

Resveratrol

Description: Resveratrol is a compound found in red wine that has potent antioxidant activity. Preliminary research has demonstrated cardiovascular benefit and possible anticancer properties.

Indications:	Antioxidant	Diabetes
	Cancer prevention	Weight loss
	Cardiovascular disease prevention	

Precautions: There have been no reported side effects.

Dosage: Take 500 mcg to 50 mg daily.

Royal Jelly

Description: Royal jelly is the substance that worker bees secrete to feed the queen bee. It contains B vitamins and other nutrients. Holistic doctors use it for energy support. It has been shown in studies to lower cholesterol.

Indications: Fatigue   Stress
                   High cholesterol

Precautions: People who are allergic to bee pollen or honey should not use royal jelly.

Dosage: The typical adult dosage is 50 to 100 mg daily.

Rye Pollen

Description: Rye pollen is a supplement used for the treatment of chronic prostatitis and benign prostatic hyperplasia.

Indications: Benign prostatic hyperplasia   Chronic prostatitis

Precautions: There are no reported side effects.

Dosage: Take 3 tablets twice daily.

SAMe (S-Adenosylmethionine)

Description: SAMe is a naturally occurring substance in the body that is made from combining the amino acid methionine with ATP. It is regarded as a methyl (CH3) that enables a variety of biochemical reactions to occur properly. SAMe is mainly used for the treatment of osteoarthritis, depression, and fibromyalgia.

Indications: Depression   Hepatitis
                   Detoxification   Liver cirrhosis
                   Fibromyalgia   Osteoarthritis

Precautions: SAMe is very safe. However, it is not recommended for people with bipolar disorder. It can be used in conjunction with pharmaceutical antidepressants as long as you are being monitored by a physician.

Dosage: Take 400 to 1,200 mg daily.

Shark Cartilage

Description: Shark cartilage is used as a supplement for the treatment of cancer and arthritis. It has been reported that shark cartilage prevents the growth of new blood vessels that feed tumors. The health benefits of shark cartilage lack scientific validity. However, some practitioners report obvious clinical improvement in patients.

Indications: Arthritis   Cancer

Precautions: Pregnant women and breast-feeding mothers should avoid the supplementation of shark cartilage.

Dosage: Take 50 to 100 mg daily.

Soy Isoflavones

Description: Phytoestrogen compounds that are extracted from soy, such as daidzein, genistein, and glycitein, are known as soy isoflavones. They are commonly used to reduce menopausal, PMS, and other female hormone–related conditions. They have been shown to help improve bone density, protect against bone loss, and reduce cholesterol levels. Interestingly, men with prostate problems are also helped.

Indications: High cholesterol   Prostate enlargement
                   Menopause   Vaginitis
                   PMS

Precautions: Women with a history of breast or uterine cancer should avoid isolated-soy-isoflavone supplementation until further research shows benefit.

Dosage: Take 100 to 300 mg daily.

Tyrosine

Description: This amino acid is derived from another amino acid known as phenylalanine. L-tyrosine is a precursor for the formation of the neurotransmitters L-dopa, dopamine, norepinephrine, and epinephrine. The skin also converts tyrosine into melanin, the pigment that protects the skin against harmful UV radiation. In addition, this amino acid is required for the synthesis of thyroid hormone.

Indications: Depression   Parkinson's disease
                 Hypothyroidism   Phenylketonuria

Precautions: People with liver or kidney disease should not supplement amino acids unless under the direction of a health care professional.

Dosage: Take 250 to 500 mg twice daily between meals.

Vinpocetine

Description: Vinpocetine is an extract from the leaf of the periwinkle plant. It has been shown in studies to dilate blood vessels, enhance circulation in the brain, improve oxygen utilization, make red blood cells more pliable, and inhibit aggregation of platelets. Studies have shown it to benefit cognitive function for people with dementia.

Indications: Dementia   Memory problems
                 Hearing loss   Tinnitus

Precautions: Pregnant women or breast-feeding mothers should not take vinpocetine. Use caution if you are currently taking blood pressure medications.

Dosage: Take 10 to 20 mg daily.

Whey Protein

Description: Whey is a component of cow's milk and is a good source of branched-chain amino acids, which are required for the maintenance and the building of muscle mass. Whey protein has also been shown to increase the body's levels of glutathione, a very important antioxidant.

Indications: Athlete's support   Meal replacement

Precautions: People with kidney or liver disease should check with their physicians before supplementing whey protein.

Dosage: Take 25 grams daily.

Xylitol

Description: This substance is found naturally in fruits, vegetables, the bark of some trees, and the human body. It is approved as a food additive by both the World Health Organization and the FDA. Xylitol has 40 to 50 percent fewer calories than sugar.

Indications: Bone-density support   Ear-infection prevention
                 Cavity prevention   Natural sweetener

Precautions: Higher dosages may cause loose stool.

Dosage: Take 1 to 8.5 grams daily.

Zeaxanthin

Description: This nutrient is a carotenoid in foods such as kale, fruits, and corn. It is a powerful antioxidant found predominantly in the eyes (particularly the retina) and brain.

Indications: Age-related macular degeneration   Inflammation

Antioxidants

What are antioxidants? The use of antioxidant supplements has become very popular with consumers and health professionals. Researchers are continuing to find that many diseases are prevented or improved with the help of antioxidants, either from a healthful diet or from supplementation. The role of antioxidants is to prevent or control oxidation—hence the prefix "anti-" (meaning "against"). Oxidation refers to the burning of oxygen as fuel in cells and the subsequent creation of substances known as free radicals. Free radicals are unstable molecules that are very reactive and can damage cell DNA and various tissues. Researchers estimate that our cell DNA receives anywhere from seventy-five thousand to one hundred thousand hits from free radicals every day. A free radical is missing an electron (a charged particle) and seeks out another molecule to pair up with, to gain an electron. This process actually creates more free radicals. It should be noted that free radicals also have beneficial effects, such as being used by the body to destroy foreign invaders like viruses.

THE PROCESS OF OXIDATION

A good example of the oxidation process is an apple that has been sliced open. Within a short amount of time, the flesh of the apple will turn a brownish color. This occurs because of oxygen interacting with the exposed apple. If you were to slice an apple and immediately squirt lemon juice on it, you would find that the brownish discoloration (oxidation) occurs over a much longer period of time. This protective effect occurs from the antioxidants vitamin C and bioflavonoids that exist in lemon juice. Within our bodies, similar reactions are occurring all the time. For example, antioxidants protect cholesterol from becoming oxidized. Researchers have found that cholesterol really becomes a villain only when it becomes oxidized and makes the process of atherosclerosis more likely. For people who consume a diet that's high in fruits and vegetables, our richest sources of antioxidants, the risk of cardiovascular disease is reduced. The same is true for a variety of cancers and other chronic diseases.

SOURCES OF FREE RADICALS

Besides the free radicals that are produced in the life-giving process of energy production within our cells, a variety of other factors also increase our free-radical exposure. Common sources include radiation from the sun and X-rays. Too much exposure from these sources may result in skin cancer, wrinkles, and cataracts. Industrial pollution contributes to the burden by producing toxic metals (arsenic, mercury, and others), smoke, and many other toxins. Many pharmaceutical medications trigger the production of free radicals in users. In addition, people with chronic diseases such as diabetes generate more free radicals than healthy individuals. Athletes produce a higher amount of free radicals, as a by-product of exercise. Smoking, alcohol, fried foods, and high-fat diets all are notorious sources of toxic free radicals.

ANTIOXIDANT ENZYME SYSTEM

Our bodies have a built-in antioxidant system. It includes key enzymes such as catalase, superoxide dismutase (SOD), and glutathione peroxidase. Minerals such as selenium, manganese, zinc, and copper are required to keep these enzyme systems working efficiently.

COMMON ANTIOXIDANTS

Since the typical North American diet is deficient in antioxidant-rich plant foods, it is important for people to supplement additional antioxidant nutrients. Well-known antioxidants include vitamins A, C, and E, as well as selenium, glutathione, CoQ10, and beta-carotene. Additional ones include lutein, lycopene, and other carotenoids. Grapeseed extract, N-acetylcysteine, alpha lipoic acid, and tocotrienols are also great antioxidants. Phytonutrients, found in herbs such as green tea, turmeric, ginkgo, and milk thistle, have some of the most potent antioxidant activity ever discovered. Each of the antioxidants plays a key role in neutralizing free radicals and optimizing immune-system function. These are just a few examples of the antioxidants that are available in foods and supplements.

TESTING ANTIOXIDANT STATUS

There are several different ways you can test your antioxidant status. One is to have a blood test that measures the levels of key antioxidants found in your blood. Another is to have a blood or urine test that measures the level of oxidative stress in your body. This gives an assessment of your body's oxidative-stress status and antioxidant reserves.

References

Anderson, R. A. 1997. Chromium as an essential nutrient for humans. *Regulatory Toxicology and Pharmacology* 26(1 Pt 2):S35–41.

Bower, C., F. Stanley, and D. Nicol. 1993. Maternal folate status and risk for neural tube defects. *Annals of the New York Academy of Sciences* 678:146–55.

Fairfield, K. M., and R. H. Fletcher. 2002. Vitamins for chronic disease prevention in adults: Scientific review. *Journal of the American Medical Association* 287:3116–29.

Ferslew, K. E., et al. 1993. Pharmacokinetics and bioavailability of the RRR and all racemic stereoisomers of alpha-tocopherol in humans after single oral administration. *Journal of Clinical Pharmacology* 33(1):84–88.

Recker, R. R., et al. 1988. Calcium absorbability from milk products, an imitation milk, and calcium carbonate. *American Journal of Clinical Nutrition* 47:93–95.

Werler, M., S. Shapiro, and A. Mitchell. 1993. Preconceptual folic acid exposure and risk of occurent neural tube defects. *Journal of the American Medical Association* 269:1257–61.

Herbal Medicine

History

Herbal medicine is the oldest therapy in world history, predating by tens of thousands of years the rich herbal remedies of ancient China, India, and Egypt. Herbs have been found in archaeological explorations in the most ancient of civilizations.

Much later on, around 400 BC, the Greeks began to systematize and codify medical principles. Hippocrates, whom we recognize as the father of Western medicine, and the doctors who followed him believed that there were four basic types of body fluids and that health was maintained by keeping each of these types in its proper balance. They relied upon herbs such as rosemary, fennel, and saffron, in conjunction with exercise, massage, and other gentle therapies, not just to treat the symptoms of an illness, but to stimulate a person's inner healing powers and to bring the unbalanced fluid back to its appropriate level.

Roman physicians took their cues from the Greeks. Before Roman soldiers went into battle, doctors painted the soles of the soldiers' feet with garlic oil as a way of stimulating the immune system in case of injury and promoting quick healing. One doctor, Dioscorides, detailed four hundred herbal remedies in his work *De Materia Medica*. Another doctor, Galen, expanded upon the body-fluid theories of the Greeks and further encouraged the idea of health as a matter of balance.

As the Romans conquered most of the Middle East and Europe (thanks to the garlic, no doubt), they brought their doctors, their medical treatises, and their remedies with them. By the time the Roman Empire fell, an herbal healing system had been firmly established throughout the continent. Garlic was recognized as an effective guard against colds and fever, and peppermint was widely known to encourage good digestion. Europeans knew that basil eased their cramps and that parsley acted as a diuretic. More important than the use of any one herb was the idea that plants in general were agents that, with the proper application, could be used to stimulate the body's natural healing response.

But by the medieval era, European medical practice had grown much more aggressive and invasive. Doctors began to rely upon emetics and purgatives for treating most illnesses—strategies that probably killed more patients than healed them. Worse, these doctors began to attack the local healers who used herbs. It's now thought that the witch hunts of early modern Europe were really ways for the medical establishment to remove the women who had knowledge of herbs and healing from their positions of power within the villages.

One fifteenth-century physician, Paracelsus, was so disgusted by the state of medical practice that he devoted his career to gentle, natural herbal therapies. He not only studied European sources, but also took care to include the considerable work of Middle Eastern herbalists. He learned which herbs could cure disease, and he taught other physicians that foods and herbs contained energy that could be absorbed and utilized by the body. Paracelsus didn't have everything right—he believed that a plant's shape was indicative of the part of the body it could cure—but he was a strong, credible voice that brought serious attention back to herbal treatment.

Since the time of Paracelsus, European medicine has been a battle between the holistic philosophy of herbalism and an increasingly mechanized view of the body. And as Europeans began to explore and colonize, this battleground spread to North America, where Native Americans had been using herbal remedies for centuries, if not millennia. Nevertheless, herbalism remained an important and respected tradition in Europe, as well as in America, up through the early 1900s.

By the middle of the twentieth century, however, herbal remedies were almost completely eclipsed by the development of synthetic "wonder drugs." Scientists learned how to isolate the active ingredients in herbs and patent them as medications like morphine and aspirin. Pharmaceutical companies made huge profits from the sales of their products and used the money in part to fund medical schools that shunned teaching herbalism. Soon herbs—the very source of many of the "legitimate" pharmaceuticals—were ridiculed as ineffective and untested.

It's not hard to understand the deep distrust that exists between pharmaceutical companies and many natural health-care doctors and practitioners. Pharmaceutical companies can't put a patent on a natural remedy like herbs, and, therefore, they can't control profits in the same way they can with synthetic drugs.

But it's deeper than mere greed. We've grown only too familiar with Western medicine's approach to disease, which views the body as a machine with parts to be either fixed or replaced. Symptoms of disease—fatigue, cough, constipation, and so on—are treated with drugs or procedures, while the cause, which is often improper living, goes ignored. In the United States, health is too often considered the absence of any obvious disease. Get rid of the symptoms, you have gotten rid of the disease. Right? Not really!

Since the days of Hippocrates, Western herbalism has taken a radically different approach. Although we no longer believe in Hippocrates' theory of body fluids, we continue his emphasis on balance, on building and protecting our natural constitutions. With a strong constitution, the regular waves of viral diseases, like the flu epidemics that hammer so many of us over and over again, can be successfully resisted. And while disease may afflict us from time to time, many herbs in nature's pharmacy can treat the root cause of the ailment—an essential part of preventing its reoccurrence. With herbs, we not only cure periodic illness, but also prevent fresh onslaughts from weakening our constitutions and unnecessarily shortening our lives.

Keep in mind that 80 percent of the world's population relies on herbs as a primary form of medicine. Many cultures use herbal therapies as a first line of treatment for illness. For example, hospitals in China train doctors to specialize in herbal medicine for all the different categories of disease (cardiology, dermatology, etc.). Most medical doctors in Germany utilize herbal therapies in their practices. As herbal therapy enters mainstream medicine, more doctors are becoming educated and willing to recommend these treatments to their patients. By following the guidelines in this chapter, you can strengthen the various organ systems of your body and feel a difference in your health. If you are new to herbal medicine, start with common herbs, such as peppermint for an upset stomach or echinacea for the common cold. Your confidence will grow with each successful use of these wondrous herbs.

Mixing Herbs and Pharmaceuticals

As herbals became America's fastest-growing branch of alternative medicine, the Western medical community was the last to find out. Herbs are ignored in medical school and have only recently begun to make occasional appearances in medical journals. When doctors are oblivious to the benefits of herbal remedies, patients are often reluctant to reveal that they are taking herbals because of embarrassment at the prospect of a stern lecture on the subject.

Sometimes, the only time a doctor finds out about an herbal-pharmaceutical mix is when a patient suddenly exhibits strange symptoms not seen with the pharmaceutical alone. At times, that mix can be deadly. Add a commercial stimulant to ginseng, and we now know that we are increasing the likelihood of a potential bad reaction. Cardiac glycosides, herbal ingredients that act on the heart, can cause arrythmia—an irregular heartbeat—when taken with a prescription diuretic. The side effects of certain selective serotonin reuptake inhibitors (SSRIs) that are used to treat cases of major depression—marketed under names such as Prozac, Paxil, or Celexa—may be magnified by Saint-John's-wort, a popular herb intended for mild to moderate cases of depression.

But most often, herbs can be an effective complement to conventional therapies. Ginger, for example, has been shown in clinical trials to limit nausea from chemotherapy. Reports from Europe—where herbs have been used longer and studied much more thoroughly than in the United States—indicate that pharmaceutical–herbal interactions are unusual. The symptoms of an adverse reaction are likely to be muted, if you consider the generally mild nature of herbs. When there is a reaction, it's first likely to surface as an upset stomach or a feeling of discomfort. Your first response should be to stop the remedies and get in touch with a health care professional.

The use of standardized extracts, which are made up of specified quantities of herbal ingredients in commercially prepared remedies, is a good thing, but is likely to further complicate the use of pharmaceuticals combined with herbals. As herbal remedies are better prepared and quantified, they become more effective—and more dangerous when unknowingly mixed with pharmaceuticals.

Pharmaceutical companies have been quick to pick up on the popularity of herbs and have been careful to note which herbs and which pharmaceuticals may provoke harmful side effects. On the positive side, that has helped educate the public on the dangers of mixing. On the negative side, I've noticed that pharmaceutical companies are also quick to take the knee-jerk position of warning against all mixing—no doubt, at least in part to avoid any potential litigation, as well as a result of the age-old grudge match at work between pharmaceutical giants, which are a virtual global cartel now, and the herbal companies.

Even as doctors are being advised in a growing flood of special alerts about herbs to watch for, don't rely on your physician to make the connection. Too often, doctors are still struggling to understand the basics of herbal remedies. Medical schools typically avoid the subject of herbs in medicine. Pharmacists may understand little or nothing about herbalism, even if they can make the connection between herbs and the active ingredients in many prescription medications.

That means you have to make the connection yourself. Before mixing any herbs with any prescription medication, err on the side of caution. Aggressively go after the facts for yourself, and then go in prepared to ask your doctor questions. For more information on mixing herbs and pharmaceuticals, see our book *Prescription for Drug Alternatives*.

Don't take "no" for an answer. If your doctor flatly rules out an herbal remedy, ask why. If you're not satisfied with your doctor's response, why not track down another physician? Wait until you find a qualified physician who has taken the time to learn how herbs work. Even if he or she may be suspicious of herbs' long-term health effects, you need to see a doctor or a qualified herbalist who can review the potential interactions and help weed out beneficial herbal remedies from the questionable ones.

Always keep in mind that there may be several different herbal and pharmaceutical remedies to choose from, and seeing how each will interact can offer you some healthful substitutes while enabling you to avoid any toxic reactions. In some cases, you may decide to take a mix of herbs, supplements, and vitamins instead of a drug. Instead of an SSRI tranquilizer, for example, you may decide on a mix of DHA, which is included in the omega-3 fatty acids derived from seafood, and vitamin-B complex (containing B12, B6, and B5) along with Saint-John's-wort.

In this new world of digital information, millions of people are turning to the Internet to gain an unprecedented education in medicine. Use it to its full advantage, and bring a skeptical attitude to help find the most authoritative answers to your health questions. Health is the number-one category for searches on the Internet, and this curiosity on the part of the public will force doctors to spend more time on continuing education or risk falling behind many of their patients on the latest advances in their field.

Safe Use

The proper use of herbal preparations should pose no health dangers to you. There are herbs that are toxic and should not be used by the public. Most toxic herbs are not available in your typical health food store, drugstore, or supermarket supplement section. If you are unfamiliar with an herb or a combination of herbs and cannot find any valid literature, then simply do not use it. Please pay particular attention to how you should calculate a specific dosage for your child, which is discussed later in this section. This is important to help you achieve a therapeutic effect with the herbs.

When purchasing quality herbal products:

- Make sure the label provides easy directions and recommended dosages.
- The label should list all ingredients in order of potency.
- Look to see if the specific parts of the plants used are identified. For example, some herbs work better when their leaves are used; other herbs house their medicinal ingredients in the roots, not the leaves.

- Purchase products that are wrapped in safety seals to prevent tampering and preserve freshness.
- Make sure the label lists an expiration date and a lot number.
- Buy products that are certified to be organic. This ensures that no synthetic pesticides or herbicides were used in farming, harvesting, and preparing.
- Cautions should be listed on the container.
- The company should be known for high standards in quality control.

Herbal Preparations

TINCTURES

A tincture, or liquid extract, is the preservation of herbs in water and alcohol. This is one of the most common forms of herbal medicines, along with capsules and teas. Since it is in a liquid form, tinctures are easy to absorb and assimilate. Some herbs require an alcohol-extraction process so that certain medicinal constituents are pulled out of the plant and made available to the user. Some people do not like the taste, due to the alcohol. The taste can be improved by adding the herbs to a small cup of hot water and letting it sit for a few minutes, allowing some of the alcohol to evaporate, and then adding it to juice. Glycerine-based tinctures have had the alcohol removed and are more palatable for children and people averse to a product that contains alcohol.

CAPSULES

Capsules contain the dry powder of the herb. They are popular because of their convenience— they're easy to take, because no taste is involved, and easy to store in containers. The downside is that they can be used only by older children or adults who can swallow capsules. If the herb(s) you purchase are available only in capsule form and your child cannot swallow capsules, you can open the capsules up and mix the contents in water, juice, or food.

TABLETS

Tablets contain powdered herbs that have been compressed with binders and substances that make the tablet smooth and easy to swallow. The advantage is that more material can be compressed into a tablet. The downside is that many children and some adults cannot swallow tablets.

LOZENGES

Herbs can be made into a dissolvable lozenge. A common example is echinacea/zinc lozenges.

COMPRESSES

A compress involves the application of a hot or cold herbal extract to the skin. The herb can be put directly on the skin, or it can be applied to the skin using a cloth that has been saturated with the herb.

TEAS (DECOCTION/INFUSION)

A tea consists of an herb or an herbal combination soaked in water. There are two main methods of doing this. A decoction is used for harder plant parts, such as the bark, the root, and the seeds. These require more time and heat in order to extract the medicinal ingredients. First, you heat the herb (1 tablespoon of the dry herb or 3 tablespoons of the fresh herb) in water until it boils, then let it simmer (covered with a lid) for fifteen to twenty-five minutes. Next, let it sit for ten minutes, strain, and serve. An example of a tea that would involve making a decoction is one made from raw ginger root.

The more common preparation for a tea is an infusion. This uses the softer parts of herbs, such as leaves and flowers. It is effective for herbs like peppermint leaf; the tea can be drunk more quickly to capture the volatile oils. Commercial preparations of tea bags are available, or you can use dry or fresh herbs. If using a tea bag, add 1 bag to a cup of boiling water and let it sit for ten to fifteen minutes. For dry or fresh herbs, bring 1 cup of water to a boil in a kettle and add 1 tablespoon of the dry herb or 3 tablespoons of the fresh herb to the water. Cover it with a lid, and let it sit for ten to fifteen minutes. Strain and serve.

FOMENTATIONS

With this method, a cloth is soaked in a prepared infusion or a decoction. The wet cloth is then applied to the affected area. This preparation is good for skin rashes or local inflammation.

GLYCERITES

This is an herbal extract in a glycerin base. Glycerin is made from soaps and oils. It preserves herbs and is great for kids. It has no toxicity and can be sweetened easily for a taste kids love.

ESSENTIAL OILS

Medicinal herbs are preformulated to be highly concentrated and the volatile oils are extracted. They can be applied topically or smelled for a therapeutic effect.

CREAMS

The desired herb is blended with an emulsion of water in oil. This allows the oily mixture to blend with skin secretions and penetrate the skin for healing purposes.

SALVES

This is a mixture of herbal oils or extracts with beeswax.

LINIMENTS

This is a topical herbal preparation in oil.

POULTICES

A poultice consists of plant material applied to the skin by first mixing the herb into a paste and then applying it to the affected area between two thin pieces of cloth.

STEAM

Herbs or herbal (essential) oils are added to steaming hot water. This therapy is useful for ailments of the upper respiratory tract.

SUPPOSITORIES

Herbs are inserted into the rectum (e.g., for hemorrhoids) or the vaginal opening for a local treatment. Suppositories also provide a good way to get the herb into the bloodstream.

SYRUPS

Syrups can be added to sweeten decoctions and infusions.

BATHS

Adding herbal preparations to a warm bath can be effective. An example is an oatmeal bath for itchy skin breakouts or rashes.

STANDARDIZED EXTRACTS

This is an herbal extract that has been standardized to certain levels of active compounds. It can be important to duplicate the level of active compounds that were used in positive studies. At this time, many herbs have unknown active constituents.

Herbal Terms

The following terms are used to describe the properties and the actions of herbs. We have avoided most of these terms in this book and have instead used common terms. However, this list can be helpful when you consult other works on herbal medicine.

abortifacient   A plant that causes miscarriage or expulsion of the fetus. It is important that a pregnant woman avoid this type of plant. An example is the herb pennyroyal.

adaptogen   Helps the body adapt to stress, whether it be physical, mental, or emotional. It is often referred to as a "tonic." It supports energy levels. Many adaptogen herbs work in part by supporting adrenal-gland function. Ginseng is a classic example.

alterative An herb that helps improve general health by balancing and tonifying body functions. Alteratives boost nutritional status through improved digestion and elimination. They are sometimes referred to as "blood purifiers." Alteratives generally have a low potential for toxicity and can be used on a long-term basis. A good example is burdock root.

analgesic   Pain reliever. Also termed an anodyne (e.g., white willow).

anticatarrhal   Decreases mucus production (e.g., goldenseal, mullein).

antidepressant   Relieves feelings of depression (e.g., Saint-John's-wort).

antidote   Counteracts the effect of a poison.

antiemetic   Prevents vomiting (e.g., ginger).

antifungal Destroys or prevents fungal infections.

antigalactic Reduces or stops breast milk secretion (e.g., sage).

antihelmintic An herb that destroys parasites (e.g., garlic, wormwood, black walnut).

anti-inflammatory Reduces inflammation in the body (e.g., licorice root, bromelain, boswellia, white willow, black cohosh).

antimicrobial Prevents or destroys microbe (virus, bacteria, fungus, etc.) growth.

antioxidant Prevents the damage of cells by free radicals (e.g., ginkgo, astragalus, hawthorn berry, milk thistle, thyme, wild oregano).

antiparasitic Prevents the growth of or destroys parasites (e.g., black walnut, clove, garlic, wormwood).

antipyretic Reduces fever (e.g., yarrow).

antiseptic Prevents the growth of microbes on the skin (e.g., calendula, propolis).

antispasmodic Prevents or reduces muscle spasms (e.g., black cohosh, chamomile, kava, valerian, wild yam).

antitussive Relieves or suppresses coughing (e.g., horehound, wild cherry bark).

antitumor Fights or suppresses tumor growth (e.g., astragalus, echinacea).

astringent An herb that causes contraction of the tissues. It's useful in conditions such as bleeding or diarrhea (e.g., geranium, sage, witch hazel, yarrow).

bitters Bitter-tasting herbs that stimulate the digestive-organ secretions and actions—stomach, liver, gallbladder, pancreas. They can also help increase an abnormally low appetite (e.g., gentian root, burdock, goldenseal, dandelion root).

bronchodilator An herb that causes relaxation and dilation of the bronchial tubes (respiratory passageway). They're often used for coughs, bronchitis, and asthma (e.g., peppermint, ma huang, yerba santa).

calmative An herb that gently calms the nerves (e.g., chamomile, hops, kava, passionflower, valerian).

carminative Prevents or reduces gas (e.g., ginger root, fennel, anise, peppermint).

cathartic An herb that stimulates bowel evacuation (laxative; e.g., cascara sagrada, senna, rhubarb).

cholagogue Stimulates bile flow from the gallbladder (e.g., dandelion root).

choleretic Stimulates bile production in the liver (e.g., milk thistle, burdock, dandelion root).

demulcent An herb that has a soothing and healing effect on the mucous membranes of the body (e.g., slippery elm is a demulcent for the digestive tract).

diaphoretic An herb that causes perspiration. This can be useful with a cold, to help the immune system expel the virus (e.g., yarrow, boneset).

diuretic Promotes urination (e.g., dandelion leaf, parsley).

emetic An herb that causes vomiting (e.g., ipecac).

expectorant An herb that promotes the expulsion of mucus from the respiratory tract (e.g., horehound, lungwort, yerba santa).

febrifuge An herb that reduces fever (e.g., white willow).

galactagogue Stimulates milk flow (e.g., blessed thistle, fennel, fenugreek).

hemostatic An herb that stops bleeding (e.g., cinnamon, yarrow).

hepatic An herb that acts on the liver to stimulate bile flow (e.g., burdock, milk thistle, licorice, dandelion root, yellow dock, artichoke).

hypnotic An herb that induces sleep (e.g., valerian).

hypotensive An herb that lowers blood pressure (e.g., hawthorn berry, garlic).

immunomodulator   An herb that supports the action of the immune system (e.g., astragalus, echinacea, garlic, lomatium, Oregon grape, osha).

laxative   An herb that promotes fecal expulsion (e.g., cascara sagrada, senna, aloe, rehmania).

lymphagogue   Stimulates activity of the lymphatic system (e.g., burdock, ceanothus, pokeroot).

mucolytic   An herb that thins mucus secretions.

nervine   An herb that relaxes and calms the nerves (e.g., chamomile, passionflower, valerian, skullcap, lavender).

nutritive   An herb that is nourishing to the body (e.g., nettles).

palliative   Relieves symptoms but does not cure the disease (e.g., a child sleeps well when taking passionflower before bedtime, but cannot sleep unless he or she uses passionflower).

prophylactic   Herbs used to prevent a disease or a condition.

rubefacient   Herbs that are irritating to the skin and the mucous membranes. They're used to increase blood flow to the affected area (e.g., horseradish opens up the sinuses).

sedative   A calming herb (e.g., valerian, passionflower, chamomile).

stimulant   Increases energy or has an exciting action (e.g., ginseng).

synergist   An herb that acts to increase the effectiveness of another herb or herbs in a formula so that the sum of the herbs is greater than its parts (e.g., licorice root).

tonic   Nourishes and restores normal function (e.g., Siberian ginseng).

vermifuge   Promotes the expulsion of intestinal worms (e.g., wormwood).

vulnerary   Promotes tissue healing (e.g., calendula applied topically on cuts and scrapes or aloe for burned skin).

Storing Herbs

Most of the herbs used today come in commercial packaging. Therefore, it is easy to store them. General guidelines to remember:

- Tinctures—Store in the cupboard so that they are not exposed to light.
- Capsules and tablets—Make sure the lid is closed at all times, and do not store them in an area with high humidity.
- Teas—Bagged teas should be kept in an area that is dry and out of the light.
- Herbs bought in bulk should be stored in airtight glass containers. The temperature should be between 55 and 65 degrees F. Make sure to keep bulk teas out of the light as well.

Safety note: As with pharmaceutical medications, make sure to store herbal products out of the reach of children.

Helping Your Child with Herbs

The following information offers creative ways to administer herbs to children. Medicine doesn't have to taste bad to be good. In fact, many herbal medicines not only work better than conventional medicines but also taste better!

For example, if a tincture that has an alcohol base is used, put the desired amount of herb in a quarter cup of hot water for five minutes to let the alcohol evaporate, let it cool, and then add the tincture to water or juice. One of our favorites is to mix herbal teas with juice. Other strategies include:

1. Mixing herbal capsules in foods, such as oatmeal, applesauce, or jam.
2. Using a dropper to put the desired amount of tincture in the child's juice (dilute juice with 50 percent water). Concord grape juice hides bad-tasting herbs well.
3. For children who are stubborn, who refuse to eat or drink anything with herbs, or who will not take any medicine, there is one aggressive solution left. Use a dropper and squirt the desired amount in the side of the child's mouth. This way, the child can't spit it out. Be careful that the child does not bite the glass dropper while you use this technique.

PRECAUTIONS

As with any substance, whether it is a food, a drug, or a pollen, allergic reactions can occur with herbs. Although it is rare, you could be allergic to a single herb or an herbal formula. When using an herb or an herbal formula for the first time, take a small amount—such as 3 drops or a dab of the powder form, and see whether an adverse reaction happens in the next two hours. Chances are, there won't be a problem. If a severe allergic reaction does occur, such as wheezing, difficulty breathing, or hives, seek medical attention immediately and discontinue any further use of the herb. If more mild reactions occur, such as itching or a mild rash, choose another herb that has a similar action.

Quality Herbs

We feel that it is important to use only high-quality herbs. Organically grown herbs are recommended. Consult with a naturopathic doctor or a reputable herbalist, a nutritionist, or a holistic doctor to find out which brands are of the highest quality. Many health food store and pharmacy employees will be able to help you as well.

Frequency of Use

This book provides detailed information on how to take the recommended herbs and supplements for each condition. Following are general guidelines on how frequently you should take herbal supplements.

Acute conditions: Take the recommended dosage every two to three waking hours to relieve symptoms and support the body's response. For infectious conditions, continue the herbal treatment for two days after the symptoms have resolved to prevent a relapse.

Chronic conditions: Take the recommended dosage two to three times daily.

Note: Herbs can be taken with or between meals. If you are prone to digestive upset, take the herbs with meals. If the herbs are being used to strengthen digestion, we recommend that they be taken close to mealtime.

Dr. Stengler's Quick Dosage Guide for Children

Here is a simplified calculation that parents can use to calculate the dosage for their children:

Body weight: 5 to 30 pounds: ⅕ the adult dosage
              30 to 60 pounds: ¼ the adult dosage
              60 to 90 pounds: ⅓ the adult dosage
              90 to 120 pounds: ½ the adult dosage
              120 to 150 pounds: ¾ the adult dosage

HERB CHART

Note: Common medicinal uses for children are listed. More uses may be indicated for adults.

Alfalfa (Medicago sativa)

Medicinal Uses: Arthritis, indigestion, menopause, high cholesterol, ulcers, anemia, skin disorders

Parts Used: Mainly the leaves, but the seeds are used also.

Forms Used: Capsules, tablets, bulk herb

Potential Side Effects: Caution for people with systemic lupus erythematosus. High doses should not be taken by people on blood-thinning medications.

Comments: It's used for detoxification, hormone balancing, and alkalinizing properties.

Aloe Vera (Aloe vera)

Medicinal Uses: Externally for burns, scrapes, canker sores, and general wound healing.

Take internally for inflammatory bowel disease, ulcers, candida, intestinal infections, constipation, and other disorders of the digestive tract; psoriasis; diabetes; HIV

Parts Used: Leaves

Forms Used: Gel, cream, salve, and aloe-juice preparation (taken internally)

Potential Side Effects: Aloe latex form (not commonly available) should not be taken by people with inflammatory bowel disease, pregnant or nursing mothers, or children.

Comments: One of nature's top healing herbs for the skin and the digestive tract. Use food-grade juice when taking internally.

Anise (Pimpinella anisum)

Medicinal Uses: Intestinal gas, colic, parasites, bronchitis, and coughs

Parts Used: Seeds

Forms Used: Tea or tincture

Potential Side Effects: None known

Comments: It has a sweet taste that children like; often blended with bad-tasting herbs.

Artichoke (Cynara scolymus)

Medicinal Uses: High cholesterol and triglycerides, indigestion, poor fat digestion, constipation, poor liver function

Parts Used: Leaves

Forms Used: Capsule, tincture

Potential Side Effects: Too high a dose may cause loose stools.

Comments: Avoid it if you have an obstructed bile duct.

Ashwagandha (Withania somniferum)

Medicinal Uses: Stress, immune support, memory enhancement, osteoarthritis, aging, anemia, fatigue

Parts Used: Root

Forms Used: Tincture, capsules

Potential Side Effects: None known

Comments: It's an excellent stress-hormone balancer.

Astragalus (Astragalus membranaceus)

Medicinal Uses: Supports immune system (common cold, sore throat, preventative purposes), adaptogen, fatigue, hepatitis, heart function, chronic diarrhea, chemotherapy and radiation support

Parts Used: Root

Forms Used: Tincture, capsule, tea

Potential Side Effects: Do not use if you have a fever.

Comments: It can be used on a long-term basis for immune support.

Barberry (Berberis vulgaris)

Medicinal Uses: Candida, intestinal infections, parasites, diarrhea, immune support, skin ailments (psoriasis, eczema)

Parts Used: Root and stem bark

Forms Used: Tincture, capsule, ointment

Potential Side Effects: Avoid during pregnancy and when breast-feeding. Not to be used by infants.

Comments: It has very similar properties to goldenseal.

Basil (Ocimum basilicum)

Medicinal Uses: Constipation, indigestion, diabetes, hypothyroidism

Parts Used: Seeds and leaves

Forms Used: Tablet, capsule, tincture

Potential Side Effects: Avoid during pregnancy and when breast-feeding. Do not supplement if you have kidney or liver disease.

Comments: It has potent antioxidant properties.

Bilberry (Vaccinium myrtillus)

Medicinal Uses: Diabetes, retinopathy, macular degeneration, cataracts, diarrhea, eyestrain, glaucoma, hemorrhoids, night vision, varicose veins

Parts Used: Berries

Forms Used: Tincture, capsule, tablet, tea

Potential Side Effects: None known

Comments: It's one of the best herbs for the eyes.

Bitter Melon (Momordica charantia)

Medicinal Uses: Diabetes, indigestion

Parts Used: Fruit

Forms Used: Tea, capsule, tablet, tincture

Potential Side Effects: Excessive amounts may cause abdominal pain and diarrhea.

Comments: It's a great herb for people with diabetes.

Black Cohosh (Cimicifuga racemosa)

Medicinal Uses: Arthritis, fibromyalgia, depression, menopausal symptoms, menstrual

cramps, PMS

Parts Used: Root and rhizome

Forms Used: Tincture, capsule, tablet

Potential Side Effects: Do not use during pregnancy or when breast-feeding.

Comments: It's one of the best herbs for menopausal symptoms.

Bladderwrack (Fucus vesiculosus)

Medicinal Uses: Hypothyroidism, constipation

Parts Used: Algae stem

Forms Used: Tincture, capsule, tablet, tea

Potential Side Effects: None known, but choose a product screened for toxins and contaminants.

Comments: It supports thyroid function.

Black Walnut (Juglans nigra)

Medicinal Uses: Prevent or treat infections from parasites, worms, and yeast

Parts Used: Husk

Forms Used: Tincture, capsule

Potential Side Effects: Large doses can be sedating to the circulatory system; not to be used during pregnancy.

Comments: Use under the guidance of a health professional for the treatment of worms, parasites; short-term use only.

Blessed Thistle (Cnicus benedictus)

Medicinal Uses: Constipation, indigestion, insufficient milk supply of breast-feeding mother

Parts Used: Tincture, capsule, tea

Forms Used: Leaves, stems, flowers

Potential Side Effects: None known, but use with caution during pregnancy.

Comments: It's an excellent herb to promote milk production for breast-feeding mothers.

Blue Cohosh (Caulophyllum thalictroides)

Medicinal Uses: Amenorrhea, dysmenorrhea, labor pains

Parts Used: Root and flower

Forms Used: Tincture, capsule

Potential Side Effects: Amounts that are too high may cause headaches, nausea, high blood pressure. Only use during pregnancy under the guidance of a doctor.

Comments: It's a hormone balancer that is best used under the care of a knowledge-able practitioner.

Boswellia (Boswellia serrata)

Medicinal Uses: Arthritis, sports injuries, ulcerative colitis, asthma, bursitis

Parts Used: Resin of the tree branch

Forms Used: Capsule, tablet
Potential Side Effects: Very safe
Comments: It's a tremendous natural anti-inflammatory.

Bromelain

Medicinal Uses: Arthritis, burns, cancer, cardiovascular disease, protein digestion, injuries, respiratory mucus, surgery recovery, thrombophlebitis, varicose veins, sinusitis, and prostatitis
Parts Used: Stem of pineapple
Forms Used: Capsules, tablet
Potential Side Effects: Avoid combining with pharmaceutical blood thinners.
Comments: It's a natural anti-inflammatory when taken between meals and aids protein digestion when taken with meals.

Bugleweed (Lycopus virginicus)

Medicinal Uses: Hyperthyroidism
Parts Used: Leaves and flowers
Forms Used: Tincture, capsule
Potential Side Effects: Avoid if you have hypothyroidism. Do not use if you are pregnant or nursing.
Comments: It's one of the most effective supplements for cases of hyperthyroidism.

Burdock (Arctium lappa)

Medicinal Uses: Skin conditions such as rashes and acne, to improve liver function, detoxification, antimicrobial
Parts Used: Root
Forms Used: Tincture, capsule
Potential Side Effects: None known
Comments: It's a good general detoxifier, especially for skin conditions.

Butcher's Broom (Ruscus aculeatus)

Medicinal Uses: Hemorrhoids, varicose veins
Parts Used: Roots and stems
Forms Used: Tincture, tablet, capsule
Potential Side Effects: Nausea in rare cases
Comments: It's excellent for hemorrhoids and varicose veins.

Calendula (Calendula officinalis)

Medicinal Uses: Cuts, scrapes, rashes, burns, antiseptic
Parts Used: Flowers
Forms Used: Tincture (applied topically), creams, salves
Potential Side Effects: None
Comments: It's an excellent herb to promote healing and prevent infection of the skin.

Cascara (Rhamnus purshiana)

Medicinal Uses: Laxative
Parts Used: Bark
Forms Used: Tincture, capsule
Potential Side Effects: For short-term use only; long-term use can lead to electrolyte loss.

Comments: It's best used under the guidance of a health care professional if taken long term.

Catnip (Nepeta cataria)
Medicinal Uses: Colic, fevers, restlessness, and digestive aid
Parts Used: Leaves and flowers
Forms Used: Tea, tincture
Potential Side Effects: None
Comments: Only a few drops are needed for colic and restlessness for infants and children.

Cayenne (Capsicum frutescens)
Medicinal Uses: Improves circulation, antiseptic, stimulates sweating in the first stages of colds, heals sore throats, and relieves pain
Parts Used: Fruit
Forms Used: Tincture, capsule, and topical ointment
Potential Side Effects: Digestive upset
Comments: The topical ointment is used as a pain reliever. It's a powerful cardiovascular tonic.

Chamomile (Matricaria recutita)
Medicinal Uses: Indigestion, nervousness, colic, eczema, gingivitis, diarrhea, insomnia, anxiety, ulcers, and inflammatory bowel disease
Parts Used: Flowers
Forms Used: Tea, tincture, capsule
Potential Side Effects: Rare allergic reaction
Comments: It's helpful for a wide variety of digestive ailments.

Cinnamon (Cinnamomum zeylanicum)
Medicinal Uses: Colds, diarrhea, digestive upset, bleeding, heavy menstruation
Parts Used: Inner bark
Forms Used: Tincture, tea, as a food
Potential Side Effects: None in normal dosages
Comments: It's a warming herb that improves circulation.

Clove (Syzgium aromaticum)
Medicinal Uses: Topical anesthetic for teething
Parts Used: Flower buds
Forms Used: Essential oil
Potential Side Effects: Too high a dosage can be irritating to the mucosa
Comments: Apply 1 or 2 drops of clove essential oil to gums during teething to reduce pain.

Comfrey (Symphytum officinalis)
Medicinal Uses: Externally for sprains, burns, wounds, fractures
Parts Used: Root
Forms Used: Poultice
Potential Side Effects: Not to be taken internally, due to toxic alkaloids
Comments: It speeds healing of wounds and skin conditions.

Cornsilk (Zea mays)
Medicinal Uses: Bedwetting, urinary tract infections
Parts Used: Golden silk of corn
Forms Used: Tea or tincture
Potential Side Effects: None
Comments: It's used as a tonic for the urinary tract.

Corydalis (Corydalis turtschaninovii, Corydalis yanhusuo)
Medicinal Uses: Pain, insomnia, dysmenorrhea
Parts Used: Rhizome
Forms Used: Tincture, capsule
Potential Side Effects: Vertigo, nausea, and fatigue; should be avoided by pregnant
    and nursing women
Comments: It's an excellent natural pain reliever.

Cranberry (Vaccinium macrocarpon)
Medicinal Uses: Prevention and treatment of urinary tract infections
Parts Used: Ripe fruit
Forms Used: Unsweetened juice or capsule
Potential Side Effects: None
Comments: It has potent antioxidant properties.

Damiana (Turnera diffusa)
Medicinal Uses: Low libido, erectile dysfunction, depression
Parts Used: Leaves
Forms Used: Tea, tincture, capsule, tablet
Potential Side Effects: Higher amounts may cause loose stools. Avoid during pregnancy.
Comments: Historically, it was used as an aphrodisiac for both men and women.

Dandelion (Taraxacum officinale)
Medicinal Uses: Stimulates gallbladder and liver function; stimulates general diges-
    tion; leaf has a diuretic effect for edema; constipation; chronic skin problems
Parts Used: Root and leaf
Forms Used: Tea, tincture, capsule, tablet
Potential Side Effects: Diarrhea; do not use if gallstones are present.
Comments: It's an excellent liver tonic.

Devil's Claw (Harpagophytum procumbens)
Medicinal Uses: Arthritis, lower-back pain, indigestion
Parts Used: Root
Forms Used: Tincture, tablet, capsule
Potential Side Effects: Avoid if you have an ulcer or gallstones.
Comments: It's an effective natural anti-inflammatory.

Dong Quai (Angelica sinensis)
Medicinal Uses: Anemia, dysmenorrhea, irregular menses, PMS, menopause
Parts Used: Root
Forms Used: Tincture, capsule, tablet, tea
Potential Side Effects: Sun sensitivity. Avoid if you are pregnant or nursing.
Comments: It's used for many female conditions.

Echinacea (Echinacea purpurea or angustifolia)

Medicinal Uses: Immune-system enhancement, antiviral, antibacterial, antifungal

Parts Used: Roots and flowers

Forms Used: Tincture, tea, capsule, tablet

Potential Side Effects: Caution for people who are allergic to the daisy family. Do not use on a long-term basis if you have an autoimmune condition.

Comments: It's effective for colds, flus, sore throats, and respiratory tract infections; nature's antibiotic.

Elderberry or Elder Flowers (Sambucus nigra)

Medicinal Uses: Colds, flus, coughs, and sinusitis

Parts Used: Berries, flowers

Forms Used: Tincture, tea

Potential Side Effects: None

Comments: It's one of the best herbal medicines for the flu.

Elecampagne (Inula helenium)

Medicinal Uses: Respiratory tract infections, digestive support

Parts Used: Root

Forms Used: Tea, tincture

Potential Side Effects: None in normal doses; high doses can cause vomiting and digestive upset.

Comments: Use it as a lung tonic.

Ephedra or Ma Huang (Ephedra sinica)

Medicinal Uses: Cough, asthma, hay fever, sinusitis

Parts Used: Stem

Forms Used: Capsule, tea, tablet

Potential Side Effects: Hypertension, insomnia, heart arrhythmias or palpitations, dry mouth

Comments: Avoid during pregnancy or when breast-feeding. Best used under the guidance of a holistic doctor and never for long periods. Not available over the counter since 2004.

A study conducted by the Hospital for Sick Children in Toronto, in conjunction with the Canadian College of Naturopathic Medicine, looked at the safety of echinacea during pregnancy. In the study, 206 women who used echinacea during pregnancy for upper respiratory tract infections were analyzed, along with a control group of 198 pregnant women who had upper respiratory tract infections but never used echinacea. The researchers found no association between the use of echinacea and birth defects. There were also no differences in the rates of live births or spontaneous abortions between the two groups.

Another concern patients have is whether echinacea will affect fertility. This question is asked because of a 1999 press release about the topic. A study suggested that common herbal supplements, such as Saint-John's-wort, ginkgo, and echinacea, might adversely affect fertility. Researchers took hamster eggs, removed the outer coating, and exposed the eggs to the herbs. They then mixed in human sperm, which will usually penetrate the egg. At higher dosages, the herbs either impaired or prevented the sperm's ability to penetrate the eggs. High concentrations of *Echinacea purpurea* interfered with sperm enzymes.

Based on this, some researchers have prematurely concluded that echinacea may interfere with fertility. Is this a valid conclusion? No. There are several problems. In the body, any herb is first broken down by the digestive system. In this study, the researchers used the whole herb in relatively high concentrations, which would never contact sperm in real life. Also, the experiment was done in a laboratory petri dish. To be valid, human studies would have to be done. We have no problem recommending echinacea for short-term use in pregnancy or as needed for infections in people trying to conceive.

Eyebright (Euphrasia officinalis)
Medicinal Uses: Conjunctivitis, pink eye, allergies affecting the eyes, sinus and nasal congestion, cough
Parts Used: Whole herb
Forms Used: Tincture, capsule
Potential Side Effects: None
Comments: It can be used as an eyewash or taken internally.

Fennel (Foeniculum vulgare)
Medicinal Uses: Reduces intestinal gas, colic, respiratory tract infections; increases nursing mother's breast milk supply
Parts Used: Seed
Forms Used: Tincture, tea, capsule
Potential Side Effects: None in normal doses
Comments: It's an excellent digestive tonic; sweet tasting.

Fenugreek (Trigonella foenumgraecum)
Medicinal Uses: Digestive tract inflammation, colic, blood sugar imbalances, high cholesterol, constipation
Parts Used: Seed
Forms Used: Tincture, tea
Potential Side Effects: None
Comments: It's one of the better herbs for diabetes.

Feverfew (Tanacetum parthenium)
Medicinal Uses: Migraine headaches, arthritis
Parts Used: Leaves
Forms Used: Capsule, tincture
Potential Side Effects: Not recommended for children under two years of age or for pregnant and nursing women.
Comments: It's an excellent remedy for the prevention of migraine headaches.

Flaxseed (Linum usitatissimum)
Medicinal Uses: Inflammatory skin conditions, dry skin, constipation, arthritis
Parts Used: Seeds
Forms Used: Ground-up seeds (powder) or oil
Potential Side Effects: Too much can cause diarrhea.
Comments: Excellent for chronic skin conditions as it supplies essential fatty acids.

Garlic (Allium sativa)
Medicinal Uses: Immune-system support—antiviral, antibacterial, antifungal; ear infections; high cholesterol
Parts Used: Cloves
Forms Used: Fresh cloves, tincture, capsule, tablet
Potential Side Effects: Digestive upset
Comments: It's commonly used as eardrops for ear infections; excellent for elevated cholesterol levels; anticancer.

Gentian (Gentian lutea)
Medicinal Uses: Digestive stimulation, poor appetite
Parts Used: Root
Forms Used: Tincture, capsule
Potential Side Effects: Can aggravate preexisting heartburn, gastritis, or ulcers.
Comments: It's useful for malabsorption and low appetite after an illness.

Ginger (Zingiber officinalis)
Medicinal Uses: Reduces intestinal gas; sore throats; colds; anti-inflammatory; stimulates digestion
Parts Used: Root
Forms Used: Tea, tincture, capsule
Potential Side Effects: None in normal doses
Comments: It's one of the best herbs for intestinal gas; a warming herb.

Ginkgo (Ginkgo biloba)
Medicinal Uses: Poor memory, attention-deficit disorder, improves circulation (Raynaud's disease), intermittent claudication, depression, high blood pressure, impotence, PMS, radiation toxicity, tinnitus, stroke recovery/prevention, macular degeneration, cataracts, retinopathy, vertigo, Ménière's disease, migraine headaches
Parts Used: Leaf
Forms Used: Tincture, capsule
Potential Side Effects: Headache, digestive upset, blood thinning
Comments: It's one of the best herbs to improve circulation.

Ginseng: American ginseng (Panax quinquefolius), Siberian Ginseng (Eleutherococcus senticosus), and Chinese ginseng (Panax ginseng)
Medicinal Uses: Counteract stress—physical, mental, and emotional; immune-system support; fatigue. American ginseng is used for asthma.
Parts Used: Root
Forms Used: Tincture, capsule, tea
Potential Side Effects: Chinese ginseng can cause overstimulation.
Comments: American ginseng is cooling, Siberian ginseng is cooling, and Chinese ginseng is warming.

Goldenseal (Hydrastis canadensis)
Medicinal Uses: Colds, sore throats, flu, ear infections, digestive tract infections, fungal infections, sinusitis, diarrhea, urinary tract infections, parasites, vaginitis
Parts Used: Root
Forms Used: Tincture, capsule
Potential Side Effects: Digestive upset. Avoid if you are pregnant or nursing. Not to be used on a long-term basis.
Comments: It's very bitter; one of the best herbs to use for infections of the mucus membranes.

Gotu Kola (Centella asiatica)
Medicinal Uses: Poor memory, connective-tissue healing, varicose veins, burns, arcoidosis
Parts Used: Roots and leaves
Forms Used: Tincture, capsule

Potential Side Effects: None known

Comments: It decreases scar-tissue formation after an injury.

Green Tea (Camellia sinensis)

Medicinal Uses: Cancer prevention, cardiovascular-disease prevention, detoxification, digestive health, tooth-decay prevention, weight loss

Parts Used: Leaves

Forms Used: Tea, capsule, tablet, tincture

Potential Side Effects: Insomnia, anxiety

Comments: It contains some of the most potent antioxidants known.

Guggul (Commiphora mukul)

Medicinal Uses: Atherosclerosis, elevated triglycerides and cholesterol, hypothyroidism

Parts Used: Resin from plant stem

Forms Used: Capsule, tablet

Potential Side Effects: Digestive upset; pregnant or breast-feeding women should not use it.

Comments: It's an effective and popular natural remedy for high cholesterol levels.

Gymnema (Gymnema sylvestre)

Medicinal Uses: Diabetes, insulin resistance

Parts Used: Leaves

Forms Used: Tincture, tablet, capsule

Potential Side Effects: None known, but should be avoided during pregnancy or breast-feeding.

Comments: It's an excellent natural remedy for both types of diabetes.

Hawthorn (Crataegus oxycantha)

Medicinal Uses: Heart conditions (congestive heart failure, angina, cardiomyopathy, arrhythmia), hypertension

Parts Used: Berry

Forms Used: Tincture, capsule, tea

Potential Side Effects: Seek medical consultation when combining it with heart medications.

Comments: It's an excellent heart tonic.

Hops (Humulus lupulus)

Medicinal Uses: Stomachache due to anxiety, restlessness, insomnia, colic

Parts Used: Fruiting bodies (strobile)

Forms Used: Tincture, tea, capsule

Potential Side Effects: None known

Comments: It gently calms the nerves.

Horehound (Marrubium vulgaris)

Medicinal Uses: Bronchitis, asthma, coughs

Parts Used: Flowering herb

Forms Used: Tincture

Potential Side Effects: None known

Comments: It helps discharge mucus from the respiratory tract.

Horse Chestnut (Aesculus hippocastanum)
Medicinal Uses: Back pain, hemorrhoids, varicose veins
Parts Used: Seeds
Forms Used: Capsule, tablet, tincture
Potential Side Effects: Rare cases of digestive upset, headaches, and skin itching
Comments: It's an excellent remedy for varicose veins and hemorrhoids.

Horsetail (Equisetum arvense)
Medicinal Uses: Urinary tract infections
Parts Used: Stems
Forms Used: Tincture, tea, capsule
Potential Side Effects: None
Comments: Good source of silica.

Huperzia (Qian ceng ta, Huperzine A)
Medicinal Uses: Memory (Alzheimer's disease, age-related cognitive decline)
Parts Used: Moss
Forms Used: Capsule, tablet, tincture
Potential Side Effects: No known side effects. Use under a doctor's guidance if you are taking a medication that affects acetylcholine metabolism.
Comments: It's a specific herbal remedy for poor memory.

Interesting herbal facts:

- The Latin name for goldenseal, *Hydrastis canadensis*, means "a Canadian plant that accomplishes water." This refers to goldenseal's beneficial effect on the flow of mucus.
- The name "passionflower" is believed to come from its beautiful flowers, which are thought to represent the passion of Christ, the story of the crucifixion. The flowers look like a cross.
- An old-time remedy for sleeplessness in children is to stuff the pillow with hops before bedtime.
- Studies have shown that ginger is one of the most effective treatments for nausea and vomiting after surgery.
- *Ginkgo biloba* is the world's oldest living tree species. Fossil records date back more than two hundred million years. The tree can live as long as one thousand years. Medicinal Use of ginkgo dates back to its use in Chinese herbal medicine thirty-five hundred years ago.
- Garlic not only reduces "bad cholesterol" while increasing "good cholesterol," but regular use is also associated with a lower risk of stomach and colon cancer.
- Cranberry prevents bladder infections by stopping *E. coli* (the most common bacteria involved in bladder infections) from adhering to the bladder wall.
- Chamomile is a very popular medicine in Germany. In 1987, it was named "plant of the year." They, of course, use German chamomile, not Roman chamomile.
- According to Rudolph Weiss, M.D., the bitter taste of gentian root persists even in a dilution of 1:20,000! Gentian can help increase the appetite in people who are weak and have lost their desire for food. It does not increase food cravings in people with a normal, healthy appetite.
- Horehound has been used as an herbal cough expectorant for over two thousand years.
- Hawthorn berry improves the contractions of the heart muscle and improves blood flow through the coronary arteries.
- Milk thistle has been shown to help protect and regenerate liver cells.

Kava (Piper methysticum)

Medicinal Uses: Anxiety, insomnia, hyperactivity, muscle spasms

Parts Used: Root

Forms Used: Tincture, capsule, tea

Potential Side Effects: Skin rash rarely occurs. Avoid if you have liver disease or when consuming alcohol. Do not use while nursing or breast-feeding. Do not use if you are taking antianxiety or antidepressant pharmaceutical medications.

Comments: It's an excellent remedy for anxiety.

Lavender (Lavendula angustifolia)

Medicinal Uses: Stress, anxiety, headache, muscle spasms, insomnia, indigestion

Parts Used: Flowers

Forms Used: Tea, tincture, essential oil

Potential Side Effects: Best used externally

Comments: It's calming to the nervous system and the mind.

Lemon Balm (Melissa officinalis)

Medicinal Uses: Respiratory tract infections, fevers, depression, antiviral, cold sores, genital herpes, hyperthyroidism (Graves' disease)

Parts Used: Whole herb

Forms Used: Tincture, salve

Potential Side Effects: Not to be used if you have hypothyroidism or glaucoma.

Comments: It's a gentle calming herb.

Licorice (Glycyrrhiza glabra)

Medicinal Uses: Immune-system support, antiviral, coughs, sore throats, digestive tract inflammation, heartburn, adrenal-gland support, liver support, antispasmodic, anti-inflammatory, asthma, chronic fatigue syndrome, ulcers, reflux, hepatitis, shingles

Parts Used: Root

Forms Used: Tincture, tea, capsule, cream

Potential Side Effects: Large amounts can lead to water retention and thus increase blood pressure, so avoid if you have high blood pressure. Avoid during pregnancy.

Comments: It's sweet tasting. It reduces toxicity and increases the effectiveness of other herbs. Use as a topical gel for cold sores.

Lomatium (Lomatium dissectum)

Medicinal Uses: Immune-system support, antiviral, antibacterial, colds, urinary tract infections

Parts Used: Root

Forms Used: Tincture, capsule

Potential Side Effects: Skin rash in a small percentage of users. Do not use during pregnancy.

Comments: It's an excellent antiviral herb for colds and flus.

Maitake (Grifola frondosa)

Medicinal Uses: General immune support, antiviral, antitumor, HIV, diabetes, high cholesterol, cancer, hepatitis

Parts Used: Fruiting body
Forms Used: Tincture, capsule
Potential Side Effects: None known
Comments: It provides long-term immune support.

Marshmallow (Althea officinalis)

Medicinal Uses: Urinary tract infections, respiratory infections, diarrhea, asthma, cough, ulcer, and inflammatory bowel disease
Parts Used: Root
Forms Used: Tincture, capsule, tablet, tea
Potential Side Effects: None
Comments: It's a soothing herb for the mucus membranes of the body.

Milk Thistle (Silybum marianum)

Medicinal Uses: Liver congestion and cirrhosis, hepatitis, gallstones, alcohol and drug addiction recovery, constipation, PMS, indigestion, skin conditions (acne, eczema)
Parts Used: Seed
Forms Used: Tincture, capsule, tablet
Potential Side Effects: None known
Comments: It's the best-studied herb for hepatitis; protects and regenerates liver cells.

Motherwort (Leonurus cardiaca)

Medicinal Uses: Amenorrhea, menopause, heart palpitations, anxiety
Parts Used: Leaves and flowers
Forms Used: Tincture, capsule, tablet, tea
Potential Side Effects: Avoid during pregnancy.
Comments: It's used during menopause to reduce heart palpitations and anxiety.

Mullein (Verbascum thapsus)

Medicinal Uses: Coughs and bronchitis, upper respiratory tract infections, externally for ear infections, asthma, chronic obstructive pulmonary disease
Parts Used: Flowers, leaves
Forms Used: Tincture, capsule, oil for ear infections (topical), tea
Potential Side Effects: None known
Comments: It's a soothing herb for the respiratory tract.

Myrrh (Commiphora myrrha)

Medicinal Uses: Sore throats, urinary tract infections, gingivitis, mouth sores, parasites
Parts Used: Resin from the stems of the plant
Forms Used: Tincture
Potential Side Effects: Large doses taken internally may cause kidney irritation and diarrhea.
Comments: It's commonly used for infections of the throat and the mouth.

Nettles (Urtica dioica)

Medicinal Uses: Anemia, detoxification, rashes, arthritis, prostate enlargement, hay fever, brittle hair, edema
Parts Used: Leaves and root
Forms Used: Tincture, capsule, salves, tea

Potential Side Effects: None known

Comments: Very nutritive, very high in minerals. The root is used for the prostate and the leaves used for all other conditions.

Oatstraw (Avena sativa)
Medicinal Uses: Stress, depression, restlessness, fatigue, itchy skin
Parts Used: Seeds
Forms Used: Tincture, capsule, seeds
Potential Side Effects: None
Comments: An oatmeal bath is used for itchy skin.

Oregano (Origanum vulgare)
Medicinal Uses: Candidiasis, most infections
Parts Used: Leaves and dried herb
Forms Used: Tincture, capsule
Potential Side Effects: Do not use during pregnancy.
Comments: It's a powerful antifungal herb.

Oregon Grape (Mahonia aquefolium)
Medicinal Uses: Respiratory tract and urinary tract infections, diarrhea, psoriasis, parasites
Parts Used: Root and stem bark
Forms Used: Tincture, capsule
Potential Side Effects: Avoid during pregnancy.
Comments: It's often used as an alternative to goldenseal for infections of mucus membranes.

Passionflower (Passiflora incarnata)
Medicinal Uses: Insomnia, anxiety and restlessness, heart palpitations
Parts Used: Flower
Forms Used: Tincture, capsule, tea
Potential Side Effects: None known
Comments: It's a gentle nerve relaxer.

Pau d'Arco (Tabebuia aellanedae, Tabebuia impestiginosa)
Medicinal Uses: Candida, infections, parasites, prostatitis, cancer
Parts Used: Bark
Forms Used: Tea, capsule
Potential Side Effects: Large amounts may cause nausea, bleeding, and digestive upset. Avoid during pregnancy and breast-feeding.
Comments: It's commonly used for candida overgrowth; anticancer.

Peppermint (Mentha piperita)
Medicinal Uses: Colic, indigestion, nausea, fevers, irritable bowel syndrome, head aches, gallstones
Parts Used: Leaf
Forms Used: Tea, tincture, oil
Potential Side Effects: Heartburn in some individuals
Comments: It provides acute relief from digestive complaints.

Plantain (Plantain spp.)

Medicinal Uses: Antiseptic, anti-inflammatory, urinary and respiratory tract infections, topically for wounds and bites

Parts Used: Leaf

Forms Used: Tea, tincture

Potential Side Effects: None known

Comments: It works well topically for insect bites.

Pygeum (Pygeum africanum)

Medicinal Uses: Prostate enlargement, prostatitis

Parts Used: Bark

Forms Used: Capsule, tablet, tincture

Potential Side Effects: Mild digestive upset

Comments: It's a specific herb for prostate enlargement; works well combined with saw palmetto.

Red Raspberry (Rubus idaeus)

Medicinal Uses: Diarrhea, nausea, vomiting, sore throat, pregnancy support

Parts Used: Leaf and berry

Forms Used: Tincture, tea, food

Potential Side Effects: None known

Comments: Historically, it has been used by herbalists and naturopathic doctors as a uterine tonic before or during pregnancy.

Reishi (Ganoderma lucidum)

Medicinal Uses: Allergies, bronchitis, tumors, HIV, viral infections, immune support during chemotherapy and radiation treatments, hypertension, poor memory, liver detoxification, hepatitis

Parts Used: Fruiting body

Forms Used: Tincture or as a food

Potential Side Effects: None that are common; use caution during pregnancy.

Comments: It's used for long-term immune support.

Rosemary (Rosmarinus officinalis)

Medicinal Uses: Soothes nervous system, antioxidant, memory, lice, candida, hypothyroidism

Parts Used: Leaf

Forms Used: Tea, tincture

Potential Side Effects: Avoid during pregnancy.

Comments: It's generally used in a condition-specific combination herbal formula.

Sage (Salvia officinalis)

Medicinal Uses: Antimicrobial, reduces secretions, intestinal gas, hot flashes, sore throats, gingivitis, dries up breast milk

Parts Used: Leaves

Forms Used: Tea, tincture

Potential Side Effects: Very high amounts may cause neurological symptoms. Best used short term (less than two weeks).

Comments: This herb has a drying quality.

Sarsaparilla (Smilax spp.)
Medicinal Uses: Eczema, acne, psoriasis
Parts Used: Root
Forms Used: Tincture, capsule
Potential Side Effects: Stomach upset. Do not take during pregnancy or breast-feeding.
Comments: It's used to clear up skin conditions.

Saw Palmetto (Serenoa repens, Sabal serrulata)
Medicinal Uses: Acne, baldness, prostate enlargement, bladder infection prevention (men), polycystic ovarian syndrome, prostatitis
Parts Used: Berries
Forms Used: Tincture, capsule, tablet
Potential Side Effects: Rare digestive upset
Comments: It's the most well-researched herb for the prostate.

Senna (Cassia senna)
Medicinal Uses: Constipation
Parts Used: Leaves and pods
Forms Used: Tincture, capsule, tea, tablet
Potential Side Effects: Chronic use may cause bowel sluggishness; diarrhea.
Comments: It's best used short-term.

Shiitake (Lentinus edodes)
Medicinal Uses: General immune system support, HIV, hepatitis, cancer, bronchitis
Parts Used: Fruiting body
Forms Used: Tincture or food
Potential Side Effects: Rare digestive upset
Comments: It provides long-term immune support.

Skullcap (Scutellaria lateriflora)
Medicinal Uses: Nervousness, insomnia, anxiety, hyperactivity, poor digestion
Parts Used: Aerial part (above ground)
Forms Used: Tincture, capsule, tea
Potential Side Effects: None
Comments: It's one of the best herbs to use for insomnia.

Slippery Elm (Ulmus fulva)
Medicinal Uses: Soothes mucus membranes of respiratory tract, digestive tract, and urinary tract; bronchitis; colitis; ulcers; heartburn; gastritis; sore throats; and urinary tract infections
Parts Used: Inner bark
Forms Used: Tincture, capsule, tea, and lozenge
Potential Side Effects: None known
Comments: It's a soothing herb for the mucus membranes.

Soy (Glycine max)
Medicinal Uses: Cancer prevention, high cholesterol, menopausal symptoms, osteoporosis, PMS
Parts Used: Bean

Forms Used: Capsule, tablet, powder

Potential Side Effects: Digestive upset. Do not use isoflavone extracts if you have cancer, unless instructed to do so by your doctor. Use with caution if you have hypothyroidism.

Comments: It's a great estrogen balancer.

Spirulina (Spirulina)

Medicinal Uses: Anemia, cancer, high cholesterol, detoxification, immune support, radiation poisoning

Parts Used: Algae

Forms Used: Capsule, tablet, powder

Potential Side Effects: None known

Comments: It's an excellent detoxifier and full of minerals.

Saint-John's-wort (Hypericum perforatum)

Medicinal Uses: Anxiety; depression; viral infections; topically for burns, scrapes, nerve pain, bruises; seasonal affective disorder

Parts Used: Flowers, whole herb

Forms Used: Tincture, capsule, oil

Potential Side Effects: Small percentage of users develops sensitivity to light. Should not be combined with pharmaceutical antidepressants.

Comments: It's a great herb for mild to moderate depression.

Stevia (Stevia rebaudiana)

Medicinal Uses: Natural sweetener

Parts Used: Leaf

Forms Used: Tincture, powder, crystals

Potential Side Effects: None known

Comments: It's a safe natural sweetener.

Tea tree (Melaleuca alternifolia)

Medicinal Uses: Topically for skin fungus, burns, and acne, cold sores, mouth and gum infections, skin infections, vaginitis, warts

Parts Used: Leaves

Forms Used: Tincture, oil

Potential Side Effects: Too high a concentration can be irritating to the skin. Use cautiously on the face. Do not ingest internally (except for mouthwashes), unless under the guidance of a doctor.

Comments: It's excellent for athlete's foot.

Thuja (Thuja occidentalis)

Medicinal Uses: Externally for warts

Parts Used: Branches, leaves, bark

Forms Used: Oil, tincture

Potential Side Effects: Not to be taken internally by children

Comments: It's an excellent topical treatment for warts.

Thyme (Thymus vulgaris)

Medicinal Uses: Respiratory tract infections (bronchitis) and urinary tract infections, topically for skin fungus, bad breath

Parts Used: Leaves and flowers
Forms Used: Tincture, capsule, tea
Potential Side Effects: Too much of the essential oil can cause abdominal pain.
Comments: It's mainly used in respiratory tract infection formulas.

Turmeric (Curcuma longa)
Medicinal Uses: Anti-inflammatory, antitumor, arthritis, indigestion
Parts Used: Rhizome (the part of the plant that's above ground)
Forms Used: Tincture, capsule
Potential Side Effects: Do not take high amounts during pregnancy. Use with caution if you have gallstones.
Comments: It's one of the best anti-inflammatory herbs.

Usnea (Usnea barbata)
Medicinal Uses: Cough, cold, infection
Parts Used: Entire lichen
Forms Used: Tincture, capsule
Potential Side Effects: Use with caution during pregnancy and breast-feeding.
Comments: It helps clear up respiratory tract infections.

Uva ursi (Arctostaphylos uva ursi)
Medicinal Uses: Urinary tract infections
Parts Used: Leaves
Forms Used: Tincture, capsule
Potential Side Effects: None in normal doses, but higher doses may cause cramping, nausea, or vomiting.
Comments: It's one of the best herbs for urinary tract infections.

Valerian (Valeriana officinalis)
Medicinal Uses: Insomnia, restlessness, spasms, pain
Parts Used: Root
Forms Used: Tincture, capsule
Potential Side Effects: A small percentage of users feel drowsy in the morning if it's used as a sleep aid.
Comments: It's one of the stronger nerve-relaxing herbs.

Vitex (Vitex agnus-castus)
Medicinal Uses: Acne, amenorrhea, fibrocystic breast syndrome, infertility, irregular menses, dysmenorrhea, improved lactation, hot flashes, ovarian cysts, PMS, uterine fibroids
Parts Used: Dried fruit
Forms Used: Tincture, capsule, tea, tablet
Potential Side Effects: Occasional digestive upset, headaches, skin rash. Do not use if you are taking the birth-control pill. Avoid during pregnancy unless specifically prescribed by a practitioner.
Comments: It's the most versatile female hormone–balancing herb.

Wheatgrass (Triticum aestivum)
Medicinal Uses: Detoxification, halitosis, inflammatory bowel disease
Parts Used: All

Forms Used: Juice

Potential Side Effects: Bad breath, immune enhancement, ulcers, ulcerative colitis

Comments: Wheatgrass is rich in chlorophyll, a phytonutrient that has potent anti-oxidant properties. It contains vitamin K, so do not combine it with Coumadin (warfarin), a blood-thinning medication.

Wild Cherry (Prunus serotina)

Medicinal Uses: Cough, bronchitis

Parts Used: Bark

Forms Used: Tincture

Potential Side Effects: None known

Comments: Not to be used in large amounts or for prolonged periods of time.

Willow (Salix alba and spp.)

Medicinal Uses: Headaches, pain, fever, arthritis

Parts Used: Bark

Forms Used: Tincture, capsule, tea

Potential Side Effects: Do not use if you are on blood-thinning medications or have hemophilia, as it thins the blood. Not to be used during viral infections.

Comments: It's a natural alternative to aspirin.

Witch Hazel (Hamamelis virginiana)

Medicinal Uses: Gingivitis, eczema (topically), inflamed veins, cold sores, wound healing

Parts Used: Bark

Forms Used: Tincture

Potential Side Effects: Internal use may cause stomach cramping.

Comments: It's excellent when used topically for hemorrhoids and varicose veins.

Wormwood (Artemisia absinthium)

Medicinal Uses: Parasites, indigestion

Parts Used: Leaves, flowers, oil

Forms Used: Tincture, capsule, tea

Potential Side Effects: High amounts used over long periods of time may cause digestive upset, diarrhea, and tremors. Do not use during pregnancy or when breast-feeding.

Comments: It's excellent for parasites and digestive tract infections.

Yarrow (Achillea millefolium)

Medicinal Uses: Fevers, toothaches, digestive upset, improves circulation, cold, inflammatory bowel disease

Parts Used: Flowers, leaves

Forms Used: Tincture, tea

Potential Side Effects: External application may result in a rash. Do not use during pregnancy or breast-feeding.

Comments: It's mainly used for feverish conditions.

Yellow Dock (Rumex crispus)

Medicinal Uses: Sore throat, iron-deficiency anemia, liver tonic, poor digestion

Parts Used: Root

Forms Used: Tincture, capsule

Potential Side Effects: None

Comments: It's great for iron-deficiency anemia; contains a small amount of iron and enhances the absorption of iron.

Yerba Santa (Eriodictyon californicum)

Medicinal Uses: Bronchitis, laryngitis

Parts Used: Leaves

Forms Used: Tincture, tea

Potential Side Effects: None

Comments: It helps to expel respiratory mucus.

References

Gallo, M., et al. 1999. Pregnancy outcome following gestational exposure to echinacea, a prospective controlled study. The Motherisk Program, Division of Clinical Pharmacology, Hospital for Sick Children and the University of Toronto, Canadian College of Naturopathic Medicine.

Ondrizek, R. R., et al. 1999. Inhibition of human sperm motility by specific herbs used in alternative medicine. *Journal of Assisted Reproduction and Genetics* 16(2):87–91.

Homeopathy

What Is Homeopathy?

Homeopathy is one of the fastest-growing alternative forms of medicine in North America. This form of medicine uses ultradiluted amounts of plant, mineral, and animal substances to stimulate the healing systems of the body. Homeopathy is effective for a wide range of conditions and is available in health food stores, pharmacies, and and some large grocery stores. Homeopathy can be used to strengthen the defense systems of the body and to stimulate healing of mental or emotional imbalances. Homeopathic remedies are an excellent therapy to stimulate or help repair a damaged immune system. Since homeopathic medicines are ultradiluted, they are extremely safe for children. (No side effects or toxicity!)

Homeopathic researchers are finding that each homeopathic remedy has its own "fingerprint" on the electromagnetic spectrum. It appears that homeopathic remedies work on a vibrational/energetic level. Unlike most pharmaceutical or natural medicines, homeopathic remedies appear to work directly at the electromagnetic level. In some ways, each remedy has a different electromagnetic frequency and thus action, similar to the various actions of different acupuncture points.

History of Homeopathy

> *"Like cures like."*
> —Samuel Hahnemann

Few therapies owe as much to one man as does homeopathy. While many people have gone on to study and practice homeopathy, virtually everyone in the field bows to an influential eighteenth-century physician named Samuel Hahnemann.

Born in Germany and raised to practice medicine, Hahnemann was an enigmatic, easily angered man—and an entirely original thinker. At a time when bloodletting was still a commonly exercised and often fatal "cure," Hahnemann railed against the medieval quality of Western medicine, which often hurt or killed patients instead of healing them.

Disgusted by the harmful effects of the practice, Hahnemann quit medicine. But later, he hit upon a unique—and now widely practiced—therapy. His healing methods grew out of a heated public dispute with a Scottish herbalist over the medicinal powers of Peruvian bark, known as cinchona, which we now know contains quinine.

Spanish conquerors had brought cinchona back to Europe after discovering that it could be used to cure malaria, which was then ravaging much of the continent. According to an oft-told story, the Scottish professor William Cullen attributed cinchona bark's powers to its bitter taste. Cullen theorized that the bitterness acted as a tonic to the body and reduced malaria's often-fatal fever—a key symptom. Cullen's ideas fit neatly into medical thought at that time, when researchers looked for ways to eliminate the symptoms of a disease as a method for treating the illness itself.

Hahnemann decided to test the theory, using his own body as a guinea pig. While completely healthy, he started taking doses of cinchona, carefully keeping notes as his body began to experience many of the same symptoms as a malaria patient.

"My feet, finger ends, etc., at first became cold; I grew languid and drowsy; then my heart began to palpitate, and my pulse grew hard and small; intolerable anxiety, trembling, prostration throughout all my limbs; then pulsation, in the head, redness of my cheeks, thirst, and, in short, all these symptoms which are ordinarily characteristic of intermittent fever."

When he stopped taking cinchona, the symptoms stopped, only to be triggered again by a fresh dose.

Out of this one experience grew the entire field of homeopathy, now one of the most widely practiced forms of complementary medicine in the world. Hahnemann believed that the bark's curative power was reflected by its ability to create the same set of symptoms as the disease itself. From this, he established the "law of similars," maintaining that "like cures like." It's important to understand the concept, as it lies at the heart of homeopathic cures.

First, Hahnemann was an early believer that the human body typically comes fully equipped with the ability to fight off disease. It's the role of medicine, he felt, to facilitate that great internal healer with fresh cures that would make our bodies even better disease fighters.

Symptoms weren't the problem, Hahnemann wrote, but were signs that the body's powerful immune system was fighting a disease. When his fellow doctors were busy attacking the symptoms, he felt that they were using treatments that acted only to eliminate the symptom and thereby suppress the disease. Hahnemann believed that doctors, rather than helping a patient recover, were in fact damaging the body's natural ability to fend off disease, leaving the patient even less prepared to fight off an illness the next time it occurred.

When a body responded to a cold with a nasal discharge, Hahnemann saw it as a sign that the body's immune system had gone to work. He believed that the best course wasn't to devise drugs that would stop the nose from running, which wasn't the real problem to begin with, but to find new cures from substances that, in their crude form, re-create the same symptoms.

Today homeopathy is widely practiced in Europe and the United Kingdom and is rapidly gaining popularity in North America.

If these substances mimic the symptoms in a healthy body, he said, you'll find the source of new medicines that will help the immune system combat illness. It's important to understand that what causes symptoms in large doses can act as a remedy when administered in tiny amounts.

It wasn't the first time this thought had been expressed. The father of Western medicine, Hippocrates, wrote, "Through the like, disease is produced, and through the application of like it is cured." The word *homeopathy* is derived from the Greek—homois (similar) and pathos (suffering). This is exactly the same thinking that goes into the development of new vaccines and allergy medications. When we take small amounts of the virus that can cause disease and inject them into the body, we improve the immune system's ability to fight off that illness. Addressing immunity is one of the few areas of traditional Western medicine that homeopaths can completely agree with.

The Law of Proving

Using himself and his large family as his original test subjects, Hahnemann went on to test—or, as he called it, "prove," based on the German word for "test"—dozens of remedies drawn from minerals, herbs, and animal parts. "The Law of Proving," that you can determine a substance's medicinal effect by testing it on groups of people, is still practiced today much as it was in 1790.

In the beginning, Hahnemann and the early advocates of homeopathy would take small doses of different substances until they provoked a set of symptoms that could be recorded. At that time in history, animals were never used in proving, as the difference between animal and human physiology would lead to a different set of symptoms. The only major difference between proving today and proving two hundred years ago is that now homeopaths will conduct a classic double-blind test, splitting a group in two and giving half the group a placebo and the other half the remedy under examination.

Hahnemann started by journeying into some dangerous areas. He experimented with belladonna, or deadly nightshade, and even arsenic, along with a whole range of toxic substances that could provoke a violent response in a patient when administered in their concentrated crude forms. During this proving process, the homeopath would carefully write down the symptoms that were caused by each substance. The most common symptoms were written in bold face, any symptoms experienced by a large group were written in italics, and infrequently experienced symptoms were written in plain text. The fact that homeopaths still find that people respond uniformly to many of these substances underlines the clinical accuracy that has characterized homeopathy from its beginning.

Once Hahnemann and his followers found a substance that would create the classic symptoms of a disease, they felt that they could use trace amounts of the material to fight the disease itself.

The Law of Potentization

The most meticulous of men, Hahnemann began to prepare various doses of his chosen substances, weakening and strengthening the remedies and carefully noting the symptoms produced with different concentrations. During this process, he found that he could improve the results by dissolving the substances in water or alcohol and vigorously shaking the mixture—a method he called "sucussion."

By successively diluting his remedies, a process he called "potentization"—the third law of homeopathy—Hahnemann showed in his home trials that the resulting remedy would grow in potency. Hahnemann found that patients started to recover from their illnesses, usually within forty-eight hours of beginning treatment. It was a slow and methodical process. Hahnemann would take 1 drop of his remedy and start by mixing it with 99 parts of a neutral liquid—alcohol, milk, or water—then he would shake it thirty times. That first dilution of the medication is ranked 1C. Then he would take the diluted substance and dilute it again into 99 parts of the neutral liquid, a routine he repeated as many as 30 times (30C) before he reached the desired amount of potentization.

Now here is an important point to remember, since the strengths of homeopathic medicines are still ranked by this same scale. In some cases, a homeopathic doctor will recommend a remedy diluted to 6C, at other times to 30C, and many other potencies are available. By the way, Hahnemann's home kitchen recipes have been entirely replaced by modern manufacturers' precise methods of sucussion and potentization.

Hahnemann's critics, and there were many, scoffed at the idea that such minute quantities of the original substance could have a therapeutic effect on a patient. But Hahnemann maintained, as his followers do today, that the process of sucussion released the vital energies inherent in the remedies. He theorized that those primary energies were most effective in bolstering the immune system.

Most often, if there is no improvement after two days with an acute illness, the homeopath is likely to switch to another remedy. Each person's body is unique (age, weight, hereditary predispositions, allergies, etc.), so remedies need to conform to each individual. Patients who continue to take the medication for a prolonged period run the risk of staging an accidental proving, where they begin to provoke more of the same symptoms. Homeopathy seeks a rapid recovery. No one is asked to take homeopathic medicines the way he or she might take daily doses of vitamins.

The Hard Way

It was never an easy therapy to defend, though Hahnemann rarely seemed to do anything the easy way. Suffering in extreme poverty for much of his life, he remained a caustic critic of medicine as it was practiced in the nineteenth century.

In 1812, Hahnemann's theories were put to the extreme test when Napoleon allowed him to treat 180 people suffering from typhoid, a disease that was rampaging through France, killing thousands and confounding most physicians. Only one of this group died, a remarkable result at that time, and homeopathy began to take hold in European medical practices as a well-regarded complementary practice.

In 1832, homeopaths were given credit for successfully combating a cholera epidemic. The epidemic helped to usher homeopathy into America, where it became one of the most popular therapies available in nineteenth-century American medicine.

Before he died in 1843, Hahnemann and his growing band of colleagues "proved" ninety-nine remedies. These medicines are now the core of more than five hundred medicines outlined in modern homeopathy's *materia medica*.

Homeopathy continued to thrive in Europe. It is one of the most common alternative therapies available in Germany. In Britain, homeopathy has even been adopted by the royal family to treat much of what ails them. And in America, the last decade has seen a definite increase in awareness of homeopathic remedies. These remedies are now taking their place at checkout counters in grocery and health food stores across the country.

If we look back to Hahnemann's time, it is easy to see in retrospect that any therapy that relied on the power of the body's natural immune system was often vastly superior to the toxic array of treatments then in vogue. In the eighteenth and early nineteenth centuries, people's chances of making a full recovery were often markedly higher if they trusted their bodies' natural recuperative powers rather than any of the elixirs prescribed by physicians—a cause of considerable controversy then and now. Even in the present day, homeopaths often find themselves at loggerheads with conventional medicine, denouncing its reliance on suppressing drugs to wipe out symptoms without addressing the reasons why people get sick in the first place.

Most modern critics of homeopathy focus on its foundation stone: Toxic substances that can harm or kill a patient when taken in full strength will cure when weakened to the point that only trace elements remain. To the conventional physician who laughs at the healing powers of homeopathy, such a premise is illogical, even absurd.

But pharmacology has long recognized that while some poisons can kill, a reduced potion may only debilitate, and a tiny dose can stimulate a body and help fight disease. Recent research is showing that smaller doses of chemotherapy are more effective (and healthful) for people with certain cancers. Arsenic has emerged back on the scene, with small doses showing benefit against certain cases of cancer. In regard to the small doses of homeopathics, any doctor can tell you that epinephrine, which is often used for life-threatening allergic reactions, is quite effective at a dilution of 1:100,000. More recently, physicists have begun to explore the role of sucussion, speculating that the repeated shaking of the dose creates an internal electromagnetic pattern that can be duplicated ad infinitum in our bodies or that can influence our electromagnetic fields in positive and healthful ways. Several published studies have proven the effectiveness of homeopathy.

> Homeopathic remedies are aimed at balancing your body's immune system and all other healing systems of your body.

Reasons for Using Homeopathy

There are five main reasons why homeopathy is gaining popularity among doctors and the public:

1. Homeopathy is highly effective for both chronic and acute diseases, including epidemics. It works to strengthen the immune and other healing systems of the body. It can be used to treat conditions for which conventional medicine has no effective treatment.
2. It is cost effective. Compared to pharmaceutical medications, homeopathic remedies are quite inexpensive.
3. It is a preventative medicine. One does not have to have a disease to be treated with homeopathy. It can be used to optimize health.
4. It can be used to treat the whole person. Homeopathy takes into account all the

factors of a person's health, even a child's—the mental, the emotional, and the physical.

5. Side effects are not an issue, which is especially important when it comes to children and seniors, who are more prone to toxic side effects of medications.

Homeopathy, as with many of the natural therapies, works with the healing systems of the body. As we will see in the remedy chart located in this chapter, homeopathic medicines are prescribed not only for the disease itself (such as the flu or anxiety), but also for symptoms that are expressed by the person. This allows for an actual improvement in chronic health conditions, rather than just merely suppressing symptoms. Symptoms are used to differentiate the homeopathic remedy for the individual, thus allowing for the "whole" person to be treated.

Homeopathic Studies: Scientific Evidence

Researchers have been studying homeopathy for decades. There can be some challenges to studying homeopathic treatment. Pharmaceuticals and nutritional supplements can be matched to specific problems and studied accordingly. For example, the medication Celebrex and the natural supplement glucosamine both are used to treat osteoarthritis, so studies focus on the effectiveness of those therapies for that particular disease. However, homeopathic treatment is highly individualized according to a patient's overall profile. If a patient comes to me for relief of migraines, we can choose from among several dozen homeopathic remedies, taking into account the type and location of his migraines, how the weather affects him, his diet and exercise habits, etc. With so many variables affecting the choice of remedy and the patient's response to it, we are not surprised that study results sometimes are contradictory or inconclusive.

Even so, there is lots of evidence to support the effectiveness of homeopathy—even from its earliest days. For instance, this therapy was extremely successful in treating infectious disease outbreaks in the nineteenth century. Recorded death rates in homeopathic hospitals that treated cholera, scarlet fever, typhoid, and yellow fever typically were less than one-half or even one-fourth those of conventional medical hospitals.

Overall, more than one hundred clinical trials have demonstrated homeopathy's benefits. Following is a sampling:

A 2014 study lasting four years researched the benefits of complementary homeopathic treatment for those who were receiving conventional cancer therapy. Those who had received at least three homeopeathic consultations in four years had a median overall survival was prolonged for those with a variety of types of cancer.

A randomized, double-blind study conducted in 2005 at the University of Vienna involved fifty patients with chronic obstructive pulmonary disease (chronic bronchitis and/or emphysema) and a history of smoking. Compared with participants who received placebos, those who took homeopathic remedies had very significantly reduced levels of the mucus secretions that impair breathing, and their average hospital stay was just 4.2 days, compared with 7.4 days for the placebo group.

In 2000, researchers at the University of Glasgow conducted a study involving 550 patients with allergic respiratory symptoms, such as asthma and rhinitis—then compared the results to those of three other studies involving a total of 253 patients. Findings: participants who took homeopathic treatments experienced a 28 percent improvement in symptoms, compared with a 3 percent improvement in the placebo group.

A study published in the *Archives of Otolaryngology Head and Neck Surgery* involved 119 people with various types of vertigo (dizziness), half of whom were given a combination of four homeopathic medicines and half of whom were given a leading conventional drug, betahistine hydrochloride. The homeopathic medicines were found to be similarly effective as and significantly safer than the conventional drug.

A study in the *Journal of Pediatrics* that appeared in the 1980s was the first on homeopathy to be published in an American medical journal. The study compared individualized high-potency homeopathic preparations against a placebo in eighty-one children, between ages six months and five years, suffering with acute diarrhea. The treatment group benefited from a statistically significant 15 percent decrease in duration. The authors noted that the clinical significance would extend to decreasing dehydration and postdiarrheal malnutrition and a significant reduction in morbidity.

A study published in *Biomedical Therapy* that involved 131 children allowed parents to choose homeopathic or conventional medical care from their ear, nose, and throat doctor. Of those, 103 children underwent homeopathic treatment, and 28 underwent conventional care. Of the group receiving homeopathic care, 82.6 percent had a positive response to the treatment; recipients of the conventional treatment had a positive response rate of 67.3 percent. Of the "homeopathic" children who had another earache, 29.3 percent had a maximum of three recurrences, while 43.5 percent of the "antibiotic" children had a maximum of six recurrences.

A 2006 study in the *Archives of Facial Plastic Surgery* found that homeopathic remedies significantly reduced bruising. The double-blind, placebo-controlled trial involved twenty-nine women who were undergoing facelifts and were randomly assigned to receive homeopathic arnica 12C or a placebo beginning the morning of surgery. The treatment was repeated every eight hours for four days. Facial swelling and bruising were evaluated by doctors and nurses, as well as through a computerized digital image of analysis of photographs taken before and after surgery. The area of bruising was significantly smaller for the group of people who took arnica. I know of plastic surgeons in the San Diego area who routinely give homeopathic arnica to their surgery patients and find less bruising and swelling and pain.

Finally, a study published in the *Lancet* analyzed eighty-nine studies and found that homeopathic treatment was 2.45 times more likely to have clinical benefit compared to placebo.

Prescribing Homeopathy

There are two basic ways that patients and practitioners can use homeopathy.

1. Combination remedies. This refers to homeopathic formulas that contain two or more homeopathic remedies. If the remedy a person needs is in the formula, then it will be helpful. If the homeopathic remedy one requires is not one of the ingredients, then usually nothing will happen or only minor improvements that do not last will occur. Combination remedies are available in most health food stores or

pharmacies. They are prepared for certain conditions, including colds, flu, teething, colic, diarrhea, rashes, headaches, and others.

2. Single remedies. This is the system that's used by trained homeopathic practitioners. The one remedy that best matches the patient's symptoms is prescribed. In general, this system is more effective than combination remedies, but it requires a knowledgeable practitioner to pick the correct homeopathic. If the single remedy choice is obvious (as described in the remedy summary), then go ahead and use single remedies for yourself or a loved one.

Administering Homeopathics

Homeopathic remedies are generally available in a pellet, tablet, liquid, or cream form. They are best taken ten to twenty minutes before eating or drinking. For infants, pellets or tablets can be mixed in an ounce of purified water, and then a few drops are put in the child's mouth with a dropper or a teaspoon. Children like the sweet taste of the pellets and the tablets. The remedies are also best taken when the patient isn't in the presence of strong-smelling odors, such as eucalyptus or essential oils.

For acute conditions, homeopathic remedies are often taken every fifteen minutes or every two hours, depending on the severity of the condition. For chronic conditions, homeopathics are usually taken one to two times daily, or less frequently, depending on the strength of the remedy prescribed.

Which Potency to Use

Potency refers to the strength of the remedy. The number behind the name of the homeopathic indicates the dilution and the strength of the medicine. The higher the number, the stronger the action of the remedy. For example, 30C is stronger than 12C, and 12x is stronger than 6x.

There are two common scales of homeopathy available in the marketplace. "X" means the lowest potencies used. X stands for a 1 in 9 dilution. So 1x is equal to 1 part of the original substance diluted in 9 parts solvent. Many stores carry the 6x and 12x potencies for the remedies.

In keeping with the third law of homeopathy, in which remedies become stronger the more they are diluted, C is more diluted and stronger than the X potencies. The first dilution—that is, 1C—is equal to 1 part of the original substance in 99 parts of solvent. Many stores carry the 12C and 30C potencies of the remedies.

Constitutional Homeopathic Remedies

One fascinating area of homeopathy consists of constitutional remedies, which are linked to physical, mental, and emotional characteristics. Based on a person's symptom profile, a homeopathic practitioner can accurately choose a constitutional homeopathic remedy to treat or prevent an imbalance by strengthening the person's overall healing and defense systems. This section describes common constitutional remedies. They are prescribed by homeopathic practitioners to improve a person's overall health and to treat chronic illness. If a remedy matches up closely to your constitution, then you can try taking a 30x, 12C, or 30C potency twice daily for a week and see if there are any changes. Once improvement has begun, stop the remedy unless progress halts, in which case take it again as needed. Otherwise, it is best to follow the advice of a qualified homeopathic practitioner.

Note: Some acute remedies, such as Sulfur, are also useful as constitutional remedies.

Common Constitutional Remedies

CALCAREA CARBONICA

Physical symptoms: People who fit this constitutional type tend to be plump or obese, tire easily, and be susceptible to infections, especially ear or upper respiratory infections. In general, they are chilly. For children, there can be a delay in development, such as a slow onset of walking or talking. People's nails may break or be brittle. They tend to sweat profusely on the back of the head when sleeping. They often crave eggs, sweets, and dairy products. The remedy is also indicated for people with chronic constipation.

Mental and emotional symptoms: They are easily overwhelmed; work oriented and organized; worriers; independent, stubborn, and curious.

LYCOPODIUM

Physical symptoms: People who fit the Lycopodium remedy picture have problems with the digestive system—bloating, gas, and burping—that get worse between 4 and 8 P.M. They often have large appetites and crave sweets. They are also prone to respiratory problems and tend to get problems on the right side of their bodies.

Mental and emotional symptoms: They like having authority, are domineering but have low self-esteem.

NATRUM MURIATICUM

Physical symptoms: People who require this remedy often complain of headaches, some of which can be severe. Symptoms are usually worse between 10 A.M. and 3 P.M. They have a strong craving for salty foods. Their cold sores break out from sun exposure. Their skin and eyes are extremely sensitive to the sun.

Mental and emotional symptoms: They tend to be depressed and prefer to be alone. They often have a history of emotional grief, such as the death of a loved one or a divorce. They do not like to cry in front of others. It is important to them to be very neat and tidy in appearance.

PHOSPHORUS

Physical symptoms: People who fit this constitutional type often have reoccurring nosebleeds for no apparent reason. Their colds have a tendency to turn into respiratory tract infections. Many people with asthma benefit from this remedy. Digestive upset, such as "tummy aches," can be common. They have a great thirst for cold drinks and crave sweets and ice cream.

Mental and emotional symptoms: The personality type is outgoing and very sociable. They like attention. They have sympathy for others and do not like to be alone, especially in the dark.

PULSATILLA

Physical symptoms: Their bodies get warm easily, and they desire to be outside in the fresh air. Children and adults are prone to getting ear and respiratory infections and sinusitis, which often has a greenish-yellow discharge. They crave sweets, especially pastries, and have little thirst.

Mental and emotional symptoms: They are generally shy, yet they crave attention. Their feelings are easily hurt.

SILICA

Physical symptoms: This remedy is for people with a very low resistance to infections, such as ear infections, colds, sinusitis, sore throats, and bronchitis. They are always coming down with an infection and have poor stamina. People who require Silica are often very thin and underweight and may have brittle skin, nails, and hair. They are chilly and cannot stand drafts of cold air.

Mental and emotional symptoms: They are usually stubborn and irritable, yet very shy and sensitive to criticism.

SULFUR

Physical symptoms: People who require this remedy are prone to getting skin rashes and have bad body odor. They have a great thirst (cold drinks) and appetite, with strong cravings for sweets and spicy foods. They get overheated and sweat easily.

Mental and emotional symptoms: They tend to be very curious (always asking why and how something works) and are very sociable. They like to be the leaders in groups of people. They also tend to be messy and unorganized.

A Guide to the Twelve Cell Salts

WHAT ARE CELL SALTS?

Cell salts are simplified forms of homeopathic remedies that quickly and simply alleviate many childhood health problems. Dr. Schussler, of Germany, discovered that twelve inorganic minerals were key constituents of cells. His theory was that a deficiency or an imbalance of these cell salts led to disease. By supplementing these naturally occurring biochemical cell salts, one can stimulate the cells to assimilate nutrients more efficiently. Replenishing and balancing these minerals restores the proper structure and the function of each cell, tissue, and organ. Ferrum Phosphoricum cell salt, for example, is a homeopathic dilution of iron, making it an excellent treatment for anemia because it bolsters iron assimilation in the cells, increasing the oxygen-carrying capacity of red blood cells.

HOW TO USE CELL SALTS

Cell salts are used similarly to other homeopathics. Just like other homeopathics, they are available in pellet, tablet, or liquid form. The most common potencies available are the 6x. They are best taken ten to twenty minutes before eating or drinking. For infants, cell salt tablets can be crushed and mixed in an ounce of purified water; then a few drops are put in the child's mouth with a dropper or a teaspoon. They are best taken when the patient is not in the presence of strong-smelling odors, such as eucalyptus or essential oils.

For acute conditions, take cell salts every fifteen minutes or every two hours, depending on the severity of the condition. For chronic conditions, cell salts are usually taken one to three times daily. Since they are of a low potency, cell salts are often used on a long-term basis.

CELL SALTS

Name	General Theme	Indications
Calcarea Fluorica	connective tissue	ligament and tendon sprains/weakness, brittle teeth and gums, abnormal spine curvature
Calcarea Phosphorica	bone health	fractures, teething, growing pains, osteoporosis
Calcarea Sulphurica	wound healer	abscess, boils, acne
Ferrum Phosphoricum	iron metabolism, bleeding	anemia, stops bleeding, fever
Kali Muriaticum	mucus	fluid in ears, sore throat
Kali Phosphoricum	nerves	nerve injury, brain tonic, concentration, anxiety
Kali Sulphuricum	skin	discharges
Magnesia Phosphoricum	muscles and nerves	muscle spasms, cramps, stomach cramps, relaxes nervous system, seizures, hyperactivity
Natrum Muriaticum	water balance	skin dryness, hay fever, grief, cold sores
Natrum Phosphoricum	acid-base balancer	heartburn, vaginitis
Natrum Sulphuricum	detoxifier	jaundice of newborn, hepatitis, head injury, colitis
Silica	tissue cleanser	acne, boils (with pus discharge), sinusitis, weak immunity

References

Frass, M. et al. 2005. A. Influence of potassium dichromate on tracheal secretions in critically ill patients. *Chest* March 127:936–941.

Friese, K. H., et al. 1997. Acute otitis media in children: A comparison of conventional and homeopathic treatment. *Biomedical Therapy* 15(4):113–22. 462-66.

Gaertner, K, et al. 2014. Additive homeopathy in cancer patients. Retrospective survival data from a homeopathic outpatient unit at the Medical University of Vienna. *Complementary Therapies in Medicine* 22(2):320–32.

Jacobs, J., et al. 1994. Treatment of acute childhood diarrhea with homeopathic medicine: a randomized clinical trial. *Nicaragua Pediatrics* 93(5)719–25.

Linde, K., et al. 1997. Are the clinical effects of homeopathy placebo effects? A meta-analysis of placebo-controlled trials. *Lancet* 350(9081):834–43. Erratum in: *Lancet* 1998 351(9097):220.

Seeley, B. M., et al. 2006. Effect of homeopathic Arnica montana on bruising in face-lifts: results of a randomized, double-blind, placebo-controlled clinical trial. *Archives of Facial and Plastic Surgery* 8(1):54–9.

Taylor, M., et al. 2000. Randomised controlled trial of homoeopathy versus placebo in perennial allergic rhinitis with overview of four trial series. *British Medical Journal* 321(7259):471–76.

Weiser, M., et al. 1998. Homeopathic vs. conventional treatment of vertigo: a randomized double-blind controlled clinical study. *Archives of Otolaryngology— Head and Neck Surgery* 124:879–85.

Aromatherapy

Introduction

We've all experienced the rush of feeling that can accompany a familiar, long-forgotten smell. Whether it's the aroma of banana bread just like grandmother's or the scent of the cologne our first love wore, smells have the power to take us back in time. Suddenly, we remember the anticipation we felt that long-ago day in grandmother's kitchen or the heartache of saying good-bye to our lover. We feel the same way, all over again.

If its sole effectiveness lay in harnessing that power of remembrance, aromatherapy would doubtless be a useful tool. But the strength of aromatherapy goes even beyond this. The essential oils used in aromatherapy are extracted from plants and impart their healing powers to the body through the sense of smell, certainly, but also through their ability to permeate the bloodstream. They have antibiotic, antibacterial, and tonic qualities that can relieve pain and stress, help balance the body and the mind, and even prevent disease. Besides, aromatherapy is enjoyable, whether you visit an expert aromatherapist for a massage or soak at home in a bath scented with your favorite essential oils.

Specific essential oils have specific properties that can alleviate particular symptoms or conditions. For example, eucalyptus oil helps to clear congestion, while peppermint oil is good for relieving nausea. Familiarity with the characteristics of just a few essential oils and with the different ways they can be used gives a person the power to self-treat many common ailments. Whether your trouble is physical, mental, or emotional, you may find relief in the use of aromatherapy.

History

Long before humans discovered the processes for extracting essential oils from plants, they found ways to use aromatic plants and other perfumes to enhance their lives. Picture an ancient Egyptian temple. Incense is burning, infusing the air with frankincense, myrrh, and sandalwood. A cadre of priests anoints the faithful with scented oils. Many of these pilgrims are already covered with various scents from their aromatic baths and perfumed cosmetics. And when they return to their homes, many of them will burn juniper or thyme to freshen the air and ward off evil spirits.

The Egyptians were among the first to indulge in aromatherapy. The same botanical knowledge that helped them embalm their dead was also used in daily life. But they were not the lone aromatherapists in the ancient world. While Egyptian priests and perfumers practiced their craft, to the east in India, Ayurvedic healers were recording the healing properties of such aromatic plants as coriander, ginger, and rose.

Farther east in China and Japan, aromatic woods and perfumes were used in religious rites and for personal beauty and hygiene. The ancient Greeks learned the secrets of aromatherapy from the Egyptians, and they became enthusiastic partakers of scent. They often used huge quantities of aromatic substances during religious rituals and adorned their bodies daily with perfume from head to toe, in hopes of gratifying the gods. But they also made the connection between scent and health. They believed that certain perfumes had therapeutic properties. Emotional or mental ailments could be healed with medicinal perfumes, and once the mind was healed, physical health would follow.

Hippocrates, the "father of medicine," prescribed perfumed therapies; Greek medical practice also yielded the label *iatralypte*, a physician who cured through the use of aromatic ointments. They passed their knowledge on to the Romans, who in turn spread the use of botanicals to each new land they conquered.

After the fall of Rome, aromatherapy in Europe dwindled. But the Arab world continued to add to the knowledge of perfumes' healing powers. By the tenth century, an Arabian physician, Avicenna, had discovered a way to distill the essential oils from rose petals. Soon, many other essential oils were available, and by the time trade resumed between Europe and the East, the use of essential oils was widespread. Oils such as juniper and pine were used to combat illness and keep it from spreading, and the use of perfumes for personal adornments and hygiene was commonplace.

Aromatherapy met an enemy with the Puritan movement, which lumped perfume and incense in with paganism and witchcraft. And with the advent of modern science, aromatherapy fell further from favor. The natural essential oils, so prized for generations, were replaced with synthetic scents in cosmetics, perfumes, and foods.

It wasn't until the 1920s that aromatherapy began a resurgence. The French chemist and perfumer René-Maurice Gattefoss actually coined the term *aromatherapy* after an accident in his laboratory left his hand badly burned. He immersed his hand in lavender oil and later noticed that the burn healed quite quickly and left no scar. This personal experience led him to delve further into the possibilities of healing with essential oils.

Dr. Jean Valnet, a French physician and a scientist, built upon the knowledge of Gattefoss by using essential oils as part of his medical practice to treat physical and psychiatric problems. Valnet later published a guide to the use of essential oils called *Aromatherapie*. One of his converts, Madame Marguerite Maury, established the first aromatherapy clinics in Paris, England, and Switzerland. There, she used essential oils in beauty therapies that were personalized for each subject. Her aromatherapy sought to rejuvenate clients with scents directed at their personalities and health problems. She published the fruits of her research in 1964 in *The Secret of Life and Youth*.

Today, their knowledge is passed on through aromatherapy courses, institutes, and seminars in North America and Europe. Many certified aromatherapists practice the same healing arts that Gattefoss and Valnet first used, and the availability of many books on the subject allows people to try it for themselves at home.

Aromatherapy Basics

Essential oils are not oily or greasy; they evaporate readily, leaving no residue. As they evaporate, their aromatic molecules permeate the air. When we inhale the aroma, these molecules travel into the nose and to the olfactory receptors where our sense of smell originates. These receptors then transmit information about the odor to the limbic system in the brain.

The limbic portion of the brain not only processes smells, but also handles emotions, which may be one reason why smells can so easily trigger our feelings. In addition, the limbic portion of the brain influences the production of hormones, the immune system, and the nervous system. As such, aromatherapy can affect basic bodily functions and mental fitness.

The essential oil molecules do not stop in the nose, however. They travel on into the lungs and, from there, into the bloodstream, where they can improve health by acting on individual cells. They are also readily absorbed into the skin, but they are most often diluted in a carrier oil—such as almond oil—before application to prevent skin irritation.

Once the tiny essential oil molecules penetrate the skin, they can stimulate circulation and encourage cell regeneration. Some oils relieve muscle soreness, while others can help release tension and spasms. They can enter the bloodstream here, too, and go on to the internal organs and the lymphatic system.

Whether inhaled or absorbed through the skin, essential oils can fight bacteria, fungi, viruses, and other microbes inside the body and can stimulate the immune system to help renew health. Essential oils can also be taken internally, but this must be done only under the supervision of a qualified aromatherapy practitioner. Never ingest essential oils on your own, and make sure to keep your supply out of reach of children.

Many essential oils are extracted from their plants in stills. No, this isn't the kind of still used in the back woods to make moonshine. It's a specially constructed piece of equipment for distilling essential oils using pressurized steam. Fresh or dried plant material is placed in a special compartment, and steam is circulated through it. The heat forces open tiny pockets in the plants to release the essential oils, which evaporate and move into a condensation chamber. As the mixture cools, the steam condenses into water and the essential oil—which does not dissolve in water—floats on top. The oil is then skimmed off and packaged for sale.

Some plant materials don't lend themselves to steam distillation, so their essential oils are extracted by other means. Citrus oils, such as orange, lemon, and bergamot, are obtained by cold pressing.

Flowers with low concentrations of essential oils, such as jasmine, are put through a complex process called enfleurage. Their petals are placed in animal fat, which absorbs the essential oil; alcohol is then added to separate the essential oil from the fat. The alcohol evaporates, leaving the essential oil—more properly called an absolute, in this case—behind.

Alcohol is also used in solvent extraction, with tree sap that's too thick to use otherwise or with flowers when enfleurage is considered too inefficient.

A solvent such as hexane saturates the plant material and chemically extracts the essential oils; the resulting material is then dissolved in alcohol to remove the solvent. These essential oils often contain residue from the solvent. For this reason, we suggest that you avoid essential oils that were extracted with solvents other than alcohol.

One of the best places to apply oil is on the bottom of the feet; the oils will be absorbed into the bloodstream immediately. Other places to apply essential oils are the crown of the head, the temples, the forehead, the nape of the neck, behind the ears, and the earlobes (never inside the ears). Additional areas are on the abdomen, the tops of the feet, and the ankles. It is also good to work the reflexology points with the essential oils.

How Oils Can Be Used

Remember when you were a child and your mother rubbed a menthol ointment on your chest to relieve chest congestion? She may also have put some of the ointment into a vaporizer to fill the room with a cloud of menthol-scented steam, to help you breathe more easily. This was a form of aromatherapy, and your mother was practicing it in different ways to maximize its healing powers. Likewise, aromatherapists not only match essential oils to particular symptoms; they also carefully choose the method of delivering aromatherapy.

There are several different ways for essential oils to be used, and different application methods are best suited to different ailments. Respiratory problems, such as sinusitis and bronchitis, respond well to steam inhalation and chest massage, while nervous complaints are best assuaged by a combination of massage, baths, and inhalation. Indigestion can be eased by directly inhaling the aroma of peppermint oil, while constipation responds to an abdominal massage with a blend of fennel and marjoram. In addition, different people respond to different oils in unique ways.

With a little practice and some common sense, you will soon learn how you can best treat yourself and your family with aromatherapy.

Massage

Aromatherapy massage combines two therapies into one very effective therapy for a multitude of complaints, whether physical, mental, emotional, or a combination of each. Besides, it's one of the most pleasurable experiences around. If you're given a prescription for a massage with sage and geranium for depression, or with eucalyptus and rosemary for a backache, you can rest assured that the treatment will be delightful all by itself—and its healing aftereffects will be an even greater bonus.

Massage alone stimulates circulation, releases toxins from the muscles, relaxes breathing and muscle tension, and soothes the nervous system.

With aromatherapy, massage becomes a multifaceted healer. It delivers aromatic molecules into the body through the skin and the nose to relax or stimulate the body as needed, while providing all the benefits of a full-body massage.

Although there's no substitute for a full-body massage from an experienced practitioner, the benefits of self-massage are well documented. A daily self-massage with a carrier oil that's infused with essential oils will not only moisturize the skin and boost circulation, it can also improve your overall well-being through aromatherapy.

And when you're experiencing a problem, massage can be used to help heal specific parts of the body. You can mix your own blend to use every day; add ½ to 1 teaspoon of essential oil to 1 pint of unscented body lotion or botanical oil, such as sweet almond oil or sunflower oil. For specific ailments, use 1 ounce of a carrier oil to 10 to 20 drops of essential oil, follow a recipe recommended by a trusted expert, or follow the directions of your aromatherapist.

Here are some suggestions to get you started. A muscle sprain or strain can be massaged gently with lavender, juniper, or cypress oil, while varicose veins can be helped with a massage around the affected area with cypress or geranium oil.

Constipation can be treated with a gentle abdominal massage using black pepper, fennel, or marjoram; be sure to massage the area clockwise, from right to left, to follow the path that wastes take through the intestines.

A chest massage with eucalyptus, peppermint, or lavender oil can relieve chest infections, while a neck massage with one of these oils can calm a cough.

Massaging the face with eucalyptus or rosemary oil will clear the sinuses (make sure not to get close to the eyes).

Aromatherapy with massage can also focus on the face to improve circulation and reduce facial tension, bringing greater beauty to the skin. Using oils such as bergamot can help combat acne, while sandalwood is good for dry, dehydrated, or aging skin. Facial massage should be done gently and with upward motions only.

Bathing

Scented baths are a perfect way to enjoy the healing powers of essential oils.

You can take a page from Cleopatra's history and soak in a soothing, rose-infused tub, or get ready to face the day with an uplifting blend of black pepper and juniper.

If your skin is sensitive, or if you are preparing a bath for a child, dilute the essential oil in 1 ounce of carrier oil first, and then add up to 6 drops of the mixture to the tub.

Caution: Skin Irritants

Several of the essential oils are known to irritate the skin when used in baths or massages. People with sensitive skin should avoid these oils when bathing or receiving massages. Other people can use these oils if they are first diluted in a carrier oil. Mix 5 to 10 drops of essential oil with 1.4 cups of bath gel or epsom salts. In massage, these oils should be used in concentrations of no more than 2 percent essential oil to carrier oil.

Irritants in baths and massages include basil, cinnamon leaf, lemon, sweet fennel, lemongrass, Siberian fir needle, verbena, parsley seed, melissa, pimenta leaf, peppermint, thyme, and tea tree.

A Simple Way to Use Aromatherapy

One of the easiest ways to use aromatherapy is to simply smell the essential oils, whether directly from the bottle, with steam, in your home with the help of a diffusor or an aromatherapy air freshener, or on your body with a personal perfume. In each case, the aroma is pleasant, and its healing properties are inhaled into the lungs and diffused throughout the body.

Grandma's smelling salts were aromatherapy of a kind; their strong smell of ammonia could rouse almost anyone from a faint. Luckily, using essential oils as inhalants is much more pleasant. Direct inhalation works particularly well for respiratory complaints, stress, emotional conditions, and nausea. You can use a suggested blend or simply select one or more of the oils recommended for treating your specific condition and mix them together in a small glass bottle. Make sure to choose oils with aromas you enjoy. You can either open the bottle and inhale the scent, or you can place 2 or 3 drops on a tissue or a cotton ball to inhale periodically throughout the day. Sinus problems respond especially well to steam inhalations, although a mixture of steaming water and essential oils can also be used to treat other respiratory ailments, such as colds and the flu, sore throats, and nervous complaints, such as anxiety and stress.

The easiest and fastest way to directly inhale essential oils is to apply 2 or 3 drops of the oil of your choice to the palm of one hand. Rub your palms together. Cup your hands around your nose and mouth and inhale deeply.

To prepare a steam inhalation, use a large heat-proof bowl that's been placed securely on a tabletop. Fill it about halfway with steaming water and add between 3 and 6 drops of an essential oil or a blend. Lavender is a good one to start with, because it is effective for anxiety and depression, as well as respiratory problems. Sit comfortably, and place a towel over your head to trap the steam. Inhale deeply for five to ten minutes.

Steam is also an effective way to use essential oils to cleanse the complexion.

For normal skin, use frankincense, geranium, jasmine, rose, vetiver, or a combination of several.

For dry skin, bergamot, fennel, geranium, myrrh, and sandalwood are recommended.

Oily skin can benefit from cedarwood, cypress, lemon, orange, peppermint, tea tree, and ylang-ylang.

Sensitive skin responds best to chamomile, rose, and rosewood.

Air fresheners and diffusers allow you to perfume your home with healing essential oils.

For everyday use, choose an essential oil or a blend that the whole family enjoys.

In sickrooms, antiseptic, antibacterial, antiviral, and antifungal oils, such as tea tree, eucalyptus, bergamot, and geranium, can help purify and cleanse the air to help control germs.

In the office, you might want to select an antianxiety or antistress aroma, such as lavender, chamomile, or lemon.

For an aromatherapy air freshener, mix distilled water with 4 to 10 drops of essential oil per ounce of fluid, and pour into a spray bottle. Spray the mixture into the room just as you would any air freshener. Make sure to shake well before each use. Diffusers distribute essential oil molecules into the air. Many of these devices work on electricity; you simply add your chosen oil or blend and plug it in.

Making your own personal perfume ensures that you can carry your favorite essential oils anywhere you go. You can choose a suggested blend or create your own by adding up to 20 drops of essential oils that you like to ⅛ ounce of jojoba oil. Dab the mixture on your pulse points and enjoy.

Compresses

Hot and cold compresses are often suggested for physical injuries, as well as for aches and pains due to chronic conditions, such as arthritis. By adding appropriate essential oils, you can increase a compress's power to heal.

Compresses can relieve pain and reduce swelling and inflammation. Hot compresses are best for chronic conditions, particularly for backaches, arthritis, toothaches, and earaches. Cold compresses are an important first-aid measure for sprains; they also help to relieve headaches and, when used on large portions of the body, can help bring down a fever.

Often practitioners suggest alternating hot and cold compresses, once the initial injury care with cold compresses is complete. This helps sprains and strains to heal.

To make a hot compress, fill a bowl with water as hot as possible while still being bearable to the touch. Add 5 to 7 drops of an essential oil—try black pepper, chamomile, coriander, or a blend. Dip into the bowl a clean cloth folded several times to absorb more fluid, making sure to absorb the essential oils floating on top of the water. Wring the excess water from the cloth and apply it to the affected area and cover with a dry towel. Replace with a fresh compress when the first one cools to room temperature.

For a cold compress, substitute ice water for the hot, and prepare the same way. Change compresses when the one in use warms up to body temperature.

Mouthwashes and Gargles

Aromatherapy mouth treatments are helpful for a variety of problems, including mouth ulcers and gum disease. They can also be used on a daily basis for oral hygiene. Oils such as myrrh, rose, and tea tree are good for gingivitis, while cypress and tea tree oils can help heal and prevent bleeding gums. Myrrh, basil, bergamot, and tea tree oils are helpful for healing mouth ulcers. Clove oil is helpful for toothaches.

The appropriate oils can be used either as a mouthwash/gargle or in oil for a gum massage.

To make a mouthwash, dissolve 3 to 5 drops of oil into a teaspoon of vodka, and then stir the mixture into ½ cup of warm distilled water. You may want to add a drop of peppermint oil to your recipe to improve the flavor. After brushing your teeth, or as needed, swish the mouthwash around in your mouth. To supplement the mouthwash, you may use a gum-massage oil. In a glass bottle with a dropper, mix ¼ ounce of carrier oil with 20 to 25 drops of the desired essential oils, including 1 drop of peppermint or fennel for flavor. Before each use, turn the bottle upside down several times to mix, and then rub a few drops onto your gums.

Custom Hair and Skin Care

Women and men can easily include aromatherapy in their everyday cleansing routines by adding a few drops of essential oils to unscented shampoos, conditioners, lotions, and cleansers. The proper oils can help ease dryness or oiliness in your skin or scalp, assist in the regeneration of skin cells, improve the circulation of blood to your skin, and improve the condition of your hair. Make sure to choose high-quality base products, with no fragrance already added. Then add 8 to 10 drops of essential oil per ounce of product. Rose, jasmine, lavender, and neroli are good oils for normal or dry skin; dry skin can also benefit from fennel, benzoin, and cedarwood.

Oily skin is best treated with juniper, patchouli, peppermint, tea tree, and ylang-ylang.

Aging skin responds well to myrrh and helichrysum; for sensitive skin, stick to chamomile, jasmine, rose, or rosewood.

For use on the hair, people with oily hair have the most choices; they can try bergamot, cypress, clary sage, juniper, pine, rosemary, tea tree, and lemon.

Dry hair responds well to chamomile, lavender, and rosemary; try a mix of the three. Normal hair can use lavender, chamomile, thyme, and ylang-ylang.

To clear up dandruff, add tea tree, cedarwood, rosemary, and pine.

Besides using essential oils in prepared products, you can also add your chosen varieties to jojoba oil for a deep-conditioning treatment. Use 10 drops in 1 ounce of jojoba oil and leave on the hair overnight, if possible, or for at least half an hour. Then shampoo.

Using Essential Oils

To get started in aromatherapy, you, of course, need essential oils. But which to choose? High-quality oils can be expensive, and it's worthwhile to select oils that both meet your personal needs and are as versatile as possible.

For general use, focus on ten basic oils: rose, rosemary, peppermint, tea tree, lemon, eucalyptus, lavender, sandalwood, juniper, and rose geranium. These ten oils can be blended or used singly, as you desire. Of course, if you have a specific condition that calls for a special oil in treatment, add that one to the list. One caveat is worth mentioning here. Generally, if you do not like the scent of an essential oil, do not use it. Trust your nose to guide you to the essential oils that will be most beneficial to you.

Certain oils should not be applied topically before going into the sun. Wait twenty-four hours after using all citrus oils and angelica. Wait forty-eight hours after using bergamot.

And, as with any treatment, care is called for in aromatherapy. As previously mentioned, never ingest essential oils on your own initiative. Consult a health care professional. Always dilute essential oils before applying them to the skin. And if you experience any discomfort, skin irritation, or sensitivity, stop using that particular oil.

Certain medical conditions require extra caution. If you are pregnant, consult your doctor before using aromatherapy. Likewise if you have cancer, asthma, high or low blood pressure, or epilepsy, or if you are taking any medications—prescription or over-the-counter. In addition, if you are using homeopathic remedies, aromatherapy can diminish their effects. Avoid using essential oils if you are under homeopathic care, or check with a homeopathic practitioner.

Whether you choose to use aromatherapy occasionally or every day, we think you'll find that it's a welcome addition. Sinking into a relaxing aromatherapy bath at the end of a long day's work or indulging in a weekly aromatherapy massage will not only help your body and mind, it will also soothe your spirit.

Of course, even frequent aromatherapy can't counteract the effects of a poor diet, a sedentary lifestyle, or a stressed-out approach to life. Whether you're trying to overcome a specific physical or mental problem or you're just seeking greater overall health, use aromatherapy to complement your good eating and exercise habits.

Choosing and Storing Aromatherapy Supplies/Buying Oils

Because the key ingredient in aromatherapy is the essential oil, properly selecting your oils is paramount. Here are a few tips for buying wisely: Choose only pure essential oils. Though scientists have learned to create quite lifelike aromas in the laboratory, these substances are made from petroleum by-products, not plants. If that isn't enough to convince you of their uselessness in aromatherapy, consider this: In each essential oil are dozens of chemical compounds, many of which are present in only trace amounts. Synthetic scents may imitate the smell but can never replicate the exact molecular makeup of healing essential oils. And don't be fooled by "nature-identical" labels. If it doesn't say "pure essential oil," don't buy it.

Trust your nose. It sounds simplistic, but it's true: If you don't like the smell of an essential oil, it isn't likely to help you—even if it is recommended for your particular ailment. God has been gracious in giving us alternatives. Simply choose another recommended oil that's more pleasing to you.

Consider the source. Buy only from reputable suppliers; well-established natural food stores are one good choice. You can find good oils at www.youngliving.org/robinyoung. If you're in doubt, consult a qualified aromatherapist for suggestions. Consider the price. Sadly, some manufacturers dilute essential oils with carrier oils or mix them with synthetics, without labeling them as such. A tip: A drop of pure essential oil placed on a tissue will evaporate completely without leaving any trace of oil. If a greasy spot is left behind, the oil has been adulterated. But you may be able to tell the difference without even opening the bottle. The prices of true essential oils vary widely, according to the difficulty of extracting the pure plant oils from their host plants. Rose oil, for example, should be quite a bit more expensive than lavender oil because many pounds of rose petals are required to make just one ounce of rose oil. If a manufacturer sells all of its oils for the same price, or if its prices are substantially lower than those of other manufacturers, chances are the products are adulterated or otherwise inferior.

Essential Oil Care

Once you've bought your precious essential oils, be sure to store and use them properly to preserve their healing properties. Most oils will keep well for a year or more.

Keep your oils in a cool, dry place in dark glass bottles. Never allow your oils to stand in a damp environment or near light or heat.

Avoid touching the inside of the bottle cap, the rim of the bottle, or the dropper to your skin or to any other surface. This will help prevent contamination.

Uncap your oils only long enough to release the amount of oil you need. The oils are extremely volatile and will evaporate quickly.

Choosing Carrier Products

Second only to the quality of the essential oils in aromatherapy is the quality of the carrier oils, the lotions, and other products you use. As with essential oils, buy from a reputable supplier and read the labels carefully. Store all of your aromatherapy oils in the refrigerator, and allow them to come to room temperature before use.

Make sure to choose products that contain no additives.

Choose unscented, cold-pressed, organic vegetable oils.

Unrefined oils are preferred over refined oils.

Avoid mineral oil, which is a petroleum product, and coconut oil, which has molecules too large to be absorbed into the skin.

Be aware of the shelf life of the oils you purchase. Buy small quantities of oils that go rancid quickly and larger quantities only of those with a longer life. Different types of carrier oils are preferred for different uses.

Following is a selection of carrier oils and their properties:

Almond oil is often used in aromatherapy massage; it also relieves itching and inflammation. It spoils quickly, however.

Apricot kernel oil is a rich oil full of vitamin A, which is often used for dry, mature, sensitive, and dehydrated skin.

Avocado oil contains lots of vitamins A and E, so it is very helpful for skin problems. Its richness makes it especially valuable for mixing with other oils. It goes rancid quickly.

Canola oil is a light, penetrating oil that keeps well and works well in blends for massage and the skin.

Evening primrose oil is often used in beauty products because it promotes skin repair and health and helps prevent premature aging. It does spoil easily, however.

Flaxseed oil is full of vitamin E, making it valuable for skin healing and regeneration. It spoils quickly.

Grapeseed oil is a good choice for oily or acne-prone skin because it is light and slightly astringent.

Hazelnut oil helps skin maintain firmness and elasticity. It is expensive.

Jojoba oil, which is actually a wax ester, softens and moisturizes skin while helping to control acne and oily skin. Its antioxidant benefits extend to other oils with which it is mixed; it can extend the shelf life of your blends.

Olive oil has been used for centuries to beautify the skin and the hair, and its benefits are still recognized today. It mixes well with other carrier oils.

Sunflower oil is high in vitamin E and is good for sensitive skin.

Vitamin E oil is renowned for its skin-healing properties. It is best blended with other carrier oils; make sure to buy natural vitamin E, not synthetic.

Medical Conditions and Pregnancy

If you have a serious medical condition or if you are pregnant, nursing, or trying to get pregnant, consult with a health care professional before using essential oils.

Emergency Situations

Irritated skin: To relieve skin irritated from essential oils, wash with soap and water or a mild detergent. If a rash occurs and does not clear up in a few days, seek medical attention. If there is blistering, seek medical attention right away.

Essential oil in the eyes: Place a small drop of plain carrier oil (e.g., olive oil) into the affected eye(s). The carrier oil helps to absorb the essential oil. Rinse with water and pat with a cloth. Seek medical attention immediately to have the eyes examined. Essential-oil residue on fingers may damage contact lenses and cause eye irritation.

Sick and nauseated: If you become sick, nauseated, confused, or get a headache from the essential oils, then breathe some fresh air. Your symptoms should improve immediately and over the next couple of hours. If there is no improvement, seek medical attention.

If a child swallows an essential oil: Call 911 immediately. Do not try to induce vomiting.

REFERENCES

Essential Oils Desk Reference, 2007. 4th ed. Essential Science Publishing.

Higley, C., and A. Higley. 2006. *Reference Guide for Essential Oils*, 10th ed. Olathe, KS: Abundant Health.

Traditional Chinese Medicine: Acupuncture and Acupressure

Introduction

Traditional Chinese medicine (TCM) is rooted deep in China's ancient past and has developed entwined with one of the world's oldest and most profound philosophies. At first glance by a Westerner, much of it may seem puzzling and alien, but a student of Chinese medicine can quickly gain an understanding of its basic tenets, as well as learn many practical remedies to ensure better health and prevent disease.

Few branches of alternative health care offer the wealth of experience associated with Chinese medicine. More than four thousand years ago, the healers in Chinese society began to experiment with various herbs to see which could cure physical and mental complaints. And not all their remedies came from plants. The medicines included a variety of minerals and animal extracts woven into a fantastic set of potions that were thought to have "magical powers."

Over the ensuing years, Chinese medicine grew up hand in hand with Chinese philosophy, following the Way, or the Tao, in search of simplicity and harmony in all things. For the Chinese physician, it was as important to understand the works of the philosopher Lao Tzu ("The Old Master," considered a contemporary of Confucius) as it was to study the collected masterworks of medicine. Central to this philosophy was the inevitability of change.

Meanwhile, in the laboratory of human experience, Chinese practitioners were able to test various remedies, losing much of the so-called magic as they improved their knowledge of medicine. But they made progress without using dissection, which was forbidden in Chinese society. As a result, TCM's anatomy is more figurative than literal and does not correspond to the body in ways that Westerners expect.

Through experimentation, they built a complex and rich tradition that extends to acupuncture, acupressure, qigong, and tai chi. New methods of care were developed and systematically inscribed in their vast *materia medica*, the encyclopedic volumes listing TCM remedies.

From this combination of philosophy and trial and error, Chinese practitioners developed a holistic approach to treating patients that is all too often lacking in the West. By learning more about human nature and emphasizing harmony and balance as the source of good health, they were able not just to treat an illness, but to teach the patient about the importance of good nutrition, preventive remedies, and a balanced outlook on life that would help prevent disease from recurring.

Contemporary practitioners of Chinese medicine begin the diagnostic process in much the same way Chinese physicians did thousands of years ago: watching, asking questions, observing the tongue and the skin, assessing personality traits, and listening carefully to the patient before making a diagnosis and devising a treatment.

Today we know that traditional Chinese medicine offers many practical and long-proven safe remedies for some of our most common ailments. Over the last generation, we've seen a number of these practices gain widespread respect in the West for the benefits they offer everyone the world over. Chinese physicians' work on nutrition plays an important role in Chinese medicine, and we're seeing a growing number of independent clinical studies back up their claims. In addition, we're routinely discovering new uses for TCM that would surprise even an ancient practitioner.

The growing confidence in this field in the West has led to important attitudinal shifts in the uses of Chinese medicine. While Westerners were glad to begin using Chinese remedies for conditions like the flu, allergies, or menstrual cramps, only recently have we begun to see the possibilities in acute cases, such as heavy bleeding, appendicitis, and dangerously high fevers.

History

By the time Hippocrates began laying down the basic philosophy of Western medicine 2,500 years ago, Chinese medicine was already widely accepted and practiced. A coherent Chinese history, in both politics and medicine, reaches back to some 3,000 years BC.

The oldest record of herbal remedies dates to the beginning of the Han Dynasty (206 BC to AD 220). *Huang Di Nei Jing*, or *The Yellow Emperor's Inner Classic*, now almost two thousand years old, is one of the oldest medical texts still in use today. Scholars believe that it was compiled over a period of centuries. Written as a dialogue between the Yellow Emperor and Qi Bo, his leading minister, it is required reading for the serious student of Chinese medicine.

Like the *Huang Di Nei Jing*, the other weighty volumes that form the backbone of Chinese medical practice reflect many centuries of compilation and review. As leading healers tried new variations of herbal remedies, they carefully noted the effects and developed new forms of treatment.

Early on, Chinese medicine included many exotic remedies to cure people afflicted by demons. Magical potions mixed from herbs, minerals, and animal parts were concocted to influence the spirits. Remedies were often linked with alchemy and astrology. Many were based on astrological observations or relied on numerology to provide answers to a patient's health problems.

By the time of the Han Dynasty, such primitive magic had given way to a new system of medicine, based on careful observation. But TCM was not separated completely from its ancient past. Consider the number five. Han astronomers could identify five planets circling the earth. Five vital elements—fire, wood, earth, water, and metal—constituted the primary building blocks of the planet. And five developed into one of the most important numbers in Chinese medicine as physicians sought to understand the complex interaction of forces that influenced their patients' health. They often would mix five different herbs to treat a disease, a practice that extends to the present day.

Near the end of the Han Dynasty, Zhang Zhong-Jing wrote *Discussion of Cold-Induced Disorders and Miscellaneous Diseases*. Many of the herbal remedies included in this classic of Chinese medicine are still in use today.

New volumes examining various remedies, herbal and otherwise, came along, and today those books are part of the classic TCM library. Chinese medicine grew to encompass not only herbal remedies for illnesses, but also forms of exercise and massage that could help heal the sick and prevent disease. Acupuncture developed into its own highly technical discipline.

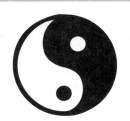

The Yin/Yang Symbol

The curve dividing the circle indicates that yin and yang continuously flow together. They blend and transform into one another, creating peace and harmonic homeostasis. The small dots of opposite color indicate that nothing is strictly yin or yang, but rather there is a small element of the opposite in each entity, creating balance in life.

After the Chinese Communists seized power fifty years ago, TCM experienced a brief period of decline, as its emphasis on the Tao and classic remedies came in confrontation with Western medicine. But within a decade, the Communists bowed to history and accepted TCM as an important practice.

In recent years, TCM has gained acceptance in the West as well. The areas of TCM that have translated best in the West include therapies that are widely respected for their clear health benefits.

Over the past two thousand years, Chinese herbalism has grown from a handful of notations in the *Inner Classic* to more than five thousand substances listed in the *Encyclopedia of Traditional Chinese Medicinal Substances*, gathered at the Jiangsu College of New Medicine.

Adherents of tai chi and qigong, ancient methods of exercise aimed at restoring the natural balance in body and mind, are believed to have developed many of their key movements after observing them in the animal world. Practiced by millions around the globe, they are daily rituals for people seeking to restore physical and mental harmony.

Acupressure and acupuncture were subjected to the same system of trial and error as Chinese physicians experimented to see which remedies carried lasting cures. Gradually, the sharpened bones used by the first acupuncturists were replaced by more carefully designed instruments.

Today, acupuncture and acupressure have gained widespread use in the West, even gaining the blessing of some insurance companies.

No other medical system in the world has the same wealth of historical experience to draw upon. And although many Western observers find the symbolic nature of TCM too fanciful, we are drawn back to Chinese medicine because of its repeatedly proven ability to heal the sick and keep the healthy well.

For many millennia, Chinese physicians relied on empirical research to back up their claims, cataloguing cures of chronic pain through acupuncture or the effect of Chinese herbal remedies on fever or fatigue. Of course, we're also learning through repeated clinical studies that many of TCM's herbal remedies, acupressure, and acupuncture have scientifically provable benefits. TCM has, in turn, had a profound effect on Western herbalism.

In TCM and Chinese philosophy, this balance is represented by yin and yang, complementary qualities that exist together in all things. Yin is cool or cold, fall and winter, wet and passive. Yang is its opposite: warm or hot, spring and summer, dry and vibrant. Yin is also bright and light; yang is dark. Yin is light; yang is heavy.

Just as the seasons change, cooling and heating the earth in turn, so do other elements. In each case, yin and yang are constantly transforming as the pendulum swings from one to the other. This concept is represented in the symbol for yin and yang, black and white that flow around and into each other.

Meridians

TCM teaches that qi (pronounced *chee* and also spelled "chi") energizes both us as individuals and also the world around us; it is constantly in motion. Within our bodies, Chinese physicians have identified channels, or meridians, that circulate qi in much the same way that blood is circulated through veins.

But don't go looking for any physical evidence of meridians. These meridians are invisible, yet within TCM, they are the most important elements in a person's health. TCM views meridians, or *jing luo*, as crucial, because they are responsible for transmitting the essential life force, qi, throughout the body.

Over the centuries, Chinese physicians identified twelve main meridians and supporting channels that branch throughout the body. Each of the main meridians corresponds to a major organ and links organs, muscles, and all the body's many parts.

The Chinese physician relies on these meridians to treat the body. Herbal remedies are processed initially by the stomach, but their essential force is channeled through meridians to reach an affected organ. The energy created there improves the function of related organs and in so doing improves one's health.

Acupuncturists are trained to play the harmonic nature of the meridians with needles, seeking particular points that will in turn lead to a vital organ. In this way, they play your body much the same way you might use a bow to play the violin, and they seek to tune your system so that it plays the sweetest music. Or you may choose to treat yourself with acupressure, using fingers in place of needles to find the points that lead you to peace and rejuvenation.

Many Westerners have sought to tie the meridians to the body's nervous system, hoping to explain the clear benefits of acupuncture in clinical terms. Unfortunately for the literal minded, Chinese physicians are quick to point out that meridians are charted through areas where the nervous system could not be affected. Even without the link, though, Western acupuncturists have gained widespread acceptance for their treatment measures.

Acupuncture

Acupuncture quickly assumed a vital role in Chinese medicine, offering a way to regulate the flow of qi in the meridians. Acupressure and acupuncture are very similar in the way that they stimulate the same points to encourage the flow of energy and relief from stress and pain. But acupuncture picks up where the milder acupressure leaves off and can offer lasting relief for people with chronic pain.

In the early days, acupuncture needles were made from sharpened slivers of bone or bamboo, inserted into one of many acupuncture points linked along the meridians to the organs and identified because of their therapeutic properties in certain disorders. Today those needles are made from stainless steel or come with copper-coated tops. Some physicians prefer to use silver or gold needles. Most practitioners, in fact, have adopted the Western practice of using disposable needles. In the West, disposable needles are the preferred choice.

Today acupuncture is used to treat a whole range of modern maladies. The uses of acupuncture extend to backaches, colds, angina, headaches, tinnitus, glaucoma, tonsillitis, sunstroke, asthma, impotence, and psoriasis, to name only a few conditions. While it may not offer a cure-all for cancer or AIDS, acupuncture can help relieve many of the painful symptoms and the effects of the modern therapies used for those diseases. More and more of our colleagues are adding it to their list of useful therapies.

Acupuncture is most often used in the West to treat chronic conditions, but it is occasionally used to treat certain acute disorders. Within TCM, though, acupuncture is routinely used to help fine-tune the system and restore balance. Think of an acupuncturist as a piano tuner, carefully checking each of the ivory and ebony keys and adjusting any sour note to conform to its harmonic whole. In our view, this is even more important today, as we deal with an ever-rising level of stress in our modern world. We need "new," yet tested, ways to dissolve the damaging array of stressors to which we are continually subjected.

Some sites on the body's map of meridians and acupuncture points, particularly at our extremities, are associated with treatments for specific disorders. The most commonly punctured points are between the elbows and the fingertips and between the toes and the knees.

Extremely fine needles are used for thin-skinned patients, while someone who is particularly fleshy may call for somewhat thicker needles. Needles also vary in length, from half an inch to three inches. In no case should the procedure cause pain. Most patients describe the feeling as a tingling sensation, though some people remark that a numbness may set in at the insertion point. In all cases, a variety of points will be selected and needles inserted, often leaving the hand or some other extremity looking like a pincushion.

In order to help stimulate energy flow, a practitioner may occasionally stroke a needle, rotate it, or flick it with a finger. Some acupuncturists have elected to connect their needles to a small electric stimulator, which sends a slight electric charge through the needles into the tissue. The technique varies from one acupuncturist to the next, and for each patient.

There are now several Western theories to explain the undeniable benefits of acupuncture. Under the neurotransmitter theory, Western scientists postulate that these needles inhibit spinal cord nerve cells and release beta-endorphins and other substances that deaden pain and relieve patients.

Acupuncture, they theorize, also helps to stimulate

Qualifications

When seeking an acupuncturist, look for someone who's thoroughly trained and certified. In China, acupuncturists are expected to complete a five-year course, which includes two years of herbal medicine. In the West, an acupuncturist should have completed at least a three-year course.

anti-inflammatory cell activity, increase skin temperature, and stimulate the flow of blood. Other scientists have studied the interaction of copper and steel needles, suggesting that these metals create an electromagnetic field that can stimulate positive and negative ions. Acupuncturists refer to this as tonification and dispersal. Treatment times will vary, according to the patient. A healthy adult may be left with needles inserted for up to twenty minutes. A child may be in and out in a matter of minutes. In the East, some acute cases will be treated daily. Chronic conditions may call for visits once a week or every other week.

Of course, periodic visits will allow the acupuncturist keep qi in harmony and prevent other disorders that lead to disease.

Acupressure

Never underestimate the healing power of human hands. The doctrine of the laying on of hands is based on sound principles. Who among us hasn't massaged our temples to soothe a headache or asked a spouse to rub our back or feet to relieve tension and ease pain? Naturally, in the empirical system of Chinese medicine, this type of treatment would come in for a significant amount of study.

Thousands of years ago, Chinese doctors noticed that something beneficial was happening with massage. These traditional physicians wanted to define this benefit and harness its powers into an understandable therapy that could be taught to others. Over the years, this therapy became known as acupressure, which is closely related to acupuncture.

Understood properly, acupressure will help you treat many of the most common complaints of the modern age. We spend long hours at work, often sitting in uncomfortable chairs that encourage bad posture. We suffer from stress-related tension, bad diets, and virtually no exercise. It's no wonder, then, that the body responds with back and stomach aches and a whole gamut of additional pains, from head to toe.

Acupressure is one of the oldest, if not the oldest, self-practiced form of therapy in the world. And just as someone in China saw the benefits of acupressure more than four thousand years ago, you can also be helped by this ancient brand of TCM.

One of the most frequently diagnosed problems in Chinese medicine is stuck or stagnant qi, indicating a blockage in the healthy flow of vital energy through the network of meridians. This disharmony is manifested by all the aches and pains that I've just described. Utilizing the same knowledge of meridians and diagnostic methods used in all branches of TCM, acupressure treats these symptoms by manipulating the acupressure points that will ease pain and release stagnant qi. By manipulating these points with the hands and the fingers, applying pressure along crucial meridians, you can release endorphins and other natural substances in your body that block pain. By stimulating the flow of blood, you will also soothe sore muscles and relax the body, promoting the body's natural ability to heal itself.

One of the most frequently observed symptoms of stress is chest tension and difficulty breathing. An acupressurist knows which points need to be manipulated to relieve the tension and restore healthy breathing. In the process, acupressure releases toxins that are built up in the body's tissues. It is always a good idea to flush these toxins with plenty of fluids after each session.

As the traditional Chinese physician always sought to treat the whole person and not just a particular disease, it was quickly noted that someone receiving acupressure not only found his or her body become relaxed but also felt day-to-day cares slip away as the mind was freed from immediate distractions and could resume its former acuity with peace.

The applications of acupressure are too numerous to list here, but let's consider a few. Sports medicine, for example, often incorporates acupressure to relieve the damage caused during a game or in practice. Many of these techniques date back to Chinese battlefields, when warriors noted that certain types of body contact would actually relieve some chronic pains. Acupressure is an ancient form of beauty therapy as well. Certain facial massages can relax your features, easing old worry lines and preventing new ones from forming.

To begin, you may want to apply either firm pressure, a slow circular massage, or a hard rubbing motion to stimulate the point, depending on the desired physical response. When you apply pressure, you can use your fingers, knuckles, palm, or thumbs. As you gain more experience, you can try various methods to see which works best for you. By applying pressure for about thirty seconds to one minute, you help ease pain, relieve stress, and calm your nervous system. Slower circular motions are used on pressure points to sedate or stimulate them. By rhythmically squeezing and releasing these muscle groups (like kneading bread), you relieve stiffness and work on constipation and muscle spasms.

When you want to increase the flow of qi, use a harsh rubbing motion. It helps to heat the body and reduce swelling. Anyone who's been out in the cold too long and has come inside rubbing his or her frozen hands knows what we are talking about here.

Finally, you may find that tapping an acupressure point will stimulate the muscles in that area. You may want to use your fingers or a loosely balled fist, depending on how close the muscle groups are to the body's surface.

Basic Acupressure Techniques

- Locate the pressure point(s) from the illustrations provided in the next several pages.
- Go to the designated area and feel for the tender point.
- Use the corner of your thumb pad for rotating procedures or the entire pad to apply direct pressure. Also, fingers and knuckles can be used to apply direct pressure. You can tap on points using the index finger, instead of applying direct pressure, or you can knead muscle areas as if kneading dough.
- Use a slow, steady movement.

- Work the pressure points on both the right and the left corresponding positions, when applicable.
- Each pressure-point treatment should last from ten to thirty seconds. Repeat the procedure five times.
- If the problem is acute (quick onset, short term), you can massage these points two to three times a day until symptoms subside.
- If it is a chronic problem, you can treat it once a day for a longer period of time for relief of pain or for respiratory or nervous disorders.

Common Acupressure Points

Over the years, Chinese physicians came to identify 365 acupressure points, the same ones used in acupuncture, which in turn lie along the body's meridians. In the meticulous fashion of TCM, each point was named according to the benefit it offered.

You might start with the Sea of Vitality Points (B23, B47). Seat yourself comfortably and manipulate this point, located at the lower left of your back. Meanwhile, you may find it helpful to focus on your energy reserves filling up again. In addition, Sea of Vitality can help alleviate acne or the ache of bruises elsewhere on your body.

Under each cheekbone, directly under the eyes, lies the Facial Beauty Point (St3). Massaging this area can relieve acne, stimulate your facial skin, and improve the tone of your skin.

On the top of your head between the cranial bones lies the One Hundred Meeting Point (GV20). You find it by tracing your fingers from the back of each ear to the top of the back of your head. Press at this point to help relieve stress and headache pain while restoring clear thinking and concentration.

Below the base of the skull lies the Gates of Consciousness Point (GB20), which can improve concentration and memory and relieve pain.

Joining the Valley Point (LI4) offers some quick relief for frontal headaches and shoulder pain. It is also effective for labor pain, which is why you need to avoid it if you may be pregnant; it can stimulate premature contractions. In the angle that lies at the top of the hand between the thumb and the forefinger lies the Joining the Valley Point. Apply appropriate pressure to bear on this point, and you can feel your headache draining away.

In one of the simplest and most effective maneuvers in the books, you can take your forefinger and place it firmly between your eyebrows, pressing for several minutes. This Yintang Point will clear your head and relieve many headaches. Oftentimes, the affected pressure point is tender to touch. In this case, massage around this spot.

If you ever visit an acupressurist, you'll see that the physician doesn't just use the muscles in his hand to apply pressure. An experienced practitioner will lean into the massage point, using body weight to apply pressure. You'll find that this is just as effective when you work on your own points, as you are being asked to apply strong pressure for several minutes to each point.

You're not asked to deal with a lot of pain here. If you experience too much discomfort, ease up on the pressure or the rubbing.

A session can last anywhere from a few minutes to a full hour, and you may want to experiment by practicing acupressure in a sitting or lying-down position. Take long, deep breaths as you engage in acupressure. By balancing your breath, you help balance the body. Open yourself to the healing powers of acupressure, and clear your mind of daily clutter.

In order to give yourself the full benefits of acupressure, develop your own schedule for healing-touch sessions. You can designate a spot in your office or at home. Make sure you follow through with a routine session at least once a day— more often, if it helps. Just exactly what kind of schedule you keep will be up to you and what you hope to achieve, whether it's reducing mild stress or dealing with chronic pain.

Standard Meridian Abbreviations

Lu Lung
LI Large Intestine
Sp Spleen
TW Triple Warmer
St Stomach
SI Small Intestine
H   Heart
CV Conception Vessel
K   Kidney
P   Pericardium
B   Bladder
GB Gallbladder
Lv Liver
GV Governing Vessel
EX Extra Point

If you'd like to gain some help with acupressure, consider tracking down a specialist in acupressure massage. An acupressure masseur will start at the top of the back and gradually work downward, applying pressure with the thumb or the whole hand. As with any professional massage, the subject experiences the exquisite pain of strong hands and is often left spent and rested.

As always, there are plenty of don'ts to be considered along with the do's.

- Don't get too strenuous while pregnant. You should check with a qualified acupressurist before using any points to see which exercises are helpful, though, as acupressure can relieve many of the aches and pains associated with pregnancy and childbirth. Make sure you moderate the finger pressure during pregnancy as well. Acupuncture at this time is not an option, as overstimulation of these points can trigger contractions.
- Certain sensitive areas, like portions of the throat or the groin, should be either avoided or only gently touched. Remember, you should never experience any excessive pain from this procedure.
- Burns, injuries, or any other physically damaged region should be allowed to heal before treating the area with acupressure. That is particularly true for fractured or broken bones, as well as for disk injuries and severe back pain. A physician should deal with injuries.
- Always remember that you're more vulnerable to cold after each session. You may need to put on an extra sweater or a sweatshirt to guard against the cold while staying comfortable.

Other than taking commonsense precautions, though, I think you'll find that acupressure can often be useful as an ongoing method of self-treatment. It's just as relevant today as it was to the ancient Chinese.

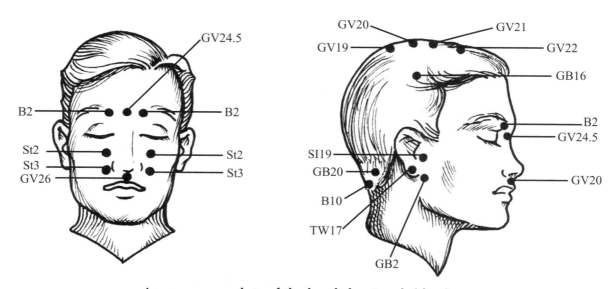

Acupressure points of the head, front and side views

Many acupressure experts suggest that you keep a diary of your activities: by tracking your symptoms, you will be able to log your progress. Obviously, many conditions, like cancer or appendicitis, can only be peripherally treated by acupressure. But don't underestimate its long-term healing powers.

While Western pharmaceutical companies compete in the hunt for ever-more-expensive drugs, this is one class of treatment that is free for all.

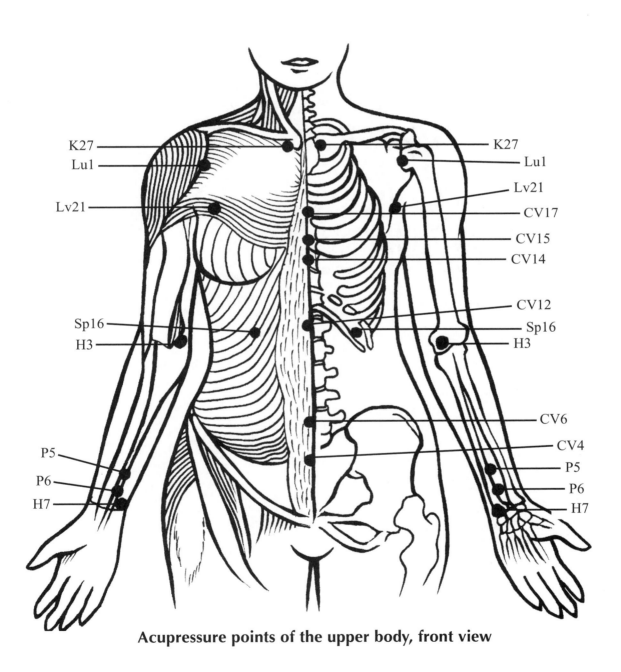

Acupressure points of the upper body, front view

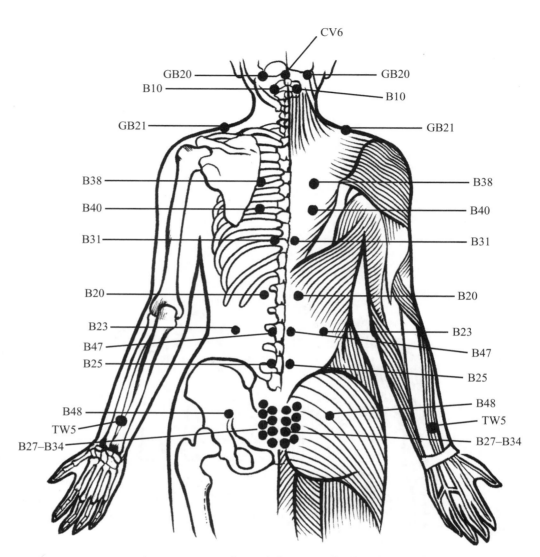

Acupressure points of the upper body, back view

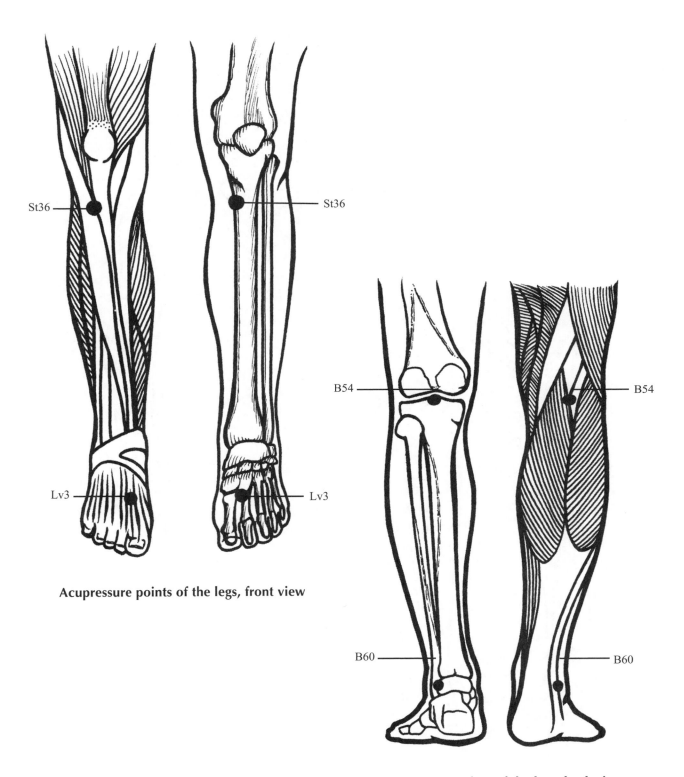

Acupressure points of the legs, front view

Acupressure points of the legs, back view

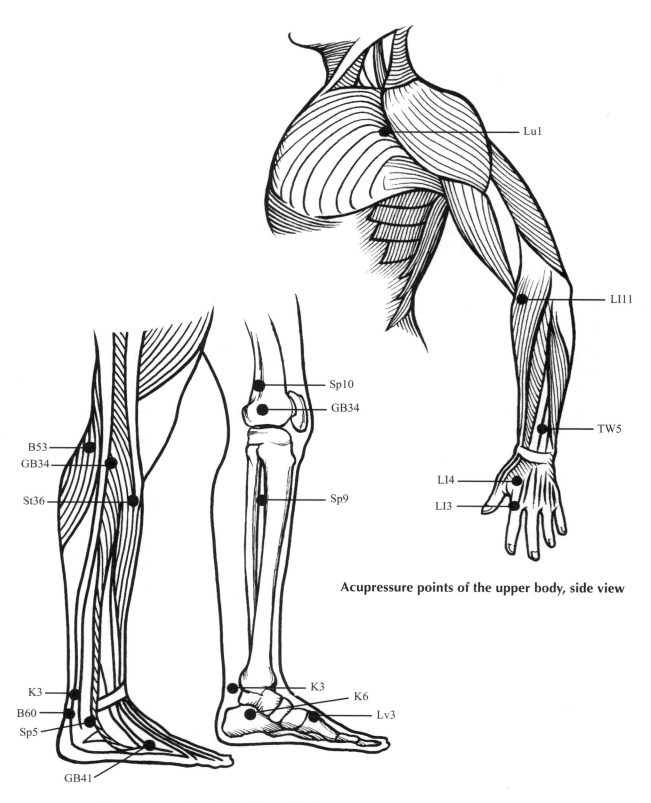

Acupressure points of the upper body, side view

Acupressure points of the legs, side view

Hydrotherapy

Hydrotherapy is a type of bodywork that uses water as a healing agent. It can involve water in the form of a liquid, a solid, or a vapor. Water is used as a stimulus to improve energy levels and resistance to disease. The manipulation of your blood's circulation by using hydrotherapy can help many ailments, such as fevers, bronchitis, headaches, sinusitis, colds, insomnia, and various other conditions. Although a gentle treatment, hydrotherapy can have profound health benefits. In addition, hydrotherapy is an effective way to stimulate the immune system, optimize circulation, and promote detoxification.

History

The use of water as a healing tool has been recorded since ancient times. Records found from the Egyptians and the Babylonians are filled with descriptions about various forms of hydrotherapy. Ancient Greeks and Romans placed a high priority on baths for healing and disease prevention. Vincent Priessnitz, who lived from 1799 to 1852, was one of the most influential people in the hydrotherapy movement. As a boy, he observed how injured animals instinctively went to a nearby creek to let the cold, flowing water heal their injuries. Priessnitz experimented with various forms of hydrotherapy as a boy growing up on a farm in Europe. At age seventeen, he was run over by a wagon and pronounced untreatable by a local surgeon. Using hydrotherapy, he was able to recover from his broken ribs. From that point on, people came from around the country for his famed hydrotherapy treatments. Later in life, the Austrian emperor gave him a gold medal for civic merit. Father Sebastian Kneipp (1821–1897) was also a famous advocate of hydrotherapy, devising approximately 120 different uses of water for healing. His hydrotherapy treatments are still used by spas and clinics in Europe today.

Constitutional Hydrotherapy

The most powerful of the hydrotherapy treatments is constitutional hydrotherapy. It has been named constitutional since it has benefits to the entire constitution of a person.
1. Optimizes circulation
2. Detoxifies and purifies the blood

3. Enhances digestive function and elimination
4. Tonifies and balances the nervous system
5. Stimulates and enhances the immune system
6. Is particularly helpful for people suffering from digestive problems; respiratory problems, such as sore throats and bronchitis; or infections, such as a cold or the flu

Note: If a child has asthma, this procedure should be used only under the guidance of a physician.

FREQUENCY OF TREATMENT

Acute conditions: one to two times daily
Chronic conditions: five to seven times weekly

DIRECTIONS

Note: This treatment is best done with the help of an assistant.

1. The person lies in bed on his or her back.
2. An assistant covers the bared chest and the abdomen with two thicknesses of towels that have been placed in hot water and wrung out (wet towels can be heated in the microwave). Towels should be hot, yet tolerable, for children. Place a small section of the towel on the child first to make sure it is not too hot.
3. Cover the hot towels with a dry towel.
4. Cover the person with blankets to prevent him or her from getting chilled. Leave the towels on for five minutes.
5. After five minutes, remove the hot towels and replace with a single thickness of a thin towel that has been run under cold water and then wrung out (with some moisture left in the towel).
6. Place the cold towel on the bared chest and the abdomen. Cover with a dry towel and blankets. Leave on for ten minutes. The towel should be warm after ten minutes. If not, leave it on longer, or do not make the towel so cold or wet next time.
7. Take cold towel off, and have the person turn over and lie on the stomach. Repeat the same procedure on the back. Five minutes of hot towels, followed by ten minutes of a thin cold towel.

HOW IT WORKS

The alternation in hot and cold increases the immune system's white blood cells to help fight off infections. It also increases circulation to the digestive organs and other organs of elimination.

Foot Hydrotherapy

A more simple treatment than constitutional hydrotherapy, foot hydrotherapy helps to relieve respiratory congestion, headaches, and insomnia.

FREQUENCY OF TREATMENT

Acute conditions: one to two times daily

Chronic conditions: once daily

DIRECTIONS

1. Sit on a chair or a couch and place both feet in a bucket of warm water (make sure it is tolerable, if for a child) for five to ten minutes.
2. Remove your feet from the water and dry them.
3. Put on a pair of cotton socks that have been placed in cold water and wrung out.
4. Cover with a pair of wool socks (or cotton, if wool is not available).
5. Leave the socks on for a half hour or longer. You should be resting now and can even go to sleep with the socks on.

Comment: The foot hydrotherapy works by diverting blood flow to the feet and away from the upper body, thus reducing congestion.

Headache Treatment

You can alleviate a headache simply by putting your feet in warm water and placing an ice pack around your neck. This hot-cold water strategy causes blood to move away from the head toward the feet, relieving the head of congestion and pain.

Natural Hormones

Introduction

Hormones have been used as a form of medicine for centuries. Ancient Chinese texts describe how the elderly rejuvenated their sex lives with the use of natural hormones. Today, specific hormones are available as dietary supplements, and many holistic doctors recommend a variety of natural hormones in the prevention and the treatment of disease. Throughout this book, you will find specific conditions that can be prevented or improved with the help of natural-hormone therapy. This section explains what natural hormones are and how to best use them.

The Study That Awakened the Establishment

Natural hormones have gained a lot of attention since July 2002, when the *Journal of the American Medical Association* reported on a study known as the Women's Health Initiative. The study involved over sixteen thousand healthy women and was originally scheduled to run until 2005. However, it was stopped prematurely when investigators found significant increases in the women's risk of developing coronary heart disease, stroke, blood clots, and breast cancer if they were receiving synthetic-hormone treatment for their menopausal symptoms. The only positive note for the patients on hormone therapy was a reduction in the risk of colorectal cancer and in fracture rates. Researchers concluded that the harm from using the synthetic-hormone replacement Premarin and Provera combination, known as Prempro, outweighed the benefit. After this information was released, many doctors and medical establishments recommended that women strongly consider discontinuing its use as a hormone replacement. This left many women in a quandary about what to do, because most of them were not offered any other options.

The Natural Choice

Holistic physicians have used natural hormones for several decades now. We define the term *natural hormone* as a hormone that is identical to what is produced and utilized in the human body. It is that simple. If a hormone does not have the identical structure to the one found in the human body, we classify it as "synthetic." The cells in our bodies were designed to be compatible with the hormones we naturally produce. By contrast, synthetic hormones are recognized differently by our cell receptors and may initiate a different reaction than they would to a natural version of the same hormone.

Perhaps the best example to illustrate this is to look at the widely prescribed estrogen hormone Premarin. This estrogen prescription is derived from the urine of horses—pregnant mares, to be exact. Now, one may think that the estrogen from a horse is natural, seeing as it is found in "nature." However, many of the estrogens in Premarin are foreign to the human body. According to the *Physician's Desk Reference*, Premarin contains a group of estrogens known as equilins. This includes equilin, 17-dihydroequilin, equilenin, and 17-dihydroequilenin. These types of estrogens are not found in the human body. How the human body metabolizes and copes with these foreign estrogens is not exactly known. Yet in vitro studies have shown that Premarin metabolites damage the DNA of cells. This may be one reason why users of Premarin have an increased cancer risk.

Natural Hormones Available as Supplements

Currently, five natural hormones are available over the counter. This includes androstenedione, DHEA, melatonin, progesterone, and pregnenolone. All other hormones such as estrogen, testosterone, thyroid, and others, require a prescription from a doctor. Following is a summary of the hormones that are currently available as dietary supplements. Please note that we feel it is best to work with a knowledgeable doctor when using these hormones instead of self-experimenting with them.

DHEA (Dehydroepiandrosterone)

Description: DHEA is the most abundant hormone produced by the adrenal glands. It has several functions, including but not limited to supporting the body's reaction to stress, control of inflammation, libido, cognitive function, immune modulation, and metabolism. DHEA is a precursor hormone to testosterone and androstenedione.

Indications: Alzheimer's disease
　　　　　　　　　Arthritis
　　　　　　　　　Chronic fatigue syndrome
　　　　　　　　　Depression
　　　　　　　　　Diabetes
　　　　　　　　　Erectile dysfunction
　　　　　　　　　Heart-disease prevention
　　　　　　　　　Immune support
　　　　　　　　　Inflammatory bowel disease
　　　　　　　　　Lupus
　　　　　　　　　Menopause
　　　　　　　　　Osteoporosis
　　　　　　　　　Prednisone withdrawal

Precautions: Too high a dosage may cause facial-hair growth and acne breakout. Pregnant women and breast-feeding mothers should avoid using DHEA. People with existing cancers should also avoid it.

Dosage: A starting dose of 5 to 15 mg for women and 15 to 25 mg for men is recommended and is increased depending on the clinical situation and laboratory testing.

Melatonin

Description: Melatonin is produced in the pineal gland, which regulates the body's biological clock and sleep cycles. Melatonin is produced in response to darkness. This hormone has been shown to be helpful for insomnia, seasonal affective disorder, and other mood disturbances. It has potent antioxidant properties and protects against radiation damage.

Indications: Aging
Cancer (breast and prostate)
Cluster headaches
Insomnia
Jet lag
Radiation exposure
Seasonal affective disorder
Tardive dyskinesia

Precautions: Pregnant women or nursing mothers should avoid supplementing melatonin unless instructed to do so by their physician. People with cancer should also consult with their doctors before supplementing melatonin. Children should not supplement melatonin unless instructed to do so by their doctors. People on steroid medications should avoid taking melatonin unless their doctors feel it is appropriate.

Dosage: Take 0.3 to 5 mg as the starting dosage for insomnia and jet lag.

Pregnenolone

Description: Pregnenolone is a steroidal hormone produced in large part by the adrenal glands. It is a precursor hormone that the body uses to manufacture DHEA and progesterone. Holistic doctors commonly recommend it for arthritis and autoimmune conditions such as lupus.

Indications: Arthritis (especially rheumatoid form)
Depression
Lupus erythematosus
Poor memory
Psoriasis

Precautions: Pregnenolone should be avoided by people who have seizure disorders or a history of hormone-related cancers.

Dosage: Take 10 to 50 mg daily.

Progesterone

Description: Progesterone is a hormone found in both men and women. For women, it is involved in regulating the menstrual cycle and reproductive function. Progesterone is mainly produced and secreted by the ovaries during ovulation. It is also manufactured by the adrenal glands, the brain, and the placenta in pregnant women. Natural progesterone cream is a popular supplement for the treatment of PMS, menopausal symptoms, endometriosis, and several other conditions.

Indications: Autoimmune conditions
Endometriosis

Fibrocystic breasts
Infertility (female)
Irregular menses
Menopausal symptoms
Osteoporosis
Ovarian cysts
PMS
Uterine fibroids

Precautions: Natural progesterone cream has a good safety record. Women with a history of cancer should consult a doctor before using it. Women using the birth-control pill or synthetic progestin should avoid it.

Dosage: The dosage depends on the condition being treated (see the corresponding sections in this book, such as Premenstrual Syndrome or Menopause). Menopausal women generally apply a quarter teaspoon (20 mg) to their skin one to two times daily.

Prescription Natural Hormones

Most natural hormones, such as thyroid, testosterone, growth hormone, estrogen, and others, require a prescription. Holistic doctors generally prescribe these hormones with the help of a compounding pharmacy. Pharmacists at these specialized pharmacies are trained in formulating natural-hormone prescriptions exactly to the requirement of each individual patient.

Testing Your Hormone Balance

Before using any of the natural hormones (or any hormones, for that matter), we recommend that you consult with a doctor to test your hormone levels. There are several ways that you can do this. They include blood tests, urine testing, and saliva testing. All three methods have their strengths and weaknesses.

References

Physician's Desk Reference, 52nd ed. 1998. Montvale, N.J.: Medical Economics Company, p. 311.

Pisha, E., et al. 2001. Evidence that a metabolite of equine estrogens, 5-hydroxyequilenin, induces cellular transformation in vitro. *Chemical Research in Toxicology* 14(1):82–90.

Writing Group for the Women's Health Initiative Investigators. 2002. Risks and benefits of estrogen plus progestin in healthy postmenopausal women: Principal results from the Women's Health Initiative Randomized Controlled Trial. *Journal of the American Medical Association* 288(3):321–33.

Bodywork

Since the dawn of humankind, bodywork has been used to heal people's injuries and illnesses and to promote relaxation. Bodywork refers to external therapies, applied to the outside of the body, that create relaxation and healing. The most common form of bodywork is massage. Almost everyone is familiar with massage, as it involves rubbing and pressing muscles and soft tissues. Yet many other forms of bodywork can help a person prevent illness and recover from it. *Prescription for Natural Cures* includes specific recommendations in the areas of massage, acupressure, reflexology, craniosacral therapy, osteopathy, chiropractic, hydrotherapy, physiotherapy, magnet therapy, and others.

Healers have long realized that the external surface of the body can be used as a conduit or a reflex center to positively influence the internal organs. The body is a complex and intelligent network of muscles, soft tissues, and nerve structures that communicate with each other. A disruption or an imbalance in the soft tissues can lead to or contribute to an imbalance elsewhere in the body.

Everyone experiences injuries to the muscles, the bones, and the connective tissue many times in his or her life. In more serious cases, pharmaceutical medication may be required to treat severe pain and inflammation, but most cases require only stimulation of the body's healing mechanisms. Various forms of bodywork improve circulation and lymphatic flow, which allow the body's cells to detoxify and the tissues to recover from injury. Studies also show that bodywork enhances healthy immune cells that fight infection. An increasing number of people are turning to practitioners of bodywork to decrease the effects of stress on their bodies and minds.

The forms of bodywork described herein (and many others that are too numerous to mention) are very compatible with the dietary guidelines and nutritional supplements recommended in this book. As a matter of fact, most people will do better with a synergistic combination of natural healing methods. Also, for people who need to use prescription drugs, bodywork is usually compatible with these and will speed the healing process. For a referral to various bodywork associations, please see the appendix, A Natural Health Care Resource Guide, on page 813.

Following are descriptions of the types of bodywork recommended throughout the book.

Acupuncture/Acupressure

These therapies are based on the ancient Chinese medicine concept that the body contains twelve main channels of acupuncture/acupressure points. Through these channels runs the energy referred to as qi (pronounced *chee*, also written as "chi"). Disease arises when one or more of these channels (meridians) are blocked. Using needles (acupuncture) or pressing on specific points (acupressure) will reestablish energy flow and balance in the body. There are hundreds of acupuncture/acupressure points. Each point has one or more indications. Practitioners of Oriental medicine use acupuncture and acupressure in their practices.

Chiropractic

This is a system of healing based on the premise that poor spinal health (subluxations) leads to improper nerve flow and disease. Through specific adjustments of the spine and the extremities, one can restore spinal health and normal body function. Doctors of chiropractic are trained as primary health care physicians.

Craniosacral Therapy

Craniosacral therapy is regarded as a gentle, noninvasive type of bodywork. The craniosacral system consists of the membranes and the fluid that surround and support the brain and the spinal cord. The craniosacral system extends from the bones of the head (cranium) down to the bones at the base of the spine (sacrum). The fluid within the membranes is continuously draining and refilling. The filling and draining create gentle, rhythmic, expanding and contracting movements that can be felt and monitored by a craniosacral therapist. The therapist then applies gentle manipulations to correct imbalances and reestablish proper fluid movement. Specific training is required to become a craniosacral therapist.

Hydrotherapy

Hydrotherapy is a type of bodywork that uses water as a healing agent to stimulate healing. It can involve water in the form of a liquid (such as a bath), a solid (ice), or a vapor (steam sauna). Various practitioners are trained in many forms of hydrotherapy.

Laser Therapy

The use of low-level lasers have been shown in research to reduce pain and inflammation and to stimulate tissue healing. Joint and muscular conditions respond well to this type of therapy.

Magnet Therapy

Magnets are used on or near the skin to positively influence the magnetic field of the body to stimulate healing. They have been shown to reduce pain and inflammation.

Massage

Massage is the therapeutic use of external pressure applied to the skin and the muscles of the body. Many different techniques are used by massage therapists.

Osteopathic Medicine

Osteopathy or osteopathic medicine is a system of medicine based on the premise that the bone structure (the spine and the extremities) is related to the internal health of the body. Osteopathic doctors may use spinal manipulation (osteopathic manipulative treatment) to help patients with musculoskeletal and systemic disorders. They are also trained in drugs and surgery, and they practice as primary-care doctors.

Physiotherapy

Physiotherapy is the use of external therapies to prevent and treat health conditions. It may involve the use of heat, cold, light, and physical and mechanical means to enhance healing within the body. Physiotherapists are health care specialists. Many holistic doctors incorporate physiotherapy techniques and methods into their practices.

Reflexology

Reflexology involves the use of therapeutic pressure on the reflex points of the foot to enhance the innate healing mechanisms of the body. It is based on the premise that internal organs can be positively influenced by the proper application of pressure applied to specific reflex points on the hands and the feet. Many massage therapists are trained in reflexology.

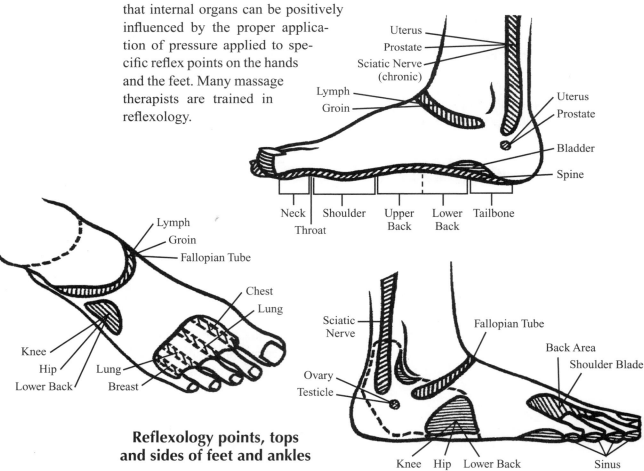

**Reflexology points, tops
and sides of feet and ankles**

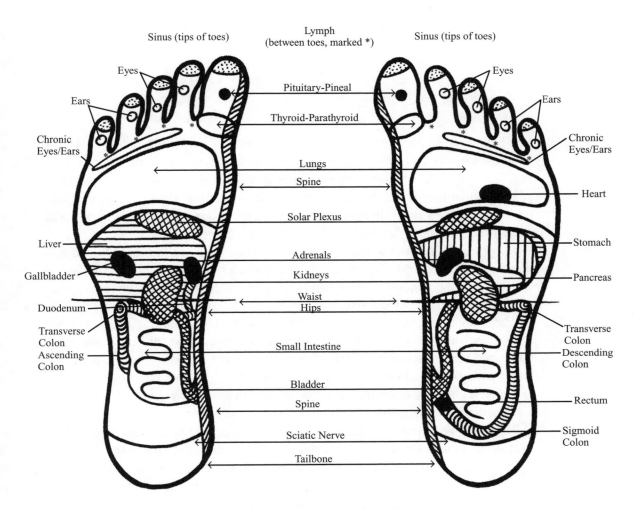

Reflexology points, soles of feet

Exercise and Stress Reduction

You have heard the expression "Stress kills." There is some truth to this statement, although the way you perceive and respond to stress is more important. One crucial thing we can do as doctors and educators is to help people realize how stress is affecting their health and then recommend stress-reduction techniques to help them better handle their stress. In many instances, we have found that how patients handle stress makes all the difference between their healing or remaining ill.

Many people fail to see the connection between their health problems and how they handle their stress. Unfortunately, many doctors fail to see the connection as well. Research continues to show that how one handles stress is paramount to one's physical, mental, and emotional health.

The body responds to stress by releasing adrenal hormones, such as cortisol, DHEA, and other hormonal and neural chemicals, into the bloodstream. These "stress hormones" are powerful chemicals. When they are heightened or depressed for too long a period of time, as a result of stress, a person becomes susceptible to disease. For example, high levels of cortisol are associated with an increased risk of Alzheimer's disease, diabetes, heart disease, certain cancers, and other serious illnesses.

The stress-reduction techniques in this chapter will help you to lessen the effects of stress on your body. Keep in mind that everyone is different, so you should choose the technique(s) that interest you most. As with anything, the more you practice them, the more helpful they will be in preventing and treating health problems. Many professionals in these areas can be of assistance.

You can use the following techniques to reduce the effects of stress and improve your health.

Deep Breathing

Proper breathing is key in reducing the effects of stress and improving your energy and concentration levels. Every time you breathe in, cells are replenished with the oxygen that sustains life. When you breathe out, carbon dioxide and other toxins are released from the lungs. Numerous studies have shown that deep breathing relaxes the mind, calms the nervous system, improves mental focus, and improves energy.

When you look at a young child, you can observe the proper way to breathe. Children breathe from the belly, not the chest. This allows for maximal oxygen intake and carbon dioxide release, because the diaphragm comes into play. During deep breathing, this muscular covering over the top of the abdominal cavity has a massaging effect on the internal organs.

To deep-breathe properly, you should first find a quiet, comfortable place. Stand or sit up straight, with your belly and chest relaxed. Breathe in through your nose slowly for a count of five, hold for two seconds, and then exhale through your mouth. Please note that when you inhale, your stomach, not your chest, should expand outward. This is how to assess whether you are breathing deeply and using your diaphragm. As you breathe out, your stomach should flatten.

Exercise

Exercise is one of the simplest and most underrated ways to reduce the effects of stress on the body. Few people would argue that exercise calms the mind, improves energy, and makes one more resilient to stress. Exercise has been shown in numerous studies to be very effective in reducing anxiety and depression, two conditions that millions of Americans deal with. Exercise also offers an opportunity to enjoy more social contact, which is healthful for the mind and the spirit.

One key we have found to long-term exercise commitment is choosing exercise(s) that you truly enjoy. Too many people join a local gym or begin an exercise regimen with a friend, but it is short lived since they really don't enjoy it. Think of a type of exercise that makes you excited enough to get out and do it. It may be something as simple as walking or biking, or it may be more involved, such as joining a gym or a sports team.

Before you begin a new exercise, get evaluated by your doctor. With all forms of exercise, start with a warm-up period, in which you loosen up and perform mild stretches. Then, after the activity, spend even more time stretching and cooling down to prevent injury and soreness. You should try to exercise a minimum of three times a week for twenty minutes. If you have not been physically active for a while, start with a lesser amount of time and gradually increase it every week. As long as you can recover from your exercise and do not remain stiff and sore for more than a day or two, you are on the right track.

Optimally, it is most beneficial to choose exercises that target the cardiovascular system (such as walking, biking, jogging, swimming, hiking, dancing, etc.), along with those that build lean muscle and bone density (weight lifting).

Laughter

A good laugh can go a long way toward reducing the effects of stress. Research shows that laughter prevents inflammatory triggers that lead to heart and artery damage, and it reduces the effects of stress. Research done at the University of Maryland School of Medicine found that laugher and a good sense of humor resulted in protection against heart disease. In this study, researchers evaluated the responses of three hundred people to potentially humorous situations. For example, one questionnaire asked how they would respond to a specific scenario that could cause a stress response, such as having a drink accidentally spilled on them by a waiter while dining with friends, or arriving at a party dressed in clothing identical to that worn by one of the other guests. People with the highest "humor scores" had a 48 percent lower risk of heart disease, independent of their age or sex. However, those with heart disease were much less likely to use humor as an adaptive mechanism.

Music Therapy

The human brain has been programmed to be responsive to music. Examine any culture throughout the world, and you are sure to find music being used as a way to relax and combat the effects of stress. Certain types of music induce a relaxation state. This, of course, depends on each individual's music interests. On the other hand, some types of music are stimulating and should be avoided when you are trying to achieve a relaxation response.

Prayer

The most powerful mind-body relaxation technique, in our opinion, is prayer. It offers an opportunity to communicate with the Creator and cast your doubts and cares upon Him. This is the time to "Be still" and hear from God. Make prayer a daily habit, and it will help you relax and achieve a more healthful life.

Progressive Muscle Relaxation

A popular technique to help people relax is to tighten and relax muscles throughout the body. People do not realize how tight their muscles are until they consciously tighten and relax them.

Starting by curling your toes and holding them tightened for three seconds, then relax them. Work your way up the body, focusing on how each muscle group feels as you tighten and relax it. This is a great technique for unwinding at the end of the day or reducing anxiety that is troubling you.

Tai Chi and Qigong

Tai chi and qigong are two aspects of traditional Chinese medicine that have become popular in the West as forms of exercise and stress reduction. They involve specific body movements and deep breathing. Videos and public classes are readily available to help you learn these two systems of movement and relaxation.

Visualization

The use of positive imagery is a potent tool in the war against stress. The visualization of positive images invokes a relaxation response. Find a quiet, comfortable place and visualize images that make you feel relaxed and content. You can also visualize yourself feeling relaxed and healthy.

Yoga

Yoga has become a popular way to relax the body. It involves deep breathing and stretching Take classes from a yoga instructor whom you are comfortable with. There are many different types of yoga, so research the styles to see what you prefer.

References

Clark, A., A. Seidler, and M. Miller. 2000. Coronary disease and reduced situational humor-response: Is laughter cardioprotective? [Abstract] Presented at the 73rd Scientific Session of the American Heart Association, November 15, New Orleans.

PART THREE

Appendix

A Natural Health Care Resource Guide

Acupuncture/Acupressure

These therapies are based on the ancient Chinese medicine concept that the body contains twelve main channels of acupuncture/acupressure points. Through these channels runs the life-giving energy referred to as qi (pronounced *chee*, also written as "chi"). Disease arises when one or more of these channels (meridians) are blocked. Using needles (acupuncture) or pressing on specific points (acupressure) will reestablish energy flow and balance in the body. There are hundreds of acupuncture/acupressure points. Each point has one or more indications. Practitioners of Oriental medicine use acupuncture and acupressure in their practices.

American Oriental Bodywork Therapy Association
1010 Haddonfield-Berlin Road, Suite 408
Voorhees NJ 08043
(856) 782-1616

American Association of Acupuncture and Oriental
  Medicine
PO Box 96503 #44114
Washington DC 20090-6503
(866) 455-7999
www.aaaomonline.org

Aromatherapy

The use of essential oils made from plants, leaves, bark, roots, seeds, and flowers can treat a wide range of conditions. Aromatherapists use essential oils that have specific properties to prevent or alleviate symptoms or conditions. The scents from these essential oils stimulate the healing mechanisms of the body.

National Association for Holistic Aromatherapy
PO Box 27871
Raleigh NC 27611-7871
(919) 894-0298
www.naha.org

Ayurvedic Medicine

Ayurveda is a Sanskrit word that is translated as "science of life" or "knowledge of how to live." Ayurveda is an ancient East Indian system of healing that seeks to promote balance through a healthful lifestyle and various natural healing methods. Ayurveda practitioners tailor treatments to each person's unique condition.

Biofeedback

Biofeedback consists of information supplied instantaneously about an individual's own physiological processes. Data concerning cardiovascular activity (blood pressure and heart rate), temperature, brain waves, or muscle tension are monitored electronically and returned, or "fed back," to each person via a gauge on a meter, a light, or a sound. It has been shown that an individual can be taught to use biofeedback to voluntarily control the body's reactions to stress or "outside-the-skin" events. An individual learns through biofeedback training to detect his or her physical reactions (inside-the-skin events) and establish control over them. An example would be a child with anxiety who learns to calm his or her nervous system by using biofeedback. Clinical psychologists, counselors, and some health practitioners use biofeedback in their practices.

Chelation Therapy

Chelation therapy is the use of certain agents or nutrients to help pull toxic substances out of the body (e.g., heavy metals such as lead). This can be done intravenously, with chelating agents, such as ethylenediaminetetraacetic acid (EDTA), or with oral agents (e.g., DMSA, or certain vitamins and minerals).

American College for Advancement in Medicine
380 Ice Center Lane, Suite C
Bozeman MT 59718
(800) LEADOUT
www.acam.org

The American Association of Naturopathic
    Physicians
818 18th Street NW, Suite 250
Washington DC 20016
(866) 538-2267
www.naturopathic.org

Chiropractic

This is a system of healing based on the premise that poor spinal health (subluxations) leads to improper nerve flow and disease. Through specific adjustments of the spine and the extremities, one can restore spinal health and normal body function. Doctors of chiropractic are trained as primary health care physicians.

American Chiropractic Association
1701 Clarendon Boulevard
Arlington VA 22209
(703) 276-8800
www.acatoday.org

Craniosacral Therapy

Craniosacral therapy is regarded as a gentle, noninvasive type of bodywork. The craniosacral system consists of the membranes and the fluid that surround and support the brain and the spinal cord. The craniosacral system extends from the bones of the head (cranium) down to the bones at the base of the spine (sacrum). The fluid within the membranes is continuously draining and refilling. The filling and draining create gentle, rhythmic, expanding and contracting movements that can be felt and monitored by a craniosacral therapist. The therapist then applies gentle manipulations to correct imbalances and reestablish proper fluid movement. Specific training is required to become a craniosacral therapist.

Guided Imagery

This is the use of imaging techniques in one's mind to enhance health and well-being. Studies have shown a benefit to the immune system from guided imagery. For example, many people with cancer are taught to visualize their immune cells becoming active and fighting cancer cells. Clinical psychologists, counselors, naturopathic and medical doctors, and various health practitioners recommend guided imagery.

Herbal Medicine

Herbal medicine is the therapeutic use of plant extracts for the prevention and the treatment of illness. Herbalists and naturopathic doctors are trained extensively in the therapeutic uses of herbs as medicine.

American Botanical Council
PO Box 144345
Austin TX 78714-4345
(512) 926-4900
www.herbalgram.org

Holistic Dentistry

Holistic dentists view the body as a whole. They utilize nontoxic materials whenever possible—for example, by avoiding the use of amalgam fillings.

Holistic Dental Association
1825 Ponce de Leon Blvd. #148
Coral Gables FL 33134
(305) 356-7388
www.holisticdental.org

Homeopathy

Homeopathy is a system of natural healing based on the premise that "like cures like." Homeopathic remedies are highly diluted medicines that stimulate the healing response of the body. Homeopaths, homeopathic doctors, and naturopathic doctors have had extensive training in this field.

National Center for Homeopathy
7918 Jones Branch Drive, Suite 300
McLean VA 22102
(703) 506-7667
www.hanp.net

Homeopathic Academy of Naturopathic Physicians
1607 Siskiyou Blvd
Ashland OR 97520
(541) 708-1827
www.hanp.net

Hydrotherapy

Hydrotherapy is a type of bodywork that uses water to stimulate healing. It can involve water in the form of a liquid (such as a bath), a solid (ice), or a vapor (steam sauna). Various practitioners are trained in many forms of hydrotherapy.

The American Association of Naturopathic Physicians
818 18th Street NW, Suite 250
Washington DC 20016
(866) 538-2267
www.naturopathic.org

Massage

Massage is the therapeutic use of external pressure applied to the skin and the muscles of the body.

American Massage Therapy Association
(877) 905-0577
www.amtamassage.org

Naturopathic Medicine

Naturopathic medicine is a system of natural medicine that focuses on working with the healing systems of the body. Naturopathic doctors are trained as primary health care providers. As general practitioners, they work to restore health by using clinical nutrition, herbal medicine, homeopathy, physical medicine, counseling, nutritional supplementation, natural hormones, hydrotherapy, and other forms of natural healing. They are also trained in the use of pharmaceutical medicines and minor surgery.

The American Association of Naturopathic
  Physicians
818 18th Street NW, Suite 250
Washington DC 20016
(866) 538-2267
www.naturopathic.org

Canadian Association of Naturopathic Doctors
(CAND)
20 Holly St., Ste. 200
Toronto ON, Canada M4S 3B1
(800) 551-4381
www.cand.ca

Nutrition

The use of clinical nutrition means the therapeutic use of foods as medicine. Many practitioners of holistic and natural medicine use nutrition as the basis for their treatment.

Osteopathic Medicine

Osteopathy or osteopathic medicine is a system of medicine based on the premise that bone structure (the spine and the extremities) is related to the internal health of the body. Osteopathic doctors may use spinal manipulation (osteopathic manipulative treatment) to help patients with musculoskeletal and systemic disorders. They are also trained in drugs and surgery, and they practice as primary-care doctors.

American Osteopathic Association
142 East Ontario Street
Chicago IL 60611
(800) 621-1773 | (312) 202-8000
www.aoa-net.org

Physiotherapy

Physiotherapy is the use of external therapies to prevent and treat health conditions. Physiotherapy uses heat, cold, light, and physical and mechanical means to enhance healing within the body. Physiotherapists are health care specialists. Many holistic doctors incorporate physiotherapy techniques and methods into their practices.

Reflexology

Reflexology involves the use of therapeutic pressure on the reflex points of the foot to enhance the innate healing mechanisms of the body. It is based on the premise that internal organs can be positively influenced by the proper application of pressure applied to specific reflex points on the hands and the feet. Many massage therapists are trained in reflexology.

Reflexology Association of America
PO Box 1235
Evart MI 49631
(980) 234-0159
www.reflexology-usa.org

Yoga

The word yoga means "to join or yoke together," and this discipline is said to bring the body and the mind together. Yoga involves exercise, breathing, and sometimes meditation. There are many different types of yoga.

Glossary

absorption   The process of assimilation, whereby nutrients are absorbed through the digestive tract and into the bloodstream, then into the body's cells.

acetylcholine   A neurotransmitter that's involved in nerve-muscle activity and memory.

acidophilus   A species of healthful or friendly bacteria found throughout the body, especially in the digestive tract.

acupressure   The use of pressure and massage techniques along the meridians and at acupressure points to promote balance and good health.

acupuncture   The use of needles inserted in specific spots along the body's meridians to relieve pain or create balance in the body.

acute illness   An illness that may cause relatively severe symptoms but is of limited duration; a type of disease or disorder having a sudden onset, with severe symptoms, and generally a short or self-limited duration (such as a head cold or a sprain). The opposite of chronic.

adaptogen   An agent, such as an herb, that helps the body adapt to various stressors, whether they be physical, mental, or emotional. Often referred to as a "tonic." Many adaptogen herbs work, in part, by supporting adrenal-gland function. Ginseng is a classic example.

additive   A substance added to food as a preservative to extend the shelf life or the nutritional value. It can be made from natural sources or synthetically.

adrenal glands   A pair of glands situated above the kidneys that secrete the stress hormones epinephrine (adrenaline) and cortisol, as well as the sex steroids DHEA and pregnenolone.

aggravation   When symptoms worsen for a short time after a patient begins a homeopathic or natural treatment. Also known as a healing crisis.

allergen   A substance that provokes an allergic response.

allergy   Hypersensitivity caused by a foreign substance, small doses of which produce a bodily reaction; an immune-system response to a normally harmless substance, which can affect any of the tissues in the body.

alopecia   Baldness, loss of hair.

alternative medicine   Health care existing outside the established medical system—for example, herbalism, nutritional, chiropractic, naturopathic medicine, and so on.

amino acids   The individual building blocks of protein. There are approximately twenty different amino acids. Ten of the amino acids are known as "essential amino acids," which means that our bodies cannot manufacture them, so it is essential that we consume them in our diets. The remaining ten nonessential amino acids can be manufactured in the body.

analgesic   A substance that reduces or relieves pain.

anemia   A blood condition in which there are too few red blood cells or the red blood cells are deficient in hemoglobin. The most common form of anemia is caused by iron deficiency, although B12 and folic acid deficiencies occur as well.

aneurysm   An enlarged dilated artery that results from a weakened artery wall.

antibiotic   A substance (natural or synthetic) that destroys or reduces the growth of bacteria or fungi.

antibody   A protein molecule made by the immune system that intercepts and neutralizes a specific invading organism or other foreign substance.

anticoagulant   A substance that thins the blood. Used to prevent blood clots.

antigen   A substance that can cause the formation of an antibody when introduced into the body.

antihistamine   A substance that reduces or blocks the histamine response.

anti-inflammatory   A substance that is used to relieve inflammation.

antimicrobial   A substance or a treatment that destroys or neutralizes microorganisms (bacteria, virus, fungus, etc.).

antioxidants   Substances that neutralize or reduce the effects of cell-damaging free radicals. Common examples include vitamins A, C, and E and selenium.

antiparasitic   A substance (natural or synthetic) that kills or reduces the growth of parasites.

antispasmodic   Protects against muscle spasms.

aromatherapy   The use of essential oils and other pure plant extracts to treat a variety of conditions through inhalation and/or absorption through the skin.

arrhythmia   An abnormal or irregular heart rhythm.

arteriosclerosis   Hardening of the arteries created when plaque and calcium attach to the interiors of the arterial walls. This causes a loss in elasticity and flexibility of the artery, resulting in reduced circulation.

artery   A blood vessel through which blood is pumped from the heart to all the organs, glands, and other tissues of the body.

ascorbic acid   Vitamin C.

aspartame   An artificial sweetener that is used as a sugar substitute.

atherosclerosis   The most common type of arteriosclerosis, in which fatty deposits accumulate within the walls of medium and large arteries.

autoimmune disease   One of several conditions in which the immune system attacks and damages its own tissues. A common example is rheumatoid arthritis.

bacteria   Single-celled microorganisms. Some bacteria can cause disease; other ("friendly") bacteria are normally present in the body and perform such useful functions as aiding digestion and protecting the body from harmful invading organisms.

benign   Literally means "harmless"; it refers to cells, especially cells growing in inappropriate locations, that are not malignant (noncancerous).

bile   A greenish-yellow substance that the liver releases into the intestines; it assists in the digestion of fats, the elimination of toxins, and the absorption of fat-soluble vitamins.

biofeedback   Information supplied instantaneously about an individual's physiological processes. Data concerning a person's physiological processes (blood pressure, heart rate, temperature, brain waves, muscle tension , etc.) are monitored electronically and returned to that person by a gauge on a meter, a light, or a sound. This information is used to help a person learn how to voluntarily control body reactions to stress or related events.

bioflavonoid   Biologically active flavonoids that act synergistically with vitamin C; they are not technically vitamins but are often referred to as vitamin P.

bitters   An herbal term for a substance that tastes bitter and stimulates stomach and digestive activity.

bronchi   The two branches of the trachea (windpipe) that transport oxygen to and carbon dioxide from the lungs.

bronchodilator   A substance that relaxes and dilates the airway passages.

candida   A fungus that normally inhabits the human body. Overgrowth of this organism can lead to a systemic infection, including immune-system suppression, fatigue, and a multitude of other symptoms. Women experience vaginal infections caused by candida.

Candida albicans   A type of fungus that normally inhabits the digestive tract and the body and results in systemic disease when it overwhelms the body's immune system.

capillaries   The smallest vessel that connects small arteries with small veins for the exchange of nutrients and waste products.

carbohydrate   A food compound that contains carbon and water molecules, and which provides an energy source for the body.

carcinogen   A substance or an agent that is known to cause cancerous changes in the body.

cardiac   Of or relating to the heart.

cardiovascular disease   Disease of the heart and the blood vessels.

carotenoids   A group of fat-soluble pigments (i.e., colors) found in plants or nutritional supplements and that are known to have antioxidant properties.

carrier oil   A pure plant oil, such as sweet almond oil, used to dilute essential oils for aromatherapy. Cold-pressed, unrefined oils are preferred.

cell   The smallest independently functioning unit in the structure of an organism.

cellulose   The indigestible portion of a carbohydrate (plant food).

cerebral   Of or relating to the brain.

cervical   Of or relating to the neck.

cervix   The portion of the vagina that connects to the uterus.

chelation therapy   The use of certain agents or nutrients to pull toxic substances out of the body; commonly used for toxic metals (e.g., lead, mercury, etc.).

chemotherapy   The use of chemical agents to treat disease—most commonly, cancer.

chiropractic   A system of healing based on the premise that poor spinal health (subluxations) leads to improper nerve flow and disease. Through specific adjustments of the spine and the extremities, one can restore normal health.

chlorophyll   A green plant pigment that's responsible for capturing the light energy needed for photosynthesis. It is used in natural medicine for detoxification, red blood cell support, and antioxidant properties.

cholesterol   A yellow, waxy substance that is necessary for life; an important component of cell walls. It is used to manufacture hormones and other life-giving substances.

chronic illness   When a patient experiences gradually eroding health associated with a long-term illness.

coenzyme   A substance that works with enzymes to activate a specific reaction in the body. For example, coenzyme Q10 is required for energy production within cells.

collagen   A protein matrix that holds connective tissue and skin together.

contagious   A disease or condition that is spread from one person or animal to another person.

craniosacral therapy   The use of gentle manual techniques to correct or balance the flow of fluid through the craniosacral system and relieve undue pressure on the brain and the spinal cord, resulting in a healthier nervous system.

CT scan (computerized axial tomography)   A diagnostic image involving X-rays and a computer that allows for a three-dimensional picture inside the body.

decoction   The heating of herbs to make a tea.

dementia   The deterioration or the impairment of mental functioning.

detoxification   The process of eliminating toxins and waste products from the body.

diffuser   A device used to spread essential-oil molecules through the air. It may operate on electricity or with a heat source, such as a candle or a lightbulb.

digestion   The chemical and physical process of breaking down and assimilating food.

digestive enzyme   A supplement that acts as a catalyst in the breakdown of food.

diuretic   A substance or a drug that increases the amount of urine flow.

DNA (deoxyribonucleic acid)   A nucleic-acid molecule that contains the "genetic blueprint" for protein synthesis and cell reproduction and is responsible for passing along hereditary characteristics from one generation to the next.

dysmenorrhea   Menstrual cramps or pain around the time of menses.

dyspepsia   Indigestion.

dyspnea   Shortness of breath.

edema   A buildup of fluid in the tissues that results in swelling.

electrolytes   Minerals that are required for body functioning, especially sodium, potassium, calcium, magnesium, and chloride. Electrolytes help to control fluid levels in the body, maintain normal pH levels, and ensure the transmission of nerve signals.

endorphin   A substance produced in the brain that reduces pain.

enema   An aid to move the bowels and eliminate waste material. It involves the administration of water or a solution into the rectum.

enteric-coated   Refers to a supplement that has a special coating on the exterior so that it does not become inactivated by stomach acid and can then be absorbed in the small intestines.

enzyme   A protein produced by cells or taken in supplement form that acts as a catalyst for a specific biochemical reaction, such as digestion or energy production.

essential amino acids   Amino acids that the body requires but cannot manufacture. They must therefore be consumed in the diet. Of the twenty amino acids, ten are "essential."

essential fatty acids   Fats that the body cannot manufacture and that are required by every cell in the body. The two essential fatty acids are alpha linolenic acid (ALA), of the omega-3 family, and linoleic acid (LA), from the omega-6 family.

essential oils   A material that is present in plant cells and that is extracted by various physical processes and used in aromatherapy.

fat soluble   Dissolves in fats and oils. Fat-soluble vitamins require a source of dietary fat for optimal absorption.

fermented food   A biochemical process in which a microorganism breaks down a substance into a simpler one, using enzymes from bacteria, yeast, or molds. Examples of fermented foods include cheese and yogurt.

fiber   The indigestible portion of plant food. It helps us to eliminate waste from the body.

free radicals   Unstable, negatively charged molecules that are potentially damaging to the organs and the tissues of the body. They are formed by the normal process of energy production within cells, as well as from pollution, toxins, and radiation. Antioxidant enzyme systems within the body, as well as antioxidants from foods or supplements, protect against free radicals. Free radicals can also have beneficial properties, as part of the immune response to destroying microbes.

fungus   A single-celled or multicellular organism that reproduces by spores and lives by absorbing nutrients from organic matter. Examples include mildews, molds, mushrooms, and yeasts.

gastrointestinal tract   Collectively, the stomach, the small intestine, and the large intestine.

genetic Having to do with one's genes or inherited traits.

gland An organ or a group of cells that secretes substances such as hormones. Endocrine glands such as the thyroid are ductless and secrete directly into the bloodstream, while exocrine glands—for example, the salivary glands—secrete via ducts to a surface.

glucose A simple sugar that is the body's preferred fuel source.

gluten A protein combination found in many grains, such as wheat, spelt, barley, rye, and oats.

glyconutrients Food and supplements that contain some or all of the eight essential saccharides.

guided imagery The use of imaging techniques in one's mind to enhance health and well-being.

hair analysis A laboratory technique used to identify mineral balance and heavy-metal toxicity from a person's hair.

heavy metal A metal with high relative density (relative density of 5.0 or higher) that is often toxic to humans. Examples include lead, mercury, copper, and cadmium. Also referred to as toxic metals.

hemoglobin The iron-containing portion of red blood cells that transports oxygen to cells.

hemorrhage Excessive or uncontrollable bleeding.

hepatic Refers to the liver.

herbicide A class of chemicals used to kill weeds.

histamine A chemical released by the immune system (from mast cells) in response to an allergen, resulting in allergy symptoms (runny nose, watery eyes, sneezing, skin rash, etc.).

holistic From the Greek term *holos*, for "whole." Pertaining to the "whole" person in mind, body, and spirit. Often used in the term *holistic medicine*.

hormone A substance produced by an endocrine gland that regulates the function of cells and organs.

hydrogenation A chemical process that uses hydrogen to turn liquid oils into solids. This results in trans-fatty acids that are harmful to the human body. Examples include margarine and shortenings.

hydrotherapy A type of bodywork that uses water as a healing agent. It can involve water in the form of a liquid, a solid, or a vapor.

hypoallergenic A substance that is unlikely to cause an allergic reaction.

hypoglycemia Low blood sugar levels.

hypothalamus Gland located in the brain and involved with the regulation of body temperature and other metabolic processes.

immune system The body's complex defense system, which recognizes and protects against disease. It is also involved in the healing of damaged tissues. It's composed of a variety of white blood cells, the lymphatic system, and other specialized substances.

infection The invasion and the proliferation of microorganisms within the body.

inflammation The immune system's reaction to an illness, an irritation, or an injury that results in heat, pain, redness, and/or swelling.

infusion The use of hot water to make an herbal tea.

insulin A hormone that is secreted by the pancreas for the function of regulating blood sugar levels by transporting glucose into the cells.

International Unit (IU) A unit of potency for certain vitamins, such as A and E.

intolerance An adverse but not life-threatening reaction to a food, a chemical, or another substance.

intravenous Refers to the administration of drugs, nutrients, fluids, or other substances directly into a vein.

IU See International Unit.

Lactobacillus acidophilus A species of "friendly bacterium" found throughout the digestive tract and other mucus-membrane areas of the body. The bacteria are involved with digestion, vitamin synthesis, and immunity.

laxative A substance that promotes bowel movements.

lesion Abnormal tissue due to an injury, an infection, or a cancerous growth.

ligament The connective tissue that connects bones to each other.

lignans Plant substances that have hormone-balancing, cholesterol-lowering, and immune-enhancing properties. The lignans found in flaxseeds are a common example.

lipid A group of compounds consisting of fats or oils; also used to describe cholesterol and triglycerides in medical terms.

liver The primary filter for cleansing the blood. It metabolizes hormones, toxins, and other substances that enter the bloodstream, and it also stores carbohydrates, vitamins, and minerals.

lumbar The lower back area.

lymph Part of the lymphatic system, which carries lymphocytes and nutrients to cells and expels toxins.

lymph node A small structure located in lymphatic vessels that produces white blood cells, known as lymphocytes, that fight infection and remove toxic debris.

magnetic resonance imaging (MRI) A diagnostic image that uses electromagnetic radiation to obtain images of the body's soft tissues—for example, the brain and the spinal cord.

malignant A medical term that refers to cancerous cells.

melatonin A natural hormone produced by the body at night to promote sleep. It's also available in supplement form.

meridian In Chinese medicine, a conduit that can be compared to an imaginary line (or a channel) linking points on the body's surface with internal organs, in which qi (chi) flows. Traditional Chinese medicine defines twelve main meridians and several supporting meridians. The surface points are used in acupuncture.

metabolism The chemical and physical interactions taking place in the body that provide the energy and the nutrients needed to sustain life.

metabolite A substance that is a by-product of metabolism.

mg See milligram.

microgram (mcg) A measure of weight equivalent to $\frac{1}{1000}$ mg or one millionth of a gram.

micronutrient A substance, such as a mineral, that is required in minute amounts by the body.

microorganism An organism that is not visible to the naked eye, such as a bacterium, a virus, a fungus, or a parasite.

milligram A measurement of weight that is $\frac{1}{1000}$ of a gram.

minerals Inorganic substances that are important components of tissues and fluids. They are necessary for the proper functioning of vitamins, enzymes, hormones, and other metabolic activities in the body.

monosodium glutamate (MSG) An additive commonly used to increase the flavor of foods. It is known to cause allergic reactions, such as headaches, in some sensitive individuals.

MRI See magnetic resonance imaging.

MSG See monosodium glutamate.

naturopathic medicine A system of natural medicine that focuses on working with the healing systems of the body. Naturopathic doctors are trained as primary health care providers. As general practitioners, they work to restore health by using clinical nutrition, herbal medicine, homeopathy, physical medicine, counseling, nutritional supplementation, natural hormones, hydrotherapy, and other forms of natural healing. They are also trained in the use of pharmaceutical medicines and minor surgery.

nerves The body's complex wiring, which carries messages to and from the brain.

neural Of or relating to the nerves.

neuralgia Pain along a nerve.

neuropathy A disease or a disorder that affects the nerves.

neurotransmitter A chemical that carries messages between nerve cells of the brain and the nervous system.

nonsteroidal anti-inflammatory drug (NSAID) A class of drug used to reduce pain and inflammation.

NSAID See nonsteroidal anti-inflammatory drug.

nucleus The central part of the cell containing the DNA and the RNA (genetic information), which are necessary to control cell growth and reproduction.

nutraceutical A natural substance that is usually of plant origin, which is taken as a dietary supplement for therapeutic use.

nutrition-oriented doctors Doctors who place an emphasis on the role of nutrition in treating patients.

organic Foods grown without the use of artificial chemicals, such as pesticides, herbicides, or hormones.

oxidation A chemical reaction between oxygen and another substance.

parasite An organism that requires a host to receive nourishment. Certain parasites cause diseases in humans and animals.

parotid gland A salivary gland located below each ear.

pathogen Something that causes disease.

peristalsis A series of wavelike muscle contractions that moves food and waste material through the digestive tract.

pH A scale of measurement of the acidity or the alkalinity of a substance. The scale runs from zero to fourteen. A pH of seven is considered neutral, anything below seven is acidic, and anything above seven is alkaline.

pharmacognosy A study of the biochemistry and the pharmacology of plant drugs, herbs, and spices.

pharyngitis A sore throat.

phytochemicals See phytonutrients.

phytonutrients Naturally occurring substances that give plants their characteristic flavor, color, aroma, and resistance to disease. Thousands of phytonutrients have been identified in fruits, vegetables, grains, seeds, algae, and nuts. They have tremendous benefits for people because they help prevent and treat disease. They are also referred to as phytochemicals.

pituitary gland An endocrine gland located at the base of the brain that controls growth, metabolism, and other glands in the body. The "master endocrine gland."

placebo A "sugar pill" or another inactive substance that helps researchers determine the effects of a drug or substance being tested.

platelets Blood cells that are responsible for clotting.

prebiotic A substance that assists in the formation of a probiotic. For example, fructooligosaccharides are a type of sugar that promotes the growth of the friendly bacteria *Lactobacillus acidophilus* and *Bifidobacterium*.

precursor   A substance required for another substance to be formed or utilized. For example, beta-carotene is a precursor to vitamin A, and DHEA is a precursor hormone that the body converts into testosterone.

preservative   An additive that extends shelf life or preserves color.

probiotic   A substance that contains friendly flora such as *Lactobacillus acidophilus* and *Bifidobacterium*.

protein   A nitrogen-containing compound found in plant and animal foods. The body uses protein as a fuel source and to form or repair tissues, organs, and muscles. Protein comprises enzymes and hormones and is found in every cell in the body. Amino acids are the individual building blocks of protein. There are approximately twenty different amino acids.

proteolytic enzymes   Enzymes that break down protein when taken with food. They also have an anti-inflammatory effect when taken between meals.

pustule   A small, raised lesion that usually contains white or yellow pus.

qi (chi)   In Chinese medicine, the body's vital energy.

radiation therapy   The use of radiation to treat certain types of cancers; also known as radiotherapy.

RDA   See Recommended Daily Allowance.

Recommended Daily Allowance (RDA)   The average daily dietary intake level that is sufficient to meet the nutrient requirement of nearly all (97 to 98 percent) healthy individuals in a group. In other words, the RDAs are the amounts of vitamins and minerals that a healthy person requires to stay healthy. This standard is regarded as woefully inadequate for optimal health by most nutrition-oriented doctors.

saturated fat   Refers to a fat that is full or "saturated" with hydrogen molecules. Saturated fats are semisolid to solid at room temperature. Examples include butter and lard. Dairy products and red meat products contain higher percentages of saturated fats than most foods. Too much saturated fat in the diet is associated with various diseases, such as arthritis and cancer.

sebaceous glands   Glands located in the skin that secrete sebum.

sebum   An oily lubricant secreted by the sebaceous glands of the skin. This lubricant is necessary for protecting the skin from the elements and for keeping it moist.

secondary infection   An infection that occurs after an initial infection. For example, a cold that turns into bronchitis.

sedative   Promoting sleep or a deep sense of relaxation.

sensitivity   An adverse but not life-threatening reaction to a food, a chemical, or another substance.

serotonin   A neurotransmitter that influences mood and sleep, as well as other mechanisms in the body.

simple carbohydrate   A carbohydrate that is broken down and absorbed quickly in the body. Examples include table sugar, honey, and fruit sugars.

steam inhalation   An aromatherapy technique that uses steamy water to carry essential oil molecules into the nose, the mouth, and the sinuses and into the body to heal. It's especially useful for respiratory ailments.

sublingual   A supplement that dissolves beneath the tongue and is absorbed directly into the bloodstream.

systemic   Of or relating to the entire body.

tendon   Connective tissue that joins bones and muscles together.

thrombus   A blood clot.

tincture   Herbs preserved in water and alcohol. Also referred to as "liquid extract."

tonic   A substance, such as an herb, that renews and supports the body as the body rebuilds its strength.

tonify   Strengthen and restore.

toxin   Any impure, poisonous substance that impairs the body's functions.

trace element   A substance, such as a mineral, that the body requires in minute amounts. An example would be chromium.

trans-fatty acids   Harmful fatty acids that are formed during a chemical process that uses hydrogen to turn liquid oils into a solid.

triglyceride   A chemical compound formed from a molecule of the alcohol glycerol and three molecules of fatty acids. Triglycerides constitute many of the fats and the oils in the diet.

tumor   An uncontrolled growth of cells or tissues. Benign tumors are generally harmless, while malignant tumors can interfere with body functions or, in more advanced cases, cause death.

unsaturated fat   Fat that is liquid at room temperature. These fats come from vegetable oils. An example is olive oil.

uric acid   The by-product of protein metabolism. High levels are associated with gout and kidney stones.

urticaria   The medical term for hives.

vaccine   The administration of a substance to stimulate immunity to a particular disease.

vasoconstriction   The constriction of blood vessels, resulting in less blood flow.

vasodilation The relaxation of blood vessel walls, resulting in increased blood flow.

venous return Blood flow from the extremities through the veins back to the heart.

virus A large class of parasitic structures, each of which consists of a nucleic acid core and a protein covering. A virus requires a host to replicate itself.

vitamin An organic substance that is essential ("vital") for life. Most vitamins cannot be synthesized in the body and so must be attained through the diet or from supplements. Vitamins fall into two main groups. Fat-soluble vitamins require some amount of fat to be absorbed. They are also stored longer in the body. Common examples of fat-soluble vitamins include vitamins A, D, K, and E. The second major group of vitamins are the water-soluble vitamins. These vitamins do not need fat to be absorbed and are excreted out of the body much more readily than fat-soluble vitamins are. Vitamin C and the B vitamins are water-soluble.

volatile oil An easily evaporated oil. Essential oils are volatile oils. They evaporate and leave no oily residue.

water-soluble A substance that dissolves easily in water.

white blood cells Immune cells that prevent and fight against infection and tissue damage.

withdrawal A period during which someone who is addicted to a drug or another addictive substance stops taking it, which results in uncomfortable symptoms.

yeast A single-celled organism that can cause infection in the body.

Index

About the Authors

MARK STENGLER, N.M.D.

Mark Stengler, N.M.D., is a licensed naturopathic medical doctor and an author. He is considered one of the leaders in the field of integrative medicine, in which the best of holistic and conventional medicine are combined. Dr. Stengler is the author/coauthor of more than thirty books, including several bestsellers. He has served on a medical advisory committee for the Yale University Complementary Medicine Outcomes Research Project. Dr. Stengler has been interviewed on dozens of television shows on Fox, CBS, NBC, and PBS. He is the author of one of the nation's largest newsletters, *Health Revelations*. He maintains a private practice in Encinitas, California. His Web site is www.markstengler.com.

JAMES BALCH, M.D.

Dr. Balch has been a physician and a surgeon for over thirty-five years. A Certified Nutritional Consultant, a member of the American Medical Association, a Fellow in the American College of Surgeons, and a leading authority on integrative medicine and nutritional healing, Dr. Balch visits clinics worldwide, sharing his ideas with doctors in various disciplines. He has written several books and has coauthored two best-selling books, including *Prescription for Nutritional Healing*, which has sold over eight million copies. He has appeared on ABC, Fox, and CBS, and has been interviewed on various national radio talk shows. Dr. Balch continues to produce publications that address a broad range of health and nutrition topics. He has lectured extensively across the United States, Canada, and overseas, encouraging patients to seek wise counsel in order to maintain good health and prevent disease, which he believes is wisdom in action.

ROBIN YOUNG BALCH, N.D.

Robin Young Balch, N.D., has been an alternative–health care provider for twenty years and is credentialed as a naturopathic doctor, certified professional health consultant, and master Chinese herbalist. She has expertise in aromatherapy, reflexology, acupressure, herbal remedies, and iridology. She is the coauthor of *Prescription for Drug Alternatives*, with Dr. James Balch and Dr. Mark Stengler, and was a consultant, collaborator, and researcher for *The Super Anti-Oxidants* and *Ten Natural Remedies That Can Save Your Life*. Dr. Robin Young Balch has done many radio programs and infomercials with her husband.